To the memory of my father, Glenn J. Lawlor; to my mother, Erma; my wife, Sondra; and my children, Stephanie and Glenn

G. J. L., Jr.

To the memory of my father, Paul Fischer; to my mother, Marcella; my wife, Kathy; and my children, Christopher, Matthew, Elizabeth, and Julia

T. J. F.

Contents

Preface to the Second Edition

We are pleased with the success of the
first edition of *Manual of Allergy and
Immunology*. In this second edition we
have maintained the same theme of
presenting all the basic information,
collected in a single source, required in
the practice of allergy and
immunology. In an attempt to keep
pace with this rapidly advancing field
we have updated each chapter
appropriately and added new material
when necessary.
We again thank our contributors for
their dedication and effort applied to
their respective chapters. We
acknowledge with regret the passing of
our colleague and contributor Manley
McGill and express our sincere
sympathy to his family.
We also thank our editor, Susan Pioli,
for her patience and consistent
cooperation and our project editor,
Elizabeth Willingham, who guided the
book to its final form.

G.J.L., Jr.
T.J.F.

Preface to the First Edition

Manual of Allergy and Immunology is designed to serve the health care professional in the diagnosis and management of allergic diseases and other conditions associated with immunologic dysfunction. We have attempted to present this material in a clear, direct manner, anticipating questions that occur during decision making and providing specific information to allow an individualized approach to diagnosis and treatment. Contributors to this book were chosen for their specific expertise and interest in their respective areas. Only currently accepted therapeutic regimens and dosages are presented; all material that we think is investigative is so identified.

Didactic material has been minimized; what is included has been carefully edited to allow a basic understanding of each subject. More definitive reference material is indicated for each chapter under Suggested Reading. We feel the Manual contains all the basic information, collected in a single source, required in the practice of allergy and clinical immunology. The specialist will find it a convenient handbook while the generalist can use the Manual as a helpful guide in formulating a diagnostic and therapeutic approach to patients suspected of having an allergic or immunologic disorder or in choosing immunologic studies generally available (e.g., for patients with infectious diseases, hematologic disorders, or rheumatoid diseases). Students and house officers will find the Manual a useful introductory guide to the clinical practice of allergy and immunology.

We wish to thank all our contributors for unselfishly giving a considerable amount of time and effort to prepare their respective sections. We also want to thank Little, Brown and Company for providing us the opportunity of publishing the Manual; our editors, Lin Richter, who initially authorized the Manual; Diana O'Dell Potter, who provided initial support; Jim Krosschell, who supervised copyediting and production; and especially Kathleen O'Brien, who patiently gave editorial assistance throughout the preparation. We also wish to thank Ms. Andrea Lippelman for her secretarial help in preparing the typed manuscript. We have enjoyed this undertaking and have found the writing and editing of this book a personal learning experience. We hope that others will find it equally informative.

G.J.L., Jr.
T.J.F.

Contributing Authors

Robert F. Ashman, M.D.   Professor of Medicine and Microbiology, University of Iowa College of Medicine; Attending Physician and Director, Division of Rheumatology, Department of Internal Medicine, University of Iowa Hospitals, Iowa City, Iowa
Chapter 14

Robert W. Ausdenmoore, M.D.   Clinical Professor of Pediatrics, University of Cincinnati College of Medicine; Attending Staff, Allergy/Immunology Division, Children's Hospital Medical Center, Cincinnati, Ohio
Chapter 3

I. Leonard Bernstein, M.D.   Clinical Professor of Medicine and Environmental Health Science, University of Cincinnati College of Medicine; Co-Director, Allergy Research Laboratory, Department of Medicine, Division of Immunology, University of Cincinnati Medical Center, Cincinnati, Ohio
Chapter 4

Gregory N. Entis, M.D.   Assistant Clinical Professor of Pediatrics, University of Cincinnati College of Medicine; Attending Pediatrician, Children's Hospital Medical Center, Cincinnati, Ohio
Chapter 4

Michael K. Farrell, M.D.   Associate Professor of Pediatrics, University of Cincinnati College of Medicine; Director, Nutrition Support Team, Children's Hospital Medical Center, Cincinnati, Ohio
Chapter 13

Stanley M. Fineman, M.D.   Clinical Assistant Professor, Department of Pediatrics, Allergy Division, Emory University School of Medicine, Atlanta, Georgia
Chapter 9

Thomas J. Fischer, M.D.
Associate Professor of Pediatrics, University of Cincinnati College of Medicine; Director, Division of Allergy/Immunology, Children's Hospital Medical Center, Cincinnati, Ohio
Chapters 1, 4, 8, 11, 17

Joseph E. Ghory, M.D.
Clinical Professor of Pediatrics, University of Cincinnati College of Medicine; Emeritus Director, Division of Allergy/Immunology, Children's Hospital Medical Center, Cincinnati, Ohio
Chapter 5

Henry Gong, Jr., M.D.
Associate Professor of Medicine, University of California, Los Angeles, UCLA School of Medicine; Associate Chief, Pulmonary Division, UCLA Medical Center, Los Angeles, California
Chapter 7

Alfredo A. Jalowayski, Ph.D.
Director, Pediatric Respiratory Unit, University of California, San Diego, School of Medicine, La Jolla, California
Appendix IIB

Hemant H. Kesarwala, M.D.
Clinical Associate Professor of Pediatrics, University of Medicine and Dentistry of New Jersey-Robert Wood Johnson Medical School; Attending Physician, Robert Wood Johnson University Hospital and St. Peter's Medical Center, New Brunswick, New Jersey
Chapters 1, 19

Alan P. Knutsen, M.D.
Assistant Professor of Pediatrics, Saint Louis University School of Medicine; Director of Pediatric Allergy/Clinical Immunology, Cardinal Glennon Children's Hospital, Saint Louis, Missouri
Chapter 17

Glenn J. Lawlor, Jr., M.D.
Associate Clinical Professor of Pediatrics, University of California, Los Angeles, UCLA School of Medicine; Director, UCLA Student Health Allergy Clinic, UCLA Center for Health Sciences, Los Angeles, California
Chapters 6, 8, 10, 11

Anne W. Lucky, M.D.
Associate Professor of Dermatology and Pediatrics, University of Cincinnati College of Medicine; Director, Division of Pediatric Dermatology, Children's Hospital Medical Center, Cincinnati, Ohio
Chapter 8

Manley McGill, Ph.D.*	Associate Professor of Transfusion Medicine and Scientific Director, Hoxworth Blood Center, University of Cincinnati College of Medicine, Cincinnati, Ohio Chapter 15
Michael H. Mellon, M.D.	Clinical Associate Professor of Pediatrics, University of California, San Diego, School of Medicine, La Jolla, California; Staff Pediatric Allergist, Kaiser Permanente Medical Center, San Diego, California Chapter 12
Roy Patterson, M.D.	Chairman and Professor of Medicine, Northwestern University Medical School; Chairman, Department of Medicine, Northwestern Memorial Hospital, Chicago, Illinois Chapter 12
Howard M. Rosenblatt, M.D.	Assistant Professor of Pediatrics, Baylor College of Medicine; Attending Pediatrician, Department of Allergy/Immunology, Texas Children's Hospital, Houston, Texas Chapter 10
Andrew Saxon, M.D.	Professor of Medicine, University of California, Los Angeles, UCLA School of Medicine; Chief, Division of Clinical Immunology/Allergy, UCLA Medical Center, Los Angeles, California Chapter 2
Michael Schatz, M.D.	Associate Clinical Professor of Medicine and Pediatrics, University of California, San Diego, School of Medicine, La Jolla, California; Staff Allergist, Kaiser Permanente Medical Center, San Diego, California Chapter 12
Mary J. Spencer, M.D.	Associate Clinical Professor of Pediatrics, University of California, San Diego, School of Medicine, La Jolla, California; Attending Pediatrician and Infectious Disease Specialist, Palomar Hospital, Escondido, California Chapter 18
Donald P. Tashkin, M.D.	Professor of Medicine, University of California, Los Angeles, UCLA School of Medicine; Attending Physician, UCLA Medical Center, Los Angeles, California Chapter 6

*Deceased

John G. Winant, Jr., M.D.   Associate Staff, Department of
Pediatrics, Medical Center at Princeton,
Princeton, New Jersey
Chapter 4

Kwan Y. Wong, M.D.   Associate Professor of Pediatrics,
University of Cincinnati College of
Medicine; Associate Director of
Hematology/Oncology, Children's
Hospital Medical Center, Cincinnati,
Ohio
Chapter 15

Robert S. Zeiger, M.D., Ph.D.   Clinical Assistant Professor of
Pediatrics, University of California, San
Diego, School of Medicine, La Jolla,
California; Chief, Allergy and Clinical
Immunology, Kaiser Permanente
Medical Center, San Diego, California
Appendix IIB

Paul M. Zeltzer, M.D.   Associate Professor of Pediatrics,
University of Southern California School
of Medicine; Director, Brain Tumor
Program, Childrens Hospital of Los
Angeles, Los Angeles, California
Chapter 16

Manual of Allergy and Immunology

Diagnosis and Therapy

Introduction to the Immune System

Hemant H. Kesarwala and
Thomas J. Fischer

The function of the immune system is to distinguish self from non-self and to eliminate the latter. Such a system is necessary for survival in all living creatures. In humans, a functioning immune system is required to prevent attack by internal forces (e.g., tumor cells, autoimmune phenomena) as well as external forces (microorganisms or toxic substances). Deficiency or dysfunction of the immune system in humans leads to a variety of clinical diseases of varying expression and severity, from such disorders as allergic rhinitis to severe rheumatoid arthritis, severe combined immunodeficiency, or malignancy. This chapter is a brief introduction to the complex immune system. Added explanations are found in subsequent chapters and in the suggested reading lists at the end of each chapter.

Organs of the Immune System

Several tissues and organs play roles in host defense and are functionally classified as the immune system.

I. **Primary lymphoid organs** are the thymus and the bursa of Fabricius in birds and the thymus and bone marrow (and/or fetal liver) in mammals.

   A. The **bone marrow** is the source of pluripotent stem cells, which differentiate into lymphocyte, granulocyte, erythrocyte, and megakaryocyte populations. In mammals, the bone marrow also supports differentiation of lymphocytes. Deficiency or dysfunction of the pluripotent stem cell or the various cell lines developing from it can result in immune deficiency disorders of varying expression and severity.

   B. The **thymus,** derived from the third and fourth embryonic pharyngeal pouches and located in the mediastinum, exercises control over the entire immune system. Its reticular structure allows a significant number of lymphocytes to migrate through it to become fully immunocompetent thymus-derived cells (T cells). A large number of cells also die within the thymus and are apparently phagocytosed, a mechanism to eliminate lymphocyte clones reactive against self-antigens. The thymus also regulates immune function by secretion of multiple soluble hormones. Absence of the thymus or its abnormal development results in T-lymphocyte deficiencies (e.g., DiGeorge syndrome).

II. **Secondary lymphoid organs** in mammals (lymph nodes, spleen, and gut-associated lymphoid tissue) are connected by blood and lymphatic vessels. Through these vessels, lymphocytes circulate and recirculate, responding to antigen and spreading the specific experience of this antigen exposure to all parts of the lymphoid system.

   A. **Lymph nodes** are the peripheral organs of the immune system that attempt to localize and prevent the spread of infection. Lymph nodes have a framework of reticular cells and fibers that are arranged into a cortex and medulla. Bursal equivalent lymphocytes (B cells), the precursors of plasma cells, are found in the cortex (the follicles and germinal centers) as well as in the medulla. T-lymphocyte areas are primarily found in the medullary and paracortical areas of the lymph node (Fig. 1-1).

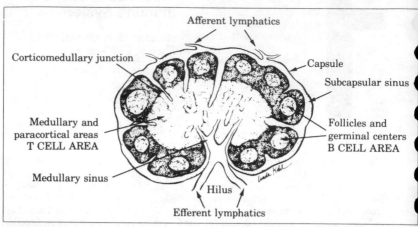

Fig. 1-1. Lymph node structure indicating primary T cell and B cell areas. (From M. S. Thaler, R. D. Klausner, and H. J. Cohen. Foundations of the Immune Response. In *Medical Immunology*. Philadelphia: Lippincott, 1977. With permission.)

    B. The **spleen,** functionally and structurally divided into T-cell and B-cell areas like those of the lymph nodes, filters and processes antigens from the blood.

    C. **Gut-associated lymphoid tissue** (tonsils, Peyer's patches of the small intestine and the appendix) shows a similar separation into T cell–dependent and B cell–dependent areas. Many lymphocytes are also seen within the lamina propria of the small intestinal villi and between the epithelial cells of the intestinal mucosal surface. Gut-associated lymphoid tissue may play a role in the differentiation of stem cells into B lymphocytes.

Cells of the Immune System

I. Lymphocytes are responsible for the initial **specific** recognition of an antigen. They are principally divided into B lymphocytes (bursal) and T lymphocytes (thymic) on the basis of surface marker identification and several functional tests, the most obvious being the production of antibody as a measure of B-lymphocyte function and cell-mediated cytotoxicity for T-lymphocyte function. B cells and T cells also have distinguishable surface structures. The B cell is coated with surface membrane–bound immunoglobulin (SmIg) and also has receptors for complement and the Fc portion of immunoglobulins. T cells are quantitated by the ability to cause adherence of sheep red blood cells to their surface (E rosettes). Structurally, T and B cells cannot be distinguished from each other under the light microscope. About 80% of circulating blood lymphocytes are T cells, and 10–15% are B cells. Approximately 10–15% of circulating blood lymphocytes are not labeled with either marker (null cells).

Further separation of T-lymphocyte subpopulations is accomplished by immunofluorescence using **monoclonal antibodies** reactive with individual cell surface antigens. Monoclonal antibodies are produced by hybridoma cell lines. Each antibody-forming cell and its clones are capable of forming an antibody that is highly specific and always identical. This hybrid is created by fusing a myeloma cell and the antibody-forming cell. The myeloma cell infers immortality on the cell line, and the antibody-forming cell confers its ability to form antibodies in large quantities. The hybridoma cells can be stored and retrieved to obtain the same antibody whenever needed. Using T cells as antigens, a variety of monoclonal antibodies have been created, enabling identification of T-cell subsets such as helper (T4), suppressor (T8), and cytotoxic cells. The monoclonal antibody technique has provided valuable reagents used both in the clinical laboratory and for immunologic research.

T cells mediate a number of functions, notably the **cell-mediated immune responses,** such as delayed (tuberculin-type) hypersensitivity, graft rejection, and immune surveillance of neoplastic cells. Quantitative and functional differences distinguish the principal T-cell subsets. T4 cells predominate over T8 cells in the circulating blood by a ratio of 2:1. T4 cells provide helper signals for B lymphocytes, T lymphocytes, T8 cell–mediated cytotoxicity, and macrophages. T8 cells, when influenced by T4 cells, suppress B-lymphocyte immunoglobulin production and T-lymphocyte response to major histocompatibility antigens and enhance cytotoxicity and natural killing.

Null cells probably include a number of different cell types, including a group of cells called **natural killer (NK)** cells. These cells do not possess the typical appearance of a lymphocyte: they are slightly larger with a kidney-shaped nucleolus. NK cells are capable of binding IgG with an Fc receptor. When a cell is coated with an antibody and destroyed by an NK cell, this phenomenon is called **antibody-dependent cell-mediated cytotoxicity (ADCC).** Alternatively, NK cells can destroy cells without involvement of antibody (e.g., virally infected cells or tumor cells). Other characteristics of NK cells include recognition of antigens without major histocompatibility restrictions, lack of immunologic memory, and regulation of activity by interferons and prostaglandins of the E series.

B cells are the direct precursors of mature antibody-secreting cells (plasma cells). Although ongoing investigations indicate an array of complex interactions between B and T cells and tend to obscure distinctions between these two systems, the division into B and T cells with different developmental and functional characteristics allows for an operational understanding of the immune system.

II. **Phagocytic cells** (polymorphonuclear leukocytes, eosinophils, and monocyte-macrophages) reach maturity in the bone marrow, circulate in the blood for a short time, and enter the tissue spaces by diapedesis through capillary walls in response to chemotactic factors released by inflammation.

    A. **Macrophages** play a central role in the immune response. Derived from the blood monocytes, they circulate for a few days in the blood and then leave the vascular compartment to become active tissue macrophages. Macrophages have the following important functions: chemotaxis (cell movement), phagocytosis (antigen engulfment), antigen-processing, and presentation of the antigen in an immunogenic form to the lymphocytes. (However, macrophages have no antigen specificity, as do lymphocytes.) Macrophages are important for their function as secretory cells. More than 50 secretion products of macrophages are known, including enzymes, plasma proteins, active metabolites of oxygen (e.g., superoxide anion), bioactive lipids (e.g., prostaglandin E_2), nucleotide metabolites (e.g., cyclic adenosine monophosphate [AMP]), and factors regulating cellular functions (e.g., interleukin-1 [IL-1]). In particular, IL-1 has important properties such as augmentation of lectin-stimulated thymocyte proliferation, which promotes expansion of lymphocyte populations.

    B. **Polymorphonuclear leukocytes** originate from the bone marrow. These cells circulate in the blood and tissue, and their primary function is phagocytosis and destruction of foreign antigens.

    C. **Eosinophils** are often found in inflammatory sites or at sites of immune reactivity, but they phagocytose and kill less efficiently than do polymorphonuclear leukocytes. Although eosinophils show certain functional characteristics similar to those of neutrophils, their role has still not been completely determined. They appear to have a modulatory or regulatory function in various types of inflammation. However, eosinophils may also have a destructive effect in the inflammatory process by the release of cytolytic proteins such as the eosinophilic major basic protein.

III. **Basophils and mast cells** release the mediators of immediate hypersensitivity, e.g., histamine, leukotrienes, eosinophil chemotactic factor of anaphylaxis (ECF-A), and platelet-activating factor (PAF) (see Chap. 2), which have significant effects on the vasculature and on the inflammatory response. Basophils are present in the circulation, while mast cells are present only in tissue, but in much larger numbers.

Development of the Immune System

I. Phylogenetic development. In unicellular animals, nonspecific mechanisms of host defense consist of phagocytic processes and hydrolytic enzymes, while primitive prevertebrate organisms acquire external and internal surface barriers as well as specialized phagocytes. In primitive vertebrates with notochords, immunocytes with primitive recognition and memory capacity are added, which help to amplify and direct the phagocytic process. With progressive evolution, the immune system in higher animals and humans has evolved with increasing complexity in terms of its specific antibody and cell-mediated immune response capacity. Despite the complexity of the human immune system, host defense is still highly dependent on surface barriers and phagocytic mechanisms. Absence of phagocytic function (e.g., severe neutropenia) or loss of surface barriers (e.g., extensive surface burns) can present a tremendous risk of fulminant, life-threatening invasion by microorganisms that normally are not pathogenic.

II. Ontogenetic development

  A. Cellular precursors of **T cells** are derived in early fetal life from the fetal yolk sac. By 4–5 weeks of gestation, they arise from the liver and thereafter from the bone marrow. T-lymphocyte precursors undergo differentiation and maturation (identifiable by changes in cell membrane surface markers) under the influence of the thymus, which is formed from the third and fourth pharyngeal pouches at 6–8 weeks of gestation. Functional cellular responses, heavily dependent on T cell immunocompetence, are not fully developed in the fetus, neonate, and young infant as compared with the adult.

  B. Precursor B cells, derived from the same sources as T-cell precursors, demonstrate IgM or IgM and IgD immunoglobulins on their cell membranes. After antigenic stimulation, B cells differentiate into plasma cells, which are responsible for antibody formation. The antigenically stimulated human fetus is able to synthesize IgM antibody by 10½ weeks of gestation, IgG antibody by 12 weeks, and IgA antibody by 30 weeks. The normal human infant, usually born without antigenic stimulation unless infected in utero, has little circulating IgA and IgM antibody. IgG antibody is almost completely derived from the mother by active and selective transport across the placenta. Adult serum levels of IgG, IgM, and IgA immunoglobulins are attained separately (Fig. 1-2) (see Appendix VII).

  C. Phagocytic cells are seen in the human fetus at 2 months of gestation as a few myelocytes and histiocytes, present in the early yolk-sac stage of hematopoiesis. Monocytes first appear in the spleen and lymph nodes at 4–5 months of gestation, with gradual maturation of macrophage function with advancing fetal age. Isolated newborn polymorphonuclear leukocytes have normal phagocytic activity when tested in vitro in the presence of adult serum. However, cells from a premature infant phagocytose less effectively than do those from a term infant. Chemotaxis (cell movement) of leukocytes and monocytes appears to be deficient in the newborn.

  D. Complement components are synthesized by the fetus early in gestation either at the same time as or just before the beginning of immunoglobulin synthesis. There is almost no placental transfer of complement components from mother to fetus. The levels of individual complement components C1q, C2, C4, C3, and C5 and the total hemolytic complement in the newborn are low. Such deficiency and dysfunction may be responsible for the relative opsonic deficiency in newborns.

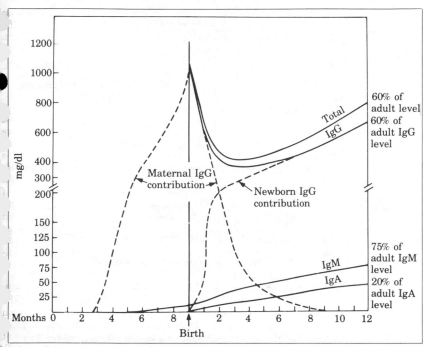

Fig. 1-2. Immunoglobulin (IgG, IgM, IgA) serum levels in the fetus and infant in the first year of life. The IgG in the fetus and newborn infant is solely of maternal origin. The maternal IgG disappears by the age of 9 months, at which time endogenous synthesis of IgG by the infant is well established. The IgM and IgA at birth are entirely neonatal in origin (no placental transfer). (From E. R. Stiehm. Immunoglobulins and Antibodies. In E. R. Stiehm and V. A. Fulginiti [eds.], *Immunologic Disorders in Infants and Children.* Philadelphia: Saunders, 1973. With permission.)

Immune System Components

The immune system consists of specific and nonspecific components that have distinct but overlapping functions. Antibody (humoral) and cell-mediated immune systems provide specificity and a memory of previously encountered antigens. Phagocytic cells and complement proteins are **nonspecific** cellular mechanisms and **nonspecific** humoral factors, respectively. Despite their lack of specificity, these components are essential because they are largely responsible for the natural immunity to a vast array of environmental microorganisms.

I. **Antibody immunity.** Lymphocytes passing through the bursa-equivalent organ in humans acquire the characteristics of B cells that undergo transformation into plasma cells. The plasma cell has an increased endoplasmic reticulum, indicating active protein synthesis.

A. **Immunoglobulin structure.** All immunoglobulin molecules have a certain structural similarity, with four polypeptide chains divided into two light and two heavy chains linked by disulfide bonds (Fig. 1-3). Disulfide linkages are also present on each chain. There are five classes of immunoglobulins, termed **IgA, IgG, IgM, IgD,** and **IgE,** based on the structure of their heavy chain (alpha [α],

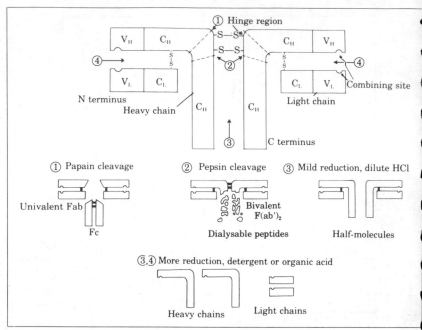

Fig. 1-3. Basic immunoglobulin structure with immunoglobulin subunits produced by enzyme, acid, or wetting agents. Interchain disulfide bonds are shown (large S-S), but intrachain bonds have been omitted for clarity. The number of H-H disulfide bonds varies with each class and subgroup of immunoglobulin. Numbers 1 through 4 show points of attack of various agents, with the cleavage products noted in smaller diagrams in the bottom half of the figure (V_H and V_L indicate variable regions of heavy and light chains, respectively; C_H and C_L indicate constant regions of heavy and light chains). Polymeric forms of IgM and IgA are not shown but are joined at the Fc region near the carboxy terminus. (From R. Hong. Immunoglobulin Structure and Function. In E. Middleton, C. E. Reed, and E. F. Ellis [eds.], *Allergy: Principles and Practice,* 1978. St. Louis, The C. V. Mosby Co. With permission.)

gamma [γ], mu [μ], delta [δ], and epsilon [ϵ], respectively) (see Table 1-1). There are only two classes of light chain: kappa (κ) and lambda (λ). Each immunoglobulin molecule has only one class of light chain and only one class of heavy chain, although each class of immunoglobulin can have either kappa or lambda light chains. Accordingly, the structural formula for each immunoglobulin molecule can be written $\alpha_2 \kappa_2$, $\alpha_2 \lambda_2$, etc. Monomers consist of a single immunoglobulin, e.g., IgG antibody, while polymers have multiple basic units e.g., IgM antibody, which consists of five basic units of 10 light chains and 10 heavy chains. In addition to the polypeptide chains, other structures can be incorporated into the immunoglobulin molecule, e.g., J chains and the secretory piece of IgA.

B. Structural-functional correlates. Study of the immunoglobulin subunits can help to localize and specify the function of biologically active sites.

    1. Agents used in cleaving the immunoglobulin molecule include enzymes such as papain and pepsin, dilute acids, or wetting agents such as urea (see Fig. 1-3). The enzymes papain and pepsin break the immunoglobulin molecule into different fragments. Papain breaks the molecule into two Fab fragments and one Fc fragment. Pepsin breaks the molecule into a single $F(ab')_2$ fragment and multiple Fc fragments.

Table 1-1. Characteristic features of the five classes of immunoglobulins

Immunoglobulin	Heavy chains	Light chains	Molecular weight (daltons)	Serum concentration (mg/dl)	Localization in secretions	Presence of other structures	Serum half-life (days)	Placental transfer	Classic complement activation	Alternate complement activation	Biologic activity (function)
IgG	Gamma (γ_1) (γ_2) (γ_3) (γ_4)	Kappa or lambda	150,000	1200	−	−	23	+	+*	−	Neutralization, opsonization, bacteriolysis, agglutination, hemolysis
IgM	Mu (μ)	Kappa or lambda	900,000	150	±	J chain	5	−	+	−	Neutralization, hemolysis, agglutination, bacteriolysis, opsonization, first detectable antibody, receptor on B lymphocyte
IgA	Alpha (α_1) (α_2)	Kappa or lambda	160,000 (secretory IgA, 370,000)	300	+	J chain and secretory component for secretory IgA	6	−	−	+	Neutralization, present in body secretions
IgD	Delta (δ)	Kappa or lambda	180,000	3	−	−	3	−	−	+	Receptor on B lymphocyte
IgE	Epsilon (ϵ)	Kappa or lambda	200,000	0.03	±	−	2	−	−	+	Mast-cell binding and increased vascular permeability on antigen exposure

Key: + = present; − = absent; ± = possibly present.
*Except IgG$_4$.

    a. The **Fab end** of an immunoglobulin molecule is called the amino-terminal end, which, with the presence of both light and heavy chains, i the antibody-combining site. The amino-terminal end possesses marked variability in the amino acid sequence. This variability enables the immunoglobulin molecule to combine with a variety of antigens.

    b. The **Fc end** is the carboxy-terminal end, which contains only heavy-chain components. This Fc, or constant, region (fixed amino acid se quence) is responsible for conferring biologic activity on the immuno-globulin molecule, such as placental transfer, complement fixation binding to skin and cells (macrophages, platelets, granulocytes, mast cells), and determining its rate of synthesis and catabolism. The Fc fragment is not involved in specific antigen recognition.

  2. Various **genetic markers** have been demonstrated on the constant region of light and heavy chains. Genetic variations in light chains produce amino acid changes at certain positions, creating genetic allotypes. On kappa chains these are called Km (Inv) markers; a nonallelic marker on lamb-da chains is either present or absent (Oz+, Oz−). Genetic variations of heavy chains also produce allotypes called **Gm, Am,** and **Mm markers,** which are inherited by mendelian genetic ratios.

C. Immunoglobulin classes. Immunoglobulins are divided into five major classes. The characteristic features of each are summarized in Table 1-1.

  1. IgG is the immunoglobulin primarily involved in the secondary or recall immune response. IgG antibodies are composed of two light chains and two heavy chains. This molecule is further divided into four different subclasses termed **IgG$_1$, IgG$_2$, IgG$_3$,** and **IgG$_4$,** based on structural differences in the gamma heavy chain. These subclasses also have functional variations in terms of complement fixation, alternative complement pathway activation macrophage adherence, and ease of placental transfer. The ability of IgG to diffuse into body tissue facilitates combination and efficient elimination of antigens.

  2. IgM immunoglobulin is the major part of the early humoral response, espe-cially in response to nonprotein bacterial antigens. The IgM molecule con sists of five IgG-like subunits that are linked by disulfide bonds and J chains. This immunoglobulin is incapable of placental transfer, but its poly-meric structure makes for efficient agglutination or lysis of antigens.

  3. IgA is the primary immunoglobulin of all mucosal surfaces and exocrine secretions. It exists either as a monomer, dimer, or even a trimer of the basic four-chain structure. IgA can be found in the serum or in exocrine secretions. Secretory IgA is equipped with a polypeptide (a secretory piece) that permits secretion of the IgA molecule across mucous membranes, pro viding initial protection against pathogens at the mucosal level. Selectiv IgA deficiency is the most common primary immunodeficiency in humans

  4. IgD immunoglobulin is present in very small quantities in the serum. Its functional role is not well characterized. Its structure is similar to that of other immunoglobulins, i.e., either kappa or lambda light chains linked to its own distinct delta heavy chains.

  5. IgE immunoglobulin, also known as reaginic antibody, is normally present in a very small concentration, although elevated levels are seen in atopic disease and a number of other disorders (see Table 2-3). IgE antibody is made up of the basic four-chain structure of IgG, with either two kappa or two lambda light chains and two epsilon heavy chains. Mast cells and basophils have receptors for the Fc region of IgE, and the bridging of two IgE molecules by antigen results in the release of inflammatory mediators.

II. Cell-mediated immunity consists of a set of immune phenomena distinct from anti-body-mediated immunity. The differences between the two systems are outlined in Table 1-2. Cell-mediated immunity is mediated by T lymphocytes and monocytes-macrophages and requires intact cells that carry out their immune functions either by direct cell-to-cell contact or by production of soluble factors for specific im-munologic functions, e.g., recruitment of phagocytic cells into sites of inflammation.

Table 1-2. Differences between humoral and cell-mediated immunity

Humoral-mediated immunity	Cell-mediated immunity
Antibody-mediated	Cell-mediated
Responsible cell: B lymphocyte	Responsible cell: T-lymphocyte cells or cell products required for transfer of immunity
Transfer of immunity with serum	
Primary defense against bacterial infection	Responsible for host defense against viruses, fungi, intracellular organisms, tumor antigens, allograft rejection

Table 1-3. Soluble products of lymphocytes (lymphokines)

Product	Action
Migration inhibition factor	Inhibition of migration of macrophages
Macrophage aggregation factor	Aggregation of macrophages
Macrophage-activating factor	Activation of macrophages, with increase in their metabolism
Blastogenic factor	Proliferation of lymphocytes
Leukocyte migration inhibition factor	Inhibition of polymorphonuclear leukocyte migration
Bone-resorbing factor	Decalcification of bone
Chemotactic factor	Chemotaxis of various blood cells
Lymphotoxin	Inhibition of cell growth
Interferon	Interference with viral reproduction
Skin-reactive factor	Mononuclear inflammation caused by intradermal injection
Transfer factor	Transfer of delayed hypersensitivity to a nonsensitized recipient
Interleukin-2 (IL-2) (T-cell growth factor)	Stimulates the growth of helper and cytolytic T cells

Interleukin-2 (IL-2), also known as **T-cell growth factor,** plays an important role in cell-mediated immunity. Following antigen stimulation, IL-2 promotes the growth of T-cell clones, helper T cells, and cytolytic T cells. Specific receptors are present on helper T cells and cytolytic T cells that allow for binding of IL-2 to these cells. The molecular weight and the structure of IL-2 are defined, and, depending on the species involved, IL-2 is a protein of 15,000–30,000 daltons. IL-2 is used to allow long-term growth of T cells, a technique that has facilitated the study of T-cell immunity. Because of its important role, it also offers clinical applicability, e.g., tumor immunity. The actions of these soluble factors, or **lymphokines,** are summarized in Table 1-3.

A. Histocompatibility. T lymphocytes do not recognize antigens directly but do so when the antigen is presented on the surface of an antigen-presenting cell—the macrophage. In addition to presentation of the antigen, the macrophage must present another molecule (the histocompatibility molecule) for this immune response to occur. This molecule is a cell surface glycoprotein that is coded in each species by the major histocompatibility gene complex (MHC). There are two classes of histocompatibility molecules: class I molecules (regulate interaction between cytolytic T cells and target cells) and class II molecules (regulate the interaction between helper T cells and antigen-presenting cells). T cells are able to interact with the histocompatibility molecules only if they are genetically identical (MHC restriction). Cytotoxic T lymphocytes directed against class I antigens are inhibited by T8 cells; cytotoxic T lymphocytes directed against class II antigens are inhibited by T4 cells. In humans, the major histocompatibility complex is located on chromosome 6. It is divided into four major regions: D, B, C, and A. The A, B, and C regions code for class I molecules, whereas the D region codes for class II molecules.

The MHC gene products have important roles in clinical immunology. For example, transplants are rejected if performed against MHC barriers; thus, immunosuppressive therapy is required.

B. In summary, cell-mediated immunity is responsible for the following immune phenomena:
1. Delayed hypersensitivity reactions (e.g., tuberculin test).
2. Contact sensitivity (e.g., poison ivy dermatitis).
3. Immunity to intracellular organisms (e.g., *Brucella*).
4. Immunity to viral and fungal antigens.
5. Elimination of foreign-tissue grafts.
6. Elimination of tumor cells bearing neoantigens.
7. Formation of chronic granulomas.

III. Phagocytic immunity. The phagocytic system is divided into **circulating** and **fixed** components. Circulating cells with phagocytic capacity include the granulocytes, monocytes, and eosinophils; fixed-tissue phagocytes include the Kupffer's cells of the liver, splenic macrophages, pulmonary alveolar macrophages, lymph node macrophages, and the microglial cells of the brain. The fixed-tissue phagocytes together constitute the **reticuloendothelial system.** The ability of both polymorphonuclear phagocytes and monocytes to eliminate foreign material is critical for host defense. Failure of one or both of these systems invariably results in increased susceptibility to infection. Six serial steps are required for adequate phagocytosis and destruction of foreign antigens: (1) random movement, (2) chemotaxis, (3) opsonization and fixation of the bacteria or foreign material, (4) ingestion, (5) metabolic activation of the phagocytes to destroy the foreign material, and (6) destruction of the organism or foreign material.

A. Phagocytic cells migrate either in a random manner or in response to a directed signal, i.e., **chemotaxis.** Known chemoattractants include components of the activated complement pathway (C3a and C5a), bacterial products, and products of other cells.

B. Opsonization is the process by which antibody coats a bacterial cell wall or foreign material and increases its susceptibility to phagocytosis.

C. Phagocytosis is the process of engulfing foreign material into the phagocytic cell. After an intracellular phagocytic vacuole is formed around the foreign material, lysosomal enzymes are released into this vacuole, resulting in the destruction of the foreign material.

D. The important enzyme system responsible for **increased metabolic activity** is the myeloperoxidase-hydrogen peroxide-halide system. During the process of destruction, there is an increased burst of metabolic activity, with increased oxygen consumption, increased hexose-monophosphate shunt activity, and increased hydrogen peroxide production.

IV. The complement system is made up of a series of 18 plasma proteins that are sequentially activated to mediate their biologic function. The complement system plays a broad-based role in the amplification of specific and nonspecific host defense, helping to mediate such functions as immune adherence, phagocytosis, chemotaxis, and cytolysis. Normally, complement components are present in the serum in an inactive form, and biologic activities follow sequential activation. A number of control proteins (C1 inhibitor [C1 INH], factor I (C3b inactivator), factor H (beta 1H), and C4-bp (C4 binding protein) are normally present to inhibit uncontrolled complement activation.

Complement proteins can be grouped into four functional divisions according to their interaction with the third component, C3: (1) classic pathway activation, (2) alternative pathway activation, (3) the amplification mechanism, and (4) the effector mechanism (Fig. 1-4).

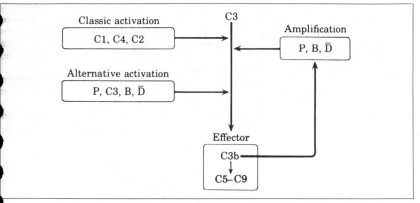

Fig. 1-4. Overview of four-compartment complement system (see text). (From D. T. Fearon and K. F. Austen. Immunochemistry of the Classical and Alternative Pathways of Complement. In L. E. Glynn and M. W. Steward [eds.]. *Immunochemistry: An Advanced Textbook*. New York: Wiley, 1977. Reprinted by permission of John Wiley & Sons, Ltd.)

A. The **classic activation pathway**, comprising the three components C1, C4, and C2, is dependent on the interaction of these three complement proteins with antigen-antibody to activate the initial cleavage of C3 and subsequent activation of the terminal components of the pathway. C1, the first complement component, consists of three subcomponents, C1q, C1r, and C1s, which form a complex in the presence of calcium. Antigen-antibody complexes (containing immunoglobulin IgG_{1-3} or IgM) can activate C1 to its enzymatically active form (C1̄). C1̄ then cleaves its two complement substrates, C4 and C2, to form a bimolecular complex, C4b2ba. This complex, the classic C3 convertase, is capable of cleaving C3 to initiate activation of the effector sequence.

B. **Alternative pathway activation.** Microbial and mammalian cell surfaces can activate the alternative pathway in the absence of specific antigen-antibody complexes. This nonspecific activation is a major physiologic advantage since host protection can be generated prior to the induction of a humoral immune response. Factors capable of activating the alternative pathway include inulin, zymosan, bacterial polysaccharides, aggregated immunoglobulins, IgG_4, IgA, and IgE. Proteins involved in this reaction include properdin, factor D̄, factor B, and C3.

C. **Amplification.** Constituent proteins of the amplification pathway include C3b, B, D̄, properdin, and two control proteins, C3b INA and C6 INA. This system extends the half-life of the C3b protein, which is responsible for activating the terminal sequence (Fig. 1-5).

D. **Effector mechanism.** The classic and alternative C3 pathways generate C3b, which serves a number of functions, including interaction of C4b2a and C3bBb to allow further activity on C5 and subsequent activation of the terminal sequence (Fig. 1-5). In the final steps, formation of membrane-bound C5b67 permits binding of C8 to the C5 fragment to cause a partial membrane lesion resulting in slow cell lysis. By complexing with C9, the cytolytic reaction is accelerated.

Antigen-Antibody Interactions

An antigen is a substance that can stimulate an immune response and react with an antibody or a sensitized T cell. The capacity of an antigen to elicit an immune

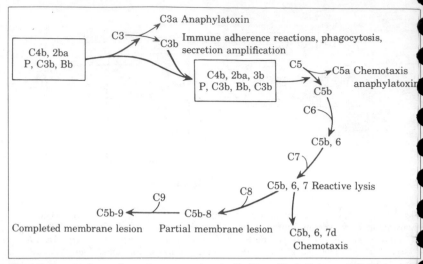

Fig. 1-5. Terminal complement sequence (see text). (From N. A. Soter and K. F. Austen. Effector Systems of Inflammation. In *Dermatology in General Medicine* by T. B. Fitzgerald et al. [eds.]. Copyright © 1979 by McGraw-Hill Book Company. Used with the permission of McGraw-Hill Book Company.)

response is termed its **immunogenicity;** its ability to react with an antibody is termed its **antigenicity.** Low-molecular-weight substances (e.g., drugs) are not immunogenic by themselves unless combined with a carrier protein. These small molecules are termed **haptens.** Although they cannot evoke an antibody response when injected alone, they can, by themselves, react with antibody. Immunogenicity is a complex phenomenon that depends not only on the physical properties of the antigen but also on the biologic system, route of administration, and method of immunization.

Antigen-antibody binding occurs by relatively weak noncovalent forces; close approximation between antigens and antibodies can facilitate their binding to each other. The reaction between antigen and antibody occurs in two stages. The **first stage** is union or a combination of antigen with antibody for interatomic, noncovalent interactions. The **second stage** of the reaction involves the **visualization** of the first stage by precipitation or agglutination. Union occurs immediately, but the second stage can require minutes, hours, or even days.

Inhibition of this complex formation is termed the **zonal phenomenon.** Reactions in which antibody is in excess are inhibited and are termed **prozones,** indicating that they occur prior to the point of reactant equivalence. Inhibition due to antigen excess is referred to as **postzone,** indicating postreactant equivalence. Although the antigen-antibody reaction is specific, it is reversible, and the reaction is not limited to fixed molar reactant ratios. Factors affecting antigen-antibody reactions also include temperature, pH, and concentration of the reactants.

Techniques for detecting an antigen-antibody reaction can vary from simple precipitation to more complex radioimmunoassays or enzyme immunoassays, which continue to assume increased importance in clinical medicine.

Classification of Immunologic Reactions

Although the function of the immune system is protection of the host from foreign antigens, abnormal immune responses can lead to tissue injury and disease. Gell

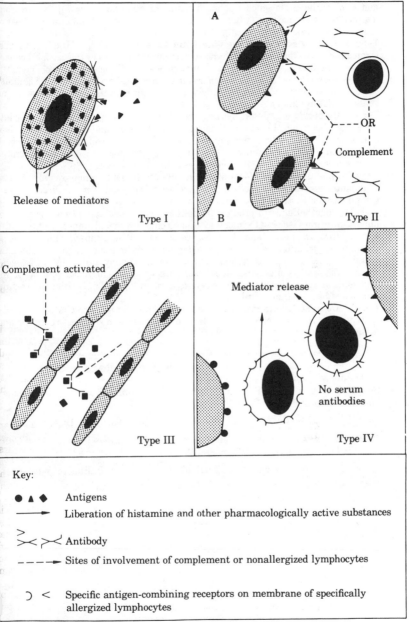

Fig. 1-6. Classification of allergic reactions (Gell and Coombs). See text for further explanation. (From M. J. Hobart and I. McConnell [eds.]. Appendix A: Classification of Allergic Reactions. In *The Immune System: A Course on the Molecular and Cellular Basis of Immunity*. Oxford: Blackwell, 1975. With permission.)

and Coombs have classified the mechanisms of immune tissue injury into four distinct types of reaction, which allows for improved understanding of the immunopathogenesis of disease (Fig. 1-6).

I. **Type I: Anaphylactic or immediate hypersensitivity.** Antigen binding to preformed IgE antibodies attached to the surface of the mast cell or the basophil causes release of mediators, e.g., histamine, leukotrienes, and the eosinophilic chemotactic factor of anaphylaxis (ECF-A), which produce the clinical manifestations. Examples of type I diseases include anaphylactic shock, allergic rhinitis, allergic asthma, and acute penicillin allergy.

II. **Type II: Cytotoxic reactions.** Cytotoxic reactions involve the binding of either IgG or IgM antibody to cell-bound antigen. Antigen-antibody binding results in activation of the complement cascade and the destruction of the cell (cytolysis) to which the antigen is bound. Examples of tissue injury by this mechanism include immune hemolytic anemia and Rh hemolytic disease in the newborn.

III. **Type III: Immune complex–mediated reactions.** Immune complexes are formed when antigens bind to antibodies. They are usually cleared from the circulation by the phagocytic system. However, deposition of these complexes in tissues or in vascular endothelium can produce immune complex–mediated tissue injury. Two important factors leading to injury by this mechanism include **increased quantity** of circulating complexes and the presence of **vasoactive amines,** which increase vascular permeability and favor tissue deposition of immune complexes. Immune complex deposition leads to complement activation, anaphylatoxin (C3a, C5a) generation, chemotaxis of polymorphonuclear leukocytes, phagocytosis, and tissue injury. Clinical examples are serum sickness, certain types of nephritis, and certain features of bacterial endocarditis.

IV. **Type IV: Delayed hypersensitivity.** Delayed hypersensitivity is mediated primarily by T lymphocytes. The classic examples are the tuberculin skin test reactions and contact dermatitis.

Selected Readings

Gell, P. G. H., Coombs, R. R. A., and Lachman, P. J. *Clinical Aspects of Immunology* (3rd ed.). Oxford: Blackwell, 1977.

Roitt, I. (ed.). *Essential Immunology* (5th ed.). Oxford: Blackwell, 1984.

Stiehm, E. R., and Fulginiti, V. (eds.). *Immunologic Disorders in Infants and Children* (2nd ed.). Philadelphia: Saunders, 1980.

Unanue, E. R., and Benacerraf, B. *Textbook of Immunology.* Baltimore: Williams & Wilkins, 1982.

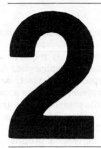

Immediate Hypersensitivity: Approach to Diagnosis

Andrew Saxon

Basic Concepts

Immediate hypersensitivity comprises a subset of the body's antibody-mediated effector mechanisms. This subset consists of the reactions primarily mediated by immunoglobulin E (IgE), a class of immunoglobulins with unique biologic properties. Although Prausnitz and Küstner, in 1921, first demonstrated the presence of a serum "reagin" in allergic persons that was capable of transferring the allergic wheal-flare reaction, it was not until 45 years later that Ishizaka and co-workers demonstrated the identity of reagin as a new class of immunoglobulin, termed **IgE**. Subsequently, the role of IgE in immediate hypersensitivity disorders has been intensively investigated.

The final expression of immediate hypersensitivity results from the culmination of the following sequence of reactions: (1) **exposure to antigen (allergen)**; (2) **development of an IgE antibody** response to the antigen; (3) **binding** of the IgE to mast cells; (4) **reexposure** to the antigen; (5) **antigen-interaction** with antigen-specific IgE bound to the surface membrane of mast cells; (6) **release** of potent **chemical mediators** from sensitized mast cells; and (7) **action** of these mediators on various organs.

I. **The antigen.** A substance must be presented to the immune system in an appropriate form to be antigenic, that is, to stimulate production of an immune response. Not all antigens will give rise to an antibody response, nor will every antigen stimulate all major classes of immunoglobulin production. For example, most so-called **T-independent antigens** (i.e., polysaccharides) in animals and humans fail to give rise to IgE antibodies. Thus, the **nature of the antigen** is important in the development of the immediate hypersensitivity state.

Most natural antigens are polar compounds with a molecular weight between 10,000 and 20,000 daltons and have a high degree of cross-linking, as indicated by their high content of sulfhydryl groups. Exposure to minute amounts of these substances (microgram quantities) will induce IgE production in **susceptible** persons. Antigens (allergens) important in immediate hypersensitivity are divided into two major groups: complete protein antigens and low-molecular-weight substances.

A. **Complete protein antigens,** such as pollen, animal danders, or exogenously administered proteins (e.g., animal hormone extracts, horse serum), are capable of eliciting a complete humoral (IgE) response by themselves. They possess a **carrier determinant** that stimulates the macrophage and T-cell arm of the IgE immune response to promote B-cell activation. They also carry an **antigenic determinant** recognized by B cells.

B. **Low-molecular-weight substances** (e.g., many drugs), which by themselves cannot elicit an IgE antibody response because they function only as **haptens,** commonly bind to tissue or serum proteins in vivo and then function as a hapten-carrier complex to elicit an IgE antibody response. This kind of reaction is typical of most cases of drug hypersensitivity. The distinction between complete antigens and those with which tissue protein combines to form a hapten-carrier complex has important diagnostic implications. Complete antigens can be readily applied in immediate skin test procedures; important metabolic haptens have been difficult to identify and manufacture for immediate hypersensitivity testing.

II. The **antibody.** The production of antigen-specific IgE antibodies requires active collaboration between macrophages, T lymphocytes, and B lymphocytes. An allergen introduced through the respiratory tract, gastrointestinal tract, or skin reacts with macrophages that "process" this antigen and present it to the appropriately responsive T lymphocytes. Then B lymphocytes, in the presence of the antigen and the responsive T lymphocytes, are stimulated to develop into plasma cells, which synthesize and secrete antigen-specific IgE (Fig. 2-1A).

A. IgE-producing plasma cells are located mainly in the **lamina propria** of the respiratory and gastrointestinal tracts and their **associated lymphoid tissues;** the spleen and the systemic lymph nodes contain few IgE plasma cells. The total serum IgE level represents the sum of IgE that has been produced in all three sites and passively diffused into the vascular compartment.

B. IgE antibodies have the unique biologic property of being able to **bind to mast cells** (i.e., homocytotropic) for prolonged periods. IgG may bind to such cells, but only for brief intervals (up to 12–24 hours). Once bound, IgE antibodies may persist for as long as 6 weeks, as demonstrated by a positive response to antigen challenge using a passive-transfer technique (Prausnitz-Küstner [P-K] test). This IgE binds to receptors on the mast cell that are specific for the **Fc (constant) region** of the epsilon heavy chain. The mast cell binding of IgE has two important consequences:

1. IgE from the serum binds to **mast cells throughout the body.** Thus, mast cells under the skin in the forearm may be found sensitive to antigens that are either inhaled or ingested. Furthermore, the majority of mast cells may be sensitive to specific allergens, and exposure to such allergens can trigger systemic mast cell activation, producing multiple system involvement (anaphylactic shock).

2. Mast cell binding gives IgE a **high fractional turnover in serum** (turnover estimates between 70 and 90% over 2–3 days). IgE, however, will not cross the placenta; therefore, the immediate hypersensitivities of the mother are not passively transferred to the fetus.

Another important activity of IgE is that when complexed to antigen, it can **activate the complement cascade** through the alternative pathway. Activation of the complement cascade results in production of anaphylatoxins (C3a and C5a) and other chemotactic substances important in the inflammatory response.

III. The **mast cell**

A. Mast cells, perivascular connective tissue cells found in all tissues of the body, are **coated with IgE antibodies** bound to receptors specific for the Fc portion of the epsilon chains. Any given mast cell will have bound IgE antibodies with many antigenic specificities and may react with a large variety of antigens. The **number** of IgE antibodies on a single basophil (the "circulating" mast cell) ranges between 5000 and 500,000 molecules/cell. Although allergic persons have a higher average number of IgE molecules on their basophils than do nonallergic persons, there is a broad numerical overlap between the two groups. The amount of cell-bound IgE is a reflection of the serum level of IgE. However, a greater total number of IgE molecules on a cell does not correlate with greater sensitivity to basophil activation.

Fig. 2-1. A. Allergen sensitization. Allergen is absorbed. A macrophage takes up the allergen, processes it, and presents it to the T lymphocyte. A B lymphocyte exposed to the allergen is influenced by the T lymphocyte to mature into an allergen-specific IgE immunoglobulin-secreting plasma cell. Allergen-specific IgE antibodies are absorbed onto the surface of a mast cell (sensitization). **B.** Allergen stimulation of mediator release. Allergen is absorbed and cross-links with specific IgE antibody on the sensitized mast cell. The mast cell degranulates and mediators are released.

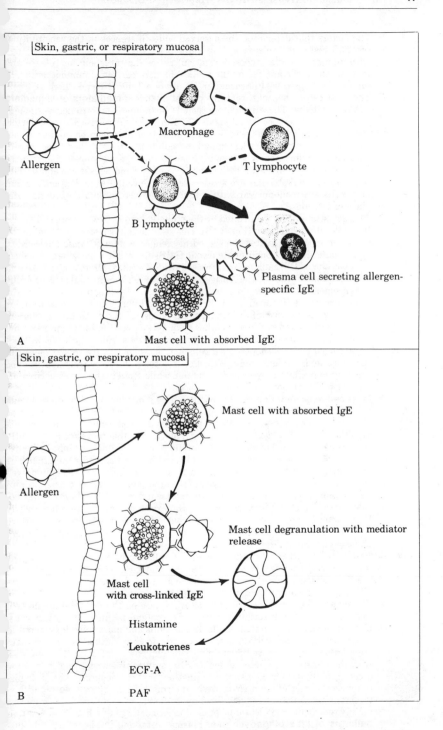

Skin, gastric, or respiratory mucosa

Allergen

Macrophage

T lymphocyte

B lymphocyte

Plasma cell secreting allergen-specific IgE

Mast cell with absorbed IgE

A

Skin, gastric, or respiratory mucosa

Mast cell with absorbed IgE

Allergen

Mast cell degranulation with mediator release

Mast cell with cross-linked IgE

Histamine

Leukotrienes

ECF-A

PAF

B

B. The factors that determine the observed wide differences in the sensitivity of basophil histamine release among individuals are unknown. Immunotherapy with allergy extracts (hyposensitization) raises the threshold for release and may be an important factor in the benefit derived from immunotherapy. A number of drugs can alter mediator release (see Table 2-1 and Chap. 4).

C. The mast cell or basophil contains **potent chemical mediators of immediate hypersensitivity.** These mediators include histamine, leukotrienes, eosinophil chemotactic factors of anaphylaxis (ECF-A), and platelet-activating factor. Mast cells are rich in heparin, whereas heparin is absent in basophils. In contrast to other animal species, human basophils and mast cells do not contain appreciable quantities of serotonin. Some mediators are stored in lysosomes (heparin, histamine) within the mast cell cytoplasm and released on appropriate stimulation. Leukotrienes are synthesized by the cell after activation. Human mast cells are mononuclear with characteristic metachromatic-staining cytoplasmic granules.

D. Allergen stimulation is initiated by the **cross-linking** of two or more cell-bound IgE molecules by antigen (Fig. 2-1B). This stimulation transmits a signal to the cell interior that activates the second messenger system of cyclic nucleotides, cyclic guanosine monophosphate (cyclic GMP) and cyclic adenosine monophosphate (cyclic AMP), causing an increased ratio of cyclic GMP to cyclic AMP and an activation of proesterase. Antigen bridging of IgE receptors also leads to the enhancement of receptor-operated calcium channels, thereby increasing the concentration of intracellular calcium ions by influx from the extracellular space (Fig. 2-2). This influx initiates the release of the preformed mediators (degranulation) and synthesis of other mediators. Cross-linking of IgE receptors is necessary for activation; univalent antigen or monovalent anti-IgE will not trigger mast cells. Although mast cells may morphologically appear identical, they may not be so functionally. Mast cells of the respiratory tract appear to be sensitive to inhibition by cromolyn sodium, while those in the skin and circulating basophils are not sensitive.

E. Mast cell degranulation can be modulated by a number of substances. Agents that **decrease** mast cell cyclic AMP or increase cyclic GMP (alpha-adrenergic stimulation, cholinergic agents, or prostaglandin $F_2\alpha$) enhance mast cell degranulation (see Fig. 2-2). On the other hand, agents that **increase** cyclic AMP, such as epinephrine (adrenergic stimulation), theophylline (phosphodiesterase inhibition), and prostaglandins E_1 and E_2, inhibit mast cell degranulation. The mechanism of **corticosteroid effect** on mast cell mediator release is unproved but may involve increased sensitivity of beta-receptors to beta-agonists. **Cromolyn sodium** appears to inhibit mediator release independent of the cyclic nucleotide system. Mast cells may also release their mediators when stimulated solely by **nonimmunologic** influences such as cold (cold urticaria), pressure (pressure urticaria or dermatographia), sunlight (solar urticaria), heat (heat urticaria), and exercise (cholinergic urticaria).

IV. Mediators of immediate hypersensitivity. Stimulation of mast cells by antigens releases powerful chemical mediators (Table 2-1 and Fig. 2-3) that trigger a sequence of physiologic events resulting in the symptoms of immediate hypersensitivity. The important known mediators include the following:

A. Histamine. The action of histidine decarboxylase on the essential amino acid histidine produces histamine. Histamine content is high in gastric cells, platelets, mast cells, and basophils. In basophils and mast cells, it is stored in lysosomes and released through exocytosis (degranulation) on appropriate stimulation. Once released, histamine causes maximal effects in 1–2 minutes, with the duration of effects as long as 10 minutes. Inactivation of histamine occurs rapidly in vivo by either deamination (through deamine oxidase or histaminase) or methylation (N-methyltransferase). Thus, the **whole blood** histamine level, which can be obtained by a number of commercial laboratories, mainly represents the histamine present in circulating basophils. **This determination is of little diagnostic use.** Plasma histamine levels reflect only histamine released immediately before the sample is obtained. Although plasma

Table 2-1. Mediators of immediate hypersensitivity reactions

Mediator	Location	Action	Inhibitor	Importance in humans
Histamine	Preformed in mast cells	Vasodilation Enhanced vasopermeability Smooth-muscle contraction Increased mucus secretion	H_1 antihistamines (e.g., diphenhydramine) H_2 antihistamines (e.g., cimetidine)	4+
Leukotrienes C_4, D_4, and E_4	Requires synthesis by cells	Smooth-muscle contraction Enhanced vasopermeability	Corticosteroids modulate production	4+
Prostaglandins PGD_2, PGI_2, PGE_2, $PGF_{2\alpha}$, thromboxanes	Requires synthesis by cells	Variable effects on smooth-muscle contraction and vasopermeability	Aspirin, nonsteroidal anti-inflammatory drugs, and corticosteroids modulate production	4+
ECF-A	Preformed in mast cells	Attracts eosinophils	Corticosteroids block effects	4+
PAF	Requires synthesis by cells	Smooth-muscle contraction, activates platelets to aggregate and release serotonin	?	3+
Bradykinin	Found as serum precursor	Enhanced vasopermeability Smooth-muscle contraction Increased mucus production Stimulation of pain receptors	?	2+
Serotonin	Preformed in platelets	Enhanced vasopermeability Smooth-muscle contraction	Lysergic acid	±
Heparin	Preformed in mast cells	Anticoagulant	Protamine	±

Key: 4+, 3+ = of major importance; 2+ = of minor importance; ± = of equivocal importance.

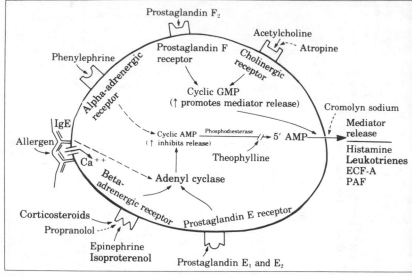

Fig. 2-2. Mast cell membrane receptors and regulation of mediator release (⟶ indicates direct stimulation; ----→ indicates direct inhibition; —/ /→ indicates inhibition of stimulation; ⟹ indicates influx).

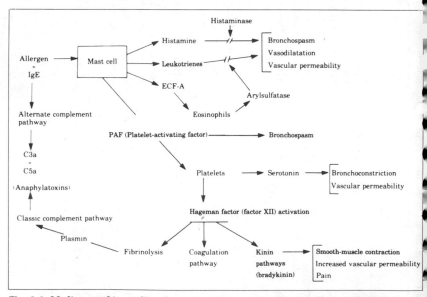

Fig. 2-3. Mediators of immediate hypersensitivity. Interaction of allergen-antibody reaction, complement system, clotting system, and kinin system (⟶ indicates stimulation; —/ /→ indicates inhibition; ECF-A = eosinophil chemotactic factors of anaphylaxis).

histamine levels may be elevated during immediate hypersensitivity reactions, they are not usually helpful as a **clinical** diagnostic tool. Plasma histamine levels can be determined only in specialized laboratories.

1. Histamine acts on many target organs through two known types of **receptors, H_1 and H_2.** H_1 receptors appear primarily on bronchiolar and vascular smooth-muscle cells; H_2 receptors appear on gastric parietal cells. Some types of antihistamines show a preference for H_1 receptors (chlorpheniramine and the other "classic" antihistamines). Other types show a preference for H_2 receptors (burimamide, cimetidine, metiamide, and ranitidine). Histamine receptors are present on different types of lymphocytes (especially on T-lymphocyte suppressor cells) as well as basophils. In addition to providing feedback to the mast cell–basophil system, histamine may play an important and previously unappreciated role in regulating the immune response.

2. The **physiologic effects** of histamine in humans can be described under the major organ systems involved.

   a. In the **lung** it causes contraction of the bronchial smooth muscle, leading to bronchoconstriction and the clinical picture of bronchospasm and wheezing.

   b. In the **vascular system,** small venules become dilated, while larger vessels show constriction from smooth-muscle contraction. Furthermore, histamine increases capillary and postcapillary venular permeability. These vascular changes lead to the classic **wheal-flare response** or **triple response of Lewis,** observed with intradermal injections of histamine. Initially, erythema (vasodilatation with flare) occurs, which is soon followed by increased permeability and edema formation (wheal) with erythema (flare) extending beyond the borders of the wheal. When these vascular changes occur systemically, the symptoms of hypotension, urticaria, and angioedema may be manifest. In the **nasal mucosa,** edema and vasodilatation are prominent.

   c. Histamine increases secretion by gastric and respiratory mucosal cells. The **intestinal smooth muscle** may respond with increased motor activity, leading to diarrhea or hypermotility, frequently observed in systemic release of histamine (anaphylaxis or systemic mastocytosis). These responses to histamine appear to be **direct** effects on the target organ and not mediated by neuron-reflex activity.

B. **Leukotrienes.** For many years, a low-molecular-weight sulfur-containing substance (slow-reacting substance of anaphylaxis [SRS-A]) had been known to be important in allergic reactions, particularly the pulmonary bronchospastic response. Recently, this material has been shown to be a family of compounds termed **leukotrienes.** These materials are generated by the action of the enzyme lipoxygenase on arachidonic acid, which is liberated from membrane phospholipids by the phospholipase A_2 enzyme in activated cells. Thus, when cells are activated, arachidonic acid is generated internally, and the lipoxygenase enzyme pathway generates a family of biologically active mediators (Fig. 2-4). There is a range of lipoxygenase enzymes, each of which appears to have preferential expression in various cell types such as neutrophils, eosinophils, monocyte-macrophages, or mast cells. The first stable leukotriene to be generated is leukotriene B_4, which primarily functions as a chemotactic factor. However, this material is then converted to leukotrienes C_4, D_4, and E_4 by a series of metabolic steps. The biologic activities of these latter leukotrienes (C_4, D_4, and E_4) are identical to the substance termed **SRS-A.** These leukotrienes possess a wide variety of biologic activities, and the latter "mediator" leukotrienes are not equal in these activities. While intradermal D_4 and E_4 cause a burning erythematous wheal-and-flare response, C_4 causes a wheal and flare that is asymptomatic. Similarly, D_4 is the most potent in causing smooth-muscle contractility, while C_4 is somewhat less active and E_4 has little activity. Overall, compared with histamine, the leukotrienes are between 100 and 1000 times more potent in causing bronchoconstriction. The effects of leukotrienes are mediated

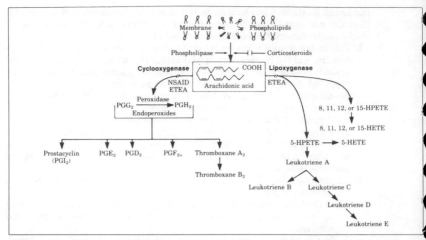

Fig. 2-4. The metabolism of arachidonic acid occurs through two pathways: the cyclooxygenase pathway, which produces prostaglandins and thromboxanes, and the lipoxygenase pathway, which produces leukotrienes. Various agents affect this metabolism. Corticosteroids inhibit the release of arachidonic acid from membrane phospholipids. Aspirin and other nonsteroidal anti-inflammatory drugs (NSAIDs) and eicosatetraenoic acid (ETEA) inhibit the cyclooxygenase pathway; ETEA inhibits the lipoxygenase pathway. Key: HPETE = hydroperoxyeicosatetraenoic acids; HETE = hydroxyeicosatetraenoic acids; PGG_2 = prostaglandin G_2; PGH_2 = prostaglandin H_2; PGD_2 = prostaglandin D_2; $PGF_2\alpha$ = prostaglandin F_2 alpha; $\longrightarrow$ indicates stimulation; $-\!/\!\!\longrightarrow$ indicates inhibition. (From "Allergy and Immunology." In *Medical Knowledge Self-Assessment Program VII*, Syllabus. Published by The American College of Physicians, 1985. With permission.)

through specific receptors. No specific antagonists of leukotrienes are available for clinical use in human beings. However, this is an area of intense research, and these antagonists will probably be developed in the near future. Furthermore, at present there are no assays of leukotrienes in either serum or biologic fluids that are of practical use for clinicians.

C. **Eosinophil chemotactic factors of anaphylaxis (ECF-A)** are preformed in human mast cell granules and released immediately on degranulation. These small polypeptides (molecular weight 400 daltons) attract eosinophilic leukocytes to sites of immediate hypersensitivity reactions (e.g., the lung in asthmatic patients or the nose in allergic rhinitis patients). At such sites, the attracted eosinophils may **degrade** antigen-antibody complexes and **inhibit** the action of leukotrienes and histamine.

D. **Other mediators**
   1. **Platelet-activating factor (PAF)** was originally found in rabbit basophils, but is now demonstrated to be generated from human macrophages, neutrophils, eosinophils, and possibly mast cells and basophils. It initiates platelet aggregation at sites of immediate hypersensitivity reactions. Platelet aggregation is then sustained by the continued release of ADP from the platelet aggregates. Platelet-activating factor may play a role in human immediate hypersensitivity. It has been identified and synthesized (acetyl glyceryl ether phosphorylcholine). Besides aggregating platelets, this material has now been shown, in very low concentrations, to cause bronchoconstriction and increased vascular permeability.
   2. Platelet-activating factor may further influence hypersensitivity states through platelet aggregation and subsequent **activation of Hageman fac-**

tor (factor XII). Activated Hageman factor will induce the formation of kinins, the most important of which is the nonapeptide **bradykinin.**

3. **Bradykinin** is not found in human mast cells. It affects numerous cell types, as does histamine. Smooth muscles of the bronchi and blood vessels respond with gradual, prolonged, and intense contraction. Bradykinin also causes increased permeability of the capillaries and postcapillary venules, which results in tissue edema. It stimulates nerve cell fibers to produce pain. Finally, mucus-secreting cells in the respiratory and gastric tract respond to bradykinin stimulation with increased mucus production. Bradykinin appears to mediate its effect through receptors on cells distinct from the receptors of both histamine and the leukotrienes.

4. **Serotonin (5-hydroxytryptamine),** an important mediator of immediate hypersensitivity in rodents, is not found in human mast cells. It is present in human platelets and released during platelet aggregation or through other mechanisms. Serotonin causes contraction of human bronchial smooth muscle, but this effect is short-lived because of the rapid onset of tachyphylaxis. Serotonin is of minor, if any, importance in human immediate hypersensitivity.

5. **Prostaglandins** are a group of compounds with effector and modulator activity on cellular functions. These compounds are produced by the action of cyclooxygenase and peroxidase enzymes on arachidonic acid liberated from cell membrane phospholipids (see Fig. 2-4). Prostaglandins may play an active role in human immediate hypersensitivity beyond the effects on mast cell cyclic nucleotides discussed previously. Prostaglandins A and F produce smooth muscle contraction as well as increased capillary permeability; prostaglandins E_1 and E_2 directly dilate bronchial smooth muscle.

6. **Activation of the complement system** may play a role in mediating hypersensitivity reactions. This process may occur either from direct alternative pathway activation by IgE-antigen complexes or through a sequence initiated by activated Hageman factor that causes the generation of plasmin, which subsequently activates the classic pathway of complement. In either case, activation of complement components from C3 onward leads to the generation of the anaphylatoxins (C3a and C5a).

The Atopic Diseases

The atopic diseases are processes mediated by or related to IgE-immediate hypersensitivity. (**The terms atopic and allergic are frequently interchanged.** In its broadest sense, the term **allergy** has been used in the past to describe any immunologic alteration in the capacity to react following contact with a foreign substance. **Atopic,** on the other hand, characterizes conditions produced only by the action of IgE.)

In the United States, 10–20% of the population suffers from atopic diseases. Genetic factors play an important role in the susceptibility to these diseases. The association of the atopic diathesis with the inheritance of histocompatibility (HLA) antigen haplotypes in families has been demonstrated and suggests that immune-response genes associated with the major histocompatibility complexes may genetically determine or define the atopic state. An IgE response occurs normally in all individuals, but the presence of immune-response genes may be needed for **antigen specificity** and **clinical manifestations** of the atopic state. The expression of this potential response may clearly be altered by factors such as dose, route, and timing of antigen exposure, drug therapy, and concomitant illnesses.

I. **Anaphylaxis,** the most dramatic and devastating form of atopic disease, is the systemic manifestation of immediate hypersensitivity. The implicated antigen is often introduced parenterally, such as by injection of penicillin or a bee sting. Oral exposure may also produce anaphylaxis, although less frequently. The activation and degranulation of mast cells systemically, with massive mediator release, results in the clinical picture of bronchospasm, urticaria, and anaphylactic shock (see Chap. 10).

II. **Allergic rhinoconjunctivitis** is the most common atopic disorder, affecting approximately 15% of the United States population. Like anaphylaxis, allergic rhinoconjunctivitis is a well-documented model of immediate hypersensitivity pathophysiology. It is mediated by IgE produced locally under the mucosal surfaces of the nose and eye. Airborne antigen comes into contact with mast cells sensitized by the locally produced IgE and produces mast cell degranulation, with the resulting picture of "local anaphylaxis" of the nasal or conjunctival membranes, or both (see Chap. 5).

III. **Urticaria and angioedema.** Immediate hypersensitivity may express itself in a cutaneous form of disease: urticaria, or angioedema, or both. Allergic urticaria-angioedema is often self-limited, lasting less than 6 weeks, and is frequently related to the ingestion or administration of foods or drugs. If urticaria persists longer than 6 weeks, the causative agent is not often determined (see Chap. 9).

IV. **Asthma** is the expression of immediate hypersensitivity reactions in the lung. Inhaled intact pollens, deposited heavily in the nose and pharynx, probably do not reach the small or even the large airways. Fragments of these materials detected by immunochemical methods may reach the smaller airways to produce direct antigen stimulation. Although bronchial challenge studies may provoke bronchospasm, they employ large doses of antigen (e.g., aerosolized aqueous extract of pollen). On the other hand, bronchospasm develops after **natural** exposure to pollen antigens. The definite role of inhaled antigens has not been completely elucidated, but reflex parasympathetic stimulation of the bronchial mucosa through the vagus nerve from afferent cholinergic receptors in the nasal and pharyngeal membrane probably plays an important role.

The antigens may also be ingested in the mucous membrane of the oropharynx, their active allergens eluted and subsequently absorbed, with hematogenous spread producing symptoms. Pulmonary manifestations alone, without cutaneous or nasal symptoms, may follow antigen exposure. The reason for this differential expression of target organs in atopic patients is unknown (see Chap. 6).

V. **Gastrointestinal allergy.** The gastrointestinal tract is a known site for the expression of localized immediate hypersensitivity disease. Nausea, abdominal cramps, vomiting, and diarrhea may follow food exposure within a matter of minutes to hours. These reactions can be mediated by IgE-type hypersensitivity, although other mechanisms are more commonly operative (e.g., enzyme deficiency as seen in lactose intolerance). The presence of increased numbers of eosinophils in the small intestine on biopsy after food challenge is suggestive, but not definitive, evidence of immediate hypersensitivity (see Chap. 13).

VI. **Atopic dermatitis** is an eczematous cutaneous eruption associated with the previously mentioned atopic disorders of asthma and allergic rhinitis. The incidence in the general population is up to 10%. Several features suggest its classification as an atopic disorder: familial association with allergic rhinitis and asthma; markedly elevated serum levels of IgE; frequent hypersensitivity to environmental allergens; eosinophilia; evidence for a beta-adrenergic-receptor defect in atopic dermatitis patients similar to that described in asthmatic patients; and the association of allergic rhinitis and asthma in patients with atopic dermatitis. In contrast, atopic dermatitis correlates less well with immediate hypersensitivity skin tests and antigen exposure, does not respond well to immunotherapy (hyposensitization), and has histopathologic features that do not resemble those of the usual atopic states (see Chap. 8).

Approach to the Patient

I. **Allergic history.** A comprehensive allergy history produces the best data base for the diagnosis and management of patients with allergic disease. A **standardized allergic history form** (Table 2-2) allows the physician to obtain a comprehensive picture of the patient's problem as it relates to allergic disease and exposures. The

Table 2-2. Allergy history guidelines

I. Name: _____ Date: _____ Age: _____ Sex: _____
II. Clinical illness
    A. Present illness
        1. Nature of illness
        2. Age of onset
        3. Frequency of attacks
        4. Duration of attacks
        5. Changes in nature, frequency, or duration of attacks
        6. Previous evaluation and treatment
        7. Present treatment
    B. Family history
    C. Past medical history
III. Environmental reactions
    A. Time of year and day of symptoms
    B. What produces symptoms?
    C. What relieves symptoms?
    D. Symptoms at home, work, vacation
    E. Reactions to dusty or moldy environments, pets, odors, foods, medicines, insects, colds, change in weather, smoke, exercise, emotion, mowing lawn
IV. Environmental survey
    A. Occupation, where employed, unusual exposures
    B. Place and type of residence, basement, heating, air conditioning, etc.
    C. Carpets or rugs in home, type and matting
    D. Pillow, blanket, and mattress, type and age
    E. Exposure to barns, dead leaves, or other moldy environments
    F. Pets in home (indoors and/or outdoors), number and type
    G. Exposure to chemicals, insecticides, etc.
    H. Hobbies
    I. Medications
    J. Tobacco smoke

---

principles of history taking are similar to those for any medical history, but certain aspects of the history require particular attention and expansion, namely, noting the **temporal** and **spatial** relationships of symptoms as related to possible allergen exposures. Historic details should include the following:

    A. The **time relationships** of symptoms should include the time of day, time of the week (all week or weekends only), and time of the year, as well as the duration of symptoms.
    B. Do the symptoms occur at home, at work, or on vacation, when the patient is away from his or her work or home environment?
    C. Does sensitivity occur to known allergens (e.g., dust, animals, grass cuttings) in addition to possible exposures to unsuspected allergens (e.g., room humidifiers, jute carpet pads)?
    D. Do symptoms relate to physical changes (cold, heat, dampness) or activities (e.g., smoking, exercise, or painting)?
    E. Does past or current use or abuse of antiallergic therapy (medication, immunotherapy, environmental controls) change allergic symptoms?
    F. Since atopic diseases have a strong propensity for familial incidence, a careful history to detect possible atopic disorders in other family members is necessary.
    G. The patient should estimate the degree of difficulty or impairment experienced from the allergic symptoms. **This is the primary factor in determining the extent of further evaluation and treatment.**
    H. The presence of any concomitant medical conditions should be noted, since these conditions may mimic allergic disease or alter its expression (e.g., pregnancy, hypothyroidism).

II. **Physical examination.** A **complete** physical examination is mandatory. Specific attention should be directed to areas where atopic diseases are manifested: the skin, the conjunctiva, the nasopharynx, and the lungs. A more complete discussion of the physical findings in each specific atopic disorder is found in subsequent chapters. However, certain principles bear emphasis at this time.

A. The **entire skin** should be examined for important physical changes (e.g., lichenification in the flexor areas or other chronic alterations of the skin) that may not be mentioned by the patient who feels that they are unimportant, unrelated, or embarrassing.

B. The **conjunctiva** should be carefully examined for hyperemia and edema (chemosis) involving both the palpebral and bulbar membranes. The presence of increased or abnormal-appearing secretions in the palpebral fissures should be noted. The fundus should be examined, because cataracts are often associated with both atopic disease and corticosteroid treatment.

C. The **middle ear** is often a site of secondary complications of allergic disease, such as serous or infectious otitis media. Similarly, the frontal and maxillary sinuses should be examined by palpation.

D. The **nose** is the most accessible area to observe the physical alterations resulting from the pathophysiologic features of immediate hypersensitivity disease.

1. A transverse line across the **top of the nose,** the **allergic crease,** may occur as a result of chronic upward nose rubbing **(allergic salute),** especially in children.

2. The **interior of the nose** should be assessed using adequate illumination and exposure as provided by a head mirror and nasal speculum. An otoscope with a large speculum provides an alternative method. The examiner must be careful **not to distort the anatomy** of the nasal vestibule. If the turbinates are swollen such that adequate visualization is impaired, a topical decongestant should be applied to temporarily shrink these structures to allow better visualization of the nasal passages.

a. The **mucosa** and the structures it overlies (septum, turbinates) should be examined carefully.

b. The quantity and quality of **nasal secretions** should be assessed.

c. The presence of **polyps** or **foreign bodies** should be noted.

d. The **patency** of the nasal passages is assessed by having the patient sniff through one nostril with the other lightly occluded.

E. The **mouth** and **oropharynx** are examined with a bright light source and tongue blade. Because the mucosa of the oropharynx is continuous with the nasal mucosa, in allergic rhinitis the posterior lateral pharynx and uvula may often be erythematous, edematous, or both. A narrow, high-arched palate, narrow chin, and elongated maxilla with overbite occasionally result from chronic allergic disease in childhood **(allergic facies).**

F. The **chest** should be examined by visual inspection, palpation, percussion, and auscultation. The findings in allergic disease vary from normal during symptom-free intervals to marked hyperinflation, accessory muscle use, and marked wheezing during acute asthma attacks. The changes of chronic lung disease (e.g., increased anteroposterior diameter) may result from severe asthma or may be a complication of repeated infections or immune injury (e.g., hypersensitivity pneumonitis). Digital clubbing is not commonly seen in patients with severe asthma and usually indicates other pathology, e.g., bronchiectasis.

III. **Laboratory procedures useful in diagnosis and management.** The results of laboratory studies do not make the diagnosis of allergic disease. They strengthen or weaken various diagnostic possibilities suggested by the history and physical findings. They are also an aid in patient management—in monitoring both the complications of allergic disease and the effects of therapy.

A. **Complete blood count with differential.** The white blood cell count is usually normal except during states of increased catecholamine input (endogenous or exogenous) or intercurrent infection. Eosinophil percentages between 5 and 15% are nonspecific but do suggest atopic disease. Corticosteroids cause eosinopenia and may mask eosinophilia.

1. **Moderate eosinophilia** (15–40% of peripheral blood leukocytes) may be found in allergic disorders, but other causes should be considered, namely, parasitic infections, drug exposure, malignancy (e.g., Hodgkin's disease), and immunodeficiencies. Radiation therapy, congenital heart disease, peritoneal dialysis, cirrhosis, periarteritis nodosa, and dermatitis herpetiformis also are associated with moderate eosinophilia.

2. **Exaggerated eosinophilia** (50–90% of peripheral blood leukocytes) is commonly observed in visceral larva migrans, seen especially in children, and in the idiopathic hypereosinophilic syndrome, more commonly seen in adults. In disorders generally associated with moderate eosinophilia (parasites, Hodgkin's disease, periarteritis nodosa, drug hypersensitivity), the eosinophilic response may occasionally be exaggerated.

B. **Total eosinophil count.** Although the number of eosinophils per cubic millimeter of blood can be estimated from the differential and total leukocyte counts, more accurate counts can be obtained by the use of special diluting fluids that hemolyze the erythrocytes and stain the eosinophils. The eosinophils can then be counted directly in a counting chamber (see Appendix III). Normal values for absolute eosinophil counts are 0–450 cells/mm^3 for adults, 50–700 cells/mm^3 for young children, and 20–850 cells/mm^3 for newborns.

C. **Smears for eosinophils.** The nasal secretions, conjunctival secretions, and sputum of atopic patients usually reveal eosinophils. During symptomatic periods, eosinophils predominate in these secretions. Intercurrent infection may produce a prominent neutrophil response. Repeat smears after treatment of the infection reveal the characteristic eosinophilic nature of the cells. Conjunctival secretions are obtained by a cotton swab. Nasal secretions are secured by having the patient blow the nose in a piece of wax or nonabsorbent paper. In younger children, nasal secretions may also be obtained with a bulb-suction apparatus, a syringe with feeding tube, or cotton-tipped applicator. Sputum is obtained by inducing a deep cough. Eosinophils are best demonstrated by Hansel's stain; alternatively, Wright's stain may be used (see Appendixes II and III for staining techniques and method for total eosinophil count). If clinically indicated, these secretions may be stained and cultured for bacteria and fungi.

D. **Total serum IgE levels.** An elevated **total** serum IgE level supports the diagnosis of atopic disease. However, there is an overlap of IgE values between atopic and normal persons; a **normal IgE level does not exclude** the diagnosis of an allergic disorder. Techniques such as the direct sandwich radioimmunoassay (paper radioimmunosorbent test [PRIST] or enzyme-linked immunoassay [ELISA]—see Appendix IV) are more sensitive, especially for low levels (< 50 units/ml). Accurate interpretation of IgE levels must be based on knowledge of the **test assay** and normal values for each laboratory (see Appendix VI). Using a PRIST method, approximately 63% of adults with asthma, hay fever, or both will have an IgE value above the 2 S.D. limit for healthy adults (*J. Clin. Pathol. [Suppl.]* 28:33, 1975). In children with high serum IgE levels, 96% are found to have significant allergy (*Clin. Allergy* 4:41, 1974). Patients with atopic dermatitis and respiratory symptoms often have a markedly elevated IgE level (> 1000 units/ml).

1. The following are the **current clinical indications** for IgE determinations (laboratory kits for IgE determinations are commercially available):

   a. Differentiation of atopic and nonatopic asthma and rhinitis (especially in young children).

   b. Differentiation of atopic and nonatopic eczema (especially in children).

   c. Prediction of allergy among children with bronchiolitis.

   d. Initial laboratory screening for allergic bronchopulmonary aspergillosis.

   e. Evaluation of immunodeficiency.

   f. Evaluation of drug reactions.

   g. Paraprotein evaluation in patients with multiple myeloma.

2. **Parasitic infections,** a common cause of marked IgE elevations, must be excluded. Diseases with known elevations of IgE are listed in Table 2-3.

Table 2-3. Disorders associated with elevated serum IgE levels

Common disorders
  Atopic diseases
  Parasitic infections
  Laennec's cirrhosis
  Mononucleosis
Less common disorders
  Selective IgA deficiency
  Gluten-sensitive enteropathy
  Pulmonary hemosiderosis
  Drug-induced interstitial nephritis
  Minimal change nephritis
  Bullous pemphigoid
  Acral dermatitis
  Mucocutaneous lymph node syndrome (Kawasaki disease)
  Wegener's granulomatosis
  Polyarteritis nodosa
  Bone marrow transplantation (immediate post-transplantation period)
Rare disorders
  IgE myeloma
  T cell deficiency (DiGeorge syndrome, Wiskott-Aldrich syndrome, Nezelof
    syndrome)
  Hyper IgE syndrome

E. Skin tests for immediate hypersensitivity. The direct introduction of an antigen into the skin of a patient provides a simple and efficient technique for determining IgE antibodies to **specific antigens.** The **clinical significance** of positive reactions (wheal and flare) depends on **correlation** with the history, physical findings, and other laboratory tests.

  1. Indications. The **principal indication** for skin testing is a reasonable suspicion that a specific allergen or a group of allergens is producing symptoms in an allergic patient. Skin tests should be undertaken with allergens to which the patient has a **probability of exposure.** Exposure to pollens demonstrates regional variations; house dust mites, molds, and animal dander are relatively ubiquitous (see Chap. 3).

  In the United States, several suppliers provide allergens for both diagnosis and treatment (see Appendix XIV) as concentrated solutions (1:10 or 1:20 weight to volume) or in dilutions if ordered by the physician. Individual antigens are available for epicutaneous testing (prick or scratch) and intradermal testing. Because stored allergen solutions lose potency within weeks to months, extracts, especially diluted preparations, must be regularly renewed.*

  2. Precautions. Several precautions should be observed during skin testing procedures.

    a. Testing should be deferred during periods of symptomatic bronchospasm to prevent worsening of the clinical status.

    b. Epicutaneous tests (scratch or prick tests) are done initially. This type of testing can detect the sensitive patient with minimal risk of systemic reaction.

---

*Most suppliers place a 2- to 3-year expiration date on concentrated allergen solutions. The half-life of an allergen solution decreases with increasing dilution and increasing temperature. Properly stored allergen solutions (2–8°C) at 1:100 dilution or stronger may maintain antigenicity up to 1 year, but more dilute (1:1000 or weaker) solutions may lose antigenicity in 2–6 months (less in very weak solutions).

    c. Emergency treatment materials (see Chap. 10, **V**), syringes, and needles should be readily available to treat systemic reactions.

    d. A trained technician or nurse may perform skin tests, but **a physician must be immediately available.**

    e. The back is preferable for prick or scratch testing because its flat surface permits the performance of many tests.

3. Methods of skin testing

    a. Prick skin tests

        (1) Procedure. Cleanse the skin with isopropyl or 70% ethyl alcohol and allow it to dry by evaporation. Using a pen or inked stamp, mark future test sites 2 cm apart to prevent coalescence of positive test reactions. Every fifth site should be coded to recheck the test order. Aseptically place a drop of allergic solution, 1:10 or 1:20 (weight to volume) dilution, at each mark, and insert a sterile 26-gauge needle, a sterile sewing needle, or a blood lancet through the drop into the superficial skin and withdraw with a slight lifting of the skin. Do not draw blood. Because blood lancets and sewing needles are not hollow, they can be simply wiped with sterile gauze after testing at each site. Alternatively, a fresh disposable needle can be used for each test site. After 15–30 minutes, observe the test sites for erythema and wheal formation. The average (greatest and smallest) or largest diameter of the wheal in millimeters should be noted and compared with controls. If a large wheal (> 10 mm) appears in less than 15 minutes, wipe the allergen solution from the test site.

        (2) A test using **diluent solution** alone (a **negative control**) should be included to assess skin reactivity to mechanical trauma. (This diluent is usually a phosphate-buffered physiologic saline at pH 7.4 with 0.4% phenol added to inhibit bacterial growth.)

        (3) If patients with **dermatographia** are detected, reactions greater than those in the control site may be considered positive.

        (4) A 0.1% **histamine solution** (histamine phosphate) can serve as a positive control. This histamine control aids in interpreting skin tests (a "standard" 3+ reaction) and demonstrates diminished or absent skin reactivity, which is commonly found in very young or very old patients or in patients taking medications such as antihistamines. Place a greater distance apart from other test sites.

    b. Scratch tests employ the same principles as prick tests but are less sensitive and more time consuming. There are, however, minor technical differences.

        (1) After the skin is cleansed and marked, a 2-mm skin scratch without bleeding is made with a small scalpel, needle, or punch scarifier.

        (2) The test controls and allergen solutions are aseptically dropped onto and gently rubbed into the scratch areas, using a clean toothpick for each allergen.

        (3) Allergen solutions are wiped off and reactions read after 15–30 minutes.

    c. Intradermal skin testing. Following scratch or prick testing, intradermal skin testing is done to allergens that did not elicit clearly positive reactions. Because intradermal skin testing employs a larger antigen challenge than does scratch or prick testing (between 100-fold and 1000-fold, depending on the concentration of antigens), marked local or systemic reactions can occur if intradermal testing is performed with the same antigens that produced positive prick or scratch reactions. In patients with five or less positive epicutaneous skin tests, intradermal tests can be done immediately following the reading of scratch or prick tests. If the number of positive epicutaneous tests is large, intradermal tests should be deferred to another day. In sensitive patients it is best to divide cross-reactive groups (especially grasses) into separate testing sessions since many strongly positive reactions may yield systemic symptoms. Careful antigen selection correlated with the geographic area and history will minimize the number of tests.

   (1) The **sequential steps in intradermal testing** are as follows:

      (a) Use a 1:500 or 1:1000 (weight to volume) dilution of allergen, a 0.01% histamine base solution (histamine phosphate) as a positive control (3+ reaction), and a buffered phenol saline diluent as a negative control. Place a greater distance apart from other test sites.

      (b) The upper half of the volar surface of the forearm and the lateral aspect of the upper arm are choice test sites. The skin of the back may be used. This site precludes the use of a tourniquet in case of systemic reactions. Intradermal skin testing in young children (2–5 years of age) is easier on the back because tests can be applied with better control than on a moving arm.

      (c) With the patient comfortably positioned, cleanse the skin and mark test sites approximately 2.5 cm apart.

      (d) Fill sterile plastic disposable 1-ml tuberculin syringes with approximately 0.1 ml of test solution. To avoid misleading "splash" reactions from injected air, **expel all air bubbles.**

      (e) Stretch the skin taut and introduce the needle into the skin at a **45-degree angle** with the bevel facing **downward.** Advance the needle until the entire bevel of the needle is into the skin.

      (f) Inject the smallest amount of allergen solution that will raise a 1- to 3-mm wheal (approximately **0.02 ml** of solution). If no wheal forms immediately after injection (either the needle is too deep, with subcutaneous fluid injection, or too superficial, with a fluid leak), withdraw the needle and repeat the injection at a different site.

      (g) Read the skin test reactions after 15–30 minutes. Measure the size of the erythema and the size of the wheal with a millimeter ruler. As in scratch or prick tests, this may be done by measuring the greatest and smallest diameter of each reaction and taking the average. Alternatively, only the greatest diameter can be used. **Pseudopods** (protrusions from the wheal) should be noted. A helpful method of measuring wheal size is to stretch the skin taut between the fingers. The wheal will appear as a definite blanched central area that can be easily measured.

   (2) Beginning intradermal skin testing with dilute solutions (1:100,000) and serially increasing them 10-fold until a wheal-and-flare reaction occurs is more quantitative than fixed dilution testing. However, in most cases, this method is not clinically advantageous or practical.

   d. The **Multi-Test applicator** (Lincoln Laboratories, Decatur, Illinois) is a disposable plastic device with multiple test heads and allows the simultaneous administration of antigen by multiple prick-puncture at different sites. This applicator provides for uniform deposition of antigen at each epidermal puncture site, and positive results (3–4+) correlate well with intradermal testing, positive radioallergosorbent test (RAST) scores, and clinical disease.

4. Grading and interpretation of skin tests

   a. Although many grading systems are used, consistency and familiarity with the particular system are most important. The grading system should be noted on the skin test sheet (Table 2-4) for later interpretation by others.

   b. **False-negative** skin tests result from improper techniques, loss of potency of allergen solutions, and prior use of drugs that suppress skin reactivity. Rarely, patients have target organ sensitivity but lack skin sensitivity to a particular allergen. These few patients may need RAST tests (see **H**) or direct **provocation** tests (see **F**). Since antihistamines,

Table 2-4. Stylized skin test sheet[a]

Allergen	Epicutaneous (Date)	Intradermal (Date)
Controls		
Diluent (0–1+)[a]		
Histamine (3+)[a]		
Tree pollen[b]		
Elm		
Oak		
Walnut		
Sycamore		
Birch		
Grass pollen[b]		
Timothy		
Bermuda		
Rye		
Brome		
Blue grass		
Weed pollen[b]		
Ragweed		
Pigweed		
Sage		
Cocklebur		
Plantain		
Molds		
Alternaria		
Hormodendrum		
Aspergillus		
Penicillium		
Monilia		
Mucor		
Helminthosporium		
Environmental allergens		
House dust mite		
Cat		
Dog		
Feathers		
Wool		
Kapok		
Jute		
Pyrethrum		

[a]Suggested reading scale (in greatest diameter): 0 = no reaction; 1+ = erythema ≤ 15 mm; 2+ = erythema > 15 mm or wheal < 3 mm; 3+ = wheal 3–6 mm; 4+ = wheal > 6 mm or pseudopod formation.
[b]Pollens should be geographically defined as important (see Appendix VIII).

especially hydroxyzine, suppress skin test reactivity, they should be withheld **48 hours** prior to testing. Hydroxyzine and newer long-acting antihistamines (e.g., astemizole*) should be eliminated for 96 hours or longer. Theophylline, oral or inhaled adrenergic drugs, sodium cromolyn, and corticosteroids do not interfere with reactivity and may be used prior to immediate hypersensitivity skin testing. (Corticosteroids, however, do suppress delayed hypersensitivity skin test reactions.)

   c. False-positive skin tests may result from improper preparation or administration (or both) of allergen solutions (deviation from physiologic pH or osmolarity, presence of low-molecular-weight irritants, intradermal injections of solutions containing a concentration of glycerine of 6% or higher, intradermal injection of too large a volume [> 0.02 ml]). Substances causing nonspecific histamine release (particularly food extracts) and dermatographia can also cause false-positive reactions.

   d. Interpretation of the clinical relevance of positive or negative skin tests requires correlation of the history, physical examination, and other laboratory studies. Important guidelines for correct interpretation include the following:

   (1) Skin tests are usually more reliable for diagnosing atopic sensitivity in patients with allergic rhinosinoconjunctivitis than in patients with asthma (many asthmatic patients who have positive skin tests cannot relate their symptoms physically or temporally to known allergen exposure or do not react to provocation challenges).

   (2) Skin testing with mixes of allergens is less reliable than with specific allergens but is useful for screening purposes, especially in small children.

   (3) Positive skin tests correlate highly with food allergy, which is manifested as acute urticaria, angioedema, or anaphylaxis.

   (4) Correlation of positive skin tests with causative factors in atopic dermatitis is usually unreliable but may correlate in some instances with ingested, inhaled, or topical allergen challenge.

   (5) The use of skin tests to diagnose immediate hypersensitivity to drugs is limited because metabolites of the drugs, not the drug itself, are usually responsible. These metabolites are usually unknown or unavailable. Skin testing with **complete protein** drug allergens (e.g., insulin or animal serum) and **penicillin** (which has been extensively studied) provides useful information (see Chap. 12).

F. Provocative testing. Direct administration of the allergen to respiratory mucosa (nasal, conjunctival, bronchial), with later observation of target-organ response, is an adjunct to skin testing in some patients (see Chaps. 5, 6).

   1. The **major advantage** of this technique is that it allows more precise identification of clinically important allergens, especially in patients with a large number of positive skin tests. Patients with positive skin tests frequently fail to react to provocation testing to the same allergens, while positive provocation tests with negative skin tests are very unusual.

   2. The **major disadvantages** of provocation testing are the limitation of one antigen per test session, the imprecise quantitation of response, especially for conjunctival and nasal provocation, the difficulty in standardization of each allergen, and the production of severe symptoms, especially marked bronchospasm following bronchial challenge in patients with severe asthma. (Because severe symptoms may occur, provocation techniques should be attempted **only** with strict precautions and by experienced personnel. Provocative testing is a relative **contraindication** in patients with clearly defined histories of immediate bronchospasm, anaphylaxis, urticaria, or angioedema.)

   3. Provocative testing is needed to confirm doubtful cases of **food allergy.**

*Astemizole is not currently available in the United States.

Because of the poor reliability of food skin tests not associated with acute urticaria, angioedema, or anaphylaxis, **double-blind–controlled** food challenges are required to document questionable sensitivity to food (see Chap. 13).

G. **Passive cutaneous transfer testing** (Prausnitz-Küstner [P-K] testing), now more of historical interest, provided the first demonstration of a substance (reagin) in the serum of allergic persons that is capable of sensitizing the skin of nonallergic persons. In the past, P-K testing was used in patients with dermatographia or generalized skin eruptions. Currently, it is contraindicated and rarely performed even in these selected patients because in vitro testing for specific IgE antibodies (RAST) provides the same information without the risk associated with transferring serum from one person to another. For historical interest, the P-K test involves the following: Allergic serum (0.1 ml) is injected intradermally into a carefully marked site on the forearm of a nonallergic person. After 24–48 hours this site is challenged with intradermal allergen (0.02 ml) and observed for an immediate positive wheal-and-flare response not present on the control site. For accuracy more than one site should be tested.

H. **In vitro tests for antigen-specific IgE**
   1. The **RAST test** is a radioimmunoassay or enzyme-linked immunoassay (ELISA) measuring **allergen-specific IgE**. RAST and other in vitro methods are further detailed in Appendix V.
      a. The assay consists of **three major steps:**
         (1) Allergen is coupled to a solid-phase support (e.g., cellulose disks or Sephadex beads).
         (2) The serum is added, and antigen-specific IgE, if present, binds to allergen on the disk or bead.
         (3) Radiolabeled anti-IgE globulin is then added, and the amount of allergen-specific IgE is quantitated by the amount of radioactivity present. Alternatively, enzyme-labeled anti-IgE globulin is added and the amount of allergen-specific IgE is quantitated by colorometric change induced by enzyme activity on a substrate. The radioactive counts or colorometric changes are compared with a reference serum with known high levels of allergen-specific IgE and are usually reported on a scale of 0–5; **2 + or greater is considered significant.** As routinely performed, RAST values **are not** absolutely quantitative in terms of nanograms of antibody.
      b. The **major advantages** of RAST testing include the lack of risk of systemic reaction; lack of dependence on skin reactivity modified by drugs, disease, or age of the patient; and stability of antigens in the solid-phase state.
      c. The **chief disadvantages** of RAST testing include the limited allergen selection (reliable correlation with pollens, epidermals, and some foods; less reliable correlation with dust, mold, and drug allergens); reduced sensitivity as compared with intradermal skin tests; lack of immediately available results; and increased expense due to added technical help, specialized laboratory equipment, and costly reagents.
      d. The RAST and RAST variant techniques are useful **research tools**, especially for allergen standardization and monitoring immunotherapy. It is **clinically helpful** in patients with severe atopic dermatitis, generalized urticaria, poor skin reactivity, or enhanced skin reactivity (dermatographia). As currently performed, it does not supplant the use of direct skin testing.
   2. The **in vitro histamine release test** is an assay that uses separated sensitized leukocytes to measure allergen-specific IgE. It is usually available only on a research basis.
      a. The bioassay involves the following steps:
         (1) A leukocyte fraction containing basophils (coated with allergen-specific IgE in allergic persons) is obtained.

    (2) After incubating the leukocyte fraction with varying concentrations of allergens, the amount and percentage of histamine released at each concentration are measured.

    (3) Comparisons are made with the leukocytes and with the maximal histamine released from leukocytes subjected to a freeze-thawing technique or treated with anti-IgE.

    (4) Cell sensitivity is calculated by determining the antigen concentration (expressed in micrograms) required to release 50% of the cellular histamine (HR_{50}).

  b. The assay correlates well with the history, RAST test results, and intradermal skin test results. Compared with RAST testing, the histamine-release method is a more biologically meaningful in vitro indication of allergic sensitivity. However, the assay's increased technical difficulty and potential for drug interference (similar to that for in vivo skin testing) make it an impractical tool for clinical use.

I. Pulmonary function testing

  1. Measurement of pulmonary function is used in patients with allergic pulmonary disease to aid in the differential diagnosis of obstructive airway disease, to evaluate bronchial challenge objectively, and to determine the clinical severity and monitor the results of therapy. Although complete spirometry before and after the use of bronchodilators is performed initially, a simple measurement such as peak expiratory flow rate or forced expiratory volume at 1 second is used to follow patients routinely. **Arterial blood gases** are the best guides to gas exchange abnormalities. In severe asthma they should be assessed frequently to predict the onset of respiratory failure (see Chap. 6, II.C).

  2. Spirometric measurements of nasal airflow and resistance are technically difficult and are not commonly used in clinical practice.

J. X-ray examinations

  1. X-ray examination of the chest is indicated during the initial evaluation of allergic pulmonary disease. The chest x-ray film in asthma is usually normal; accentuation of the bronchovascular markings, thickening of the bronchi on end, or hyperinflation may be noted in patients with chronic disease. During acute exacerbations, an x-ray can exclude complications such as pneumonia, atelectasis, or pneumothorax.

  2. Tomography, newer scanning techniques, and rarely, in selected cases, **bronchography** are helpful in patients with suspected bronchiectasis or other lesions not revealed by routine chest radiography.

  3. Sinus x-rays are indicated for suspected acute or chronic sinusitis, a common complication of upper respiratory allergy (see Chap. 5).

K. Miscellaneous studies

  1. Urinalyses and serum chemistries are usually normal in atopic patients.

  2. Stool specimens should be examined for **ova** and **parasites** in cases of unexplained urticaria, eosinophilia, or elevated serum IgE. A **duodenal or small-bowel aspirate** can uncover parasitic infection in a patient with negative stool findings (e.g., giardiasis).

  3. The **erythrocyte sedimentation rate** is normal in uncomplicated atopic disease. An elevated rate suggests an alternative or additional diagnosis or infectious complications.

  4. Alpha$_1$-antitrypsin level and phenotype should be assessed in patients showing irreversible obstructive airway disease.

  5. Serum quantitative immunoglobulins, especially IgA and immunoglobulin subclasses, can be deficient or altered in patients with symptoms suggestive of allergy. In immunodeficiency, however, wheezing, sneezing, and nasal and eye itching are not usually the predominant presenting symptoms.

  6. Quantitative sweat chloride test values are elevated in cystic fibrosis, a disease primarily affecting children but occasionally seen in adults. Symptoms of poor growth, chronic pulmonary infection, and malabsorption should prompt performance of this test.

Selected Readings

American Academy of Allergy. Position statement. Skin testing and radioallergosorbent testing (RAST) for diagnosis of specific allergens responsible for IgE-mediated diseases. *J. Allergy Clin. Immunol.* 72:515, 1983.

Geha, R. S. Human IgE. *J. Allergy Clin. Immunol.* 74:109, 1984.

Ishizaka, K., and Ishizaka, T. Immunology of IgE-mediated Hypersensitivity. In E. Middleton, Jr., C. E. Reed, and E. F. Ellis (eds.), *Allergy: Principles and Practice.* St. Louis: Mosby, 1983. Chap. 5.

Kaliner, M. Mast cell mediators in asthma. *Chest (Suppl.)* 87:2, 1985.

Nelson, H. S. The clinical relevance of IgE. *Ann. Allergy* 49:73, 1982.

Rose, M. R., Friedman, H., and Fahey, J. L. (eds.). *Manual of Clinical Immunology* (3rd ed.). Washington, DC: The American Society for Microbiology, 1986. Chap. 80.

Wasserman, S. I. Mediators of immediate hypersensitivity. *J. Allergy Clin. Immunol.* 72:101, 1983.

3

Aeroallergens and Environmental Factors

Robert W. Ausdenmoore

Aeroallergens

Aeroallergens are relatively large and complex particles, such as pollens, molds, and house dust mites, that are capable of eliciting allergic reactions in susceptible persons. These particles contain many molecular components, only some of which are antigenic. When specific antigenic components have been identified, they usually are proteins with some carbohydrate subunits and have a molecular weight of 3000–40,000 daltons.

The **antigenicity** of these molecules is fundamentally a property of their **size, spatial configuration,** and **chemical groupings.** The overall **allergic importance** of these particles is not only a function of their **antigenicity** but also of their **availability** in the environment for contact with susceptible persons and the suitability of **particle size** for impingement on the respiratory mucosa.

I. **Sources and size of aeroallergens**
   A. **Biogenic** particulate matter commonly identifiable in air samples includes pollen grains, fungal spores, plant fragments, animal dander, algae, and insect fragments. **Nonbiogenic** materials, such as hydrocarbons, salt crystals, and other types of particulate matter, may also be identified, especially near areas of industrial activity. Whether or not some of these diverse inorganic materials modify responses to acknowledged aeroallergens is unclear.
   B. Most airborne substances of allergic importance identifiable microscopically are between 2 and 60 μ in diameter. Most of these particles (particularly those > 15 μ in diameter) strike ocular, nasal, and pharyngeal surfaces because of their linear momentum. Because the majority of allergenic particles do not reach the bronchi, it has been postulated that the bronchial pathophysiologic features in asthma result from a bronchial reflex stimulated by nasopharyngeal receptors. Alternatively, active allergenic material may be eluted from the particles in the nasopharynx and aspirated, or may reach the bronchi by a hematogenous route.
   C. **Allergenic particles less than 15 μ in diameter** have been shown to exist in atmospheric aerosols by immunochemical means. These particles probably represent fragments of the identifiable particulate matter in air formed by pulverization and dissolution by moisture, with subsequent redrying and refloatation in the air.

II. **Sampling techniques**
   A. **Gravitational methods.** Solid particles suspended in the air will settle because of gravitational forces. The gravitational method (Durham sampler, Fig. 3-1) involves the placement of a glass microscope slide coated with soft glycerin jelly* in a holder between two metal plates and exposed to the air for 24 hours.

I wish to thank Dr. James Thompson and Mr. Don Claridge of Hollister-Stier Laboratories for their helpful comments and suggestions.

*Soft glycerin with fuchsin stain: 5 gm gelatin, 40 ml water, 4 gm phenol is combined with 195 gm glycerin and warmed. To facilitate pollen identification, 2 ml of Calberia's solution is combined with this glycerin mixture while warming. Calberia's solution contains 5 ml glycerin, 10 ml 95% ethanol, and 2 drops of saturated, aqueous basic fuchsin.

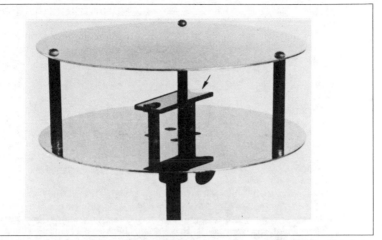

Fig. 3-1. Gravity slide (Durham) sampler with its fixed, adhesive-coated horizontal slide (arrow). Courtesy of Air Pollution Training Institute, Research Triangle Park, NC.

Particles deposited on the surface by gravity and turbulent horizontal airflow are then identified, counted, and reported as particles per centimeters squared per 24 hours. This simple, inexpensive method collects useful data but has the following limitations:

1. Wind direction and velocity, raindrops, and condensation influence the results more than with other techniques.
2. Collected quantities are low even over a 24-hour period.
3. Collection of larger particles is favored; smaller ones are less likely to be trapped.

B. **Volumetric methods**
1. With the **rotating air impactor,** a coated surface is rotated for specific periods of time at a fixed and known speed. Then the particles are counted and reported as with the Durham sampler. Such methods reduce the factors of wind velocity and direction. One adaptation, the Rotorod Sampler* (Fig. 3-2), involves the use of clear acrylic collector rods **coated** with a thin layer of **silicone grease** to enhance retention of impacted particles. Other modifications provide **timed intermittent rotation** to prevent overloading and shields to cover exposed surfaces between operating intervals. The American Academy of Allergy currently recommends the intermittent rotoslide sampler as the standard volumetric collector for larger micromic particles.
2. **Inertial suction samplers.** When a given volume of air is drawn through membrane filters with defined pore sizes or is aspirated through an orifice with a defined size, particles of a given density leave the air stream and impinge on a collecting plate as the air changes direction because of the plate. One modification, the **Burkhard (Hirst) spore trap** (Fig. 3-3), contains a collecting plate (rotated at the rate of 2 mm/hour) within the trap to allow observations of the fluctuations in the count. In addition, a rudder eliminates the factor of wind direction.

C. **Interpretation of sampling data**
1. Large particles (> 20 μ in diameter) with high seasonal levels (e.g., ragweed pollen) can be adequately and simply monitored by gravity slides. For research purposes, however, the more accurate volumetric techniques must be employed. Manuals with identification guidelines are available for pol-

*Ted Brown Associates, 26338 Esperanza Drive, Los Altos Hills, CA 94022.

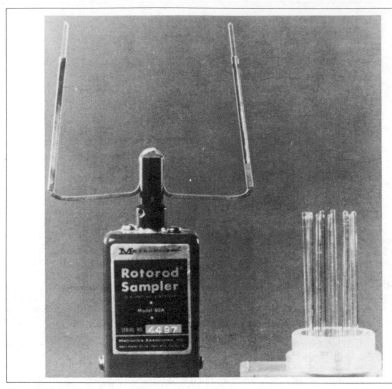

Fig. 3-2. Rotorod Sampler (rotating arm impactor), well suited to short periods of continuous collection. Field carrier for storage of additional lucite rods is shown at right. Courtesy of Air Pollution Training Institute, Research Triangle Park, NC.

lens and mold spores (see Selected Readings). Tabulation of their concentrations (by counting under the microscope) can help determine seasonal prevalences of common aeroallergens in given locales (see Appendix VIII). Correlation of particle counts with clinical symptoms on a given day must be cautiously interpreted. Unfortunately, some news agencies report daily pollen or mold counts to help promote medication advertisements to a lay public unaware of sampling limitations, the important aspects of personal exposure variations, the effects of multiple sensitivities, or complex allergen dose-response relationships.

2. **Immunochemical quantitation** of allergens in air samples can be made using radiolabeled antibody toward the allergen being measured. Fractions of these allergens are separated by collecting on progressively smaller pore-sized filters. Correlations of quantitative data derived by immunochemical means with clinical symptom scores, especially in asthma, is considerably better than the correlation with pollen or mold spore counts. Relatively few studies of this type have been carried out and, thus far, only data with respect to ragweed, *Alternaria,* ragweed antigen E, and *Alternaria* 1 fraction have been published. This new, more precise method of quantitating allergen in the air may not only provide better data to correlate with clinical symptoms, but also may increase the understanding of the effect of antigens not recognizable under the microscope, e.g., dander and insect fragments in dwellings and workplaces.

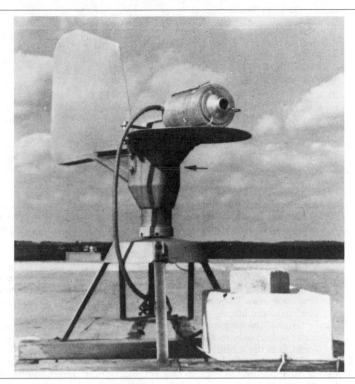

Fig. 3-3. Burkard (Hirst) spore trap serving as wind vane for exposure of Anderson sampler in free air. The intake orifice (arrow) of spore trap is 2 × 14 mm. Particles are collected on greased tape–coated drum, advanced by clock mechanism. Courtesy of Air Pollution Training Institute, Research Triangle Park, NC.

III. Pollen aeroallergens. Pollen grains are male reproductive structures of seed-bearing plants and function to carry the male gametes (sperm) to the female gametes (egg), which remain on the plant. Pollen transfer for plants with showy, colorful, and fragrant flowers is accomplished by insects (entomophily). In these instances, the pollen is often large, with an adhesive coating. Remarkable adaptations of some plants allow dissemination of pollen by birds, bats, mice, or even snails.

Most **pollens of allergic importance are windborne** (anemophily). Plants with windborne pollen transfers are typically drab, with small, inconspicuous, and odorless flowers. Their pollen is usually small and nonadhesive, with a smooth unsculptured surface.

Most pollen is shed in the early morning hours, but dispersal by wind currents usually produces maximal pollen concentrations in the afternoon or early evening. Although pollen grains are viable for only a few hours, nonviable pollen is still an active allergen. A gentle wind can carry pollen of anemophilous plants for many miles and produce high pollen concentrations in urban and metropolitan areas, far from their rural or suburban source.

A. Weeds. Although many different classes of plants may be considered weeds, plants from within the family Compositae are most important from an allergy perspective. Within this family, ragweed (*Ambrosia* species) is the single most important cause, quantitatively and qualitatively, of seasonal allergic rhinitis (hay fever) in the United States. (A regional pollen guide listing the periods of prevalence and relative importance of various pollens in various regions of the United States appears in Appendix VIII, together with a floristic map of the United States and Canada.) The highest concentrations of ragweed pollen occur in the central plains and eastern agricultural regions. Cultivation of soil as seen in the midwest grain fields allows dense ragweed growth and the greatest seasonal exposure risk for the ragweed pollen–sensitive patient.

Antigen E is a highly reactive fraction of ragweed with a molecular weight of 37,800 daltons, representing approximately 6% of the extractable protein of ragweed. It is 200 times as active as whole ragweed extract. Another fraction, antigen K (molecular weight 38,000) is somewhat less potent than antigen E, but still produces reactions in almost all ragweed-sensitive patients.

B. Grasses. It is difficult to distinguish the pollen of different grasses solely on the basis of morphology. Consequently, the importance of individual species is largely determined on the basis of total grass-pollen counts combined with knowledge of the regional presence of individual grass species.

    1. In general, **Bermuda grass** is the predominant species throughout the **southern** half of the United States and the **southern Pacific coast regions.** In the **northeastern** and **northern midwestern states, the bulk of the grass pollen usually comes from the blue grass, orchard grass, timothy grass, and red top** (see Appendix VIII for individual locales).

    2. Grass pollen is seen only during the **growing seasons,** so that seasonal patterns (spring and summer) are noted in the north, and more perennial patterns are observed in the south. As with weed pollen, **grass pollen concentrations are generally low at high altitudes such as in the Rocky Mountain area.** They are also low in the far north regions of Wisconsin, Michigan, and Maine.

    3. In terms of the **frequency** and **severity** of allergic symptoms, grass pollen ranks second only to ragweed in the United States. In other parts of the world, it is the leading aeroallergen.

C. Trees. The pollens of wind-pollinating (anemophilous) trees are the principal causes of respiratory allergy in this botanical group. Insect-pollinating (entemophilous) trees (e.g., ornamental and fruit trees) and the anemophilous conifers whose pollen has a thick exine or outer covering (e.g., pine trees) are of minor allergic significance.

    1. Each tree genus produces pollen morphologically distinct from that of any other genus and exhibits marked individual variation with respect to the duration, intensity, and seasonal pattern of pollination.

    2. Little cross-antigenicity is noted between genera. Also, clustering of certain genera often occurs within the same floristic zone. As a result of these factors, an allergic patient can have selective sensitivity (frequently only to one genus or a few different genera).

    3. In general, the period of pollination within a given locality is short, with the result that tree-sensitive patients often exhibit correspondingly brief periods of discomfort.

    4. Pollination occurs before, during, or shortly after leaves develop in deciduous trees. In more temperate climates, tree pollination concludes by late spring when the trees are fully leaved; in warmer areas this season may be extended (see Appendix VIII).

IV. Mold aeroallergens. Although some biologists consider molds (fungi) as distinct from the plant and animal kingdom, the majority classify them as simple plants lacking stems, roots, leaves, and chlorophyll. Despite the simplicity of molds, they are among the most successfully adapted organisms on earth. They exist in large numbers in almost every environment—dry areas virtually devoid of water or other life, moist areas with wide temperature extremes, or in soil and fresh water or salt water. All are either saprophytic (obtaining food from dead organic material) or parasitic (feeding on viable tissue).

A. Mold structure. In spite of the enormous number of species, only two basic structural forms exist: **Yeast forms** grow as single cells and reproduce by simple division or "budding" to form daughter cells; **hyphal forms** grow as a network of interconnecting tubes. Some hyphae are specialized to produce reproductive spores, which are dispersed by water, wind, insects, or other animals. Most fungi have hyphae.

B. Mold classification. The mode of sexual reproduction has been chosen as the basis for classification of fungi. During the life cycle of most fungal species, reproduction is accomplished by **fragmentation** of the hyphae, or by **production of spores**, or by both processes. Spores may be produced asexually (simple division of a cell) or sexually (fusion of two compatible cells to form a zygote followed by reduction-division). Most fungi reproduce both asexually (the **imperfect stage**) and sexually (the **perfect stage**). By this method, four major classes may be easily distinguished: **Oomycetes, Zygomycetes, Ascomycetes,** and **Basidiomycetes.** Many species (20,000 or more) cannot be classified in this manner, however, because they either have no perfect stage, or only the asexual spores are seen, or both. Such spores often differ morphologically from sexual spores of the same species, thus making it impossible to assign them to the correct botanic class. This unclassifiable group is called **Deuteromycetes,** or **Fungi Imperfecti.** Subclassifications within this group are based on morphologic differences of spores (form classification); such classification may be expected not to reflect true botanic groupings and probably **does not reflect antigenic similarities** (Table 3-1).

C. Mold distribution. The enormous diversity of these organisms and their remarkable adaptations result in unavoidable human exposure regardless of geographic region. However, because a small amount of moisture and oxygen is a basic requirement for fungal growth, arid regions or areas of high altitude are relatively free of fungi by conventional sampling and culture methods. Fungal dormancy is also observed in subfreezing climates. Beyond these generalities, **it is difficult to predict fungi prevalence by geographic locale.**

Molds are found in **houses** and can be a source of perennial allergic symptoms. Spoiled food, soiled upholstery, and garbage containers are favorite substrates for home mold growth. Other common sites include damp basements, shower curtains, plumbing fixtures, and contaminated cool-mist vaporizers and console humidifiers. Molds are common components of house dust.

D. Mold exposure patterns. Mold sensitivity in allergic persons is commonly characterized by sporadic exacerbations that reflect local, concentrated exposures (e.g., visiting a farm, harvesting and storing hay, picking corn, cutting weeds or grass, raking leaves, hiking in the woods) or periods of maximal mold growth (e.g., during moist, warm summers and falls, especially with leaves on the ground). Many occupations predispose to a high risk of mold exposure (e.g., grain farmers, fruit pickers, papermill workers). Heavy mold growth on cut Christmas trees brought indoors can produce a distinctly seasonal pattern in mold-sensitive patients. Combined with the irritant pine scent and dusty stored decorations, this mold exposure can initiate allergic symptoms. For general measures toward improving mold control, see Chap. 4.

E. Assessment of mold prevalence. Empiric mold-control methods are mandatory for allergic patients to prevent reactions, sensitization, or both. In selected situations, identification and semiquantitative determinations of mold exposures are helpful. These situations include: (1) patients with hypersensitivity disease requiring mold identification for more accurate diagnosis and treatment (e.g., hypersensitivity pneumonitis), (2) monitoring the success of mold eradication measures, and (3) determining mold types in locales where prevalence data are unavailable.

Measurement of airborne mold is accomplished by microscopic identification of samples obtained by volumetric collectors or by cultured mold plates. General purpose mold plates can be made with Sabouraud's glucose, potato dextrose, corn meal, or V-8 agars. Certain conditions of temperature, humidity, and barometric pressure also can favor growth of molds that are not clinically relevant. Mold identification requires time, equipment, and mycologic expertise. References are available (see Selected Readings); mold-identification services are also available through manufacturers of allergen extracts (Appendix XIV).

Table 3-1. Classification, primary sources, and allergenic importance of molds in the United States

Classification	Number of species	Primary sources	Relative allergenic importance
Deuteromycetes (Fungi Imperfecti)	20,000		
Alternaria		Plants, leaves, damp walls; ↑ outdoors on hot, dry days (July, August)	Major
Cladosporium (Hormodendrum)		Decaying plants, compost piles; ↑ outdoors on hot, dry days (July, August)	Major
Aspergillus		Spoiled food, organic debris; ↑ indoors	Major
Penicillium		Spoiled food, organic debris; ↑ indoors	Moderate
Fusarium		Soil, compost piles; ↑ in wet weather	Moderate
Helminthosporium		Plants of all types	Positive skin tests frequent; ? importance
Aureobasidium		Leaves, soil, paper, lumber	Minor
Zygomycetes	250		
Rhizopus		Soil, leaves; ↑ in dry weather; also found in damp interiors	Moderate
Mucor		Soil, leaves; ↑ in dry weather; also found in damp interiors	Moderate
Basidiomycetes	12,000		
Smuts		Grass, grain fields	Major (agricultural areas)
Rusts		Grass, grain fields	Major (agricultural areas)
Mushrooms		Damp, forested regions; ↑ in wet weather	Minor
Ascomycetes	15,000	Trees, bark, deadwood; ↑ in wood pulp mills	Regional major (central North America)
Oomycetes	250	Grass, broad-leaved plants	Minor

Table 3-1 lists important allergenic molds and their common sources. Individual mold prevalence by region in the United States can be found in Appendix VIII.

V. Epidermal allergens. Inhaled dander (epithelial scales) from animal species (other than human) can sensitize an allergic person. Any foreign animal dander could conceivably be responsible for sensitization, but the most common epidermal allergens come from dogs, cats, and fur or feathers (cattle, horse, sheep, goat, duck) used for stuffing materials. Because the soluble dander, rather than the hair, produces allergic reactions, finished material without dander is less allergenic (e.g., furs used as clothing). (The concept of dander-induced allergic reactions has been questioned recently with the demonstration of several major allergens found in other body fluids, e.g., cat allergen 1 in the saliva and urinary antigens in rats and mice. Further research is needed to better clarify the exact source or sources of the allergens.)

Sensitivity is often exquisite, requiring only a brief or unexpected exposure to create a marked allergic response. Dander concentrations may be cumulative within a home or other enclosed space; dispersal throughout the home is easily accomplished by the heating system. Vacuuming and pet cleansing are only mildly effective, temporary methods of control. Because the allergen is in the soluble dander, **short-haired breeds** or **nonshedding dogs** also cause allergy.

Occupational exposure to laboratory animals can be an important cause of difficulty for allergic individuals and can preclude their ability to function in this occupation. It is also possible that large exposures to rodent dander in tenements and other poorly kept dwellings can account for a significant amount of allergic difficulty.

VI. Miscellaneous aeroallergens

A. House dust. The term **house dust,** normally used to describe material from indoor household environments, consists of animal dander, indoor molds, vegetable fibers, food particles, insect parts and emanations, algae, and human dander. The relative concentration of indoor particles increases when the doors and windows are closed because little or no dilution with outdoor air occurs.

B. House dust mite. It has been known that dust from mattress stuffings is an important source of indoor allergens. In 1967, European investigators identified the house dust mite (*Dermatophagoides pteronyssinus*) as a highly allergenic fraction of mattress dust. House dust mites subsist on epithelial scales, reaching a seasonal peak concentration in September and October. *Dermatophagoides farinae*, a different species, is the most widespread mite in mattress stuffing samples in North America.

Mite allergenicity does not depend on viability of the mite. Therefore, preventive measures include not only destruction of the mite but also physical removal of the mite, or placing a barrier between mite antigen and the susceptible person, or both. Secondary reservoirs include overstuffed furniture, rugs, and pillows.

C. Seeds. Cottonseed, kapok, and flaxseed (linseed) are plant fibers widely used for consumer dry goods. Finished fabrics are relatively nonallergenic, but unrefined material is routinely used for stuffing materials. This unrefined material consists of large quantities of markedly allergenic seed and flower parts. Cottonseed and flaxseed can produce explosive allergic symptoms in susceptible persons. Prick testing is especially recommended before intradermal injection of these seed allergens.

D. Orris root. Bulbs of the iris family are the source of this allergen. When powdered, the pleasant odor, moderate adhesiveness, and finely granular nature make it a desirable cosmetic base. Because of its antigenicity, its use is largely limited to children's cosmetics, bubble baths, and inexpensive cosmetics.

E. Pyrethrum. The flower heads of chrysanthemums are dried and used for insecticides.

F. Vegetable gums. Karaya, acacia, and tragacanth, used in permanent wave set lotions, are infrequently implicated as allergens.

G. Insect parts. Allergic persons can show sensitivity by skin testing to a wide variety of insects, suggesting that inhalation of insect parts can play a role in symptom production. The cockroach, in particular, is known to be an important allergen, especially for allergic individuals living in crowded and poorly kep dwellings or working in warehouses or other storage facilities.

Environmental Factors

I. **Climatic factors.** It is difficult to isolate and separately study the complex interaction of temperature, humidity, and barometric pressure in producing or exacerbating allergic symptoms. Nevertheless, it appears that allergic disease, especiall asthma, tends to be adversely affected by **high humidity,** by **sudden temperatur changes** (particularly from warm to cold), and by **drops in the barometric pres sure.** Intolerance to these factors is highly individual. Dry, cold air common' precipitates exertional dyspnea.

II. **Air pollution**
  A. **Industrial smog** results from the combustion of liquid or solid fossil fuels and usually measured by the levels of carbon monoxide, particulate matter, an sulfur dioxide.
    1. **Carbon monoxide,** even at peak levels measured in urban rush-hour traffi (120 ppm), cannot be shown to affect respiratory function adversely in noi mal persons or asthmatic patients.
    2. **Particulate matter** (fog, mist, dust, smoke, soot) can cause coughing an reflex bronchoconstriction or direct stimulation of small-airway receptoi causing bronchiolar constriction. It can also potentiate the effect of othe pollutants.
    3. **Sulfur dioxide** in very high experimental concentrations (13–50 ppn causes increased airway resistance and suppression of mucosal ciliary activ ities in humans and other animals. Peak levels in the atmosphere have n exceeded 1.5 ppm. An increased incidence of asthma occurs with high poll tion, suggesting that a combination of different inhalant factors is opere tive.
  B. **Photochemical smog.** Photochemical smog is produced by ultraviolet radiatio on hydrocarbons (emitted by automobile exhaust) with the formation of **ozon nitric oxide,** and other oxidants. Average urban levels of oxidants may be in th range of 0.2–0.5 ppm, with a peak at 1 ppm. Low levels (0.25 ppm) cause ey irritation and coughing; high concentrations cause diminished vital capacit forced expiratory volume, and diffusion capacity (even in normal persons). Mos of the oxidants measured are ozone (> 90%), but **nitrogen dioxide** is ofte present in significant concentrations. Nitrogen dioxide, in addition to its direc toxic effect on the lung, may produce irreversible pulmonary changes in smol ers.

III. **Tobacco smoke.** The role of allergic sensitivity to tobacco smoke is unclear. How ever, **intolerance** to smoke exists. Tobacco smoke, because of its strong irritar effect, potentiates allergic reactions.

IV. **Volatile odors.** Many noxious chemicals, such as camphor, formaldehyde, kerosene gasoline, or wood smoke, aggravate allergic symptoms. Cooking odors, especiall fish and animal odors, in specifically sensitized people may precipitate an acut allergic crisis by an IgE-mediated mechanism.

V. **Chemicals.** Workers in certain industries (e.g., plastics manufacture) can develo asthma on exposure to a variety of chemicals including acid anhydrides (e.g phthalic anhydride) and diisocyanates (e.g., toluene diisocyanate [TDI]). TDI ar related compounds may produce asthma by both allergenic and nonallergenic mecl anisms (see Chap. 6).

Selected Readings

Agarwal, K., et al. Airborne allergens: Association with various particle sizes an short ragweed plant parts. *J. Allergy Clin. Immunol.* 74:687, 1984.

Ausdenmoore, R. W., and Fischer, T. J. Inhalant Aerobiology and Antigens. In E. B. Weiss, M. S. Segal, and M. Stein (eds.), *Bronchial Asthma: Mechanisms and Therapeutics* (2nd ed.), Boston: Little, Brown, 1985.

Batchelder, G. L. Sampling characteristics of the rotorod, rotoslide, and Andersen machines for atmospheric pollen and spores. *Ann. Allergy* 39:18, 1977.

Lopez, M., and Salvaggio, J. E. Climate–Weather–Air Pollution. In E. Middleton, C. Reed, and E. F. Ellis (eds.), *Allergy: Principles and Practice*. St. Louis: Mosby, 1983.

Ogden, E. C., et al. *Manual for Sampling Airborne Pollen*. New York: Hafner, 1974.

Smith, E. G. *Sampling and Identifying Allergenic Pollens and Molds. An Illustrated Manual for Physicians and Lab Technicians*. San Antonio, TX: Blewstone Press, 1984.

Solomon, W. R. The aerobiology of pollinosis. *J. Allergy Clin. Immunol.* 74:449, 1984.

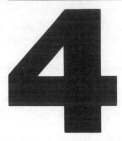

Basic Principles of Therapy for Allergic Disease

Thomas J. Fischer,
Gregory N. Entis,
John G. Winant, Jr., and
I. Leonard Bernstein

The treatment of patients with allergic disease must be individualized, based on the general principles of avoidance of allergens and irritants, judicious use of pharmacologic therapy, and, if indicated, the administration of immunotherapy (hyposensitization). This individualized approach must be adjusted according to the intensity and severity of the allergic disease, considering the discomfort, inconvenience, cost, and possible adverse effects of the treatment. This chapter is designed to serve as an outline for this individualized approach. Added information on specific diseases is found in subsequent chapters.

Environmental Controls

Avoidance of identifiable allergens and irritants is the most effective method of managing atopic disease. Many well-defined and other, less well-characterized environmental factors can induce or worsen allergic symptoms. The extent of environmental control measures must reflect the individual patient's needs.

I. **Standard environmental control methods** attempt to reduce allergic and irritant exposure in the home to a minimum without excessive alteration of life-style or purchase of expensive air-cleaning devices. Allergic patients and their families should understand that environmental control measures are essential if management of allergic disease is to be successful. Drug therapy and immunotherapy are not adequate substitutes for basic avoidance measures. Table 4-1 presents the standard environmental control measures that should be taken. Instruct the patient or family in these measures and review them regularly, especially if symptoms increase without explanation.

II. **Mechanical devices for environmental control.** In addition to standard home environmental control guidelines, three types of mechanical devices can help modify the home environment.

   A. **Air conditioners.** The beneficial effect of air conditioning on allergic symptom control is recognized, with several studies demonstrating its efficacy in reducing pollen exposure. *Consumer Reports* * is an excellent source of general information on air conditioning and ratings of individual air conditioning products. For individual or central air conditioning units, proper maintenance and cleaning are necessary to prevent dispersal of allergens (e.g., mold) through dirty filters. Air-conditioning manufacturers or service companies can provide information on the methods and frequency of service.

   B. **Air cleaners** reduce airborne particles by four different methods: impingement, straining, diffusion, or electrostatic precipitation. For purposes of rating, air cleaners have been categorized into four types by the Air Conditioning and Refrigeration Institute (ARI).†

      1. **Group RI** filters include unit or panel-type air cleaners (e.g., fiberglass home furnace filters using impingement and straining methods). Some

*Published by Consumers Union of United States, Inc., Orangeburg, NY
†1501 Wilson Boulevard, Arlington, VA 22209

Table 4-1. Standard environmental control measures

The patient's **bedroom** is most important, since a significant portion of the day is spent there. Follow these suggestions:

1. The bedroom should contain no stuffed chairs, rugs, or drapes; linoleum or wood floors, wood or metal furniture, and washable cotton curtains or curtains made of plastic or Plexiglas are preferable. Everything in the room should be washable.
2. Avoid storing blankets, woolens, felt hats, or other dust catchers in bedroom closets. Keep the doors closed.
3. If there is a furnace vent in the room, cover it with three layers of cheesecloth. (Exercise caution with flammable material in contact with metal.)
4. Doors and windows in the room must fit tightly. Close windows during major pollen seasons or during pollution alerts.
5. Once or twice a week, clean the room with a damp dustcloth (the patient should avoid the room during and for 3–4 hr after cleaning).
6. Use Dacron or foam pillows and wash monthly.
7. Vacuum mattresses and springs and completely encase in plastic with a zipper closing.
8. Wash blankets; use fuzz-free cotton or Dacron sheets next to patient's body.
9. Have only wooden, plastic, or nonallergic (not fuzzy) toys.
10. Keep pets out of the bedroom.

In the rest of the house, follow these instructions:

1. **No smoking** should be allowed.
2. The allergic patient should not sit on overstuffed furniture or on rugs. Cotton or nylon rugs backed only with rubber are best.
3. No pets should be kept indoors.
4. Eliminate all house plants (dust and molds).
5. Do not use room deodorizers, mothballs, or bug sprays (strong odors).
6. Have regular furnace cleaning, and provide covers for furnace vents if needed.
7. The allergic patient should not be in the house while the house is being cleaned.
8. Keep humidifiers and air conditioners clean; replace or, if possible, wash filters monthly during heavy use.
9. Masks are helpful during periods of unavoidable allergen exposure.
10. *Consumer Reports* is an excellent source for techniques to modify the environment.

filters also utilize viscid impingement by incorporating mineral oil or glycol, which helps to hold collected particles on the filter.

2. **Group RII** air cleaners include extended surface filters with pleats or pockets incorporated within the filtering media. Like Group RI cleaners, these filters are either cleanable or disposable and either dry or viscous-coated.
3. **Group RIII** air cleaners are electronic, using the electrostatic precipitation method (charging of particles that are then attracted and held to oppositely charged plates). These cleaners offer high air-cleaning efficiency without introducing excessive airflow resistance; however, high air velocities will decrease their efficiency. Two basic types of electronic air filters are available: charged-media filters (single-stage electronic air cleaners) and two-stage electronic air cleaners (two-stage electrostatic precipitators).
4. Several **unclassified** air cleaners have been used in industry and are now being adapted as home filtering devices. An example is the **high-efficiency particulate air (HEPA)** filter, which ranks as one of the most efficient air cleaners available. The HEPA filter is composed of various sized glass (borosilicate) fibers that can remove 99.97% of particulate matter that is more than 0.3 μ in diameter. Some clinical studies using HEPA filters have demonstrated improved control of atopic disease. Table 4-2 summarizes the advantages and disadvantages of the various types of air cleaners.

C. **Humidifiers and dehumidifiers.** The effect of humidity on asthmatic patients is not fully understood, but the evidence suggests that high humidity or low

Table 4-2. Advantages and disadvantages of air-cleaning devices

Type of device	Advantages	Disadvantages
Viscous impingement	Low initial cost	Low efficiency with atmospheric dust
Polystyrene electrostatic filters	Ability to collect smaller charged particles than typical furnace filters	Requirement that particles have previous static charge
Extended surface filter	Greater effective surface area Increased efficiency due to reduced air velocity through filter Moderate cost	More expensive than preceding devices Not readily available
Charged-media (single-stage electronic air cleaner)	More dirt-holding capacity Medium efficiency	Frequent, expensive replacement Decrease in efficiency above relative humidity of 70%
Electronic air cleaner (two-stage electrostatic precipitator)	High efficiency on both large and small particles (70–90%) Pressure drops and power required are low compared with other high-efficiency collectors Ability to collect wet or dry particles Washable	Initial expense Requirement for safeguard against high voltage
High-efficiency particulate air (HEPA) filter	Highest efficiency (95.0–99.9%)	High pressure drop Expensive Costly periodic replacement

humidity can be detrimental to them. For optimal results, maintain environmental humidity at 35–50%. Insist on proper maintenance of humidifiers to prevent mold contamination and subsequent aerosolization of mold, resulting in exacerbation of symptoms or hypersensitivity pneumonitis in mold-sensitive patients.

D. Negative ion generator. This device produces negative ions, which disperse into a room, combine with particles in the air, and give them a negative charge. These charged particles are then attracted to and held by floors and walls, which possess a positive charge. Although claims have been made as to a beneficial health effect (e.g., with asthma), studies are inconclusive and the FDA has challenged these claims.

III. Specific control measures

A. Mite control. The house mite *Dermatophagoides* (a major component of house dust, especially in moist, temperate environments) thrives on human skin scales in mattresses, furniture stuffing, and rugs. Patients with mite sensitivity should encase all mattresses, box springs, and pillows with plastic coverings to minimize exposure to either live or dead mites.* Maintenance of appropriate humid-

---

*Information on encasings can be obtained from The American Textile Company, 303 Fifth Avenue, New York, NY 10016 (212-686-3361); and from Allergen-Proof Encasings, 1450 East 363rd Street, Eastlake, OH 44094 (216-946-6700).

Table 4-3. Guidelines for the asthmatic patient during air pollution alerts

1. Avoid unnecessary physical activity.
2. Avoid smoking and smoke-filled rooms.
3. Avoid exposure to dusts and other irritants, such as hair sprays, insect sprays, or other sprays, paint, exhaust fumes, smoke from any fire, or other fumes.
4. Avoid exposure to those with colds and respiratory infection.
5. Try to stay indoors in a clean environment. Air conditioning is helpful, if available, as are charcoal filters, electrostatic precipitators, or HEPA-type filters.
6. If it appears that the air pollution episode will persist or worsen, it is desirable to leave the polluted area temporarily until the episode subsides.
7. Ask your physician to devise specific instructions to follow. Know what medication to use and when to call your physician. Remember that in case of an air pollution episode the physician may be busier than usual and harder to reach. Keep emergency telephone numbers readily available. Know where and when to go to a hospital emergency center.

Source: From R. G. Slavin et al. Guidelines for asthmatic patients during air pollution episodes. *J. Allergy Clin. Immunol.* 55:222, 1975. With permission.

ity can help control mites; these arthropods thrive in high relative humidity. No commercially available chemical is effective in killing mites.

B. Odor control. Numerous household odors can induce allergic symptoms. Such odors include cooking odors, commercial sprays (air fresheners or cleaners), perfumes, soaps, and smoke from fireplaces. The use of lids on cooking utensils and exhaust fans when cooking can reduce odors. Room deodorizers, mothballs, or bug sprays producing strong odors should be stored away from allergic patients and used only when the patient is out of the house. Plastic Christmas trees and decorations are preferable to natural Christmas trees and wreaths. These natural ornaments also promote mold growth.

C. Mold control. Most indoor molds, originating primarily from growth on outdoor vegetation, grow in moist, cool environments such as basement crawl spaces, shower stalls, and window sills. Although complete eradication of mold is impossible, the use of dehumidifiers and fungicides can produce a significant reduction in mold concentration, which can benefit the mold-sensitive patient.

    1. Dehumidification. Excess humidity (relative humidity > 60–70%) enhances mold growth, and the use of dehumidification is helpful if molds are present. Dehumidification in damp areas can complement fungicide use.

    2. Fungicides can be used either by direct application or by fumigation and repeated on a regular basis as needed.

        a. Direct application

            (1) Phenolated disinfectants (e.g., Lysol) are inexpensive, readily available as sprays or solutions, and effective in controlling mold growth.

            (2) Disinfectants containing **halogens** (Clorox) are also useful in controlling mold growth.

            (3) Benzalkonium chloride (Zephiran chloride, 1:10,000 aqueous dilution) is a representative of the cationic surface disinfectant types of fungicides.

        b. Fumigation. Significant inhibition of mold growth can be obtained by placing crystalline paraformaldehyde in an open jar on the floor of the rooms of a house. (H. C. Mansmann. Environmental Control. In E. Middleton, C. E. Reed, and E. Ellis (eds.), *Allergy—Principles and Practice.* St. Louis: Mosby, 1978.) Evaporation by sublimation results in a slight smell of formaldehyde. One or more jars can be placed in an unoccupied room. The vapor alone is nontoxic, although the chemical is a poison and irritant. The allergic patient should not enter the room until the vapor has dissipated after a few minutes of adequate ventilation.

D. Air pollution control

1. **Smoking** should be avoided in the household of patients having any respiratory disease. Passive inhalation of smoke increases asthmatic symptoms and, in all children, increases the frequency of respiratory infections compared with that in children in smoke-free households.
2. **Air pollution,** especially for asthmatic persons in urban areas, constitutes a continual threat. Advise these patients to follow the recommendations outlined by the Weather and Air Pollution Committee of the American Academy of Allergy (Table 4-3).

IV. **A home visit** by a health professional can provide important information for improvement in the home environment, especially in the allergic patient with poorly controlled symptoms.

V. **Moving to another climate** is usually unsuccessful in controlling severe allergic disease. Furthermore, an impulsive decision to make such a move can produce financial and psychological hardships that then complicate an already difficult situation. If a move of this kind is anticipated, a trial period should be attempted.

Pharmacologic Management of Allergic Diseases

Drug therapy plays a major role in the treatment of allergic diseases, both for acute symptoms and for control of chronic symptoms, and prophylaxis. In recent years new preparations and added information about established drugs (e.g., theophylline) have allowed more specific, aggressive, and safe pharmacologic management. The following section serves as a general introduction to drug therapy in allergic disease. Additional information is available in subsequent chapters.

I. **Antihistamines** are drugs that antagonize the effects of histamine. First studied in the late 1930s, they became available for clinical use in the 1940s. Since that time, a wide variety of antihistamines, either alone or in combination with decongestants, have been produced. (Currently, over 90 different preparations of antihistamines are listed in the *Physicians' Desk Reference.*)

A. Chemical structure. Antihistamines are divided into two categories, those that block **H_1 cell-membrane receptors** (the classic antihistamine used for the treatment of allergic diseases) and those that block **H_2 cell-membrane receptors.** H_2 antihistamines are used primarily to inhibit gastric secretions in peptic ulcer disease. However, they are used on an investigational basis in the treatment of allergic diseases such as chronic urticaria.

All H_1 antihistamines are modifications of a basic structure that resembles histamine. They are separated into the following chemical classes:

1. **Ethylenediamines,** including tripelennamine, pyrilamine, and antazoline.
2. **Ethanolamines,** including carbinoxamine, diphenhydramine, doxylamine, and clemastine.
3. **Alkylamines,** including chlorpheniramine, brompheniramine, and triprolidine.
4. **Piperazines,** e.g., cyclizine and meclizine.
5. **Piperidines,** including cyproheptadine.
6. **Phenothiazines,** e.g., promethazine, trimeprazine.
7. **Nonsedating agents,** e.g., terfenadine (Seldane), astemizole (investigational). Extensive pharmacologic data exist for these newer agents that do not appear to cross the blood-brain barrier, accounting for the decrease in central nervous system (CNS) side effects. The usual dose of terfenadine for adults and children 12 years and older is 60 mg twice a day. Safety and effectiveness in children below the age of 12 years have not been established.

B. Pharmacokinetics. Absorption of H_1 antihistamines occurs rapidly after oral administration, causing systemic effects in less than 30 minutes. The liver metabolizes approximately 70–90% of antihistamines, with little drug excreted in the urine in the unmodified form. Information on the metabolism and excretion of most antihistamines is incomplete.

C. **Mechanisms of action.** Antihistamines act by competing with histamine for its specific receptors on the cell surface. All H_1-blocking drugs are very similar in their ability to block histamine. (Astemizole, which is not yet FDA-approved, can have a prolonged H_1 blockade extending to 21 days after the end of therapy.) The choice of a particular type of antihistamine is chiefly related to the difference in side effects produced (e.g., somnolence). Also, antihistamines are more effective in preventing than in reversing the actions of histamine once established; prophylactic administration is preferred.

Other pharmacologic effects of H_1 inhibition include the following: local anesthetic action when applied topically; inhibition of salivary and lacrimal secretions; transient hypotension following rapid intravenous injection; possible potentiation of actions of other CNS depressants such as alcohol, barbiturates, and certain tranquilizers; sedation and somnolence at the usual doses, with convulsions at toxic doses. Monoamine oxidase inhibitors prolong and intensify the anticholinergic effects of antihistamines.

D. **Indications.** Antihistamines are the most commonly used drugs providing symptomatic relief from a number of allergic disorders. Antihistamines are often combined with decongestants in a single fixed preparation in an attempt to achieve added symptomatic relief.

1. **Seasonal allergic rhinitis** (e.g., hay fever) and **perennial allergic rhinitis** respond well to H_1 antihistamines. Most patients with seasonal allergic rhinitis obtain at least partial relief of symptoms (sneezing, rhinorrhea, and, to a lesser extent, nasal airway obstruction and congestion). The best results are obtained when antihistamines are given prior to allergen exposure. Although their efficacy is reduced in **vasomotor rhinitis,** their anticholinergic action can improve symptoms by reducing rhinorrhea.

2. In **acute allergic urticaria,** H_1 antihistamines reduce the rash and pruritus. Their effect in chronic urticaria is less dramatic.

3. In **acute anaphylactic reactions,** H_1 antihistamines are used as an **adjunct** to epinephrine, which is a mandatory treatment and frequently lifesaving. Diphenhydramine (Benadryl) is the antihistamine most commonly employed.

4. In **serum sickness,** antihistamines help to control the urticaria but have little effect on arthralgia or fever and do not shorten the course of the reaction. Prophylactic use may attenuate symptoms.

5. In **contact dermatitis** and **fixed drug reactions,** an oral antihistamine used in combination with appropriate topical therapy helps to reduce pruritus. **Avoid topical antihistamines in order to prevent sensitization.**

6. Treatment with H_1 antihistamines is sometimes used to prevent or ameliorate **allergic drug reactions** or **mild transfusion reactions.** Sole reliance on these drugs may not give protection from such reactions and can expose the patient to extreme risk (see Chaps. 12 and 15 for an approach to allergic drug reactions and transfusion reactions, respectively).

7. H_1 antihistamines are used for the prevention of **motion sickness** and the treatment of **parkinsonism.**

8. Certain antihistamines (e.g., diphenhydramine, promethazine, hydroxyzine) are used as sedatives, especially with preoperative medication. In patients with severe pruritus, the dual effects of sedation and antipruritic effect can be helpful.

9. Terfenadine and astemizole are being studied in the treatment of asthma. Terfenadine appears to attenuate exercise-induced bronchospasm with no effect on antigen- and methacholine-induced bronchospasm. Astemizole protects against histamine-induced bronchoconstriction and inhibits the immediate response to antigen. Future clinical studies are required.

E. **Adverse effects.** H_1 antihistamines are exceptionally safe drugs and are used in nonprescription preparations. Side effects do occur, the most common being sedation and somnolence (higher incidence with ethanolamine types, lower inci-

dence with alkylamine types). Dizziness and ataxia rarely occur. Warn patients
to avoid antihistamines with alcohol, which can potentiate sedative effects.

   1. H_1 antihistamines produce anticholinergic effects in susceptible patients or
when given in large doses. Excitation, nervousness, dryness of the mouth,
palpitation, urinary retention, tachycardia, and constipation can occur.
CNS stimulation can produce convulsions, especially in patients with focal
lesions of the nervous system.

   2. H_1 antihistamines rarely produce blood dyscrasias, fever, or neuropathy.
Sensitization to antihistamines can occur, resulting in urticarial, eczematous, or petechial rashes.

   3. In animals, cyclizine and meclizine have been shown to be **teratogenic.**

   4. Treatment of acute poisoning is largely supportive, consisting of efforts
maintain adequate oxygenation and circulation and control convulsions.

   5. In usual therapeutic doses, nonsedating antihistamines (e.g., terfenadine,
astemizole) produce few side effects. They rarely produce drowsiness, im-
pair psychomotor performance, or potentiate effects caused by CNS depressants such as alcohol and diazepam.

 F. Antihistamine preparations are listed in Tables 4-4 and 4-5. H_1 antihistamines
are similar in pharmacologic activity, and the selection of a particular preparation depends largely on the sedative properties of the drug, the familiarity with
its use, and successful suppression of allergic symptoms in the individual patient. In patients whose allergy is poorly controlled with one preparation,
switching to another drug, especially to another class of antihistamine, may be
beneficial.

II. Adrenergic drugs (sympathomimetic amines) are widely used in the pharmacologic
management of allergic diseases. The effects of adrenergic drugs are mediated
through at least two different receptor systems. The alpha-adrenergic receptor
primarily associated with excitatory functions, including constriction of the smooth
muscles of arteries, veins, and bronchi, and of the urinary bladder trigone sphincter,
and relaxation of the intestinal smooth muscle. The beta-adrenergic receptor is
mainly associated with inhibitory functions, such as smooth-muscle relaxation in
the bronchi, uterus, ciliary muscle, and blood vessels. An important excitatory
function of the beta-adrenergic receptor is myocardial stimulation.

The concept of the beta-adrenergic effect has been further refined by distinguishing
beta-1 agonists, which produce lipolysis and cardiac stimulation, and beta-2 agonists, which mediate bronchodilation, vasodilation, lactic acidemia, inhibition of
histamine release, and skeletal muscle tremor. The clinical responses to individual
adrenergic agents can often be predicted from their selectivity in reacting with
alpha- or beta-1 and beta-2 receptors.

 A. Alpha-adrenergic agonists are used primarily as nasal decongestants because
of their vasoconstricting effect on dilated arterioles in the nasal mucosa. Opening of obstructed nasal passages improves nasal ventilation as well as aeration
and draining of the sinuses.

   1. Clinical indications. Nasal decongestants provide temporary symptomatic
relief in acute or chronic rhinitis of allergic, vasomotor, or infectious origin.
The vasoconstrictor action of these drugs may be an adjunct to antibiotic
therapy in otitis media, or the drugs may be used as the sole medication in
serous otitis media to relieve obstructed eustachian ostia.

   2. Dosage and route of administration. Dosages and routes of administration
for alpha-adrenergic decongestants are given in Table 4-6. For acute symptomatic treatment on a limited short-term basis (< 5 days), topical decongestants (in the form of vapors, sprays, or drops) are more effective than oral
preparations. Instruct the patient to deliver nasal sprays into each nostril
in the upright position; blow the nose 3–5 minutes later as decongestion
begins in the inferior part of the middle turbinates. When using nasal
drops, instruct the patient to lie supine (not hyperextended), and, if the ears
are involved, with the head turned 15 degrees toward the affected side.
Instill the nasal drops into the affected side, allowing them to run along the

Table 4-4. Antihistamine-containing preparations, by chemical classification

Generic name	Product trade name*
Ethylenediamines	
Pyrilamine maleate	Histalet Forte tablets
	P-V-Tussin syrup
	Triaminic preparations
Pyrilamine tannate	Rynatan tablets and pediatric suspension
Tripelennamine hydrochloride	PBZ-SR tablets and PBZ tablets
Tripelennamine citrate	PBZ elixir
Ethanolamines	
Bromodiphenhydramine hydrochloride	Ambodryl cough syrup
Carbinoxamine maleate	Cardec DM drops and syrup
	Clistin tablets
	Rondec tablets, drops, and syrup
Clemastine fumarate	Tavist tablets, syrup
	Tavist-1 tablets, Tavist-D tablets
Diphenhydramine hydrochloride	Benadryl capsules, elixir, and parenteral preparations
	Multiple generic preparations
Doxylamine succinate	Contac severe cold formula night strength
	Formula 44 cough mixture
	Nyquil Nighttime colds medicine
	Unisome Nighttime Sleep-Aid
Phenyltoloxamine citrate	Atrohist Sprinkle and LA tablets
	Comhist LA capsules and tablets
	Decontabs tablets
	Histamic capsules and H/S tablets
	Magsal tablets
	Naldecon products
	Percogesic analgesic tablets
	Polyhistine D capsules, elixir, pediatric capsules
	Sinubid
Alkylamines	
Brompheniramine maleate	Atrohist LA tablets
	Atrohist Sprinkle
	Bromfed capsules
	Dimetane tablets, elixir, and Extentabs
	Dimetapp elixir, tablets, and Extentabs
	Drixoral syrup
	Dura Tap-PD
	Histatapp elixir and T.D. tablets
	Poly-Histine CS
Chlorpheniramine maleate	Alka-Seltzer Plus cold medicine
	Allerest tablets
	Allerest timed-release capsules
	A.R.M. tablets
	Brexin L.A. capsules
	Chlorafed Liquid and Timecelles
	Chlor-Trimeton tablets, syrup, and Repetabs
	Chlor-Trimeton Decongestant tablets

Table 4-4 (*continued*)

Generic name	Product trade name*
Chlorpheniramine maleate (*cont.*)	Codimal-L.A. capsules
	Comhist LA capsules
	Comtrex tablets, capsules, liquid
	Contac capsules
	Coricidin tablets, "D" decongestant tablets, Demilets
	Coricidin Extra Strength sinus headache tablets
	CoTylenol cold formula tablets and liquid
	Deconamine tablets, elixir, and SR capsules
	Demazin syrup and Repetabs
	Dristan Advanced Formula tablets and caplets
	Extendryl chewable tablets, syrup, and capsules
	Fedahist tablets, syrup, and gyrocaps
	Histalet tablets and syrup
	Histaspan D capsules
	Isoclor Timesule capsules
	Kronofed A Kronocaps and Kronofed A Jr. Kronocaps
	Naldecon preparations
	Nolamine tablets
	Novafed A capsules
	Novahistine DH
	Ornade Spansule capsules
	P-V-Tussin Syrup
	Pediacof cough syrup
	PediaCare 2 and 3
	PROTID
	Pyrroxate capsules
	Quelidrine
	Rhinolar capsules
	RuTuss liquid, tablets
	RuTuss II capsules
	Ryna liquid
	Sinarest tablets
	Sine-Off Extra Strength Tablets
	Singlet tablets
	Sinutab Maximum Strength tablets
	Sudafed Plus tablets and syrup
	Teldrin timed-release capsules
	Triaminic allergy tablets, chewables, and cold syrup
	Triaminicin tablets and chewables
	TRIND, DM
	Tussar DM, SF, 2
Chlorpheniramine tannate	Rynatan tablets and pediatric suspension
	Rynatuss tablets and pediatric suspension
Dexbrompheniramine maleate	Disophrol Chronotabs
	Drixoral sustained-action tablets
Dexchlorpheniramine maleate	Polaramine Repetabs, tablets and syrup
Pheniramine maleate	Fiogesic tablets
	Triaminic preparations
	Tussagesic tablets
Triprolidine hydrochloride	Actidil tablets and syrup
	Actifed tablets and syrup

Table 4-4 (*continued*)

Generic name	Product trade name*
Piperazines	
Chlorcyclizine hydrochloride	Fedrazil tablets
Hydroxyzine hydrochloride	Atarax tablets and syrup
Hydroxyzine pamoate	Vistaril capsules and suspension
Meclizine hydrochloride	Antivert tablets
	Bonine tablets
Phenindamine tartrate	Nolahist tablets
	Nolamine tablets
	P-V-Tussin syrup and tablets
Phenothiazines	
Methdilazine hydrochloride	Tacaryl tablets and syrup
Promethazine hydrochloride	Phenergan tablets, syrup, rectal suppositories
	Remsed tablets
Trimeprazine tartrate	Temaril tablets, syrup, and Spansule sustained-release capsules
Piperidines	
Azatadine maleate	Optimine tablets
	Trinalin tablets
Cyproheptadine hydrochloride	Periactin tablets and syrup
Nonsedating antihistamines	
Terfenadine	Seldane tablets
Astemizole	Hismanal (not FDA-approved)

*Individual products usually contain decongestant components and occasionally other drugs (aspirin, acetaminophen, dextromethorphan, guaifenesin, phenacetin, alcohol, caffeine, ascorbic acid, or belladonna alkaloids). **Antihistamines from different classes may be present in the same preparation.** Check package insert, *Physicians' Desk Reference,* or *Physicians' Desk Reference for Nonprescription Drugs* to obtain component composition, dosage forms, and dosage for adults and children.

floor of the nasal passage, pooling at the eustachian tube orifice. Ideally, keep the patient in this position for 5 minutes.

Oral preparations are preferred for chronic use (> 5 days) since prolonged or excessive use of topical agents increases the incidence of adverse effects.

3. **Adverse effects**
   a. Topical decongestants used in excess can produce local effects of rebound congestion, dryness, interference with ciliary action, and chronic swelling.
   b. Topical decongestants can produce systemic reactions, especially in infants and young children, in whom significant absorption from the nasal mucosa or gastrointestinal tract can occur. For children under 6 years of age, because of the difficulty of controlling dosage, drops are preferable to sprays.
   c. Oral decongestants are more likely than topical decongestants to cause systemic reactions since their action is not selective for the nasal vessels.

Table 4-5. Commonly used antihistamine preparations: oral dosages and characteristics

| Class[a] | Generic name[b] | Oral dosage[c] | | | Characteristics |
		Pediatric	Adults	
Ethylenediamines CH_3O — $CH_2NCH_2CH_2^+NH$ with CH_3, CH_3 groups and N (pyridine ring)	Pyrilamine maleate	Dosage not established for children	75–100 mg/24 hr in 3–4 divided doses	Low sedative and anticholinergic effects; gastrointestinal complaints common (reduced by giving drug with meals)
	Tripelennamine hydrochloride (and citrate)	5 mg/kg/24 hr divided into 4–6 doses[d]	25–50 mg q4–6h[d]	As above
Ethanolamines Cl — $CHOCH_2CH_2^+NH$ with CH_3, CH_3 groups and N (pyridine ring)	Carbinoxamine maleate	0.8 mg/kg/24 hr in 4 divided doses	12–32 mg/24 hr in 4 doses	Lowest incidence of drowsiness of all the ethanolamines; weak anticholinergic effects; gastrointestinal complaints uncommon
	Clemastine fumarate	(0.5 mg/5 ml) Children 6–12 yr, 1–2 tsp bid	1.34 mg bid–2.68 mg tid (max. 8.04 mg/24 hr)	Drowsiness most frequent complaint but no marked sedation; anticholinergic effects weak and gastrointestinal complaints uncommon
	Diphenhydramine hydrochloride	Under 12 yr, 5 mg/kg/24 hr in 4 divided doses[e]	25–50 mg q6–8h[f]	Sedative effects high; anticholinergic effects moderate; gastrointestinal complaints uncommon; most widely used antihistamine preparation for parenteral administration

Alkylamines

Brompheniramine maleate	0.5 mg/kg/24 hr in 4 divided doses (max. 6 mg/24 hr for age 2–6 yr; 12 mg/24 hr for age 6–12 yr)	4 mg q4–6h (max. 24 mg/24 hr) or 8–12 mg q8–12h using timed-release form	Alkylamines as a group have low sedative, anticholinergic, and gastrointestinal effects. Approximately 75% of prescribed or over-the-counter products contain an alkylamine, often chlorpheniramine maleate.
Chlorpheniramine maleate	0.35 mg/kg/24 hr in 4 divided doses; over 7 yr, 8 mg q12h in timed-release form	2–4 mg q6–8h; as timed-release form, 8–12 mg q12h	As above
Dexchlorpheniramine maleate	Under 12 yr, 0.15 mg/kg/24 hr in 4 divided doses	1–2 mg q6–8h	As above
Triprolidine hydrochloride	Over 6 yr, 1.25 mg q6–8h; under 6 yr, 0.3–0.6 mg q6–8h	2.5 mg q6–8h	As above
Piperazines			
Hydroxyzine hydrochloride (and pamoate)	2–5 mg/kg/24 hr in 3–4 divided doses	25–100 mg q6–8h	The piperazines, cyclizine and meclizine, are teratogenic in animals and should not be used in pregnant patients or patients likely to become pregnant.
Meclizine hydrochloride	Not recommended	25–100 mg/24 hr in 3–4 divided doses	Drowsiness is common; dry mouth is a common anticholinergic effect. Meclizine is used primarily for motion sickness and vertigo.

Table 4-5 (continued)

Class[a]	Generic name[b]	Oral dosage[c]		Characteristics
		Pediatric	Adults	
Phenothiazines	Methdilazine hydrochloride	Over 3 yr, 4 mg q6–12h	16–32 mg/24 hr in 2–4 divided doses	Sedation moderate but reduced compared with other phenothiazines; used primarily for treating pruritus
	Promethazine hydrochloride	0.5 mg/kg/dose q6–8h	25 mg hs or 12.5 mg qid	Marked sedative effects; used primarily as sedative and antiemetic
	Trimeprazine tartrate	6 mo–3 yr, 3.75 mg/24 hr in 3 divided doses; 3–12 yr, 7.5 mg/24 hr in 3 divided doses	10 mg/24 hr in 4 divided doses	Marked sedative effect; used primarily to treat pruritus
Piperidines	Azatadine maleate	Dosage not established	1–2 mg bid	Drowsiness most common side effect; chemically similar to cyproheptadine
	Cyproheptadine hydrochloride	2–6 yr, 2 mg q8–12h (max. 12 mg/24 hr); 7–14 yr, 4 mg q8–12h (max. 16 mg/24 hr)	4–20 mg/day in divided doses (max. 0.5 mg/kg/24 hr)	Drowsiness most common side effect; weight gain can occur; useful for pruritus and especially for cold urticaria. Do not use in newborn or premature infants.

[a] Chemical formula of the initial generic preparation as a structural representation of each class of antihistamine.
[b] Refer to Table 4-4 for trade names.
[c] Daily pediatric dose based on milligram per kilogram should not exceed adult doses. Bioavailability of drugs in timed-release form may be neither uniform nor reliable.
[d] Dosages based on hydrochloride salt.
[e] IV or deep IM administration: 5 mg/kg/24 hr in 4 divided doses (max. 300 mg/24 hr).
[f] IV or deep IM administration: 10–50 mg q6–8h (max. 400 mg/24 hr).

Table 4-6. Adrenergic nasal decongestants

Generic name	Product name	Route of administration	Dosage Pediatric	Dosage Adult	Comments[a]
Epinephrine hydrochloride	Adrenalin chloride solution (aqueous) (0.1%)	Topical	Not recommended	Max. in healthy adults, 1 ml over 15 minutes (not recommended)	Short duration of effect and frequent adverse reactions limit use to control epistaxis or facilitate nasal surgery; **rarely used now as nasal decongestant**
Ephedrine sulfate	Generically available capsules (25 and 50 mg), syrup (10 and 20 mg/5 ml)	Oral	3 mg/kg/24 hr in 4–6 divided doses	25–50 mg q4–6h	Rarely used as decongestant because of tachyphylaxis, CNS stimulation, hypertension, palpitations, and short duration of action
	Generically available 0.5–3% topical solution	Topical	Not recommended	Not recommended	As above
Pseudoephedrine hydrochloride	Sudafed tablets (30 and 60 mg), syrup (30 mg/5 ml) Novafed capsules, Sudafed 12-hr capsules (120 mg)	Oral Oral	4 mg/kg/24 hr in 4 divided doses Over 12 yr, 1 capsule q12h	60 mg q6–8h 1 capsule q12h	Stereoisomer of ephedrine with similar effects but less CNS stimulation and hypertensive effects; found in many antihistamine-decongestant combinations and "cold" medicines; not effective in asthma
Pseudoephedrine sulfate	Afrinol long-acting decongestant Repetabs tablets (120 mg)	Oral	Over 12 yr, 1 tablet q12h	1 tablet q12h	As above

Table 4-6 (*continued*)

Generic name	Product name	Route of administration	Dosage		Comments[a]
			Pediatric	Adult	
Phenylephrine hydrochloride	Neo-Synephrine hydrochloride solutions (0.125% [pediatric], 0.25%, and 1%), sprays (0.25% and 0.5%), and jelly (0.5%)	Topical	For infants (0.125% concentration), 2–3 gtt into each nostril q4h as needed	2–3 gtt or 1–2 sprays of 0.25–1% solution into each nostril (for older children also) q4h as needed	Adverse effects similar to those of epinephrine and ephedrine but less CNS stimulation. Avoid prolonged use to avoid rebound congestion. **Oral forms are ineffective.**
	Nostril nasal decongestant (0.25% and 0.5% spray)	Topical			
	Sinex decongestant nasal spray (0.5%)	Topical			
Phenylpropanolamine hydrochloride	Generic capsules (timed-release [75 mg]); 25- and 50-mg tablets	Oral	Not recommended in children under 6 yr except under the direct supervision of a physician[b]	25 mg q4h (max. 150 mg/day)	Similar to ephedrine but has fewer CNS effects
	Propagest (25-mg tablet)				
	Contained in multiple antihistamine-decongestant combinations				
Propylhexedrine	Benzedrex inhaler	Topical	Not recommended in children	2 inhalations (0.6–0.8 mg) into each nostril as needed, avoiding excessive use	Less toxic than ephedrine and very effective for short-term, intermittent use. If inhaler is cold, warm in hands before use, to increase volatility.
Naphazoline hydrochloride	Privine hydrochloride solution, spray (0.05%)	Topical	Not recommended under 6 yr	Over 6 yr, 2 gtt into each nostril q3h; 2 sprays into each nostril q4–6h	Imidazoles are effective topically with longer duration of action. Arrhythmias can occur. **Use with extreme caution in young children and patients with cardiovascular disease.**

Oxymetazoline hydrochloride	Afrin or Neo-Synephrine 12-hour nasal spray, nose drops (0.05%), pediatric nose drops (0.025%), or Dristan Long-Lasting nasal spray (0.05%)	Topical	2–5 yr, 2–3 gtt (0.025%) into each nostril q12h	Over 6 yr, 2–4 gtt or 2–3 sprays into each nostril q12h	As above
Tetrahydrozoline hydrochloride	Tyzine nasal solution (0.1%), pediatric nasal drops (0.05%)	Topical	2–6 yr, 2–3 gtt of 0.05% solution into each nostril q4–6h (**extreme caution required**)	Over 6 yr, 2–4 gtt into each nostril q3h	As above
Xylometazoline hydrochloride	Neo-Synephrine II nasal spray, nose drops (0.1%), pediatric nasal drops (0.05%)	Topical	2–12 yr, 2–3 gtt (0.05%) solution into each nostril q8–10h; not recommended under age 2 yr	2–3 gtt or 2 sprays (0.1%) solution into each nostril q8–10h	As above
	Otrivin adult nasal spray, drops (0.1%), pediatric nasal drops (0.05%)	Topical			

[a] Use topical decongestants only during acute stage (not exceeding 5 days); use oral agents on a long-term basis. These agents should be used with caution in patients with thyroid disease, hypertension, diabetes mellitus, or heart disease and in patients taking tricyclic antidepressants. Avoid completely in patients receiving monoamine oxidase inhibitors or demonstrating sensitivity (insomnia, dizziness, tremors, or arrhythmias) to even small doses.

[b] It is contained in multiple antihistamine-decongestant combinations. For dosage of these compounds in children, consult the *Physicians' Desk Reference* or *Physicians' Desk Reference for Nonprescription Drugs*.

    d. Oral and topical decongestants should be used cautiously in patients with thyroid disease, hypertension, diabetes mellitus, heart disease, or those receiving tricyclic antidepressants. Nasal decongestants should be avoided in patients receiving monoamine oxidase inhibitors or whose sensitivity to even small doses is demonstrated by insomnia, tremor, dizziness, or cardiac arrhythmias. Adverse reactions to individual preparations are given in Table 4-6.

B. Alpha-adrenergic antagonists. The human bronchial smooth muscle contains alpha-adrenergic receptors that, if stimulated, may induce bronchoconstriction. In investigational studies, alpha-adrenergic antagonists, including phentolamine, dibenamine, thymoxamine, and indoramin, appear to be useful in the treatment of asthma. Until further clinical trials are made, these agents are considered investigational.

C. Beta-adrenergic agonists are extensively used in the treatment of asthma by virtue of their ability to produce bronchodilatation through stimulation of beta-adrenergic receptors in the lungs.

    1. Mechanism of action. The beta-adrenergic agonist induces changes in at least three cell membrane components (beta-adrenergic receptor, guanine nucleotide regulatory protein, and the adenylate cyclase catalytic unit). These changes lead to increased cyclic adenosine monophosphate (cyclic AMP) production from adenosine triphosphate (see Chap. 2).

    2. Pharmacokinetic properties. The absorption, transformation, and excretion of the beta-adrenergic agonists are best understood by examining their structural-functional relationships and separating them into catecholamines and noncatecholamines.

        a. Catecholamines, including epinephrine, isoproterenol, and isoetharine, contain a benzene ring with two adjacent hydroxyl groups and an amine side chain (see Table 4-7). Alteration of the basic structure produces changes in relative beta-1 and beta-2 activity. Monoamine oxidase and catechol-o-methyltransferase are two enzymes responsible for metabolic transformation of the catecholamines; the former is associated with the mitochondria, while the latter is found in the soluble cytoplasmic areas of the cell. The highest concentrations of these enzymes are in the liver and the kidney. Epinephrine, isoproterenol, and isoetharine are not effective oral agents because of rapid destruction in the gastrointestinal tract and rapid conjugation and oxidation in the liver.

        b. Noncatecholamines. In contrast to catecholamines, noncatecholamines are effective when given orally and have a longer duration of action because of their resistance to the inactivating enzymes of the liver and other tissues. Although the metabolic pathways of these drugs are not fully elucidated, several pathways, including beta-hydroxylation, N-demethylation, deamination, and conjugation in the liver, are involved. A significant amount of administered drug is excreted in the urine. Noncatecholamines are further classified on the basis of chemical substitutions into resorcinols (metaproterenol, terbutaline, and fenoterol) and saligenins (albuterol) (see Table 4-7). These agents have greater beta-2 selectivity than do catecholamines.

    3. The **dosage and route of administration** for individual agents are given in Table 4-7 (see also Chap. 6).

    4. Adverse effects. Drugs with primarily beta-agonist effects can produce tachycardia, palpitation, nervousness, muscle tremors, nausea, and vomiting. Rarely, headache, flushing of the skin, tremor, dizziness, weakness, sweating, precordial distress, or anginal-type pain can occur.

    5. General guidelines for safe adrenergic use in asthmatic patients include the following:

        a. Warn patients against excessive use of these agents, particularly inhaler abuse (especially in unsupervised children and adolescents).

        b. Avoid giving nonselective beta-adrenergic agonists to asthmatic patients with hypertension, thyrotoxicosis, and cardiac disease. If such agents are used in these patients, selective beta-2 agonists by inhalation are preferable.

c. Selective beta-2-adrenergic agonists administered by inhalation may cause fewer side effects than systemically administered agents in patients suffering severe tremor, jitteriness, or a noticeable increase in heart rates.

III. Methylxanthines. Theophylline is a widely used pharmacologic agent in the treatment of acute asthma and, more important, in the control and prevention of chronic asthma. Increased knowledge of theophylline pharmacokinetics and pharmacodynamics and an improved clinical availability of determining serum theophylline concentrations permit effective dosing. Theophylline is available as anhydrous theophylline, as the salts of theophylline, or combined with sympathomimetics, mucolytic agents, or tranquilizers in fixed-dosage preparations.

A. The **chemical structure** of theophylline (Fig. 4-1) is 1, 3-dimethyl-xanthine with a molecular weight of 198. Aminophylline (Fig. 4-1) is the ethylenediamine salt of theophylline. It contains approximately 80–85% anhydrous theophylline.

B. Mechanism of action. The mechanism of action is not completely understood despite the fact that theophylline has been in use for several decades. Although the ability to inhibit cyclic AMP phosphodiesterase has been the classic explanation, this effect is clearly demonstrable only in high doses. Additional actions of methylxanthines contributing to their beneficial effects include an antagonism of adenosine receptors in the lung, adrenaline release from the adrenal medulla, effects on cell calcium distribution, inhibition of the formation of contractile prostaglandins, and improvement in diaphragmatic contractility.

C. Pharmacokinetics

1. **Absorption.** Anhydrous theophylline is well absorbed from the gastrointestinal tract and is generally 100% bioavailable. The rate of absorption depends on the disintegrative and dissolubility characteristics of the individual formulation and determines the time of peak serum concentrations; e.g., liquid preparations peak at approximately 1–1.5 hours, rapidly dissolving uncoated tablets in 2 hours, and sustained-release preparations peak at 4–6 hours (24-hour preparations peak at approximately 12 hours in adult patients).

2. **Distribution.** Absorbed theophylline rapidly equilibrates with the peripheral tissue compartment and central plasma compartment. In the circulating plasma, 53–65% of theophylline is reversibly bound to protein. Premature infants and adults with hepatic cirrhosis have reduced binding.

   The **apparent** volume of distribution in a steady state averages 0.45 liter/kg of body weight, regardless of age, sex, or a history of smoking, asthma, or acute pulmonary edema. Larger volumes of distribution for theophylline are found in premature infants and adults with hepatic cirrhosis, obesity, or acidemia.

3. **Metabolism.** Theophylline is eliminated primarily by biotransformation in the liver, with urinary excretion of its metabolites.

   a. The three-methylxanthine formation pathway is the limiting metabolic pathway responsible for the observed dose-dependent elimination kinetics of theophylline.

   b. Seven to thirteen percent of theophylline is excreted unchanged in the urine (theophylline can be safely given to patients with isolated impaired renal function).

   c. At concentrations of less than 20 μg/ml, theophylline elimination kinetics are generally first-order; i.e., the rate of elimination is directly proportional to the serum concentration. At higher concentrations, theophylline elimination becomes dose dependent and toxicity becomes more likely.

   d. There is pronounced variability among individuals in theophylline elimination; for example, the elimination half-life in healthy adults **ranges** from 3–13 hours.

Table 4-7. Adrenergic agents for the treatment of asthma

Generic name	Trade name	Route of adminis-tration	Dosage Pediatric	Dosage Adult
Catecholamines				
Epinephrine	Adrenalin chloride solution, 1:1000	SC injection	0.01 ml/kg (max. 0.4 ml) May repeat 2 times, 20 min apart	0.3–0.5 ml
	Sus-Phrine aqueous suspension for subcutaneous injection, 1:200	SC injection	0.005 ml/kg (max. 0.15 ml) May repeat q6h	0.1–0.3 ml
	Medihaler-Epi, 0.16 mg/puff	Pressurized aerosol	1–2 inhalations q4h	
	Primatene Mist, 0.2 mg/puff	Pressurized aerosol	1–2 inhalations q4h	
	Bronkaid Mist, 0.25 mg/puff	Pressurized aerosol	1–2 inhalations q4h	
Epinephrine (racemic)	Vaponefrin solution, 2.25%	Nebulization	0.25 ml (< 10 yr)–0.5 ml in 1.0–2.5 ml sterile water or normal saline q4h	
Ethylnorepinephrine hydrochloride	Bronkephrine (aqueous), 2 mg/ml	SC injection	0.02 ml/kg/ dose (max. 0.5 ml) May repeat 2 times, 20 min apart	0.3–1.0 ml
Isoproterenol (Isoprenaline[a])	Isuprel hydrochloride solution, 1:200 or 1:100	Nebulization	1:200 solution, 0.25 (< 10 yr)–0.50 ml in 1.0–2.5 ml sterile water or normal saline q4h	
	Vapo-Iso (1:200)	Nebulization	As above	
	Duo-Medihaler (isoproterenol HCl 0.16 mg/puff, with phenylephrine)	Pressurized aerosol	1–2 puffs q4–6h (for older children and adults)	
	Isuprel Mistometer (isoproterenol HCl, 131 µg/puff)	Pressurized aerosol	As above	
	Norisodrine Aerotrol (isoproterenol HCl, 0.12 mg/ puff)	Pressurized aerosol	As above	
	Medihaler-Iso (isoproterenol SO_4, 80 µg/puff)	Pressurized aerosol	As above	
	Isuprel Glossets, 10- and 15-mg tablets	Sublingual	5–10 mg tid (max. 30 mg/day)	10–20 mg tid (max. 60 mg/day)
Isoetharine	Bronkosol (isoetharine HCl, 1%)	Nebulization	0.25 (< 10 yr)–0.5 ml in 1.0–2.5 ml sterile water or saline q3–4h	
	Bronkometer (isoetharine mesylate, 340 µg/ puff)	Pressurized aerosol	1–2 puffs q3–4h for older children and adults	
Bitolterol	Tornalate metered-dose inhaler, 370 µg/puff	Pressurized aerosol	Adults and children over 12 yr, 2–3 inhalations q6–8h	

64

Onset of action (minutes)	Peak action	Duration (hours)	Commonly observed side effects
Catecholamines			
5–15	18 min	0.5–1.0	Agitation, restlessness, palpitations, tachyarrhythmias, nausea, sweating, headaches, pallor, dizziness; rarely psychoses. Administer cautiously during pregnancy, to elderly patients, and to patients with cardiovascular disease, hypertension, diabetes, hyperthyroidism, and psychoneuroses.
5–15	1–3 hr	4–6	As above
5–15	18 min	0.5	As above. This is not a drug of choice for oral inhalation.
5–15	18 min	0.5	As above. This is not a drug of choice for oral inhalation.
5–15	18 min	0.5	As above. This is not a drug of choice for oral inhalation.
5–15	18 min	0.5	As above. This is not a drug of choice for oral inhalation.
5–15	18 min	0.5–1.0	Side effects are similar to those of epinephrine.
2–5	5 min	1.5–2.0	Side effects are similar to those of epinephrine. When inhaled, can cause paradoxical response and fall in arterial oxygen concentration.
2–5	5 min	1.5–2.0	As above
2–5	5 min	1.5–2.0	As above
2–5	5 min	1.5–2.0	As above
2–5	5 min	1.5–2.0	As above
2–5	5 min	1.5–2.0	As above
	Absorption variable		Neither drug of choice nor route of administration of choice
2–5	5 min	1.5–2.0	Similar but decreased effects compared with those of epinephrine or isoproterenol
2–5	5 min	1.5–2.0	
3–4	30–60 min	5–8	As above

Table 4-7 (*continued*)

Generic name	Trade name	Route of administration	Dosage Pediatric	Adult
Noncatecholamines				
Ephedrine	Multiple preparations of 25- and 50-mg capsules; syrup, 10 and 20 mg/5 ml	Oral	3 mg/kg/24 hr in 4 divided doses	25–50 mg q4–6h
Metaproterenol sulfate (orciprenaline[a])	Alupent, Metaprel, 10- and 20-mg tablets; syrup, 10 mg/5 ml	Oral	Under 6 yr, 1.3–2.6 mg/kg/day as q6h dose; under 60 lb 10 mg q6h; over 60 lb, 20 mg q6h	
	Alupent metered-dose inhaler, Metaprel metered-dose inhaler, 0.65 mg/puff	Pressurized aerosol	2–3 inhalations q4h, not to exceed 12 inhalations/day for older children[b] and adults	
	Alupent or Metaprel inhalant solution 5%	Nebulization	0.2–0.3 ml (0.1–0.2 ml in children[b]) in 2.5 ml sterile water or saline q4h	
Albuterol (salbutamol[a])	Ventolin or Proventil 2- and 4-mg tablets	Oral	Usual starting dose for adults and children 12 yr and over, 2–4 mg tid–qid	
	Ventolin or Proventil syrup, 2 mg/5 ml	Oral	Usual starting dose for children 2–6 yr is 0.1 mg/kg tid (max. 2 mg tid); for children 6–12 yr, 2 mg tid–qid	
	Ventolin or Proventil inhaler, 90 µg/puff	Pressurized aerosol	1–2 puffs tid–qid[b]	
	Ventolin and Proventil solution 0.5%	Nebulization	0.5 ml (2.5 mg) in 2.5 ml of sterile water or saline tid–qid[b]	
Fenoterol[c]	Berotec, 2.5-mg tablets	Oral	2.5 mg bid–tid[b]	
	Berotec metered-dose inhaler, 0.2 mg/puff	Pressurized aerosol		1–2 puffs q6–8h (max. 3 in 3-hr period)
Terbutaline sulfate	Bricanyl, 2.5- and 5.0-mg tablets	Oral	12–15 yr, 2.5 mg q8h[b]	Over 15 yr, 5 mg q8h
	Brethine, 2.5- and 5.0-mg tablets	Oral	As above	
	Bricanyl subcutaneous injection (ampules), 1 mg/ml	SC injection	0.25 mg (repeat in 15–30 min, then 4–6 hr)[b]	
	Brethine ampules, 1 mg/ml	SC injection	As above	
	Brethaire metered-dose inhaler, 0.25 mg/puff	Pressurized aerosol	1–2 puffs tid–qid[b]	

[a] Approved name in the United Kingdom.
[b] The FDA does not recommend for children under 12 years of age.
[c] Not currently FDA approved.

Onset of action (minutes)	Peak action	Duration (hours)	Commonly observed side effects
Noncatecholamines			
60	2.0–3.5 hr	3–5	Same as epinephrine. Newer beta-2 selective agents preferred.
30	2.0–2.5 hr	Up to 5	Decreased effects when compared with those of epinephrine or isoproterenol. Muscle tremors, central nervous system stimulation, and increases in pulse and blood pressure can occur, especially after oral administration.
5–10	3–5 hr	Up to 5	As above
5–10	3–5 hr	Up to 5	As above
20	2–4 hr	6–8	Oral administration produces fewer side effects than less selective beta-2 agents, although muscle tremor can occur.
20	2–4 hr	6–8	As above
<5	60 min	4–6	Inhalation of usual therapeutic doses does not produce cardiovascular or other pharmacologic side effects.
<5	60 min	4–6	Same as above
20	2–4 hr	6–8	Same as albuterol
<5	60 min	6–8	Same as above
30	2–4 hr	Variable 4–8	Decreased effects when compared with those of epinephrine or isoproterenol. Muscle tremors, CNS stimulation, and increase in pulse and blood pressure can occur.
30	2–4 hr	Variable 4–8	As above
	30–60 min	1.5–4.0	Similar to epinephrine, especially in doses in excess of 0.25 mg
	30–60 min	1.5–4.0	As above
–2	15 min	6–8	As above

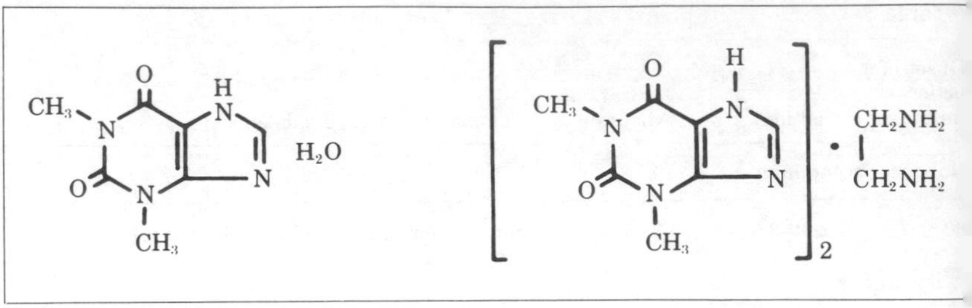

Fig. 4-1. Chemical structure of theophylline (left) and aminophylline (right).

    e. Because the volume of distribution is minimally changed under most conditions, **variations in theophylline half-life reflect alteration in plasma theophylline clearance.** Factors that alter plasma theophylline clearance are listed in Table 4-8. Rates of elimination are decreased in premature infants, and increased in children; childhood rates approach adult values in the mid-teens.

    f. **Elimination is prolonged in obese patients, and maintenance doses must be calculated from ideal body weights (IBW).** Ideal body weight is estimated from height and weight by the formulas: IBW for males = 110 lb ± 5 lb/in. above or below 5 ft; IBW for females = 100 lb ± 5 lb/in. above or below 5 ft (*Clin. Pharmacol. Ther.* 23:438, 1978).

D. Dosage. Calculate theophylline dosage in terms of **anhydrous theophylline.** Underdosing occurs if doses are based on **theophylline salt** content because of the substantially decreased anhydrous theophylline availability in theophylline salts. (See also Chap. 6.)

    1. Oral dosage. Because of the variability among individuals, dosage and frequency of administration must be individualized according to symptomatic improvement, production of side effects, and—if large doses are used—maintenance of serum theophylline levels between 8 and 20 μg/ml. (Asthma is a variable disease, and asthmatic patients may obtain benefits from theophylline at lower serum concentrations, e.g., between 5 and 10 μg/ml.)

The usual starting dose is between 10 and 16 mg/kg/day. (In infants of normal size less than 1 year of age, initiate therapy at a dose no higher than two-thirds the average dose requirements for age, calculated by the formula, mg/kg/day = 8 + 0.3 times age in weeks. If average doses are maintained or exceeded, monitor serum theophylline levels. [Nassif. *J. Pediatr.* 98:158, 1981.]) Increase the dose **if tolerated** in increments of approximately 25% at 3-day intervals to the following levels:

    a. Age 1–9 years, 24 mg/kg/day

    b. Age 9–12 years, 20 mg/kg/day

    c. Age 12–16 years, 18 mg/kg/day

    d. Age over 16 years, (≥ 45 kg), 800 mg/day

Doses above these levels may be necessary but should be followed with serum theophylline determinations. **Do not try to maintain any dose that is not tolerated. Use IBW for obese patients.** Sustained-release preparations usually require a smaller total daily dose than do short-acting forms. If larger doses are required or side effects occur, the final dose adjustment should be guided by measurement of serum theophylline levels, as in Table 4-9. (FDA guidelines for theophylline dosing in young infants, especially neonates, are found in *FDA Drug Bulletin 1985* 15:16, 1985. Comments concerning these guidelines are noted in P. Gal and J. T. Gilman

Table 4-8. Factors altering the plasma clearance of theophylline

| Factor | Theophylline elimination | |
	Decreased	Increased
Age	Prematurity Neonatal age ?Age over 50 yr (Older age decreases response to factors that usually stimulate biotransformation.)	Age 1–16 yr
Weight	Obesity (Ideal body weight must be used to calculate maintenance dose [see text].)	
Diet	High carbohydrate Dietary methylxanthines	Low carbohydrate, high protein Charcoal-broiled meats
Habits		Cigarette smoking (tobacco or marijuana)
Drugs	Allopurinol Cimetidine Erythromycin Propranolol Thiabendazole Troleandomycin (TAO) ?Long-term theophylline therapy ?Oral contraceptives ?Influenza virus vaccine ?Furosemide	Phenobarbital Phenytoin Rifampin
Disease	Liver dysfunction Congestive heart failure Acute pulmonary edema Chronic obstructive pulmonary disease Pneumonia ?Acute febrile episodes Viral upper respiratory infections Alcoholism	Cystic fibrosis Hyperthyroidism

Concerns about the Food and Drug Administration Guidelines for neonatal theophylline dosing. *Ther. Drug Monit.* 8:1, 1986.)

2. **Intravenous dosage.** The primary goal of intravenous theophylline therapy is rapid achievement of a steady-state plasma theophylline concentration in the therapeutic range of 8–20 μg/ml.

   a. If the patient has received no prior theophylline dosage, administer a loading dose of 6 mg/kg of aminophylline infused over 20–30 minutes and continue the maintenance dose as given in Table 6-4. This suggested infusion rate is used only as an initial guideline; serum levels of theophylline must be monitored.

   b. After the loading dose, **continuous infusion** therapy is preferable to bolus therapy to maintain steady-state serum theophylline levels. Serum theophylline levels should be determined at 1, 12, and 24 hours (1) after initiation of an aminophylline infusion, (2) when the patient's infusion is changed, or (3) when the patient is given another bolus dose.

Table 4-9. Final dose adjustment guided by measurement of serum theophylline concentration

Peak theophylline level (μg/ml)	Approximate adjustment in total daily dose	Comments
< 7.5	25% increase*	If patient is asymptomatic, consider trial off drug. Recheck serum theophylline level for guidance in further dose adjustment.
7.5–10	25% increase	Even if patient is asymptomatic at this level, an increased serum concentration may prevent symptoms during a viral upper respiratory infection, or heavy exposure to an inhalant allergen, or vigorous exertion.
10–20	None	Maintain dose if tolerated. Recheck serum concentration at 6- to 12-mo intervals or sooner if drug interactions or physiologic abnormalities occur.
14–20	Occasional intolerance requires 10% decrease.	If side effects occur, decrease total daily dose as indicated.
21–25	10% decrease	Decrease even if side effects are absent.
26–30	25% decrease	Even if side effects are absent, omit next dose and decrease total daily dose as indicated. Repeat measurement of serum concentration.
> 30	50% decrease	Omit next two doses; decrease as indicated. Repeat measurement of serum concentration.

*To avoid potential toxic reaction, (1) be sure that the sample represents a peak level obtained at steady state (i.e., no missed or extra doses, with close approximation of prescribed dosage intervals during previous 48 hr; at least 3 days with sustained-release products); (2) repeat laboratory determination if not initially performed in duplicate; (3) make increases of 50–100% in increments of 25% at 2-day intervals (3-day intervals for sustained-release products) for further assurance of safety and tolerance.

Source: Adapted from L. Hendeles, M. Weinberger, and R. Wyatt. Guide to oral theophylline therapy for the treatment of chronic asthma. *Am. J. Dis. Child.* 132:876, 1978; and from M. Weinberger and L. Hendeles. Slow-release theophylline; rationale and basis for product selection. *N. Engl. J. Med.* 308:760, 1983.

Another bolus dose may be required when theophylline levels are subtherapeutic. In this event, follow the dosage guidelines in Table 6-4.

   E. Theophylline preparations. A variety of oral theophylline preparations are available (Table 4-10). These preparations include short-acting liquid preparations, tablets, and capsules; sustained-release preparations; and combinations of theophylline with other medications (Table 4-11). In selecting a preparation, note the following guidelines:

      1. The presence of **alcohol** in liquid preparations offers no therapeutic advantage, does not enhance theophylline absorption, and has the potential for causing long-term adverse effects if administered in high doses for long periods of time.

      2. Avoid fixed drug combinations. The incidence of side effects is increased with the use of combined theophylline and ephedrine preparations (see Table 4-11), without clinical evidence of an added bronchodilatory effect. Similarly, phenobarbital additions may enhance corticosteroid metabolism, producing decreased effectiveness in chronic corticosteroid-dependent asth-

Table 4-10. Oral theophylline preparations

Theophylline preparation	Product	Dosage forms (mg)	Tablet or capsule color	Equivalent amount anhydrous theophylline (mg)	Percent alcohol
Anhydrous theophylline					
Short-acting tablets	Quibron-T Dividose tablets	300	Ivory	300	
	Slo-Phyllin	100	White	100	
		200	White	200	
	Theolair	125	White	125	
		250	White	250	
Short-acting capsules	Bronkodyl	100	Brown/white	100	
		200	Green/white	200	
	Elixophyllin	100	White	100	
		200	White	200	
	Quibron-300	300 (+180 mg guaifenesin)	Yellow/white	300	
	Quibron	150 (+90 mg guaifenesin)	Yellow	150	
	Somophyllin-T	100	White	100	
		200	White	200	
		250	White	250	
Sustained-release tablets	Respbid	250	White	250	
		500	White	500	
	Constant-T	200	Light pink	200	
		300	Light blue	300	

Table 4-10 (*continued*)

Theophylline preparation	Product	Dosage forms (mg)	Tablet or capsule color	Equivalent amount anhydrous theophylline (mg)	Percent alcohol
Sustained-release tablets (*cont.*)	Duraphyl Controlled Release	100	White	100	
		200	White	200	
		300	White	300	
	Quibron-T/SR Dividose	300	White	300	
	Sustaire	100	White	100	
		300	White	300	
	Theo-Dur	100	White	100	
		200	White	200	
		300	White	300	
	Theolair-SR	200	White	200	
		250	White	250	
		300	White	300	
		500	White	500	
	Uniphyl	200	White	200	
		400	White	400	
Sustained-release capsules	Aerolate Sr.	260	Red/clear	260	
	Aerolate Jr.	130	Red/clear	130	
	Aerolate III	65	Red/clear	65	
	Elixophyllin SR	250	Clear	250	
		125	White	125	
	Slo-Bid Gyrocaps	300	Opaque white	300	
		200	Opaque white (cap)/clear (body)	200	
		100	Clear	100	
		50	Clear (cap)/opaque white (body)	50	

			Description	
	125		Brown	125
	60		White	60
Somophyllin CRT	300		½ clear, ½ white, white beads	300
	250		As above	250
Theo-24	200		As above	200
	100		As above	100
	300		Red/clear	300
	200		Orange/clear	200
	100		Gold/clear	100
Theobid Duracaps	260		Blue/clear	260
Theobid Jr. Duracaps	130		Dark blue/light blue	130
Theoclear L.A.	260		Clear/white beads	260
	130		Clear/white beads	130
Theo-Dur Sprinkle	200		Clear (cap)/white opaque (body)	200
	125		Clear (cap)/white opaque (body)	125
	75		Clear (cap)/white opaque (body)	75
	50		Clear (cap)/white opaque (body)	50
Theospan SR	260		White, clear/white pellets	260
	130		White, clear/orange and white pellets	130
Theovent LA	250		Green/clear	250
	125		Green/yellow	125

Table 4-10 (*continued*)

Theophylline preparation	Product	Dosage forms (mg)	Tablet or capsule color	Equivalent amount anhydrous theophylline (mg)	Percent alcohol
Liquid preparations	Accurbron	50/5 ml		10/ml	7.5
	Aerolate liquid	150/15 ml		160/15 ml	
	Aquaphyllin syrup	80/15		80/15	
	Elixophyllin elixir	80/15 ml		80/15 ml	20
	Quibron	150 (+90 mg guaifenesin)/15 ml		150/15 ml	
	Slo-Phyllin 80 syrup	80/15 ml		80/15 ml	
	Slo-Phyllin GG syrup	150 (+90 mg guaifenesin)/15 ml		150/15 ml	
	Theoclear-80 syrup	80/15 ml		80/15 ml	
	Theolair liquid	80/15 ml		80/15 ml	
	Theostat 80 syrup	80/15 ml		80/15 ml	1
Theophylline salts					
Theophylline ethylenediamine (aminophylline)					
Short-acting tablets	Aminophyllin (Searle)	100	White	79	
		200	White	158	
Liquid preparations	Somophyllin oral liquid	105/5 ml		90/5 ml	
	Somophyllin DF oral liquid	105/5 ml		90/5 ml	
	Somophyllin rectal so-	300/5 ml		255/5 ml	

	Preparation	Composition	Color	Theophylline (mg)	Alcohol (%)
...phylline sodium glycinate					
Short-acting tablets	Asbron G Inlay-Tabs	300 (+100 mg guaifenesin)	Green/white	150	
	Synophylate-GG tablets	300 (+100 mg guaifenesin)	Red	137	
Liquid preparations	Asbron G	300 (+100 mg guaifenesin)/15 ml	White	150/15 ml	15
	Synophylate elixir	330/15 ml		150/15 ml	20
Theophylline choline (ox-triphylline)					
Short-acting tablets	Brondecon	200 (+100 mg guaifenesin)	Salmon pink	128	
	Choledyl (enteric coated)	200	Yellow	128	
		100	Red	64	
Timed-release tablets	Choledyl SA	600	Tan	382	
		400	Pink	254	
Liquid preparations	Brondecon elixir	100 (+50 mg guaifenesin)/5 ml		64/5 ml	20
	Choledyl elixir	100/5 ml		64/5 ml	20
	Choledyl pediatric syrup	50/5 ml		32/5 ml	20
Dihydroxypropyl theophylline (dyphylline)*					
Short-acting tablets	Dilor	200	Blue	Undetermined	
	Lufyllin	400	White	Undetermined	
	Lufyllin-400	200	White		
Liquid preparations	Lufyllin elixir	100/15 ml	White	Undetermined	20

*Although dyphylline is a xanthine bronchodilator, it is not a true theophylline. The *Physicians' Desk Reference* states that dyphylline is equivalent to approximately 70% theophylline.

Table 4-11. Combination oral bronchodilators

Product	Contents	Amount in mg	Tablet color	Percent alcohol
Bronkaid tablet	Theophylline Ephedrine Guaifenesin	100 24 100	White	
Bronkolixir	Theophylline Ephedrine Guaifenesin Phenobarbital	15/5 ml 12/5 ml 50/5 ml 4/5 ml		19
Bronkotabs tablet	Theophylline Ephedrine Guaifenesin Phenobarbital	100 24 100 8	White	
Marax tablet	Theophylline Ephedrine Hydroxyzine	130 25 10	White	
Marax DF syrup	Theophylline Ephedrine Hydroxyzine	32.5/5 ml 6.25/5 ml 2.5/5 ml		5
Mudrane tablet	Aminophylline Potassium iodide Phenobarbital Ephedrine	130 195 8 16	Yellow	
Primatene M tablet	Theophylline Ephedrine Pyrilamine maleate	130 24 16.6	Yellow	
Primatene P tablet[a]	Theophylline Ephedrine Phenobarbital	130 24 8	Yellow	
Quadrinal tablet	Theophylline calcium salicylate Ephedrine Phenobarbital Potassium iodide	130[b] 24 24 320	White	
Tedral tablet	Theophylline Ephedrine Phenobarbital	118 24 8	White	
Tedral SA tablet	Theophylline Ephedrine Phenobarbital	180 48 25	Coral/mottled white	
Tedral-25	Theophylline Ephedrine Butabarbital	130 24 25	Salmon pink	
Tedral elixir	Theophylline Ephedrine Phenobarbital	32.5/5 ml 6/5 ml 2/5 ml		15
Tedral suspension	Theophylline Ephedrine Phenobarbital	65/5 ml 12/5 ml 4/5 ml		

[a] Available only in states where nonprescription phenobarbital is sold.
[b] Equivalent to 65 mg anhydrous theophylline.

matic patients. If adrenergic medications are desired, use them with theophylline separately (e.g., metaproterenol, terbutaline) and titrate individually.

3. **Sustained-release** preparations are helpful in chronic asthma requiring around-the-clock theophylline. These preparations offer a steady-state serum level, and the dosage schedule of every 8, 12, or 24 hours improves patient compliance. In young children, **capsulized, beaded** sustained-release preparations can be sprinkled on soft food and followed with a drink to discourage chewing, which destroys the sustained-release properties of the preparation. **(Do not use this technique with sustained-release tablets.)**

   A variety of slow-release theophylline products are available. Clinically important differences in the extent and rate of absorption exist among these products; for example, food has different effects on different formulations. To properly use these slow-release products, the physician must select a dosing interval appropriate for both the absorption characteristics of the particular product and the rate of theophylline elimination of the individual patient (L. Hendeles and M. Weinberger. Selection of a slow-release theophylline product. *J. Allergy Clin. Immunol.* 78:743, 1986).

4. **Peak serum levels** should be monitored in chronic asthmatic patients when large doses are used. For liquid and rapidly dissolving tablets, measure levels at approximately 2 hours after administration; for sustained-release preparations, at approximately 5 hours after administration.

   Diphylline (dihydroxypropyltheophylline) is an alkylated derivative of theophylline and its presence in serum **is not** detected by the standard theophylline assay.

F. **Adverse reactions.** The incidence of adverse reactions increases as the serum theophylline level exceeds 15 µg/ml. The most common adverse reactions include gastrointestinal and CNS side effects. For other side effects, see Chap. 6 and Table 6-3.

   1. **Avoid rectal suppositories** because of unreliable and incomplete absorption. Many overdoses, especially in children, are secondary to rectal suppository administration. If vomiting precludes the oral theophylline route (making sure theophylline is not the cause of the vomiting), an accepted method is to administer **rectal solutions,** which are better absorbed.

   2. In-office monitoring of blood theophylline levels has been simplified by the introduction of AccuLevel (Syntex Medical Diagnostics, 900 Arastradero Road, Palo Alto, CA 94304). This methodology using monoclonal antibody technology does not require an instrument, employs a fingerstick blood sample, and gives a reading in 15 minutes.

   3. **Treatment of overdosage** (E. F. Ellis. Theophylline toxicity. *J. Allergy Clin. Immunol.* [Suppl.] 76:297, 1985; and M. J. Goldberg, G. D. Park, and W. G. Berlinger. Treatment of Theophylline Intoxication. In J. A. Grant and E. F. Ellis [eds.], *Update on Theophylline* [Symposium Proceedings] 78:811, 1986) includes the following:

      a. Stop the drug immediately and obtain serial serum levels.

      b. Administer orally a dose of high-surface area activated charcoal (30–100 gm, depending on the size of the patient). Additional doses may be required at 2- to 3-hour intervals, especially in patients who have ingested slow-release theophylline products. Intoxicated patients with impaired pharyngeal reflexes should be provided with airway protection to avoid pulmonary aspiration.

         Stomach-emptying procedures (Ipecac or gastric lavage) are recommended only for patients who have ingested large quantities of theophylline and are seen within the first few hours of ingestion, and only if spontaneous emesis has not occurred. The administration of a cathartic such as sorbitol may be helpful.

      c. Provide supportive care and adequate hydration for complications of the intoxication such as seizures and metabolic (e.g., hypokalemia) and cardiovascular complications (e.g., hypotension, cardiac arrhythmias).

d. Charcoal hemoperfusion is the method of choice for the rapid removal of theophylline from the serum. This technique requires experienced personnel and appropriately sized filters (50 ml in infants, 100 ml in toddlers, and 250 ml in teenagers; available from Clark Research and Development, 6 Davies Boulevard, New Orleans, LA 70121). Controversy exists concerning when these filters should be used. Goldberg et al. recommended prophylactic hemoperfusion for patients with acute theophylline intoxication if the serum concentration is greater than 80 μg/ml following an acute ingestion. For chronic intoxication, hemoperfusion is recommended (1) if the serum theophylline concentration is greater than 60 μg/ml or (2) if the concentration is greater than 50 μg/ml and the patient is 60 years of age or more, or significant liver disease or congestive heart failure and inability to tolerate oral activated charcoal therapy exists.

e. Phenobarbital administration has been shown to have potential effects as an antidote to theophylline. Prophylactic administration of phenobarbital may prevent the occurrence of tissue damage; it should be considered in patients who satisfy criteria for hemoperfusion. Additional controlled trials are necessary.

f. Maintain an airway with adequate ventilation and administer oxygen as needed. Treat seizures with IV diazepam, 5–10 mg (0.1–0.3 mg/kg in children).

IV. Anticholinergic drugs. The parasympathetic nervous system and its neurotransmitter acetylcholine help to mediate bronchial tone and may play a role in triggering bronchospasm in patients with asthma. Atropine sulfate, belladonna, scopolamine hydrobromide, methantheline bromide, and epoxymethamine bromide are effective in protecting against the bronchospastic effects of methacholine but not against histamine-induced bronchospasm. Atropine aerosols yield varying responses in antigen-induced and exercise-induced asthma.

At present, the use of atropine aerosols is limited because of the associated side effects, which include drying of the oropharynx, increased heart rate, sedation, and blurred vision. Although it is claimed that atropine increases the viscosity of bronchial secretions, there is little evidence that this effect is clinically significant. The dose for adults is 0.025–0.050 mg/kg diluted with 3–5 ml of saline and given by nebulization 3–4 times a day (maximum single dose for adults is 2.5 mg; for children, 0.05 mg/kg). Atropine can be prepared from a stock solution; it is also available commercially as a solution for nebulization (Dey-Dose Atropine Sulfate 0.2% (1 mg) and 0.5% (2.5 mg) in 0.5-ml containers).

Analogues of atropine (e.g., ipratropium bromide [Atrovent]) have fewer side effects and a longer duration of action. Ipratropium bromide is especially helpful in asthmatic patients with coexisting chronic bronchitis or cough as the predominant syndrome, in patients unable to tolerate theophylline or beta-2 agonists, and in some patients with acute asthma when treatment with beta-adrenergic drugs is inadequate. The usual adult dose is two inhalations (36 μg) by a metered-dose inhaler 4 times a day. Additional inhalations may be taken although the total number of inhalations should not exceed 12 in 24 hours. Safety and effectiveness in children under 12 years of age has not been established.

V. Cromolyn sodium is the disodium salt of 1,3-bis-(2-carboxy chromone-5-yloxy)-2-hydroxypropane (Fig. 4-2). The drug has the capacity to inhibit allergen-induced bronchospasm. Investigational drugs (e.g., doxantrazole) have cromolyn sodium-like activities but possess a wider spectrum of antiallergic properties and better oral absorption.

A. Mechanism of action. Cromolyn sodium appears to mediate its activity by inhibiting the release of various chemical mediators (e.g., histamine, leukotrienes, and serotonin) released after antigen challenge of tissue sensitized with IgE-specific antibodies. In addition to inhibiting IgE-mediated reactions, cromolyn sodium may inhibit late immune responses that possibly are mediated by

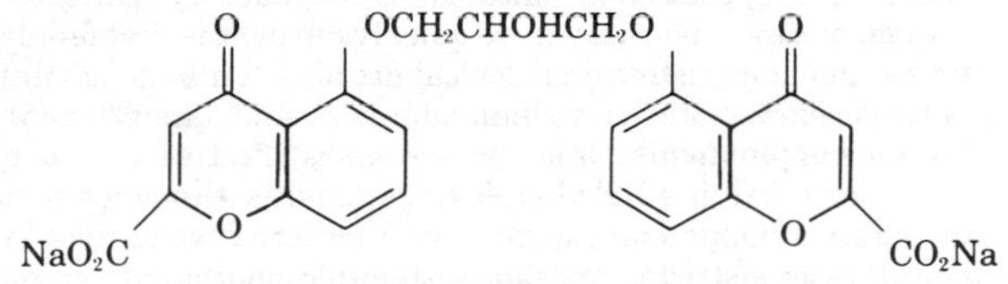

Fig. 4-2. Chemical structure of cromolyn sodium.

nonreaginic precipitating antibodies. In humans, cromolyn sodium is organ-specific since it inhibits antigen-induced mediator release from sensitized lung fragments but not from sensitized circulating basophils or dermal cell suspensions.

The exact mechanism of action is uncertain. Experimental evidence suggests that cromolyn sodium functions as a nonspecific stabilizer of mast cell membranes, stimulates cyclic AMP, inhibits phosphodiesterase, and regulates the calcium "gating" mechanism by increasing the intracellular level of cyclic AMP. Reduction of calcium transport across the mast cell membrane inhibits calcium-dependent, antigen-induced mediator release. Inhibition of calcium transport may also produce attenuation or blockade of respiratory neuronal reflexes.

B. Pharmacokinetics. Cromolyn sodium (Intal), inhaled by a turboinhaler (Spinhaler) as a dry-powder aerosol (20 mg of cromolyn sodium plus 20 mg of coarse lactose as a carrier), is absorbed, distributed, metabolized, and excreted in the following way: 25% remains in the Spinhaler; 40% can be recovered from mouth washings; 10% is absorbed into the bloodstream; and the rest is deposited in the upper airways and swallowed. Of the 2 mg absorbed into the upper airways and swallowed, 50% is excreted unchanged in the urine, and 50% is excreted unchanged in the bile. Virtually all of the drug in the gastrointestinal tract is excreted unchanged in the feces. Consequently, the antiallergic activity of cromolyn sodium in the lungs may be achieved by less than 1 mg of the drug.

C. Indications

1. **Asthma.** The long-term clinical efficacy of cromolyn sodium in the treatment of asthma has been corroborated by several well-controlled, double-blind investigations and has been used as a primary drug for prophylaxis. Approximately 70% of all patients described as clinically suffering from asthma seem to derive benefit from the drug (see Chap. 6).

   a. Although cromolyn sodium appears to be effective primarily in extrinsic asthma, asthmatic patients without demonstrable allergic sensitivities should be given a trial of cromolyn sodium since allergic factors alone do not accurately predict a favorable response. **All patients with chronic perennial asthma should be given a therapeutic trial with cromolyn sodium therapy before continuous corticosteroids are instituted.**

   b. Intermittent administration of cromolyn sodium can be used in patients with **seasonal asthma** (giving the drug 1 week before the expected appearance of the specific aeroallergen).

   c. In patients with **exercise-induced bronchospasm,** give the drug shortly before exercise to provide protection for approximately 2–3 hours. For patients already taking cromolyn sodium, give an extra dose of cromolyn sodium immediately before exercise in addition to the regular daily doses.

   d. Cromolyn sodium is an excellent choice in the prophylactic treatment of asthmatic patients sensitive to **animal danders,** especially when occupational allergens cannot be avoided (e.g., veterinarians).

2. **Allergic rhinitis.** Cromolyn sodium nasal solution (Nasalcrom) is effective for perennial and seasonal allergic rhinitis. Because it is for prophylactic rather than symptomatic treatment, cromolyn sodium should be administered to the nose on a regular basis starting 1 week before the expected

aeroallergen appears and continued throughout the patient's season. Improvement can be obtained more quickly during the first few days of cromolyn sodium administration if topical decongestants are administered 5–10 minutes before cromolyn sodium administration (see Chap. 5).

3. **Allergic conjunctivitis.** Cromolyn sodium is effective in some patients with vernal conjunctivitis and allergic conjunctivitis. Cromolyn sodium ophthalmic solution (Opticrom) can be a useful alternative to the commonly used topical vasoconstrictor and antihistaminic ophthalmic preparations (see Chap. 5).

4. **Food allergies.** Several preliminary reports suggest that cromolyn sodium can help certain cases of food allergy in which the primary manifestations are gastrointestinal (see Chap. 13).

5. **Mucous membrane ulcerations.** Cromolyn sodium has been used in patients with **aphthous ulcers** and in patients with **ulcerative proctocolitis.** Additional confirmatory evidence is needed before cromolyn sodium therapy can be recommended for these conditions.

D. **Dosage.** When using cromolyn sodium powder (20 mg 4 times/day) by the Spinhaler, **it is imperative that the patient understand the proper use of this device.** (Most children under the age of 5 years cannot use the Spinhaler.) Instruct the patient in the correct use as follows:

1. Load the colored end of the capsule firmly into the propeller cup. Avoid excessive handling of the capsule, which can cause it to soften.

2. Screw the body of the Spinhaler back into the mouthpiece, making certain it is securely fastened.

3. Keeping the inhaler vertical and the mouthpiece down, slide the colored sleeve down firmly until it stops, to pierce the capsule. Then slide the sleeve up as far as it will go. **Do this maneuver only once.**

4. Exhale with the inhaler away from the mouth.

5. Tilt the head backward slightly in order to straighten the angle between the mouth and the trachea.

6. Place the mouthpiece of the inhaler between the teeth and inhale as rapidly as is comfortable with the lips sealed around the mouthpiece.

7. Hold the breath for a few seconds and then exhale with the Spinhaler away from the mouth to avoid deposition of moist air and interference with proper functioning. A whistle device is available to help give auditory feedback for proper operation of the Spinhaler.

8. Wash the Spinhaler at least once a week with clean, warm water.

Two other dosage forms of cromolyn sodium are also available and show similar efficacy. The metered-dose inhaler delivers 0.8 mg/actuation (dose of two inhalations four times daily) and the solution form for nebulization (given with power-driven devices with a suitable face mask or mouthpiece) contains 10 mg/ml in 2-ml glass containers. The nebulized dose should be given four times a day to start and, like other dosing forms, may be reduced to two or three doses a day if symptom control is achieved. This solution is compatible with 0.25% isoetharine, metaproterenol sulfate, and terbutaline sulfate for at least 1 hour after mixing.

For optimal results when cromolyn sodium is used by any inhalational route, it is imperative that the asthmatic patient understand the appropriate use of the Spinhaler, metered-dose inhaler, or solution for nebulization. Instructions found in the package insert should be carefully followed and the patient monitored for appropriate use of these inhalational routes.

E. **Adverse effects.** Long-term surveillance for possible adverse effects of cromolyn sodium has indicated no adverse hematologic, biochemical, or urinary effects.

1. Most side effects are classified as minor and include such symptoms as irritation of the throat, hoarseness, dryness of the mouth, acute cough, and a sensation of chest tightness or bronchospasm occurring immediately after inhaling the powder. Throat irritation can be prevented by taking a drink of

water immediately after the inhalation or by gargling; bronchospasm is diminished by inhalation of a beta-2 agonist before (i.e., 15–20 minutes) the cromolyn sodium treatment. Nausea and vomiting, facial rash, and urticaria have been reported in a few patients. Nasal congestion occurring several weeks after starting cromolyn sodium has also been reported.

2. Adverse effects of a more serious nature have included a few cases of pulmonary infiltration and eosinophilia.

F. Contraindications

1. Cromolyn sodium is contraindicated in the few patients who have shown hypersensitivity to it.

2. Cromolyn sodium should not be used in the treatment of acute asthma, especially status asthmaticus.

3. Although cromolyn sodium has been used in women during the first trimester of pregnancy without an obvious increase in birth abnormalities, and although animal tests also have shown no teratogenic effects with cromolyn sodium, the advantage to the patient, as with all drugs, must be weighed against the possible risk to the fetus (FDA Pregnancy Category B).

4. There are no clinically significant interactions between cromolyn sodium and other drugs. Cromolyn sodium can be used concomitantly with other forms of asthma therapy.

VI. Corticosteroids.
Since 1948, when Hench and co-workers demonstrated that cortisone had remarkable anti-inflammatory effects on rheumatoid arthritis, corticosteroids have been employed in the management of severe bronchial asthma, chronic inflammatory diseases, and various immunologic disorders. Despite their beneficial effects, production of multiple, severe adverse side effects by corticosteroids prohibits their widespread and indiscriminate use.

Natural and synthetic corticosteroids are divided into **glucocorticoids** and **mineralocorticoids.** Mineralocorticoids primarily mediate electrolyte regulation, including potassium excretion and sodium retention. Glucocorticoids affect carbohydrate metabolism and produce suppression of the hypothalamic-pituitary-adrenal axis, an increase in resistance to stress, suppression of growth, marked anti-inflammatory effects, lymph node and thymus involution, and lymphocytopenia. Because of their anti-inflammatory and immunoregulatory actions, glucocorticoids play a major role in the pharmacologic management of allergic diseases.

A. Structural and functional relationships.
Most corticosteroids produced by the adrenal cortex are C_{21} steroids with the basic configuration shown in Figure 4-3. Three functional groups are required for **glucocorticoid** activity: a double bond between C_4 and C_5; ketone groups (= 0) at C_3 and C_{20}; and hydroxyl groups (OH) on C_{11} and C_{21}. Alteration of any of these essential groups destroys biologic activity. Other changes of the basic structure produce corticosteroids with increased glucocorticoid activity and decreased mineralocorticoid activity. Although improvement in the separation of glucocorticoid and mineralocorticoid activity occurs, synthetically produced preparations with primarily glucocorticoid activity **still possess variable mineralocorticoid activity and can cause sodium retention and potassium depletion when given in pharmacologic amounts.** (The relative potency and characteristics of systemic corticosteroids are given in Table 4-12.)

B. Mechanisms of action.
Despite seemingly diverse effects on a number of physiologic systems, corticosteroids mediate these effects by their influence on the cellular production of proteins. The steroid molecule enters cells and binds to specific protein receptors in the cytoplasm. The active steroid-protein complex enters the nucleus, where the active complex associates with DNA and alters nuclear gene expression, leading to the de novo synthesis of messenger RNA (mRNA) and ribosomal RNA (rRNA). The synthesis of messenger RNA is followed by the synthesis of proteins that mediate the effect of the corticosteroid hormone. The time course necessary for corticosteroids to accomplish their biologic function is in the range of hours.

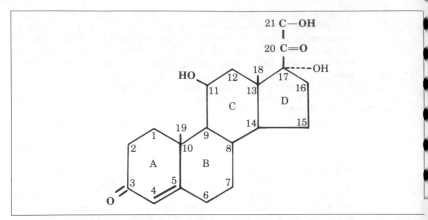

Fig. 4-3. Basic chemical structure of the C_{21} corticosteroid molecule. Components in bold type are essential for biologic activity (see text). (From H. G. Morris. Pharmacology of Corticosteroids in Asthma. In E. Middleton, C. Reed, and E. Ellis [eds.], *Allergy: Principles and Practice.* St. Louis: Mosby, 1978. With permission.)

C. Corticosteroid physiology
   1. **Secretion.** Under basal conditions the adrenal cortex secretes about 15–25 mg (12–15 mg/sq m) of cortisol and 1.5–4.0 mg of corticosterone a day.
   2. **Transport.** Most of the corticosteroid is transported in the blood reversibly bound to albumin and corticosteroid-binding globulin. The unbound hormone is the active form that is available for metabolism and exerts physiologic effects.
   3. **Metabolism and elimination.** Natural corticosteroids have short plasma half-lives (e.g., 90 minutes for cortisol); the half-lives of synthetic corticosteroids are variable, ranging from 90 minutes to over 4 hours. Although plasma half-lives usually correlate positively with tissue half-lives, **tissue half-lives determine the duration of biologic effectiveness.** Tissue half-lives range from 8–12 hours for cortisol to 3 days for dexamethasone. Metabolism of 70% or more of endogenous corticosteroid takes place in the liver, where physiologically inactive water-soluble conjugates are formed and then excreted in the urine.
D. Indications for corticosteroids in allergic diseases
   1. **Severe acute allergic reactions** can be life-threatening. They include status asthmaticus, anaphylaxis, and exfoliative dermatitis.
   2. **Self-limited allergic reactions,** although not life-threatening, can be severe and produce marked discomfort or morbidity. These conditions include severe contact dermatitis, serum sickness–like reactions, and seasonal pollen asthma.
   3. Patients with **severe chronic allergic conditions** may require corticosteroids if they are not responding to orthodox therapy, if they need temporary relief while awaiting the results of conventional therapy, or to quiet acute severe exacerbations.
   4. **Previous corticosteroid therapy,** especially if prolonged, often necessitates repeat treatment when acute exacerbations of the underlying disease occur.
   5. Corticosteroids can be used as a **diagnostic test** on a short-term basis, e.g., to differentiate reversibility of pulmonary function abnormalities in asthmatic patients from the fixed, irreversible abnormality in patients with chronic obstructive pulmonary disease.
E. Dosage. Corticosteroid dosages for specific allergic or immunologic disorders

Table 4-1. Corticosteroids for systemic administration

Preparations (dosage forms)	Trade name	Equivalent anti-inflammatory doses (mg)	Salt and water retention	Appetite increase	Muscle myopathy	Plasma half-life (minutes)	Biologic half-life (hours)	Adrenal suppression
Short-acting								
Cortisone[b]	Cortisone acetate tablets, USP	25	2+	2+	1+	30	8–12	2+
Tablets, 5, 10, 25 mg Sterile suspension (IM), 25, 50 mg/ml	Cortone acetate in a saline suspension							
Hydrocortisone (cortisol) Tablets, 5, 10, 20 mg Oral suspension, 10 mg/5 ml Sterile solution (IV), 50 mg/ml Powder (for IV reconstitution), 100, 250, 500, 1000 mg/vial Sterile suspension (IM, intra-articular, intralesional), 25, 50 mg/ml	Hydrocortisone tablets, USP, and sterile solution Cortef tablets and oral cypionate suspension Hydrocortone tablets and acetate sterile suspension Hydrocortone phosphate sterile solution A-hydroCort for injection Solu-Cortef for injection	20	2+	2+	1+	90	8–12	2+
Retention enema, 100 mg/60 ml	Cortenema							

Table 4-12 (*continued*)

Preparations (dosage forms)	Trade name	Equivalent anti-inflammatory doses (mg)	Salt and water retention	Appetite increase	Muscle myopathy	Plasma half-life (minutes)	Biologic half-life (hours)	Adrenal suppression
Intermediate-acting								
Prednisone[c] Tablets, 1, 2.5, 5, 10, 20, 50 mg	Prednisone, USP Deltasone Meticorten Orasone SK-Prednisone	5	1+	3+	1+	200	12–36	2+
Syrup, 5 mg/5 ml	Liquid Pred Pediapred							
Prednisolone Tablets, 1, 2.5, 5 mg Syrup, 15 mg/5 ml Sterile solution (IV), 20 mg/ml Sterile suspension (IM, intra-articular, intralesional)	Prednisolone tablets, USP Delta-Cortef tablets Prelone Hydeltrasol Injection Prednisolone tebutate Hydeltra-T.B.A.	5	1+	3+	1+	200	12–36	2+
Methylprednisolone Tablets, 2, 4, 8, 16, 24, 32 mg Sterile powder (for IV reconstitution), 40, 125, 500, 1000 mg/vial Sterile aqueous suspension (IM, intra-articular, intralesional), 20, 40, 80 mg/ml Retention enema, 40 mg/unit	Methylprednisolone tablets, USP, and sterile suspension Medrol tablets Solu-Medrol for injection Depo-Medrol suspension Medrol Enpak (enema)	4	0	2+	1+	200	12–36	2+

Preparation (forms)	Preparations							
Triamcinolone Tablets, 1, 2, 4, 8, 16 mg Syrup, 2 or 4 mg/5 ml Sterile suspension (IM, intra-articular, intralesional), 5, 10, 20, 40 mg/ml	Triamcinolone tablets, USP, and sterile suspension Aristocort tablets and syrup Kenacort tablets and diacetate syrup Kenalog Injection Aristocort and Aristospan suspension	4	0	0	3+	200	24–48	3+
Long-acting								
Dexamethasone Tablets, 0.25, 0.5, 0.75, 1.5, 4 mg, 6 mg Elixir, 0.5 mg/5 ml Sterile solution (IV, IM, intra-articular, intralesional), 4 mg/ml Sterile, timed-release acetate suspension (IM, intra-articular, soft tissue), 8 mg/ml	Dexamethasone tablets, USP, elixir, sterile solutions, and suspensions Decadron tablets and elixir Decadron phosphate injection Decadron-LA suspension Dalalone L.A. Decaject-L.A. Dexone tablets Hexadrol tablets and phosphate injection	0.75	0	4+	2+	300	36–54	4+
Betamethasone Tablets, 0.6 mg Syrup, 0.6 mg/5 ml Sterile solution (IV, IM), 4 mg/ml Sterile suspension[d] (IM, intra-articular, intralesional), 3 mg/ml of phosphate, 3 mg/ml of acetate	Celestone tablets and syrup Celestone Soluspan[d] (betamethasone acetate and sodium phosphate)	0.60	0	4+	2+	300	36–54	4+

[a] See Table 8-3 for topical corticosteroid preparations.
[b] Must be converted to biologically active hydrocortisone.
[c] Must be converted to biologically active prednisolone.
[d] Sodium phosphate gives rapid onset of action; acetate ester provides a sustained effect.

are found in subsequent chapters; preparations and dosage forms are listed in Table 4-12. See Chap. 6 for inhaled corticosteroids.

F. Adverse effects. Corticosteroids can produce multiple adverse side effects of varying severity (Table 4-13). Before beginning therapy, weigh the risk of adverse effects against the expected benefits using the following guidelines:

1. Adequately document the presence of an allergic or immunologic condition **responsive** to corticosteroid therapy.

2. Use corticosteroids only after **less toxic treatments** have proved inadequate, e.g., cromolyn sodium and adrenergic drugs in asthma.

3. Use the **lowest possible dose** that controls the disease. Symptom palliation is an acceptable goal (rather than complete remission of symptoms).

4. Use corticosteroid agents with **short durations of action** (see Table 4-12) and, if possible, use topical preparations with decreased absorption, e.g., creams for cutaneous disorders and inhaled corticosteroids for respiratory allergy.

5. Limit the **duration** of corticosteroid therapy (5–7 days); or, if prolonged therapy is needed, administer intermittent doses, e.g., alternate-day prednisone treatment. Divided doses (3–4 times daily) are more adrenal-suppressive than are single doses; corticosteroids administered before bedtime are more adrenal-suppressive than are morning doses.

6. **Closely monitor the patient for diseases or complications** associated with long-term corticosteroid therapy, e.g., glaucoma, cataracts, gastritis, osteoporosis (see Table 4-13).

7. Use corticosteroids with caution and attention to risk to benefit ratio in pregnancy (see Chap. 6), and avoid use when live virus vaccines are given.

8. **Do not stop long-term, high-dose corticosteroid therapy abruptly.** This can precipitate **adrenal insufficiency** or an acute exacerbation of the underlying disease. The **initial** reduction from pharmacologic doses to physiologic doses must be guided by the presence or the lack of an exacerbation of the underlying disease. Thereafter, the degree of treatment-induced adrenal suppression becomes the limiting factor in reducing the corticosteroid dose. Return to normal hypothalamic-pituitary-adrenal function can require 9–12 months or longer when corticosteroids are completely withdrawn. Until complete recovery has occurred, assume that the patient will require basal corticosteroid therapy and supplemental therapy for stress (i.e., infections, trauma, surgery, or any serious illness). A suggested protocol (Byyny, R. L. Withdrawal from glucocorticoid therapy. *N. Engl. J. Med.* 295:30, 1976) for corticosteroid withdrawal includes the following steps (alternative approaches may be used):

   a. Begin a cautious reduction (i.e., decrements of 2.5–5.0 mg of prednisone every 3–7 days or longer), carefully observing the activity of the underlying disease. If increased activity occurs, increase the dose, and thereafter attempt a more gradual reduction. If no exacerbation occurs, wean the patient to physiologic doses of corticosteroid (20 mg of hydrocortisone or 5 mg of prednisone/day; in children, 12–15 mg/sq m/day of cortisol).

   b. Begin hydrocortisone, 20 mg/day, as a single oral morning dose. Instruct the patient about the need for supplemental doses for stress situations (see f). After 2–4 weeks, obtain an 8 A.M. plasma cortisol level (omit that morning's dose of hydrocortisone). If the plasma cortisol is greater than 10 μg/dl, stop maintenance hydrocortisone therapy but supplement for stress. If the plasma cortisol is less than 10 μg/dl, taper the hydrocortisone by 2.5 mg/week until the patient is taking 10 mg each morning. Supplement for stress.

   c. For patients with levels less than 10 μg/dl, repeat the 8 A.M. plasma cortisol determinations every 4 weeks until the level is greater than 10 μg/dl, and then stop hydrocortisone supplementation. Continue supplementation for stress.

   d. To assure complete recovery of adrenal responsiveness, draw a baseline

Table 4-13. Adverse effects of corticosteroid therapy[a]

General and metabolic
  Cushingoid appearance,[b] including facial mooning
  Increased appetite with excessive weight gain[b]
  Suppression of linear growth[b]
  Negative nitrogen balance
  Hyperglycemia, diabetes[b]
  Hyperlipidemia
  Negative calcium balance
  Interference in metabolism of vitamin D
  Increased fetal risk during pregnancy
Bone
  Osteoporosis[b]
  Vertebral collapse[b]
  Fractures
  Abnormal teeth
  Aseptic necrosis
  Delayed skeletal maturation
Cardiovascular
  Hypertension[b]
  Arrhythmia
  Arteritis
  Congestive heart failure
  Edema
  Thromboembolic phenomenon
Central nervous system
  Mood changes, irritability, and depression[b]
  Insomnia
  Headache
  Cortisone habituation
  Psychosis
  Pseudotumor cerebri (rare)
  Seizures
  Neuritis
Endocrine
  Suppression of hypothalamic-pituitary-adrenal axis[b]
  Decreased secretion of antagonized effects of a number of hormones, including insulin, growth hormone, parathyroid hormone, calcitonin, thyrotropin, and luteinizing hormone
  Delayed sexual maturation[b]
  Menstrual irregularities
  Suppression of neonatal hypothalamic-pituitary-adrenal axis

Gastrointestinal
  Peptic ulceration
  Upper gastrointestinal bleeding
  Pancreatitis
  Fatty liver
Hematologic
  Agranulocytosis
  Disturbances in coagulation
  Thromboembolism
Immune
  Hypersensitivity reactions
  Decreased resistance to infections
  Activation of latent infections
  Masking infections
  Enhancement of virulence and opportunistic infection
  Diminished bactericidal activity of leukocytes
  Decreased serum IgG
Muscular
  Muscle wasting, myopathy
  Pseudorheumatism secondary to withdrawal
  Tendon rupture
Ocular
  Posterior subcapsular cataracts[b]
  Corneal lesions and glaucoma (topical administration)
Renal
  Increased urinary frequency and nocturia
  Nephrosclerosis
  Nephrolithiasis
  Uricosuria
  Hypernatremia
  Hypokalemia
Skin
  Acne[b]
  Purpura[b]
  Thinning of skin[b]
  Striae[b]
  Hirsutism[b]
  Dermatitis
  Panniculitis
  Lipomatosis
  Telangiectasia

[a] See Table 8-4 for adverse effects of topical corticosteroids.
[b] Frequently observed.

cortisol level, give 250 µg (125 µg in children under 2 years of age) of synthetic adrenocorticotropic hormone (ACTH, cosyntropin*) IM, and repeat the plasma cortisol level in 30–60 minutes. An increase in plasma cortisol greater than 6 µg/dl and to a level greater than 20 µg/dl is normal, and no further supplementation for stress is needed. A metyrapone test (in addition to a normal cosyntropin test) and an insulin challenge test can further document the integrity of the entire hypothalamic-pituitary-adrenal axis.

e. If clinical manifestations of adrenocortical insufficiency develop in a patient with a normal plasma cortisol level, repeat the cortisol level determination and give stress replacement. If the cortisol level is low, a complete reevaluation of the hypothalamic-pituitary-adrenal axis is necessary.

f. Supplemental corticosteroid dosage for stress
  (1) For **minor stress** (gastroenteritis, influenza, otitis media, streptococcal pharyngitis, or minor surgical procedures, including endoscopy and dental work), give 100 mg of hydrocortisone/day for 2 days during the stress period.
  (2) For **major stress** (major trauma or surgery), give 100 mg of **parenteral** hydrocortisone every 6–8 hours for the first 3–4 days until the stress is resolved. Taper the dose gradually.

VII. Expectorants. See Chap. 6.

Immunotherapy

Immunotherapy (hyposensitization) is a method employing subcutaneous injections of gradually increasing doses of antigenic (allergenic) materials for the purpose of altering the immunologic response of atopic patients. Since its initial introduction by Noon in 1911, multiple, controlled clinical investigations of the response to extract therapy have been done. These studies reflect a wide difference in the dosage of antigen and the response expressed by subjective self-evaluation and specific laboratory measurements. Many show that immunotherapy, especially with large doses of antigen, benefits patients with seasonal allergic rhinitis. Improvement of seasonal allergic rhinitis is better established than are claims of similar benefits in asthma. The efficacy of immunotherapy for eczema, food allergy, or urticaria is not established.

The efficacy of immunotherapy may result from a variety of immunologic modifications, including the production of IgG-blocking antibody, lowering of specific IgE antibodies, decrease in sensitivity of the basophil and the mast cell to antigen-induced histamine release, and modulation of T-cell response (decrease in lymphocyte transformation and release of macrophage inhibition factor and mitogenic factor and an increase of T-suppressor cells). Currently, the effect of these changes on clinical improvement is speculative.

I. Allergenic extracts for treatment
  A. Aqueous extracts are prepared from a variety of sources including pollens, epidermals, molds, and insect venom. The material to be extracted is usually first defatted with an organic solvent such as ether, suspended at 4°C in a measured volume of physiologic saline, and allowed to mix for 24 hours or more. This mixture is then sterilized by micropore filtration. Although physicians in the past have produced their own extracts, most practitioners now purchase concentrated stock extracts (e.g., 1:10 or 1:20 dilutions) from commercial suppliers (see Appendix XIV) and make sterile dilutions in the office. Aqueous extracts are available in four forms: phenol-preserved, glycerine-preserved, lyophilyzed, and phenol-preserved using human serum albumin as a stabilizer.
    1. Phenol-preserved extracts are commonly used for therapy. Phenol (0.2–0.5%) inhibits microbial growth. However, with phenol preservatives, ex-

*Cortrosyn, Organon Pharmaceuticals, West Orange, NJ 07052

tracts lose potency more rapidly than with glycerinated extracts, especially with increasing storage temperatures and weaker dilutions. Studies of phenolized extracts of concentrated ragweed pollen measuring the ragweed-specific antigen-E potency indicate that at 35°C, 100% of potency is lost in 30 days and 50% in 5 days. At 24°C, 50% of potency is lost in 40 days, and at 4°C, 50% is lost in 5 months. Knowledge of temperature dependency is important because physicians commonly store skin test and therapeutic extracts at room temperature (24°C) for many hours each day. **Refrigerate extracts whenever possible at 2–8°C.**
Dilution of antigenic solutions also increases the rapidity of loss of potency. Although the exact time after which potency is lost is not known, dilute preparations (> 1:1000) for testing or therapy should be changed at least every 2 months.

2. **Glycerinated extracts** (preserved with 50% glycerin with or without phenol) are superior to phenolized extracts in retention of allergen potency. They are used for epicutaneous (scratch or prick) skin testing and, if diluted to less than 5% of glycerin, can be used for intradermal tests. They can be used for immunotherapy, but high concentrations of glycerin can increase the incidence of local reactions and discomfort.

3. **Lyophilyzed extracts** are produced by a freeze-drying process that results in a stable antigenic material that retains potency when reconstituted after 2 years' storage at room temperature. After reconstitution, its potency assumes the characteristics of the diluent used for reconstitution. Because of the increased cost, lyophilized extracts are often used in low-volume practices and research settings as a means of conserving refrigeration space.

4. A solution of **0.03% normal human serum albumin** (0.9% sodium chloride and 0.4% phenol) can be used as a diluent for extracts (see Chap. 11 for use with venom extracts). Human serum albumin serves as an excellent stabilizer for allergen extracts.

B. **Alum-precipitated** preparations are aqueous extracts absorbed on an aluminum hydroxide carrier to slow the release of antigen. This slow release may afford a prolongation of the antigenic stimulus. These agents are strictly for immunotherapy and not for diagnostic testing. Doses are given less frequently than are doses of aqueous extracts for ragweed pollinosis.
Alum-precipitated extracts (Center-Al*) of grasses, trees, and weeds are commercially available. Efficacy studies for these nonragweed extracts are incomplete. Their disadvantages include the following:

1. Increased incidence of local reactions and nodule formation (compared with aqueous extracts).

2. The possibility of protracted systemic reactions because of slow allergen release.

3. Inaccurate allergen dosing with poorly mixed suspensions.

C. **Alum-precipitated, pyridine-extracted** pollen extracts (Allpyral†) use a weak tertiary base, pyridine, to extract undefatted pollen prior to alum precipitation. In studies with ragweed antigen, the pyridine extraction process appears to alter or destroy the allergenicity of the material, producing lower levels of blocking antibody and less clinical benefit but fewer local or systemic reactions.

D. **New extract forms** for immunotherapy, not commercially available at present, may reduce allergic reactions to the extracts while retaining their full potency for immunogenicity. These products include allergoid, polymerized antigen, and photoinactivated antigen.

1. **Allergoid** is produced by formalin treatment of pollen extracts. When combined with lysine as an adjuvant, it produces higher blocking antibody titers than do whole pollen extracts by allowing a greater quantity of protein to be tolerated without local reactions. Clinical improvement with allergoid is equivalent to that with whole pollen extract.

*Center Laboratories, Port Washington, NY 11050
†Hollister Stier, Box 3145, Spokane, WA 99200

2. **Polymerization** of antigen E or whole pollen extracts of ragweed and grass with gluteraldehyde produces a favorable clinical response with fewer injections required than with aqueous extracts.
3. **Photoinactivation** with ultraviolet light allows larger doses of antigen with fewer adverse effects. Clinical results with grass extracts are poor; with house dust extracts the results are improved.

II. **Standardization of allergenic extracts.** Standardization is critical for accurate diagnosis and effective therapy. Sensitive research methods can quantitate potency but are limited by the need for subjects sensitive to many different extracts (for in vivo dose-response skin testing or in vitro leukocyte histamine release) and by the need for pure allergens and monospecific precipitating serum (gel diffusion). The radioallergosorbent test (RAST), introduced as a diagnostic procedure (see Chap. 2 and Appendix V), can be adapted (RAST inhibition method) to measure potency, with the results correlating with other measures of evaluation (e.g., skin testing). A limited number of RAST standardized commercial extracts are now available. Other investigational techniques currently employed to measure physiochemical and biologic properties of extracts include isoelectric focusing, cross-immunoelectrophoresis, and cross-radioimmunoelectrophoresis.

The current commercial methods for measuring extract potency are the ratio of weight to volume and protein nitrogen units. These methods are practical for clinical purposes, but they do not measure true biologic potency accurately. The Food and Drug Administration (FDA) has developed the AU (allergy unit) system of allergen standardization based on biologic activity. Likewise, the Allergen Standardization Subcommittee of the International Union of Immunologic Societies has developed extracts of selected antigens standardized in international units (IU) and presented to the World Health Organization. Both of these systems will help improve immunotherapy treatment.

A. The **weight-to-volume ratio** represents a concentration of allergenic extracts obtained by extracting a given weight of pollen or other allergenic material in a particular volume of extracting fluid. For example, a 1:50 extract is prepared by extracting 1 gm of material in 50 ml of extracting fluid.

B. **Protein nitrogen units** express potency by measuring protein precipitated by phosphotungstic acid. The correlation of this measurement with actual biologic potency is variable.

C. Other units of potency, now primarily of historic interest, are pollen units, Freeman-Noon units, total nitrogen units, and total nitrogen. The approximate equivalents of these standards to 1 ml of a 1:50 dilution by weight-to-volume ratio (1 gm allergen in 50 ml of diluent) are as follows:

10,000   Protein nitrogen units (PNU): 1 PNU = 0.01 μg protein nitrogen
20,000   Freeman-Noon units
20,000   Pollen units
    0.26   Total nitrogen
26,000   Total nitrogen units

III. **Preparation of therapeutic extracts**

A. **Dilutions.** Commercial suppliers provide sterile aqueous, glycerinated, or alum-precipitated extracts in a variety of concentrations. These extracts can be either a single allergen or mixtures of individual allergens. For treatment purposes it is more economical to purchase 1:20 or 1:10 extracts in bulk (30- or 50-ml vials) and make appropriate dilutions from these concentrations. Dilutions are made either on the basis of the weight-to-volume ratio or protein nitrogen units (see Table 4-14 for dilution calculation).

B. The **choice of antigens for treatment** is based on the patient's clinical symptoms, geographic locale, and pertinent exposures, with confirmation of sensitivity by appropriately performed skin or provocative tests. Do **not** treat for positive skin tests that do not correlate with a careful history. (However, perform skin tests with **individual antigens** if negative skin tests occur with "mixed extracts," e.g., mixed trees and mixed grasses, especially in a patient with a suggestive history.)

Table 4-14. Allergen dilution calculation

Weight-to-Volume Ratio Method
The concentration of a given allergen is expressed as a ratio or a percentage of weight of allergen to volume of extracting fluid. For example:

> 10% concentration = 1:10 dilution
> 5% concentration = 1:20 dilution
> 2.5% concentration = 1:40 dilution
> 1% concentration = 1:100 dilution

Calculate dilutions by using the formula

$$V_1C_1 = V_2C_2$$

where V_1 = volume desired (known), C_1 = concentration desired (known), V_2 = volume needed (unknown), and C_2 = concentration available (known).

EXAMPLE: Prepare 5.0 ml of 1:100 ragweed from 1:10 ragweed.

Calculate volume of 1:10 ragweed.

> V_1 = 5.0 ml
> C_1 = 1:100
> V_2 = x
> C_2 = 1:10
> (5) (1/100) = (x) (1/10)
> x = 0.5 ml

Calculate volume of diluent required.

> V_1 − x = volume
> 5.0 − 0.5 = 4.5 ml of diluent

Therefore, 0.5 ml of 1:10 ragweed diluted with 4.5 ml of diluent yields 5.0 ml of 1:100 ragweed allergen.

Protein Nitrogen Unit Method
The concentration is expressed as protein nitrogen units per milliliter (PNU/ml), whereby 100,000 PNUs are equal to 1.0 mg of phosphotungstic acid–precipitable nitrogen.

Calculate dilutions by using the formula

$$V_1C_1 = V_2C_2 \text{ (as with weight to volume calculation)}$$

EXAMPLE: Prepare 10 ml of 10,000 PNU/ml ragweed from 20,000 PNU/ml ragweed.

Calculate volume of 20,000 PNU/ml ragweed extract required.

> (10) (10,000) = (x) (20,000)
> x = 5.0 ml

Calculate volume of diluent required.

> V_1 − x = volume
> 10.0 ml − 5.0 ml = 5.0 ml

Therefore, dilute 5.0 ml of 20,000 PNU/ml ragweed with 5.0 ml of diluent to obtain 10.0 ml of 10,000 PNU/ml ragweed.

    C. Other practical points include the following:
        1. Limit the number of antigens in an individual's extract mixture (usually to three or four antigens).
        2. Give separately antigens to which the patient is exquisitely sensitive (such an antigen can cause severe local reactions and reduce the total amount of material given).
        3. Do not mix antigens from different stock extracts in the same syringe because cross-contamination of these extracts can occur.

Immunotherapy: Practical Aspects

I. **Indications**
  A. **Pollen-induced** (grasses, trees, and weeds) **allergic rhinitis** responds well to immunotherapy (80–90% improvement).
  B. **Allergic rhinitis** caused by molds responds to immunotherapy, although the response is less successful than with pollen extracts.
  C. **Animal dander (epidermal) sensitivity** may respond to immunotherapy, but it is not recommended that it be used routinely to replace removal of the offending allergen. Special situations, such as unavoidable occupational exposure (e.g., veterinarians or laboratory workers), may warrant a trial of immunotherapy. The recent availability of standardized allergenic extracts of cat hair and dander (Aquagen SQ Allergenic Extracts, ALK America, Inc., 121 Whitney Avenue, New Haven, CT 06510) allows the use of a high-potency standardized cat extract (50,000 Allergy Units [AU]/μl) in those patients where cat exposure is unavoidable. Follow package inserts carefully on use of this potent extract.
  D. **Other environmental allergens** (e.g., kapok, jute, feathers) are of questionable value in immunotherapy and generally should not be used.
  E. **Bacterial vaccine.** Stock bacterial vaccines or autogenous bacterial vaccines (not FDA-approved) have been used in patients who wheeze with infections, but the majority of controlled studies using currently available vaccines have not shown an improved response compared with that obtained with a placebo. Such vaccines are generally not used in an immunotherapy regimen.
  F. **Allergen-induced asthma** is an indication for immunotherapy along the guidelines for allergic rhinitis when there is a poor response to environmental control or symptomatic treatment.
  G. **Urticaria, angioedema, and atopic dermatitis** are generally not indications for immunotherapy.
  H. **Hymenoptera sensitivity** (see Chap. 11).
II. **Treatment schedules**
  A. **Dosage increases.** The starting dose of an allergenic extract and the progression of the dose must be individualized for each patient. Based on the history and skin test findings, the average patient can begin with doses of approximately 1:100,000 dilution (weight to volume). Start **highly sensitive patients** with marked skin test reactivity (skin tests become rapidly positive within 3–5 minutes) at higher initial dilutions (1:1 million or 1:10 million). Dosage increases for aqueous extracts or alum-precipitated extracts are outlined in Tables 4-15 and 4-16.
  Interruption in the dosage schedule necessitates modification. If 3–6 weeks have elapsed since the last dose, repeat the same dose. For longer intervals, reduce the dose by working back on the schedule one step for each week beyond 4 weeks.
  B. **Maintenance dosage.** Large cumulative doses of antigen improve the therapeutic results. The maximal tolerated dose is dependent on the individual patient's tolerance, which is not always predictable from skin tests or a history of clinical sensitivity. **Most** patients, both children and adults, can tolerate **maintenance doses** of 0.50 ml of a 1:100 mixed aqueous extract or 5000 PNU of an alum-precipitated extract. However, certain patients can tolerate higher maintenance doses (0.5–1.0 ml of a 1:50 mixed aqueous extract or 8000 units of an alum-precipitated extract).
III. **Timing of immunotherapy**
  A. Levels of specific IgE increase during a particular pollen season. Many patients are more sensitive to immunotherapy injections at these times and cannot tolerate their regular maintenance doses. It may be necessary to reduce maintenance doses during these periods of increased allergen exposure. Similarly, in very sensitive patients receiving progressive dosage increases, hold the dosage constant during these periods.

Table 4-15. Suggested schedule of dosage increases
for immunotherapy with aqueous extracts

Extract concentration	Dosage[a] (ml)
Sensitive Patient	
1:1,000,000	0.05, 0.10, 0.20, 0.30, 0.40, 0.50, 0.60
1:100,000	0.05, 0.10, 0.20, 0.30, 0.40, 0.50, 0.60
1:10,000	0.05, 0.10, 0.20, 0.30, 0.40, 0.50, 0.60
1:1000	0.05, 0.10, 0.20, 0.30, 0.40, 0.50, 0.60
1:100	0.05, 0.10, 0.15, 0.20, 0.25, 0.30, 0.35, 0.40, 0.45, 0.50, 0.55, 0.60
1:50[b]	0.05, 0.10, 0.15, 0.20, 0.25, 0.30, 0.35, 0.40, 0.45, 0.50 (maintenance dose)
Average Patient	
1:100,000	0.05, 0.10, 0.20, 0.30, 0.40, 0.50, 0.60
1:10,000	0.05, 0.10, 0.20, 0.30, 0.40, 0.50, 0.60
1:1000	0.05, 0.10, 0.20, 0.30, 0.40, 0.50, 0.60
1:100	0.05, 0.10, 0.15, 0.20, 0.25, 0.30, 0.35, 0.40, 0.45, 0.50, 0.55, 0.60
1:50[b]	0.05, 0.10, 0.15, 0.20, 0.25, 0.30, 0.35, 0.40, 0.45, 0.50 (maintenance dose)

[a] Doses are given every 4–7 days until the maintenance dose is achieved. Frequency is then advanced by separating injections at weekly intervals every 3–4 months until a 4- to 6-wk interval is achieved. This frequency is maintained (individualization of dosage and frequency is necessary depending on each patient's sensitivity and response). If local (significant) or systemic reactions occur, modify the schedule to reflect this increased sensitivity of the patient, e.g., 0.05-ml increments instead of 0.10-ml increments.
[b] Higher concentrations (e.g., 1:33, 1:20, or 1:10) can be administered if tolerated by the patient. Use the same schedule of dosage increases as for 1:50.

Table 4-16. Suggested schedule of dosage increases
for immunotherapy with alum-precipitated extracts

Give every 4–7 days using the following suggested schedule:
  5 PNU, 10, 20, 40, 80, 150, 250, 400, 650, 800, 1000, 1500, 2000, 2500, 3000, 3500, 4000, 4500, 5000, 5500, 6000, 6500, 7000, 7500, 8000 (maintenance dose range 6000–8000 PNU)*

*The frequency of the maintenance dose is advanced as for aqueous extracts (see Table 4-15) and may be maintained at intervals of 4–8 wk (considering individual patient variation).

    B. Injections should not be given to a patient with a fever, or to asthmatic patients with upper respiratory infections, or if obvious wheezing is noted.
    C. The patient should avoid strenuous exercise immediately after an injection to avoid increased speed of absorption of antigen from the injection site.
    D. Pregnancy does not contraindicate the use of allergenic extracts (there are no reported associated teratogenic properties or other adverse effects). However, based on the premise that all medications should be used sparingly during pregnancy, immunotherapy should be used only if the severity of the symptoms warrants such treatment. If used, avoid systemic reactions by beginning at a lower dose of antigen than usual and progressing more slowly than usual as suggested for sensitive patients (see Table 4-15).
  IV. Technique of injection. Proper precautions and proper injection techniques reduce the frequency and degree of local and systemic reactions to immunotherapy.

A. A physician should be **immediately** available when allergy injections are given. (The administration of extracts **outside** the physician's office is discussed in a position statement by the American Academy of Allergy and Immunology, *J. Allergy Clin. Immunol.* 77:271, 1986.)

B. Inquire about any local or systemic reaction following the previous injection. If a reaction has occurred, follow the guidelines in **V.**

C. Preferably, use disposable 26- or 27-gauge needles and disposable plastic 1-ml tuberculin-type syringes (0.01-ml gradation).

D. Carefully select the correct antigen vial and draw the proper dose.

E. The usual injection site is the outer aspect of the upper arm, midway between shoulder and elbow in the groove between the deltoid and the triceps muscles.

F. Administer the dose **subcutaneously** after aspiration of the plunger of the syringe. Do not inject if blood is withdrawn (anaphylaxis is more common with intravenous injections).

G. Avoid rubbing the injected area to prevent rapid absorption, which can increase the chance of systemic reactions.

H. Keep the patient under observation for 20–30 minutes; check the injected area for local reaction, and, if present, record it in the patient's chart.

V. **Reactions to injections.** Most **severe** reactions to injections occur within 1 hour, the majority within the first 20 minutes. However, significant local and systemic reactions can occur up to 24 hours after an injection. These reactions must be recognized to avoid the **increased risk** of systemic reactions from subsequent doses.

A. **Significant local reactions** present with immediate redness and swelling, a wheal larger than 2 cm in diameter, or a wheal that lasts longer than 24 hours.

1. Treat symptomatically with an **oral antihistamine** and **local cold packs.** Prophylactic treatment with antihistamine and epinephrine is not recommended—this combination can mask a local reaction and allow a large local or systemic reaction at a higher dose. (Do not discontinue antihistamines given for symptomatic control of the patient's allergic symptoms.)

2. Following a large local reaction, **reduce** the amount of the allergenic extract to the previous dose that did not cause a reaction, and then repeat the same schedule of increasing dosage.

3. **Review** injection technique; poor technique and intradermal or intramuscular injection can cause large local reactions.

B. **Systemic reactions** include generalized erythema, urticaria, pruritus, angioedema, bronchospasm, laryngeal edema, shock, and cardiac arrest. Although severe systemic reactions are rare, they can be fatal, and a physician must be immediately available to give emergency treatment.

1. Administer **immediately** aqueous epinephrine, 1:1000 (0.01 ml/kg; maximum, 0.30 ml), subcutaneously or intramuscularly. Repeat the dose at 15-minute intervals as needed.

2. Administer **aqueous epinephrine,** 1:1000 (0.01 ml/kg or 0.2 ml) at the injection site to delay absorption of the antigen. If two immunotherapy injections were given, divide the epinephrine dose and give one-half at each injection site.

3. Place a **tourniquet** above the injection site and release every 15 minutes.

4. Give **diphenhydramine hydrochloride** (Benadryl) intravenously over 5–10 minutes or intramuscularly (1.25 mg/kg).

5. **Intravenous hydrocortisone** (5 mg/kg) should be given for severe systemic reactions. It may be helpful in preventing delayed anaphylaxis.

6. For further treatment—or if hypotension, laryngeal edema, or respiratory difficulty occurs—follow the regimen outlined in Chap. 10.

7. Review the administration of the antigen for a wrong dose or an error in the selection of antigen vials. If no error is found, review the dosage schedule (looking for evidence of previous large local reactions), and reduce the dose to 10% of that which elicited the systemic reaction. (For example, if the dose that elicited the reaction was 0.5 ml of a 1:100 solution, reduce to 0.05 ml of a 1:100 solution or 0.5 ml of a 1:1000 solution.) Then, the usual progression

in the dosage schedule can be resumed. However, it is wise to increase the dosage at a slower rate when the dose that elicited the systemic reaction is again approached. It is often advisable not to exceed the dose that produced this reaction.

    8. Patients receiving beta-adrenergic antagonists may be at increased risk to severe anaphylactic reactions resistant to epinephrine administration. The decision to initiate immunotherapy in these patients must be carefully evaluated. Likewise, patients with cardiovascular disease and sensitivity to epinephrine also deserve special consideration.

C. Alum-precipitated extracts infrequently produce protracted (3–4 days) systemic reactions (urticaria and bronchospasm) because of the delayed release unique to these preparations. In addition to antihistamine and epinephrine, give intravenous hydrocortisone (5 mg/kg) initially for severe reactions, or treat with oral prednisone (2 mg/kg/day, up to 80 mg with tapering over 5–7 days) to prevent delayed or recurring symptoms.

VI. Length of therapy. Maximal clinical benefit usually occurs within 12–24 months after reaching adequate maintenance doses. Continuation of treatment depends on the response of the patient. The average patient receives 3–5 years of therapy. **Do not continue treatment after 2 years if no clinical benefit is apparent.**

At present, there are no clinical or laboratory measurements that can accurately predict the probability of clinical relapse after discontinuing immunotherapy. A practical approach is to continue injections every 4–6 weeks for 1–2 symptom-free years and then discontinue. A relapse may occur within 6–12 months. The relapse can be partial and can sometimes be managed with environmental controls and occasional medication. If symptoms persist and the pattern of reactivity is the same, immunotherapy is resumed (at a reduced dose, e.g., 1:100,000) without retesting.

VII. Failure of immunotherapy. A therapeutic failure occurs when a patient does not experience a noticeable decrease of symptoms within a period of 12–24 months, an increase in tolerance to known allergens, and a reduction in the use of medication. Explanations for therapeutic failure include the following:

    A. Inadequate environmental controls.

    B. Failure to recognize and include a significant allergen for immunotherapy.

    C. Inadequate doses of allergen (high doses of antigen give better clinical results).

    D. Development of new allergies.

    E. Misdiagnosis of allergies (e.g., confusing vasomotor rhinitis or intrinsic asthma with their atopic counterparts).

    F. Unrealistic patient expectations, causing premature judgment of failure.

    G. Failure of the treatment method itself.

Selected Readings

Bernstein, I. L. Cromolyn sodium. *Chest* 87 (Suppl.):685, 1985.

Consumer Reports, Buying Guide Issue, 1987. Mount Vernon, NY: Consumers Union of United States, 1987. Vol. 51.

Drug Evaluations (6th ed.). Chicago: American Medical Association, 1986.

Fischer, T. J. Air Environmental Control. In E. B. Weiss, M. S. Segal, and M. Stein (eds.), *Bronchial Asthma* (2nd ed.). Boston: Little, Brown, 1985.

Grant, J. A., and Ellis, E. F. (eds.). Update on theophylline (Part 2). *J. Allergy Clin. Immunol.* 78:669, 1986.

Middleton, E., Jr., Reed, C., and Ellis, E. (eds.). *Allergy: Principles and Practice.* St. Louis: Mosby, 1983.

Nelson, H. S. Adrenergic therapy of bronchial asthma. *J. Allergy Clin. Immunol.* 77:771, 1986.

Sheffer, A. L., and Rachelefsky, G. S. (eds.). Asthma '84: Pharmacologic update (Part 2). *J. Allergy Clin. Immunol.* 76:249, 1985.

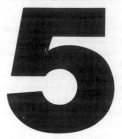

Allergy of the Upper Respiratory Tract and Eyes

Joseph E. Ghory

Allergic rhinitis, a symptom complex resulting from exposure to a specific antigen, can be seasonal or perennial, depending on the presence of the offending allergen. It may simulate a variety of chronic or recurrent nasal conditions and can result in such complications as sinusitis, recurrent ear infections, or nasal polyps.

The important antigens in allergic rhinitis are usually airborne substances to which the atopic patient becomes sensitized. High concentrations of windborne aeroallergens produce the symptoms of seasonal allergic rhinitis. In contrast, the heavier pollens from insect-pollinated plants are not as significant a cause of allergic rhinitis. Thus, allergy to flowers is rare—"rose fever" is not caused by blooming roses but by concurrently pollinating grasses. Similarly, the nasal symptoms of the ragweed-sensitive person have mistakenly been attributed to the "haying season" of late August and September.

A positive **family history** of allergy is obtained in the majority of cases. Among children with bilateral family histories of hay fever or asthma, one of these conditions will develop in 70%; among those with unilateral family histories, in 50%. The mode of inheritance in this atopic tendency has not been established, although the autosomal dominant immune-response genes, which control the antigenic response to certain antigens, appear to be linked to a major histocompatibility locus.

The onset of **upper respiratory allergy** appears to be highest in the primary-school age group, but nasal allergy develops in a large percentage of children before 5 years of age. Males predominate before age 10; females, from age 10–20 years. Three or more years of exposure to a specific pollen is usually required to produce tissue sensitization and symptoms. Seasonal pollen allergy therefore rarely appears before the third year of life. Similarly, it usually requires **3 years** for an adult moving to a new locale to become adversely affected by new pollen exposure.

Seasonal Allergic Rhinitis

I. **Pathophysiologic features.** Sensitization of atopic persons follows ingestion or inhalation of antigen. On reexposure to antigen, the nasal mucosa reacts by slowing of ciliary action, edema formation, and leukocyte infiltration, primarily of eosinophils. Continuous exposure leads to further changes, including destruction of the basement membrane and foamy cell formation. Soluble antigens are eluted from the pollen by nasal secretions and pass through the mucosa to react with IgE fixed to mast cells. Mast cell degranulation and chemical-mediator release subsequently occur.

Histamine is the major mediator of allergic reactions in the nasal mucosa. It produces tissue edema by inducing vasodilation and increasing capillary permeability. Other mediators of potential significance include leukotrienes, bradykinin, the prostaglandins, and eosinophil chemotactic factors of anaphylaxis (ECF-A).

II. **Clinical findings**
   A. **Typical symptoms** of seasonal allergic rhinitis include nasal congestion, a clear, watery discharge, paroxysmal sneezing, and nasal itching, often following a known allergen exposure. Some patients complain of itching of the throat or soft palate. Drainage of nasal mucus into the pharynx results in frequent attempts

to clear the throat, a dry cough, or hoarseness. Headache, pain over the paranasal sinuses, and recurrent epistaxis can accompany allergic rhinitis.

B. On **physical examination** the classic picture of the allergic nose is seen: enlarged, moist, pale or blue-gray turbinates and a glistening, clear, serous or watery discharge. Mucosal edema can produce a more or less prominent swelling at the floor of the nostril below the turbinates. Other common findings include the following:

1. **Allergic shiners** are dark discolorations in the orbital-palpebral grooves beneath the lower eyelids. They probably are secondary to venous stasis caused by mucosal edema of the nose and sinuses.

2. **Allergic salute,** common in children, involves using the palm of the hand in an upward thrust of the nares, thereby relieving itching and opening the nasal airway.

3. **Allergic,** or **adenoidal, facies** consists of mouth breathing, a gaping expression, allergic shiners, and often dental malocclusion.

4. The **allergic crease** is a transverse nasal skin crease or, in late stages, a hypopigmented groove at the junction of the tip of the nose and the more rigid nasal bridge. This crease, usually a pathognomonic sign developing after 2 years of constant rubbing, must be differentiated from the rarer familial transverse nasal groove. This groove, inherited as a mendelian dominant, is unrelated to allergy and, unlike the acquired crease, is not obliterated by downward pressure on the tip of the nose.

5. **Dennie's line,** a wrinkle just beneath the lower lids, is present from early infancy and is associated with atopic dermatitis and allergic rhinitis.

6. **Abnormalities of the oral cavity,** which include overriding maxillary incisors, underdevelopment of the mandible, high-arched palate, hypertrophic lymphoid follicles on the posterior pharyngeal wall, and postnasal drip.

7. A **geographic tongue,** characterized by sharply outlined bald patches on its surface, may be seen in an allergic person.

III. Diagnosis. Most cases of seasonal allergic rhinitis are easily diagnosed by history and physical examination. Should confusion exist, especially in differentiating vasomotor rhinitis, infectious rhinitis, or eosinophilic nonallergic rhinitis (ENR) (see Table 5-1) the following studies are useful:

A. Nasal smear. A specimen of nasal secretion suitable for examination is best obtained by blowing the nose directly onto wax paper or cellophane. Alternatively, a cotton-tipped applicator can be used to swab the nasal mucosa gently (leave the applicator in the nose for 2–3 minutes for best results); or the secretion can be aspirated with a small rubber bulb syringe. Instead of relying on expelled mucus, a disposable plastic scoop (Rhino-probe*) can be used to obtain an epithelial specimen from the mucosal surface of the inferior turbinate (see Appendix II). The specimen is transferred to a glass slide, the dried smear is stained with Wright's or Hansel's stain, and the types of cells are counted. The presence of clumps of eosinophils or eosinophils constituting more than **10%** of the total white cells counted indicates a probable allergic cause. During the height of the pollen seasons, the smear can show 80–90% eosinophils. A predominance of neutrophils suggests infectious rhinitis (see Appendix II).

B. Peripheral blood count. A moderate eosinophilia (> 10%) can be present, especially during the offending pollen season. Absolute total eosinophil counts (see Appendix III) can exceed 700 cells/cu mm. Although blood eosinophilia is suggestive of allergy, marked allergic symptoms can occur in its absence.

C. Total serum IgE. A measurement of total serum IgE by radioimmunosorbent methods (e.g., paper radioimmunosorbent test [PRIST]—see Appendix IV) or enzyme methods (enzyme-linked immunosorbent assay [ELISA]) can help differentiate allergic from nonallergic rhinitis in questionable cases. When measured by the PRIST, approximately 60% of adults with asthma, or hay fever, or both have IgE values 2 S.D. above healthy adult control values. Parasitic and other causes of IgE elevations must be excluded, and the IgE values obtained

*Rhino-probe Rhino Technics, Inc., P.O. Box 84058, San Diego, CA 92138.

Table 5-1. Differential diagnosis of common forms of rhinitis

Feature	Seasonal allergic rhinitis	Perennial allergic rhinitis	Vasomotor rhinitis	Nonallergic rhinitis with eosinophilia (NARES)	Infectious rhinitis
Personal history of allergy	+	+	−	±	−
Family history of allergy	+	+	−	±	−
Occurrence	Seasonal	Perennial	Perennial	Perennial	Sporadic
Fever	−	−	−	−	+
Nasal mucosa	Pale, boggy, obstructed	Variable	Pink, obstructed	Pale, boggy, obstructed	Red, obstructed
Nasal discharge	Watery, profuse	Mucoid	Minimal to mucoid	Watery, profuse	Yellow or greenish, purulent
Allergic salute	+	+	−	±	−
Ocular symptoms	+	±	−	−	−
Cause	Inhalants	Inhalants	Irritants	?	Viruses, bacteria
Nasal smear	↑ Eosinophils	↑ Eosinophils	Normal	↑↑ Eosinophils	↑ Neutrophils
Skin tests and RAST	+	+	−	−	−
Air conditioning and air cleaners	↓ Symptoms	↓ Symptoms	−	−	−
Therapeutic response					
Antihistamines	Good	Fair	Limited	Fair	Limited
Decongestants	Limited	Limited	Fair	Limited	Limited
Cromolyn sodium	Good	Good	Limited	Limited	None
Corticosteroids	Excellent	Excellent	Limited	Excellent	None
Immunotherapy	Good	Fair	None	None	None

Key: RAST = radioallergosorbent test; + = positive; − = negative; ± = questionable.

should be compared with those of normal age-matched values for each laboratory.

D. Determination of offending allergens

1. **Epidermal testing** (scratch testing, prick testing) remains the most useful method of establishing specific causative allergens (see Chap. 2). Epidermal skin testing is less helpful before 3 years of age, because skin reactivity is reduced in the very young child. In these young patients, intradermal tests of household inhalants or epidermal allergens may yield positive reactions.

2. **Intradermal tests.** In the older child or adult, scratch or prick tests are the initial procedures because of their safety, the speed with which a large number of tests are performed, and their increased specificity. Important or suspicious allergens that have elicited negative or 1+ reactions with scratch or prick tests should be verified by intradermal testing. (Exception: Intradermal food testing often gives false-positive results and has been associated with fatalities due to systemic anaphylaxis).

3. **Radioallergosorbent test (RAST).** Methods of measuring specific IgE antibodies (e.g., RAST, fluoroallergosorbent test [FAST], multiple allergosorbent test system [MAST]) against a large number of allergens are available (see Chap. 2 and Appendix V). The correlation of the findings with those of prick testing for pollens is approximately 80%. The chief advantages of these methods are the lack of risk to the patient, lack of dependence on skin reactivity, and stability of antigens in the solid phase state. The present drawbacks include more limited allergen selection, reduced sensitivity as compared with that of intradermal skin tests, lack of immediately available results, and increased expense. They can be helpful in patients with severe atopic dermatitis, poor skin reactivity, or enhanced skin reactivity (dermatographia), or in patients on antihistamines.

4. **Food elimination and challenge.** Because foods rarely cause rhinitis, they are not routinely tested. If the history suggests food allergy, prick skin tests or the RAST can help support food allergy as the cause. However, only by appropriate food elimination and a subsequent challenge that results in the production of clinical symptoms can one diagnose food allergy (see Chap. 13).

5. **Nasal provocation tests** consist of observing the patient for signs and symptoms of allergic rhinitis following the direct application of a specific allergen to the nasal mucosa. Provocative testing is occasionally helpful when allergy skin test results do not correlate with the history.

   a. The following **guidelines** are suggested for such testing:

      (1) As with all in vivo allergy tests, observe the patient carefully for signs of a systemic reaction.

      (2) Make sure that the patient is relatively free of symptoms and has not been taking antihistamines for at least 48 hours.

      (3) Spray the allergen solution (1:1000 dilution) or drop a small amount of powdered antigen on the mucosa.

      (4) Spray the diluent control into the other nostril.

   b. Nasal itching, discharge, sneezing, and pale and boggy mucosa indicate a positive result; more sophisticated equipment is available for measuring such reactions (e.g., measurement of nasal airflow resistance, rhinomanometry). Because of its expense and technical difficulty, this equipment is usually used only in a research setting.

   c. The **limitations** of nasal provocation tests are as follows:

      (1) They are time-consuming. Only one antigen can be tested at a time.

      (2) They are not useful if nasal symptoms are present.

      (3) Systemic reactions can be provoked.

IV. Treatment

A. Avoidance of allergens. Simple avoidance measures must be emphasized and environmental control measures undertaken (see Chap. 4).

1. **Air conditioning** is especially helpful to the pollen-sensitive patient because the bedroom windows can be kept closed during the summer months.

In the winter, excessive dryness may aggravate nasal stuffiness. A room or central **humidifier** will keep the humidity at an optimal level of 40%. **Electronic filters** (room or central units) remove over 90% of airborne particles passing through the unit. Air conditioners, humidifiers, and electronic filters are tax-deductible medical expenses.

2. When high allergen exposure is unavoidable, a mask may be worn over the nose and mouth to prevent inhalation of allergens. Masks reduce the intake of house dust, mold spores, animal dander, aerosol sprays, fabric fibers, and air pollution.

B. Medications

1. **Antihistamines** constitute the major class of drugs currently used for effective symptomatic control of allergic rhinitis (see Tables 4-4 and 4-5 for dosages and formulations).

   a. **Administration.** For best results with antihistamines, give before exposure to known allergens. During symptomatic periods, regular, around-the-clock administration, rather than intermittent use, should be employed.

   b. **Limitations.** There are two major limitations to antihistamine use for allergic rhinitis.

      (1) **Complete control** is not achieved in many patients because of possible inadequate tissue levels of drug at cell receptor sites, the action of other mediators not blocked by antihistamines, or other unknown factors.

      (2) **Side effects.** Somnolence is a major complaint in many patients. Other side effects include excitation, nervousness, insomnia, dizziness, tinnitus, incoordination, blurred vision, and dysphagia. Dryness of the mouth, inhibition of micturation, palpitations, and headaches can occur. Gastrointestinal side effects such as anorexia, nausea, vomiting, constipation, and diarrhea may be minimized by administration of the drug with meals. Mild drowsiness and other side effects may subside after a few days of continual antihistamine therapy. Newer antihistamines that do not cross the blood-brain barrier, such as terfenadine (Seldane) or astemizole (astemizole is not currently FDA-approved), have less sedating effects.

   c. With **prolonged treatment,** a loss of therapeutic effectiveness may occur. This effectiveness may be restored by substituting another class of antihistamine. The lack of response to an antihistamine may also result from the severity of the disease or a secondary complication, such as infection.

   d. Patients vary widely in their therapeutic response and susceptibility to antihistamine side effects. If clinically significant side effects occur, patients should reduce the dosage. In the absence of side effects and the desired clinical response, a gradual increase in dosage to double that usually recommended may afford symptomatic control.

   e. It is safe to prescribe antihistamines for allergic rhinitis in asthmatic patients. However, their use during **acute attacks** may accentuate inspissation of bronchial secretions and should be avoided.

2. **Adrenergic drugs** with primarily alpha-receptor activity are effective vasoconstrictors of mucosal vessels and are used topically (see Table 4-6) as well as orally.

   a. **Topical therapy** can be effective and can elicit fewer side effects compared with oral administration (tachycardia, insomnia, nervousness, irritability, increase in blood pressure, headache, nausea, vomiting, epigastric pain). However, topical vasoconstrictors (drops or sprays) should not be used for more than a few days to avoid rebound congestion. For best results, drops are instilled into the dependent nostril of the supine patient, and the head is held back and turned to one side for 30–60 seconds. Nasal sprays are sniffed with the head erect and tilted slightly forward. In patients with recurrent nosebleeds, 0.5% phenyl-ephrine (Neo-Synephrine) in a nasal jelly is useful.

b. Oral adrenergic preparations can be used alone or in combination with antihistamines (see Table 4-6).

3. **Cromolyn sodium** (Nasalcrom), a 4% solution delivering approximately 5 mg/spray, acts by stabilizing the mast cell membrane and inhibiting mediator release. It can be used prophylactically before antigen exposure or therapeutically in chronic allergic rhinitis. Some patients will also require antihistamines or decongestants to achieve optimal control.

a. The dose for adults and children 6 years and older is one spray in each nostril 3–4 times/day at regular intervals. If needed, increase to 6 times/day. Instruct the patient (1) to clear the nasal passages before administering the spray and (2) to inhale through the nose during administration. The effect of cromolyn sodium often does not become apparent until 2–4 weeks of treatment.

b. Adverse effects of cromolyn sodium are usually few and mild. The most frequent reactions are sneezing, stinging, burning, and irritation (< 10%). Epistaxis, postnasal drip, and rash are reported in less than 1% of patients. Its lack of sedating properties makes it attractive for those patients who are prone to this side effect of antihistamines.

4. **Topical corticosteroids** may be indicated in refractory or more severe cases of seasonal allergic rhinitis. Newer corticosteroids, such as beclomethasone (Beconase or Vancenase) or flunisolide (Nasalide), are highly potent, surface active, and rapidly metabolized. In the management of allergic rhinitis, these properties make them as effective as and safer than older topical steroids (dexamethasone). Instruct patients that, unlike antihistamines or decongestants, several days to 2 weeks can be required before full benefit is observed.

a. The usual dose of beclomethasone dipropionate for adults and children 12 years of age and over is one inhalation (42 μg) in each nostril 2–4 times/day. (This preparation is not recommended for children under age 12 years.) The recommended starting dose of flunisolide nasal solution (0.025%) for adults is 2 sprays (50 μg) in each nostril 2 times/day. For children 6–14 years, the dose is one spray in each nostril 3 times/day or two sprays in each nostril 2 times/day. After symptom control is attained, maintenance dosage can usually be reduced. Instruct the patient to direct the spray away from the nasal septum and follow the other steps listed in the patient's instruction sheet.

b. Adverse effects are mainly local and include sneezing, stinging, and burning. Epistaxis in less than 5% of patients; localized infections of the nose and pharynx with *Candida albicans* or ulceration of the nasal mucosa rarely occur. Systemic corticosteroid effects are not reported when recommended doses are used.

c. In patients with severe mucosal edema or secretions, use a topical nasal vasoconstrictor 10–15 minutes before application of the topical corticosteroids for the first 2–3 days to allow the corticosteroid to reach the intended site. Topical corticosteroids should be used with caution in patients with active or quiescent tuberculous infections of the respiratory tract, untreated fungal, bacterial, or systemic viral infections, or ocular herpes simplex. Likewise, patients who have had recent nasal septal ulcers, nasal surgery, or trauma should not use these preparations because of the inhibitory effects on wound healing.

d. The injection of long-acting corticosteroids into the nasal turbinates is not recommended because it has been associated with reported cases of blindness caused by intraarterial embolization of the particulate mixture.

5. **Parenteral corticosteroids.** Systemic adrenal corticosteroids can control the symptoms of allergic rhinitis. Prolonged use (> 7 days) is rarely, if ever,

indicated because of the possible severe side effects. Oral corticosteroids should be considered only when symptoms are severe and of limited duration, and conventional treatment measures have failed.

C. **Immunotherapy** (hyposensitization) is indicated for the treatment of allergic rhinitis only when IgE hypersensitivity is demonstrated to specific inhalant allergens the patient cannot avoid (pollens, fungi, house dust mites) (see Chap. 4). **The need for immunotherapy depends on the frequency and severity of symptoms and the ease with which they are controlled with other forms of therapy.**

V. **Prognosis.** Seasonal allergic rhinitis is a chronic, recurring condition. The expression of symptoms depends both on environmental exposure and intrinsic host responsiveness. Symptom patterns fluctuate through life; childhood symptoms often diminish during puberty, to return in the third or fourth decade. Pregnancy is often associated with a period of quiescence; menopause is associated with a recurrence of symptoms. In 3–10% of children with seasonal allergic rhinitis, asthma of varying severity can develop subsequently.

Perennial Allergic Rhinitis

Perennial allergic rhinitis is characterized by intermittent or continuous nasal symptoms resulting from an allergic reaction without seasonal variation. Symptoms generally persist throughout the year. Although perennial allergic rhinitis resembles seasonal allergic rhinitis, separate consideration of the perennial form can better clarify this complex disease, particularly with respect to diagnosis, management, and complications.

I. **Pathophysiologic features.** The alterations of normal physiology seen in seasonal allergic rhinitis are less severe but more persistent in the perennial form, often leading to the development of complications. The histopathologic changes are initially the same as those found in seasonal allergic rhinitis. With persistent disease, more chronic and irreversible changes are observed: thickening and hyperplasia of the mucosal epithelium; more intense mononuclear cellular infiltration; connective tissue proliferation; and hyperplasia of adjacent periosteum. The increase in mononuclear cell infiltration suggests a delayed hypersensitivity reaction.

Nonspecific (nonimmunologic) stimuli often increase nasal symptoms both in allergic and nonallergic (vasomotor) rhinitis. Tobacco smoke (active and passive exposure), perfumes, newspaper print, and alcohol are such examples. The supine position increases nasal resistance; in contrast, exercise reverses nasal congestion temporarily.

II. **Clinical findings.** The typical gaping facies can be seen. The intranasal findings present a variable picture—from a dry, unobstructed, almost normal airway to an airway completely blocked by severe edema, secretions, and, on occasion, polypoid tissue. There are no pathognomonic features. The classic picture of blue-gray, edematous turbinates with a copious, watery discharge seen in seasonal allergic rhinitis is the exception rather than the rule.

Other findings in perennial allergic rhinitis include mouth breathing, snoring, constant sniffing, a nasal quality to the speech, and a loss of smell and taste. The nasal congestion may interfere with sleep. Because the chronic edema involves the openings of the eustachian tube and the paranasal sinuses, dull frontal headaches or ear complaints may occur (decreased hearing, fullness, and popping of the ears). Recurrent epistaxis, especially in children, can result from the sneezing, forceful nose blowing, or nose picking that traumatizes the friable nasal mucosa. Continuous postnasal drainage of secretions can produce a chronic cough or repeated clearing of the throat. In children affected early in life, narrowing of the arch of the palate (gothic arch) and dental malocclusion can develop.

III. **Diagnosis.** Recurrent nasal congestion resulting from allergy must be differentiated from recurrent upper respiratory infections or vasomotor rhinitis. Features of the diagnosis are outlined in Table 5-1.

IV. Treatment

A. Avoidance. The home environment must be modified (see Chap. 4) to avoid factors that initiate or exacerbate the rhinitis, e.g., pollen or cigarette smoke. Control of humidity and temperature can lessen nasal instability or vasomotor hyperactivity.

B. Medications
   1. Irrigations with normal saline solutions using a bulb syringe or commercial saline spray can help liquefy mucus, moisturize mucosal surfaces, and wash away allergens.
   2. Specific pharmacologic agents are usually required to control symptoms. As with acute allergic rhinitis, start with drugs with fewer side effects and advance to additional agents if control is not achieved. Inform the patient of the potential benefits and the adverse effects and monitor accordingly, using the least amount of drugs to control symptoms.

C. Exercise can help reduce nasal obstruction by stimulating sympathetic nerve discharge, which produces vasoconstriction. The increased nasal patency occurs rapidly and lasts for 15–30 minutes.

D. Immunotherapy. Hyposensitization for perennial allergic rhinitis is not as efficacious as for acute seasonal allergic rhinitis. In perennial allergic rhinitis, house dust mites and molds probably play a greater role than do pollens; consequently, specific immunotherapy is less beneficial. However, the patient who is miserable, with a congested nose, inability to sleep because of difficulty in breathing, or lethargy from antihistamines, may benefit from a trial of immunotherapy.

E. Surgical treatment. Because breathing through each nostril normally alternates every 1 or 2 hours, a deviated septum can present additional complications to the patient with allergic rhinitis. Varying degrees of septal deviation occur in about one-third of all patients with perennial allergic rhinitis. Mild septal deviation without unilateral congestion need not be corrected. In severe cases, especially in the patient over 16 years of age, surgical correction can afford a more patent nasal airway.

Nasal Polyps

Nasal polyps can occur as a complication of perennial allergic rhinitis. They usually arise from the surface of the middle turbinate or the ostia of the ethmoid or maxillary sinuses. Both allergic and infectious factors have been postulated as the mechanisms producing polyps. Those associated with allergy appear as gray or white, glistening, gelatinous masses; those associated with chronic infection appear more erythematous, granular, and firm. Nasal polyps are rare in children. When seen in children, cystic fibrosis must be excluded, since polyps are found in approximately 6% of affected children. In adolescents and adults, the presence of polyps suggests aspirin intolerance. A classic triad has been described in patients with polyps, asthma, and aspirin intolerance. Because of the possibility of severe generalized reactions following the ingestion of aspirin and aspirin-containing drugs, they should be avoided by patients with nasal polyps and asthma (see Chaps. 6 and 12). Several tumors and neoplasms of the nose resemble polyps. These include encephaloceles, inverting papilloma, squamous cell carcinoma, sarcoma, and angiofibroma. Otolaryngologic consultation should be obtained for these conditions.

Medical treatment of polyps secondary to allergies consists of treatment of the underlying allergies by avoidance and pharmacotherapy. For bothersome polyps, a trial of topical corticosteroids (beclomethasone dipropionate or flunisolide) or a short course of oral corticosteroids (e.g., prednisone, 40–60 mg/day for 3–7 days) can be tried before surgical polypectomy. The continued use of topical corticosteroids is helpful in suppressing regrowth of polyps in intractable cases. There is no evidence that surgical removal will exacerbate asthma.

Vasomotor Rhinitis

Vasomotor rhinitis is a condition of unknown origin associated with altered vasomotor control in the nasal membrane. This altered control results in chronic nasal congestion. Many physicians use **vasomotor rhinitis** as a descriptive term and in a broader sense to include both nonseasonal allergic rhinitis and the nonallergic forms of chronic infectious rhinitis. Numerous nonspecific stimuli, such as changes in body temperature, odors, fumes, medications, humidity or barometric pressure changes, and emotional stimuli, can trigger nasal obstruction and rhinorrhea. Vasomotor rhinitis is a common ailment that often coexists with nasal allergy. Impaired smell and taste often accompany vasomotor rhinitis. The diagnostic procedures are directed toward excluding allergic or infectious components of the nasal congestion. Nonspecific treatment includes saline nasal washes and exercise programs to help increase nasal patency. Drug treatment is the same as for allergic rhinitis, but the results are poorer. Immunotherapy is not indicated.

Nonallergic Rhinitis with Eosinophilia Syndrome

Nonallergic rhinitis with eosinophilia syndrome (NARES) or, as it is also termed, **eosinophilic nonallergic rhinitis (ENR),** is responsible for 15% of noninfectious. nonstructural causes of chronic rhinitis in adults and less than 5% of chronic rhinitis in children. A proportion of patients with NARES has the aspirin triad (polyps, asthma, and aspirin intolerance). Although these patients have the same clinical picture as patients with allergic rhinitis, allergy skin tests or RAST determinations are negative. The nasal smear is strongly positive for eosinophilia. These patients generally respond well to topical corticosteroids.

Miscellaneous Forms of Rhinitis

I. **Infectious rhinitis.** Upper respiratory viral infections are frequent causes of rhinitis. The common cold is characterized initially by sneezing and clear rhinorrhea. Within several days the nasal discharge becomes purulent, with a predominance of neutrophils noted on nasal smear. The mucosal membrane is erythematous, and the patient often complains of a burning sensation. The allergic person with infection often has more intense and intractable symptoms than do those who are not allergic.

II. **Rhinitis medicamentosa** most commonly results from excessive use of **topical** vasoconstrictors. These agents should be prescribed only for short periods (3–5 days) because chronic use leads to a destruction of nasal ciliary activity, a change in the pH of nasal mucus, and transformation of the nasal mucosa into stratified squamous epithelium. Systemic drug administration (e.g., reserpine) can also cause nasal congestion. Symptoms abate when these drugs are discontinued.

III. **Endocrine rhinitis.** A chronic stuffy nose can accompany hypothyroidism, especially in young children. Other endocrine-related causes include premenstrual congestion, pregnancy, and both oral contraceptive use and postmenopausal estrogen therapy.

IV. **Cerebrospinal rhinorrhea.** Clear, watery rhinorrhea, often unilateral, can follow head trauma. Rhinorrhea secondary to a cerebrospinal fluid leak should prompt immediate neurosurgical consultation.

V. **Foreign body rhinitis.** A foreign body lodged in the nostril will produce increased rhinorrhea after a few days. The discharge is usually purulent, foul smelling, and unilateral. This problem is usually seen in small children.

Sinusitis

I. **Pathologic features.** Sinusitis is an inflammation of the mucous membranes of the paranasal sinuses resulting from bacterial or viral infection, physical or chemical trauma (e.g., barotrauma), or allergic reactions. It can be acute, subacute, or chronic; one or multiple sinuses can be affected. A variety of conditions predisposes the patient to the development of sinusitis. These include local factors (polyps, tumors, or a deviated septum), immunodeficiency, cystic fibrosis, Down's syndrome, immotile cilia syndrome, and cleft lip and palate. Asthmatic patients have a high incidence of sinusitis.

II. **Clinical findings**
   A. **Acute paranasal sinusitis.** Common symptoms include nasal obstruction, purulent nasal discharge, fever, malaise, and localized pain and tenderness over the involved sinus. Pain can be referred away from the involved sinus. Symptoms of paranasal sinusitis, especially in the acute form, can mimic pain of dental origin, migraine headache, trigeminal neuralgia, facial cellulitis, angioneurotic edema, insect bites, temporal arteritis, and neoplasms of the sinus cavities. On physical examination the nasal mucosa is hyperemic and edematous; the turbinates are enlarged and often covered with a purulent discharge.
   B. **Chronic paranasal sinusitis.** The symptoms of the chronic form resemble those of acute sinusitis, but are more persistent. They include chronic nasal congestion resistant to decongestant therapy, thick postnasal drip, thick rhinorrhea, foul odor, cough (especially at night), and loss of smell and taste.

III. **Diagnosis**
   A. **X-rays** of the paranasal sinuses showing mucous membrane thickening (> 8 mm), opacification, or air-fluid level correlate highly with positive cultures obtained by antral punctures. The maxillary sinuses are the most common site of infection and are best diagnosed with a Water's view. Although a rudimentary frontal sinus can be seen radiographically at approximately 3 years of age and a sphenoid sinus at 5 years, there is great variation from child to child. Absence of one or both frontal sinuses occurs in less than 5% of adults.
   B. **Complete blood count and erythrocyte sedimentation rate.** Acute paranasal sinusitis is usually associated with a leukocytosis. An elevated sedimentation rate, common in acute sinus infections, can occur in chronic sinusitis.
   C. **Cultures.** Normal sinuses do not yield bacteria. Cultures from sinus cavities in children with acute sinusitis yield *Streptococcus pneumoniae, Haemophilus influenzae,* and *Branhamella catarrhalis.* Cultures from adults with acute disease grow *H. influenzae, S. pneumoniae, Streptococcus viridans,* and *Staphylococcus aureus.* In chronic sinusitis anaerobic bacteria may also be cultured. Up to 40% of cultures may show no growth. There is little correlation between nasal and sinus cultures; nasal cultures are of little diagnostic value.
   D. **Ultrasonography.** Although this technique has correlated well with results of sinus irrigations in adults, it has not been helpful when evaluating young children. Further research may help define its exact role in the diagnosis of sinusitis.
   E. **Transillumination.** Recent studies have indicated that this technique is of limited usefulness in the diagnosis of sinusitis and is not an adequate substitute for roentgenography.

IV. **Treatment**
   A. **Medical treatment.** Topical decongestants can reduce nasal mucosa swelling and improve drainage (see Table 4-6). They should be used only for short periods (3–5 days) to avoid rebound congestion. Systemic decongestants (combined with an antihistamine if an underlying allergy is present) are also helpful (see Chap. 4). Analgesics should be used for pain control, especially in acute sinusitis.
   B. **Surgical treatment.** If medical management does not produce adequate drainage in acute sinusitis, nasal irrigation or needle aspiration of the frontal or maxillary sinus can help. If these simple surgical measures fail or if complica-

tions of acute sinus disease occur (osteomyelitis, meningitis, venous sinus thrombosis, cerebritis), more aggressive surgical measures are indicated.

C. Antibiotics. Because of the high incidence of *H. influenzae*, antibiotic coverage for this organism should be included for adults and children with acute or chronic disease. For unresponsive sinusitis, antral punctures may be necessary for exact bacterial identification.

D. Allergy therapy. If an underlying allergic condition is present, treatment should be appropriate for allergic rhinitis.

Ocular Allergy

Ocular symptoms resulting from immunologic mechanisms are variable in their severity, frequency, and clinical manifestations. Causes may include classic IgE sensitization, antigen-antibody complexes, or delayed hypersensitivity–type reactions. Although allergic conjunctivitis is the most common cause of ocular inflammation, other causes should always be considered to prevent severe eye damage.

I. Allergic conjunctivitis

A. Pathophysiologic features. Allergic conjunctivitis is the ocular analog of allergic rhinitis and represents the clinical manifestations of the interaction between antigen and IgE bound to mast cells located in the conjunctiva. The clinical reproducibility of this reaction is dependable and has been used as a diagnostic test for immediate hypersensitivity by instillation of antigens directly into the conjunctival sac.

B. Clinical findings. Inflammation of the conjunctiva is uncommon as the only manifestation of allergic disease and is usually associated with seasonal allergic rhinitis.

1. The **acute form** of atopic conjunctivitis is often of an explosive nature, with sudden diffuse bilateral conjunctival edema, hyperemia, and occasional superficial keratitis. The tearing and itching may become unbearable, and sleepless nights may be frequent. The presence of photophobia or pain suggests involvement of other eye structures, e.g., cornea, sclera, or uveal tract.

2. In **chronic** atopic conjunctivitis, symptoms of dryness, photophobia, itching, and blurring are out of proportion to objective evidence of inflammation. The conjunctivae may appear pale, with mild edema and hyperplasia of the papillae, giving a fine granular appearance to the palpebral conjunctivae.

C. Diagnosis

1. **Conjunctival** scrapings or eye **discharge** contain eosinophils that are demonstrated as in a nasal smear (see Appendix II).

2. **Immediate hypersensitivity skin testing** will usually demonstrate sensitivity to airborne allergens.

3. **Conjunctival testing.** It is unusual to obtain a positive result from a conjunctival test when an intracutaneous test to the same antigen has been negative. The disadvantages of this technique for routine clinical use (invalid in the presence of inflammation, time-consuming, and limited to one antigen at a time) outweigh the advantages.

D. Treatment

1. **Oral antihistamines** can provide relief both of eye symptoms and of accompanying nasal symptoms when present (see Tables 4-4 and 4-5). They should be given prior to known exposures and around-the-clock in refractory cases.

2. Sterile, nonprescription external irrigating solutions (e.g., AK-Rinse, Collyrium, Dacriose, Eye-Stream, Neo-Flo) can be used to flush the eyes to remove air pollutants as well as chemical mediators resulting from the inflammatory response. Ocular demulcents (Artificial Tears) are also used in normal eyes for temporary relief of discomfort and dryness caused by minor irritants and exposure to wind or sun.

3. **Topical ophthalmic vasoconstrictors** are adjuncts to oral antihistamines

Table 5-2. Adverse corticosteroid effects on the eye

Adverse effects	Prevention	Treatment
Systemic Administration		
Posterior subcapsular cataracts	Use of lowest possible dose for shortest duration	Ophthalmologic consultation
	Regular fundal examinations (use + 8 diopters) and visual acuity examinations	Reduce dose as low as possible.
	Semiannual or annual slit-lamp examination	
Glaucoma	Screen for family history of glaucoma. Monitor intraocular pressure.	Ophthalmologic consultation
Topical Administration		
Herpetic infections of cornea	Limit corticosteroid treatment to severe problems.	Ophthalmologic consultation
Glaucoma	Screen for family history of glaucoma. Monitor intraocular pressure.	Ophthalmologic consultation
Corneal and scleral thinning	Use carefully in rheumatoid and autoimmune diseases associated with corneal thinning.	Ophthalmologic consultation

These agents include phenylephrine hydrochloride, naphazoline hydrochloride, tetrahydrozoline hydrochloride, and a mixture of zinc sulfate and a decongestant. The usual dosage is 1–2 drops every 3 or 4 hours or as needed until symptoms subside.

4. **Cromolyn sodium** (Opticrom) solution (4%) may offer relief when 1–2 drops are given 4–6 times a day. Response may not become evident until 2–4 weeks of use. Users of soft (hydrophilic) contact lenses should refrain from wearing lenses while under treatment. (Wear can be resumed within a few hours after discontinuation of the drug.) Adverse effects are minor and few, with transient stinging and burning on instillation being the most common.

5. **Topical corticosteroids** can be used for the most severe cases. Because of the dangers of corticosteroid use, especially on a long-term basis (Table 5-2), ophthalmologic evaluation should be obtained. Such agents include cortisone, dexamethasone, fluorometholone, hydrocortisone, medrysone, and prednisolone. These topical corticosteroids are available as drops or ointment.

6. **Environmental control.** See Chaps. 3 and 4.

7. **Immunotherapy** is indicated in severe cases.

II. **Vernal conjunctivitis,** an uncommon form of chronic conjunctivitis, usually occurs in the spring and summer and is of undetermined origin. Its **clinical characteristics** suggest an allergic basis. It is common in atopic boys. The symptoms include severe itching, photophobia, blurring, lacrimation, and the presence of white, ropy secretions containing many eosinophils. In the palpebral form, hypertrophy of the papillae of the upper eyelids is present. These hypertrophic nodular papillae resemble cobblestones and consist of dense fibrous tissue with thickened epithelium and eosinophilic infiltration. In the bulbar form, these nodules are gelatinous masses, usually found at the corneal-scleral junction (Trantas' dots). With maturity, the disease generally remits and rarely is seen in adults.

The primary **treatment** is administration of topical corticosteroids. Their use should be monitored by an ophthalmologist. Although cromolyn sodium is not as effective as topical corticosteroid preparations, it is moderately helpful in relieving the symptoms of vernal conjunctivitis. Immunotherapy does not appear to be helpful.

III. Contact dermatitis of the eyelids is a common hypersensitivity skin reaction. Sensitizing substances include cosmetics and topical eye medications (most common), poison ivy, metals, and chemicals. Nail polish as a cause should not be overlooked; inadvertent rubbing of the eye can cause sensitization. Treatment is avoidance of the offending substance and short-term topical corticosteroid therapy.

IV. Uveitis. The uveal tract, consisting of the iris, ciliary body, and choroid, is a target organ for the clinical expression of many immunopathologic reactions. Uveitis can be experimentally reproduced by both Arthus-type and delayed-type hypersensitivity, and it is seen in a variety of diseases: sarcoidosis, tuberculosis, and autoimmune and rheumatoid diseases, especially ankylosing spondylitis. **Symptoms** include ocular pain, photophobia, conjunctival injection, and impairment of vision. In children, the onset can be insidious, without overt symptoms. Awareness of this complication and prompt ophthalmologic consultation are mandatory to prevent serious eye damage.

Secretory Otitis Media

Secretory or serous otitis media is commonly seen with allergic rhinitis in children, but can also occur in adults. The effusions occur most often before puberty, beginning in the newborn period in some patients (e.g., with cleft palate) and peaking in the early school or preschool years. Recurrent or persistent secretory otitis media is the most common cause of intermittent or variable childhood deafness in the United States. Approximately one-third of children with recurrent disease have an allergic component that merits investigation and treatment.

I. Etiology. Secretory otitis media is a complex disorder in which many factors can produce the observed clinical and histopathologic changes. The most common causes are anatomic, physiologic, obstructive, infectious, and allergic.

  A. Anatomic factors. The position of the nasopharyngeal ostium in relation to the angle of the eustachian tube is important for optimal drainage. In infants, the angle of elevation is only about 10 degrees, which is not conducive to adequate drainage. This angle increases with age to approximately 40 degrees in adults.

  B. Physiologic factors. Two factors play important roles: eustachian tube dysfunction (abnormal pressure changes) and abnormal middle ear mucosa (increased metaplasia of mucous glands). Measurement of middle ear pressures demonstrates the relative inefficiency of eustachian tube function during the first 7 years of life, which can be related to the lack of adequate drainage.

  C. Obstruction. The pressure of enlarged adenoidal tissue causes closure of the ostium, resulting in obstruction to normal flow and producing tubal dysfunction by limiting pressure changes.

  D. Infection becomes critical in patients with inadequately treated otitis media. This factor is particularly important in infants and toddlers who are susceptible to frequent respiratory infections or in patients with defective host defenses (see Chap. 17).

  E. Allergic factors. An allergic component is associated with approximately 35% of cases of recurrent secretory otitis media. A primary allergic reaction may occur in the ear, but it is more likely that secretory otitis media results from the obstruction and tubal dysfunction produced by an allergic reaction involving the respiratory mucosa. IgE-mediated reactions have been implicated in secretory otitis media on the basis of clinical observations, elevated total and antigen-specific IgE in middle ear effusions, and the induction of eustachian tube obstruction after nasal allergen challenge in atopic individuals.

II. Pathophysiologic features. The middle ear, normally free of fluid, contains a volume of air that is regulated by the action of the eustachian tube, which connects the middle ear and nasopharynx. Pressure is equalized on both sides of the tympanic

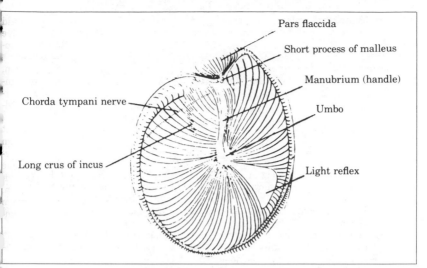

Pars flaccida

Short process of malleus

Manubrium (handle)

Chorda tympani nerve

Umbo

Long crus of incus

Light reflex

Fig. 5-1. Architecture of the normal tympanic membrane.

membrane. With tubal blockage, air cannot enter the middle ear, and the remaining air is absorbed. The resulting negative pressure causes accumulation of serous fluid, which produces the signs and symptoms of secretory otitis media. With superimposed infection, this fluid, a transudate, becomes a mucous exudate with an increased protein concentration. With continued pathologic stimulation, the cells lining the middle ear undergo hyperplasia and produce excessive secretions.

The characteristics of the middle ear fluid therefore vary with the stage of chronic secretory otitis media. In the early stages, it is usually yellow and of relatively low viscosity. With progression of the disease, the fluid darkens and becomes increasingly viscous. In the late stages, it is blue-gray and extremely viscous and tenacious, prohibiting movement of the ossicles or tympanic membrane.

III. **Clinical findings**

A. **Symptoms.** The most common and severe symptom is hearing loss. There can also be a sensation of popping of the ears, or a mild, dull earache, or a sense of fullness in the head.

The hearing loss can be intermittent and variable in severity, or insidious and often difficult to detect in young children unable to verbalize their complaints. The child often appears slow or inattentive or is disobedient. The parents may find it necessary to speak loudly or repeat what they have said. The young child is described as irritable and a poor sleeper; the older child is often called an underachiever in school. Delays in language and emotional and social development can result from this hearing deficiency.

B. **Physical signs.** The tympanic membrane in secretory otitis media can appear normal or bulging but usually is retracted, with an abnormally prominent short process of the malleus. The membrane is often dull, thickened, or wrinkled; its color can be gray, pink, amber, slightly yellow, or deep blue. Occasionally, a fluid level or bubbles are evident behind the tympanic membrane. The handle of the malleus appears chalky white, a sign considered pathognomonic of chronic secretory otitis media. At times, the bony landmarks (Fig. 5-1) may be completely obliterated. Physical signs of allergic disease may also exist, e.g., nasal crease or allergic shiners.

IV. **Diagnosis**

A. **Pneumatic otoscopy** should be part of the routine physical examination of the ear. A pneumatic otoscope can detect decreased mobility of the tympanic membrane, due to fluid or tympanic membrane retraction or both. By initial applica-

Table 5-3. Tuning fork tests

Type of hearing loss	Weber (bone only)	Rinne (air and bone)
None	Not lateralized	AC > BC
Conductive	Lateralized to poorer ear	BC ≥ AC
Sensorineural	Lateralized to better ear	AC > BC

Key: AC = air conduction; BC = bone conduction.

tion of slight pressure on the rubber bulb, positive pressure is produced. The pressure becomes negative when the seal is broken and the bulb is released. The normal tympanic membrane moves inward, away from the examiner, with positive pressure; with negative pressure it moves outward, toward the examiner. This movement is best visualized in the posterosuperior portion of the tympanic membrane.

B. **Tuning fork.** By using a tuning fork with frequencies of 500–1000 Hz (speech frequencies are roughly 500–2000 Hz), the presence of a conductive or sensorineural hearing loss can be demonstrated (Table 5-3).

   1. In **Weber's test,** place the handle of the vibrating tuning fork on the midline of the skull and ask the patient to compare the intensity of the sound in the two ears. Lateralization of the sound to one ear indicates a conductive loss on the same side, or a sensorineural loss on the other side.

   2. In the **Rinne test,** first place the handle of the vibrating tuning fork against the mastoid process while the patient covers the opposite ear with a hand. Have the patient indicate when the sound ceases. Then hold the still vibrating tuning fork near the external ear without touching the patient and have the patient indicate again when the sound ceases. Normally, air conduction persists twice as long as bone conduction.

C. **Tympanometry** is a helpful adjunct to evaluating middle ear function because i gives an accurate, sensitive measurement of abnormalities of the entire tympanic membrane–middle ear–eustachian tube system. Tympanometry is performed by inserting a small probe in the external auditory canal, delivering a fixed tone through the probe, and measuring the tympanic membrane compliance electronically as external canal pressure is artificially varied. This procedure can be performed reliably in an office setting in infants over 7 months of age and toddlers, thereby increasing the accuracy of diagnosis of middle ear disease.

   Interpretation of tympanometric curves should be correlated with clinical findings. Common patterns according to Jerger's classification (*Arch. Otolaryngol.* 92:311, 1970) are shown in Fig. 5-2.

D. The **volume test (static compliance)** uses the principles of tympanometry to evaluate the intactness of the tympanic membrane. By recording compliance as a physical volume measurement, the cause of nonmobile or flat B-type tympanograms can be determined (Table 5-4).

E. **Acoustic reflex threshold.** The stapedius muscle contracts reflexly when stimulated with a sufficiently loud sound. Even if only one ear is stimulated, the contraction occurs bilaterally. The acoustic reflex threshold is the lowest signal intensity capable of eliciting the acoustic reflex. Mild unilateral conductive hearing loss can be ascertained with this technique, even in children under 3 years of age.

F. **Audiometry.** A reliable audiogram can be obtained in most children after the age of 5 years. However, younger children with a history of recurrent ear disease or delays in language development, or whose parents suspect a hearing loss, can be tested using behavioral audiometry. If questions are still unanswered, more sophisticated evaluation such as testing for brainstem auditory-evoked poten-

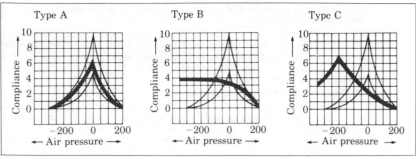

Fig. 5-2. Interpretation of tympanometry curves (pressure-compliance functions). Type A (sharp maximal compliance at pressure near 0 mm H_2O) is found in normal and otosclerotic ears. Type B (little or no maximal compliance) is found in serous and adhesive otitis. Type C (maximal compliance in negative pressure) is due to negative pressure in the middle ear. Heavy line = tympanometry curve; thin line = normal range.

Table 5-4. Static compliance measurements

Physical volume (cm³)	Probable cause
< 0.3	Cerumen or canal wall blockage
0.8–1.2	Serous otitis media
> 2.5	Perforation or ventilating tube

tials is then warranted. Such test procedures can give reliable results, even in newborn infants.

1. **Screening audiometry** is conducted in a quiet room with a screening audiometer. It measures a behavioral response to pure tones of 500, 1000, 2000, and 4000 Hz at 15- to 20-dB intensities.

2. **Threshold audiometry** in a sound booth can detect hearing losses below 20 dB and is used for patients identified by screening or with suspected speech or hearing difficulties or both.

Audiometry and tympanometry have **separate objectives:** screening for hearing loss and screening for middle ear disease, respectively. Although tympanometry is more sensitive for accurate identification of middle ear problems, a threshold hearing test is an absolute necessity for identifying a hearing loss.

G. **Myringotomy with aspiration.** The suspected presence of fluid in the middle ear can be confirmed by diagnostic myringotomy with aspiration. Although cultures of the fluid of chronic secretory otitis are usually negative, the fluid may represent an inflammatory reaction to bacterial infection originating in the nasopharynx. The organisms of importance are *S. pneumoniae, H. influenzae,* beta-hemolytic streptococci (group A), and *B. catarrhalis.* Viruses have been isolated on aspiration in approximately 5% of patients, although a significant rise in serum viral antibody titers has been noted in approximately 30%.

H. **X-ray.** A lateral x-ray view of the nasopharynx can be used to assess the degree of adenoidal hypertrophy and the possible need for adenoidectomy to relieve eustachian-tube obstruction.

I. **Allergy or immunologic evaluation.** When the history and physical findings suggest a potential atopic component, a thorough allergy evaluation as previously detailed is warranted (see Chap. 2). If the history suggests severe or refractory ear infections involving other sites in the body, as in dysgammaglobulinemia or immotile cilia syndrome, further evaluation along these lines is indicated (see Chap. 17).

V. Treatment. Although the natural course of secretory otitis media is not well characterized and the treatment modalities for it have not been subjected to controlled double-blind studies, improvement usually begins in the majority of patients when the diagnosis is made, etiologic factors determined, and treatment begun.

A. Medical treatment

1. Avoidance and environmental controls

   a. In infants, the prohibition of pacifiers, poorly vented nursing bottles, and bottle propping for self-feeding in the recumbent position can minimize the possibility of fluid aspiration into the middle ear.

   b. When allergy is implicated, environmental control measures should be instituted.

   c. Home humidification can help maintain the normal physiologic function of the respiratory mucous membrane.

2. Medications

   a. Oral **antihistamine-decongestants** may be beneficial if respiratory allergy is present.

   b. **Topical decongestants** or **topical corticosteroids** may be used intranasally, but only for short periods. Routine administration of systemic corticosteroids is **contraindicated.**

   c. **Antibiotics** are indicated if bacterial infection is present. Current recommendations for treatment in children include (1) ampicillin, 50–100 mg/kg/24 hours in 4 divided doses; (2) amoxicillin, 20–40 mg/kg/24 hours in 3 divided doses, or amoxicillin/clavulanate potassium (Augmentin), 20 mg/kg/day based on amoxicillin component in divided doses every 8 hours; (3) a combination of erythromycin, 40 mg/kg/24 hours, and sulfisoxazole, 120 mg/kg/24 hours in 4 divided doses; (4) trimethoprim-sulfamethoxazole as 8 mg/kg/24 hours of trimethoprim and 40 mg/kg/24 hours of sulfamethoxazole in 2 divided doses; and (5) cefaclor, 40 mg/kg/24 hours in 3 divided doses. All antibiotics should be given for 10 days. In older children and adults, penicillin may be used, although an increasing incidence of otitis media secondary to *H. influenzae* has been noted and the above antibiotics can be used (in appropriate adult doses). Chemoprophylaxis with antibiotics may be of benefit in preventing frequent recurrences of otitis media, e.g., three documented episodes in 6 months or four in 1 year. Sulfisoxazole offers the advantages of proven effectiveness, relative safety, and low cost. Ampicillin and amoxicillin are reasonable alternatives. Studies have used approximately one-half the therapeutic dose, given once or twice a day.

   d. **Immunization** with pneumococcal (Pneumovax) and *H. influenzae* (b-Capsa I Vaccine) vaccines are controversial in the prevention of recurrent ear infections. Unfortunately, many infections occur in the child under 2 years of age at a time when these current vaccines are not very immunogenic.

3. Immunotherapy. When allergy to unavoidable antigens (e.g., pollens, molds, or dust) is identified, immunotherapy is often beneficial. Such therapy is usually limited to older children and adults, only after environmental control measures have been adequately established.

B. Surgical treatment

1. Adenoidectomy. Hypertrophied adenoids can contribute to dysfunction of the eustachian tube by limiting pressure changes, but they probably only rarely obstruct the ostia to a significant degree. Adenoidectomy may be of temporary benefit; regrowth of adenoid tissue can occur.

2. Ventilating tubes. Procedures designed to equalize pressure on both sides of the tympanic membrane are effective in the treatment of secretory otitis media resulting from eustachian tube dysfunction. Ventilatory tubes (e.g., polyethylene tubes), in contrast to myringotomy and aspiration alone, produce sustained ventilation. This process immediately relieves the hearing

Table 5-5. Evaluation guide for recurrent secretory otitis media

Episodes of acute otitis media per year	Duration of middle ear effusion (months)	Hearing loss (months)	Behavior, language development, school performance	Personal history of allergy	Family history of allergy	Tympano-gram	Audiometry	Diagnostic approach
< 4	< 2	< 2	Normal	−	−	−	−	Observe.
> 4	> 2	> 2	Normal	±	±	Normal	<20-dB loss	Observe. Trial of antihistamines/decongestants
> 4	> 2	> 2	Poor	±	±	Flat curve	>20-dB loss	Do complete otologic and allergic evaluation.

Key: − = negative; + = possible.

impairment and reverses the underlying pathophysiologic process to restore normal middle ear function. Complications of this procedure can occur and increase as the period of tube placement lengthens. Such complications include scarring (tympanosclerosis) and localized or diffuse atrophy tha' can be accompanied by retraction, pockets of atelectasis, or both. Much less commonly, perforation at the insertion site following extrusion or cholesteatoma may result.

C. Guide for treatment. In planning therapy for chronic secretory otitis, physicians immediately confront three major areas of uncertainty about the disease: it' natural history, the degree of associated hearing impairment, and the significance of this impairment.

1. Most cases of secretory otitis in small children probably follow a benigr. course of weeks or months toward resolution. In some patients there can be a progression through various inflammatory stages to permanent middle ear damage or involvement of the cochlea, with sensorineural hearing loss. The overall prognosis for the disease in the child with recurrent secretory otitis is favorable, especially in the child over 10 years of age.

2. The ability to hear properly correlates closely with a number of aspects of normal childhood development. Critical periods exist in early life during which both auditory stimuli and perception must be optimal if the full potential for language and intellectual and emotional development is to be fulfilled. If during such periods hearing is impaired, the resulting deprivations or distortions may not be fully compensated, even if hearing acuity is restored.

Each patient must be individually considered. However, based on the general information and assumptions previously discussed, a guide for evaluation is presented in Table 5-5.

Selected Readings

Bluestone, C. D. Eustachian tube function: Physiology, pathophysiology and role o: allergy. In Pathogenesis of Otitis Media. *J. Allergy Clin. Immunol.* 72:242, 1983.

Cohen, E. J., and Allansmith, M. R. Ocular Allergy. In E. Middleton, Jr., C. Reed, and E. F. Ellis (eds.), *Allergy: Principles and Practice.* St. Louis: Mosby, 1983.

Hubbard, T. W., et al. Consequences of unremitting middle ear disease in early life *N. Engl. J. Med.* 312:1529, 1985.

Marks, M. B. Physical signs of allergy of the respiratory tract in children. *Ann Allergy* 25:310, 1967.

Meltzer, E. O., et al. Chronic rhinitis in infants and children: Etiologic, diagnostic and therapeutic considerations. *Pediatr. Clin. North Am.* 30:847, 1983.

Mygind, N., and Weeke, B. Allergic and Non-Allergic Rhinitis. In E. Middleton, Jr., C. Reed, and E. F. Ellis (eds.), *Allergy: Principles and Practice.* St. Louis: Mosby, 1983.

Northern, J. L. Advanced techniques for measuring middle ear function. *Pediatrics* 61:761, 1978.

Slavin, R. G. Upper Respiratory Tract Disease. In E. B. Weiss, M. S. Segal, and M. Stein (eds.), *Bronchial Asthma: Mechanisms and Therapeutics* (2nd ed.). Boston: Little, Brown, 1985.

Asthma

Glenn J. Lawlor, Jr.,
and Donald P. Tashkin

Asthma is the most common chronic lung disorder and affects persons of all ages. It is best defined in physiologic terms as a state of airways hyperresponsiveness leading to a reversible obstructive lung disease. The onset of asthma can occur at any age, although the peak incidence is before the age of 5 years. In childhood, asthma is about 30% more common in males than in females, and the disease tends to be more severe in male children. Beyond puberty, the sex distribution is equal. Asthma is more common in underprivileged urban areas, colder climates, and industrialized communities. There is a familial predisposition to asthma, with incidence highest among first-degree relatives, but occurrence rates are unpredictable.

Asthma of early onset carries an excellent prognosis. Marked diminution or absence of symptoms occurs in approximately 80% of asthmatic children by puberty. Primary incidence occurs in adults at any age, and about 20% of adults with childhood remission of asthma have a recurrence after the age of 45 years. Remission in adult asthma is much less common than in children. Children with respiratory allergy and eczema associated with asthma usually have a more severe course and poorer prognosis than do those who wheeze only with colds. Asthmatic patients with nasal polyps have a particularly poor prognosis, especially in association with aspirin sensitivity. The onset of aspirin sensitivity characteristically occurs in adulthood. It is more common in women than in men and is usually not associated with a history of allergies. **Mortality** varies with age. The death rate in children is under 1% and in adults, from 2–4%. The risk increases with advancing age. Other risk factors include a prolonged or recurrent record of poor control of asthma, a previous life-threatening episode, marked diurnal fluctuations, poor patient education, and poor patient-physician relationship.

The heterogeneity of asthma makes strict classification impossible. A useful method is to separate asthma according to etiologic factors into **extrinsic, intrinsic,** and **mixed.** In **extrinsic asthma,** symptoms relate to the exposure to specific environmental allergens, and onset is generally before 20 years of age. These sensitivities are usually reproducible by skin testing or bronchial provocation. In **intrinsic asthma,** symptoms are unrelated to allergen exposure and are provoked or aggravated by infection, exertion, psychological stimuli, and nonspecific climatic or environmental changes. This form is more common in adults who are more than 30 years of age. In **mixed asthma,** symptoms are aggravated by both **extrinsic** and **intrinsic** factors. This form is most common in childhood asthma.

I. **Pathophysiologic features.** The signs and symptoms of asthma are caused by anatomic narrowing of the tracheobronchial airways and the resultant (1) increased resistance to airflow, (2) overinflation of the lung, (3) uneven distribution of ventilation with regional hypoventilation in relation to pulmonary blood flow (reduced V/Q) causing hypoxemia, and (4) increased ventilation drive.

   A. **Pathologic changes** of the bronchial airways in asthma involve changes in the lumen, mucosa, submucosa, and smooth muscle of the bronchial wall, beginning with the trachea and main stem bronchi and extending to the terminal bronchioles.

      1. **Mucus plugging.** A characteristic finding in asthma is a thick, sticky mucus that contains various cellular components, including sloughed bronchial epithelium (creola bodies), eosinophils, and eosinophil by-products

(Charcot-Leyden crystals). The mucus, whose tenacity is accentuated by dehydration, partially blocks or completely occludes airways at all levels. This phenomenon is especially important in chronic and poorly reversible asthma.

2. **Changes in the bronchial mucous membrane** in chronic asthma include loss of ciliated epithelial cells, with an increase of hyperplastic mucus-secreting goblet cells, infiltration with eosinophils, edema, and thickening of the basement membrane. The **submucosa** is also edematous, with an inflammatory infiltration by eosinophils, neutrophils, lymphocytes, and histiocytes and with submucosal gland hypertrophy. Similarly, **the smooth-muscle layer** is hypertrophic.

B. **Neurogenic and immunochemical abnormalities.** The tone of bronchial smooth muscle is under the control of parasympathetic nerve fibers carried in the vagus nerve. Removal of this stimulation results in smooth-muscle relaxation and bronchodilatation. Stimulation of these fibers results in bronchoconstriction. Afferent nerve fibers arising from receptors in the lung and carried in the vagus nerve ("irritant" receptors) relay impulses affecting bronchial smooth-muscle tone. The sympathetic nervous system has a minimal effect in regulating bronchial smooth-muscle tone in normal persons but probably play a greater role in asthmatic patients.

1. It is proposed that alteration in the autonomic nervous system as well as immunochemical events leading to the release of "mediators" from sensitized cells cause the airway changes in asthma. **Hyperirritability of the airways is the most characteristic abnormality in asthma.** There is significant increase in the response of the airways of asthmatic patients to various chemical and physical stimuli as compared with normal subjects. This irritability can be reversed by blocking vagal efferent and afferent fibers, suggesting an increased cholinergic response in asthma.

2. **Bronchial smooth-muscle cells contain distinct protein membrane receptors** for alpha-adrenergic– and beta-1- and beta-2-adrenergic–mediated responses. Beta-receptors predominate throughout the airways, with beta-2 receptors in excess of beta-1 receptors by a 3:1 ratio. Stimulation of beta-2 adrenergic receptors reduces airway irritability in asthmatic patients, but blockade of beta-receptors has little effect in non-asthmatic subjects. Thus the role of a defect in beta-adrenergic response in the etiology of asthma is unclear. Alpha-adrenergic stimulation has minimal effect on bronchial smooth-muscle tone.

3. **Calcium** plays a critical role in bronchial smooth-muscle contraction. A negative resting membrane potential is maintained by an adenosine triphosphate (ATP)–dependent calcium extrusion pump. Increased membrane permeability and intracellular influx of calcium leads to smooth-muscle contraction, and extrusion of calcium leads to relaxation. Adrenergic responses appear to act through action on calcium influx as does antigen-induced mediator release from sensitized mast cells.

4. The **cyclic nucleotides adenosine monophosphate (cyclic AMP) and guanosine monophosphate (cyclic GMP)** (see Chap. 2), formed by the action of cell membrane–bound adenylate cyclase and guanylate cyclase or the purine nucleotides ATP and guanosine triphosphate (GTP), respectively, affect many cell functions, including the release of mediators from sensitized cells and the contractile process in bronchial smooth muscle. Allergen-induced mediator release is enhanced by cholinergic agents and prostaglandin $F_{2\alpha}$, presumably by increasing cyclic GMP. Enhancement may also occur with alpha-adrenergic stimulation that reduces cyclic AMP. Inhibition of mediator release occurs with beta-adrenergic stimulation that increases cyclic AMP or possibly with blockade of adenosine receptors.

5. The **immunochemical release of vasoactive mediators** from immunoglobulin E (IgE)-sensitized mast cells in the lung is responsible for symptoms in allergen-induced (extrinsic) asthma. In the mast cell, mediators are

either preformed or generated. Antigenic stimulation of IgE-sensitized mast cells initiates a chemical sequence in the cell membrane, resulting in the release of the **preformed mediators**—histamine, eosinophil chemotactic factors of anaphylaxis (ECF-A), neutrophil chemotactic factors of anaphylaxis (NCF-A), and platelet-activating factor (PAF)—and activation of the metabolism of membrane phospholipids. Membrane phospholipids are metabolized to arachidonic acid, which enters two metabolic pathways to form the **generated mediators**—the leukotrienes and prostaglandins (see Chap. 2).

When bronchial smooth muscle is sensitized, the bronchospastic effects of histamine release are immediate and short-acting, whereas the effects of the leukotrienes appear in a few minutes and act more slowly. Both constitute a part of the **immediate reaction.** The chemotactic factors and PAF attract and induce an inflammatory cell response in the bronchial mucosa with further generation of leukotrienes. This is a **delayed (late) response,** with the onset of bronchospasm from 2–8 hours after initial sensitization, and may persist for days.

Other mediators of less or undefined importance include heparin, histamine, thromboxanes, prostaglandin generating factor, serotonin, superoxides, and kinins.

C. **Physiologic changes with airway obstruction.** The characteristic physiologic feature is airway obstruction. Obstruction occurs as a result of bronchial smooth-muscle spasm, mucus plugging, and edema and inflammation of the bronchial wall. Obstruction is enhanced during expiration because of physiologic airway narrowing. Obstruction of airflow leads to air trapping and hyperinflation of the lungs and to a prolongation of expiration. The increased resistance due to airway obstruction and the greater elastic recoil at high lung volumes (hyperinflation) increase the work of breathing, resulting in dyspnea and the use of accessory muscles of respiration.

1. **Bronchospasm** is the most likely cause of acute and rapidly reversible attacks, whereas mucus plugging and edema and inflammation of the bronchial wall are more important in chronic asthma and more prolonged irreversible acute attacks.

2. The **site of involvement** can be large, medium, or small airways. In about 50% of asthmatic patients, large airway involvement predominates; in the remainder, obstruction of the smaller airways predominates. Asthma in patients with predominantly large airway involvement is more commonly characterized by wheezing than is asthma with small airway involvement. The latter tends to present with episodic dyspnea and cough rather than wheezing.

3. Obstruction of airflow in an asthma attack produces an increase in residual volume and a decrease in vital capacity proportionate to the degree of severity. The total lung capacity increases, and the increased residual volume can even supersede the total lung capacity present prior to the attack.

4. The airway obstruction in asthma is uneven in various parts of the lung, so that airflow is not uniform in each region. Pulmonary blood flow is directed away from less ventilated to better ventilated alveoli, but this shift is incomplete, and ventilation-perfusion ratios decrease in poorly ventilated areas, resulting in arterial hypoxemia (reduced PaO_2). Reduction of the PaO_2 can be the only abnormality in subclinical asthma. Arterial CO_2 tensions are directly related to alveolar ventilation. In mild to moderately severe asthma attacks, ventilation is increased and $PaCO_2$ is reduced, with an increase in pH (respiratory alkalosis). In progressively severe attacks and impending respiratory failure, alveolar hypoventilation ensues, with a rise in $PaCO_2$ and a fall in pH (respiratory acidosis).

5. Air trapping and hyperinflation have a squeeze effect on the alveolar capillaries, which, together with the constrictor effect of alveolar hypoxia on the smooth muscle of the precapillaries, causes pulmonary artery pressure to

increase. In an acute asthma attack, pulmonary hypertension occurs proportional to the severity.

II. **Clinical approach to the patient (diagnosis and assessment)**

A. **History.** The history is the most important aspect in arriving at a diagnosis and determining the appropriate therapy (see Chap. 2). The diagnosis of asthma is usually obvious; however, it should be suspected in any person with unexplained episodes of dyspnea and cough (or of cough alone) or repeated chest colds and bronchitis (especially children).

1. Information regarding the **frequency, duration,** and **intensity** of attacks indicates the severity. In the acute attack it is important to know the time of onset, possible cause (e.g., exposure, infection), present medications (type, dose, time taken), comparison with previous attacks, and presence of complicating factors (e.g., vomiting, fever, chest pain).

2. A description of **symptom-free intervals** helps to determine the degree of involvement and need for treatment. Are these periods associated with dyspnea, cough (especially at night or with exertion), sputum production, fatigue, or exercise intolerance? How often is medication for asthma taken? What preparations are used, and is the dosage appropriate? What are the side effects of the patient's medication? What factors produce attacks? How much work or school loss occurs?

3. An **environmental survey** can determine possible provocative factors, especially allergens, occupational or environmental exposure, irritant or other provocative stimuli, smoking, stress, infection, climate, activities, medication (e.g., aspirin, beta blockers), and dietary intake (e.g., metabisulfites monosodium glutamate).

4. The **family history** is frequently positive for asthma or respiratory allergy.

B. **Physical findings** depend on the frequency and severity of attacks. There are usually no specific findings in the uncomplicated, symptom-free asthmatic patient. Examination of the upper respiratory tract is helpful, and attention is given to signs associated with allergic rhinitis, sinusitis, and the presence of nasal polyps (see Chap. 5). Prior to examination of the chest, it is important to determine the patient's respiratory rate, pulse rate, and blood pressure, as well as height, weight, habitus, and attitude. In examination of the chest, attention is directed to configuration, resonance to percussion, quality and intensity of breath sounds, and fullness and evenness of ventilation on auscultation.

1. In the acute attack, the **respiratory rate and pulse rate** are increased, and the blood pressure is frequently elevated. A rapid pulse rate also reflects the effects of adrenergic medication. Other findings that indicate the severity of the attack include the use of accessory muscles of respiration (i.e., scalene and sternocleidomastoid muscles), suprasternal retractions, pursed lip expiration, and flaring of the alae nasi. Chest findings include intercostal muscle retractions and evidence of hyperinflation (increased anteroposterior diameter, hyperresonance, reduced diaphragm and chest wall excursion). On auscultation, an unevenness of ventilation with varying degrees of high-pitched inspiratory and expiratory sibilant rales, rhonchi, and wheezes accentuated during prolonged expiration can be heard.

2. **Peripheral signs of marked severity** or **impending respiratory failure** include accentuation of the findings in **1,** with cyanosis, pulsus paradoxus, asterixis, miosis, papilledema, and changes in the sensorium. Chest findings in very severe asthma include severe hyperinflation, marked reduction in respiratory excursions, and nearly inaudible breath sounds, with distant to absent wheezes (silent chest).

C. **Laboratory findings.** The diagnosis of asthma generally does not require extensive testing. The following studies are helpful in selected patients to determine the severity of an acute attack, chronicity of disease, differentiation of other conditions, selection of therapeutic measures, and response to treatment:

1. The **chest x-ray** is usually normal in uncomplicated asthma. During acute attacks the lung fields appear hyperlucent, with generalized hyperinflation of the chest and flattening of the diaphragm. Segmental or subsegmental

infiltrates or atelectasis may be present as a result of mucus plugging. In patients with more severe or chronic disease, the sternum appears bowed, with kyphosis of the thoracic spine and an increased retrosternal lucency on a lateral projection. In chronic asthma, peribronchial markings can be increased, and the hilar vessels appear enlarged.

A chest x-ray is not necessary in the initial evaluation of uncomplicated asthma. A routine film is helpful to have as a baseline for future comparison. The main **indication** for a chest x-ray is to evaluate an acute or chronic change in asthmatic symptoms. Particular attention is directed to the presence of infiltrates; atelectasis; free air in the chest, mediastinum, or soft tissue; and changes in the normal architecture in comparison with previous films. Chest x-rays should **not** be taken with each episode in patients with recurrent, acute attacks that are consistent in presentation.

2. **Sinus x-rays** are indicated when persistent upper respiratory symptoms appear to be aggravating the course of asthma. Particular attention is directed to the presence of thickened sinus membranes, cysts, polyps, cloudiness and infiltration of the sinus cavities, and air-fluid levels (see Chap. 5).

3. **Tuberculin test.** It is important to know the status of tuberculin sensitivity in the asthmatic patient, especially if corticosteroid therapy is anticipated. A tuberculin test (0.10 ml of purified protein derivative [PPD], 5 tuberculin units, injected intracutaneously on the forearm, with induration interpreted at 48–72 hours) should be done in any patient **without** a history of tuberculin positivity. The tuberculin test is especially indicated in a patient with a history of exposure to tuberculosis in the absence of a previously positive test.

4. The results of a **complete blood count** are usually normal in uncomplicated asthma, with a tendency to eosinophilia (500–1000 eosinophils/mm^3). Diurnal variation in eosinophil count (increased late at night), seasonal variation (increased during periods of allergen exposure), and suppression with corticosteroids are common. Concurrent infection will reduce the eosinophil count and can be associated with leukocytosis and a shift to immature cells. A complete blood count is usually not necessary in the evaluation of asthma, even in the presence of allergy. Its principal purpose is to aid in the diagnosis of infection. Similarly, nonspecific indicators of inflammation (e.g., erythrocyte sedimentation rate) are normal and are helpful only in suggesting a concurrent infection.

5. **Sputum analysis.** A productive cough is often not associated with mild to moderate asthma, especially in extrinsic childhood asthma. Sputum production is more common in chronic disease in adults (intrinsic asthma), especially in conjunction with chronic bronchitis.

   a. Sputum can be clear or mucopurulent. Yellow or greenish sputum can result from eosinophil or cellular debris and does not always imply infection.

   b. Sputum analysis for **cell type** is helpful in monitoring the response to corticosteroid therapy and in evaluating the presence of infection. Sputum collected from a coughed specimen can be used. If the patient is unable to cough up a specimen, inhalation of aerosolized normal saline by compressor and chest percussion or suction aspiration through a nasal or oral tracheal catheter is helpful, although these procedures can aggravate bronchospasm. Introduction of 3–5 ml of sterile saline into the trachea through a catheter will help induce an effective cough. The sputum is then placed on a slide, dried, and stained with Hansel's or Wright's stain (see Appendixes II and III). An adequate sputum specimen should contain many macrophages and bronchial epithelial cells, inflammatory cells, noncellular elements, and possibly microorganisms.

      (1) Sputum in **extrinsic asthma** usually shows 25–35% ciliated columnar epithelial cells, 5–80% eosinophils, and varying amounts of polymorphonuclear leukocytes (PMNs). In **intrinsic asthma** or **chronic bronchitis** the sputum composition is similar, with a predominance

of PMNs and eosinophils in range of 5–20%. When intrinsic asthma worsens, the ratio of PMNs to eosinophils usually remains the same, with an increase in total cell count; in extrinsic asthma, worsening is usually accompanied by an increase in total eosinophil count Corticosteroid therapy will depress the total eosinophil count—a response that can be used to assess the adequacy of the dosage.

(2) **Secondary infection** is associated with an increase in PMNs and an increased PMN-eosinophil ratio; microorganisms may also be noted. Sputum culture and sensitivities are indicated to establish further the presence and cause of infection, especially in patients with persistent or refractory symptoms.

6. **Electrocardiographic (ECG) findings** are normal in uncomplicated asthma. In acute, severe attacks or in chronic asthma, especially in conjunction with chronic bronchitis, pulmonary hypertension is common, and ECG changes such as right axis deviation, right bundle branch block, or P pulmonale, may be seen. Tachycardia is common with an acute attack and is aggravated by adrenergic medication.

7. **Serum IgE, allergy skin testing, and radioallergosorbent test (RAST).** Serum IgE levels are frequently elevated in extrinsic asthma, especially in children and in conjunction with atopic dermatitis or with upper respiratory allergy. However, serum IgE determinations are not often of practical value in the management of asthma and are usually not indicated. However, they are helpful to diagnose and monitor the effects of therapy of bronchopulmonary aspergillosis, which commonly has significantly elevated serum IgE levels.

In the extrinsic asthmatic patient in whom environmental allergens are suspected as clinically significant causative agents, allergy skin testing or RAST testing is indicated to aid in management (see Chap. 2).

8. **Pulmonary function testing**

a. **Functional abnormalities in asthma.** The principal functional abnormality in asthma is reversible airways obstruction, reflected by a reduction in forced expiratory volume in 1 second (FEV_1) or in peak expiratory flow rate (PEFR), which improves toward or to normal shortly after administration of a bronchodilator drug (Fig. 6-1). The improvement in FEV_1 is generally greater than 20% of the baseline value. This response indicates the presence of reversible bronchospasm, since narrowing of the airways by mucus or inflammatory edema would not respond so rapidly to drug therapy. However, failure of the FEV_1 to improve significantly after bronchodilator administration does not exclude the diagnosis of asthma. Lack of bronchodilator responsiveness can be due to several factors: (1) minimal or no airways obstruction at baseline during remissions of asthma, leaving little room for improvement; (2) residual effects of preceding bronchodilator therapy; (3) ineffective delivery of bronchodilator aerosol; (4) reflex bronchospastic response to airway irritation due to an ingredient in the bronchodilator aerosol; or (5) a bronchoconstrictor effect of the testing maneuvers themselves (spirometer-induced bronchospasm).

(1) During remissions of asthma, the FEV_1 is often normal. FEV_1 and PEFR generally reflect changes mainly in the large airways and are not very sensitive tests for the detection of obstruction in smaller airways. Consequently, significant narrowing of small airways (< 2–3 mm in diameter) may be present, as indicated by a reduction in the FEF rate over the middle half of the vital capacity ($FEF_{25-75\%}$), even when the FEV_1 and PEFR are still both normal; however, patients exhibiting isolated abnormalities in $FEF_{25-75\%}$ are usually asymptomatic. When the FEV_1 is reduced, the predominant site of obstruction could be in **either** large or small airways since very extensive abnormalities in the small airways can contribute to reduction in FEV_1.

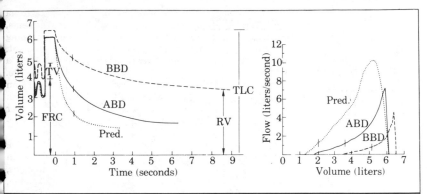

Function	Before bronchodilator		After bronchodilator	
	Obs.	% Pred.	Obs.	% Pred.
FVC(liters)	3.17	67	4.39	93
FEV$_1$(liters)	1.57	39	2.66	66
FEV$_1$/FVC(%)	49	58	60	71
PEFR*(liters/second)	4.85	46	7.60	72
FEF$_{25-75\%}$ (liters/second)	0.63	14	1.43	33
TLC(liters)	6.48	104	6.24	100
FRC(liters)	3.96	132	3.04	101
RV(liters)	3.31	215	1.85	120
DLCO(ml/minute/mm Hg)			35.0	109

*Determined from maximal expiratory flow-volume curve or by Wright Peak Flow Meter.

Fig. 6-1. Forced expiratory volume-time curve (spirogram) and maximal expiratory flow-volume curve in a 32-year-old woman with moderate asthma before and after inhalation of 250 µg isoproterenol from a pressurized hand-nebulizer. FVC = forced vital capacity; FEV$_1$ = forced expiratory volume in 1 second; FEF$_{25-75\%}$ = forced expiratory flow rate between 25 and 75% of VC; PEFR = peak expiratory flow rate calculated from maximal expiratory flow-volume curve (alternatively, may be determined using a Wright Peak Flow Meter or estimated from the maximal slope of the timed spirogram); TLC = total lung capacity; TV = tidal volume; FRC = functional residual capacity; RV = residual volume; DLCO = diffusing capacity for carbon monoxide; BBD = before bronchodilator; ABD = after bronchodilator; Obs. = observed; Pred. = predicted. Vertical lines intersecting volume-time and flow-volume curves identify volume below TLC corresponding to FEV$_1$.

(2) **Maximal expiratory flow-volume curves** obtained with the patient breathing air and a low-density gas mixture (80% helium, 20% oxygen) are required to determine the major site of airways obstruction in asthma. In those patients exhibiting substantial density-dependence of flow ($\geq$ 20% increase in flow on breathing the low-density gas mixture compared with the flow rate with air), the large airways are the major site of flow limitation. In those without density-dependence of flow, the smaller airways are the predominant site of obstruction. In mild asthmatic patients, the larger airways are generally the major site of flow limitation. More severe asth-

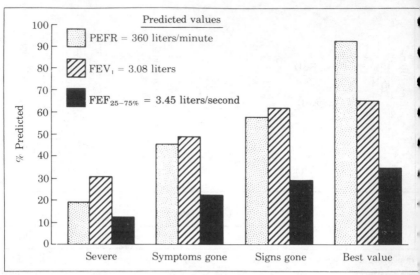

Fig. 6-2. Pattern of abnormalities in forced expiratory volume and flow rates at different stages during recovery from acute attack of severe asthma in a 25-year-old woman. Height of bars indicates percentage of predicted value. PEFR = peak expiratory flow rate; FEV_1 = forced expiratory volume in 1 second; $FEF_{25-75\%}$ = forced expiratory flow rate over the middle half of the vital capacity (maximal midexpiratory flow rate).

matic patients, especially those who smoke, cough chronically, or have frequent respiratory tract infections, are more likely to have predominantly small airways obstruction. Changes in small airways are frequently less reversible than those in large airways.

(3) During an attack of asthma, FEV_1, PEFR, and $FEF_{25-75\%}$ decrease in relation to the severity of the obstruction. During treatment of a severe attack, improvement in these indices of airflow obstruction parallels clinical improvement (Fig. 6-2). The more rapid increases in PEFR and FEV_1 toward normal (compared with $FEF_{25-75\%}$) indicate greater therapeutic responsiveness of obstruction in large than small airways; obstruction in peripheral bronchi is often due to less reversible changes of inflammatory edema and mucus plugging, which require more prolonged therapy.

(4) **Vital capacity (VC)** is often reduced during an acute attack of asthma as well as in chronic asthma. The reduction in vital capacity is due to an increase in **residual volume (RV)**, which encroaches on the vital capacity (Fig. 6-3). The increased residual volume is due to premature closure of obstructed small airways, resulting in air trapping. **Functional residual capacity (FRC),** the volume of gas in the lungs at the end of a normal breath, and **total lung capacity (TLC)**, are also frequently increased, due to air trapping and increased resistance to flow, making breathing at normal lung volumes difficult; therefore, breathing is accomplished at higher lung volumes at which the larger diameter of the airways offers a mechanical advantage. This mechanical advantage is offset, however, by the increased elastic work of breathing at higher lung volumes at which the lungs are less compliant. The abnormalities in static lung volumes (decreased VC and increased RV, FRC, and TLC) become progressively worse with increasing severity of airflow obstruction (Fig.

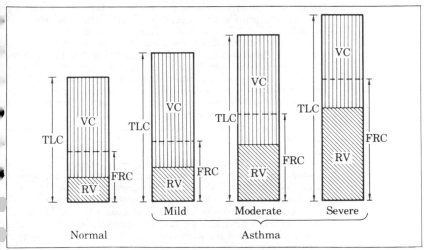

Fig. 6-3. Pattern of abnormalities in various subdivisions of lung volume in asthma of varying severity. VC = vital capacity; RV = residual volume; FRC = functional residual capacity; TLC = total lung capacity.

6-3) and are at least partially reversed by bronchodilator therapy. Complete reversal of hyperinflation after recovery from a prolonged attack of asthma may be slow. Occasional patients with severe asthma exhibit notable subjective improvement during therapy with no or little increase in FEV_1. In such patients, RV, TLC, and FRC are markedly elevated initially and fall considerably during therapy, so that the posttreatment FEV_1 is measured at a lower absolute lung volume at which the airways are relatively narrower and thus offer more resistance to flow. Relief of dyspnea in these patients is due to reduction in the FRC toward normal, with a corresponding reduction in the markedly increased **elastic** work of inspiration associated with the very high FRC that was present before treatment.

(5) The **single-breath nitrogen washout test** allows calculation of $\Delta N_2/$liter (the change in nitrogen concentration/liter of exhaled alveolar gas after a single deep inhalation of 100% oxygen) and of **closing volume (CV)** (the volume at which dependent lung zones begin to close). Abnormal increases in $\Delta N_2/$liter and CV reflect maldistribution of ventilation and obstruction in small airways. $\Delta N_2/$liter and CV are frequently abnormally elevated in asthma, even when the disease is mild, asymptomatic, and unassociated with demonstrable abnormalities in spirometry. However, these tests are of only marginal value in diagnosis and offer little assistance as guides to management.

(6) **Diffusing capacity** for carbon monoxide (D_LCO) is usually normal (or even supernormal) in asthma since, in contrast to emphysema, the alveolar-capillary membrane in the gas-exchanging portion of the lung is uninvolved in asthma. It is sometimes of value to measure D_LCO in older individuals with suspected asthma to exclude emphysema.

b. **Techniques of measurement of lung function** (see Appendix IX for normal age- and sex-matched values).

(1) **Vital capacity, FEV_1, and $FEF_{25-75\%}$** are measured with a water-seal or dry spirometer, preferably one that provides a permanent record

of forced expired volume versus time (see Fig. 6-1). Electronic spirometers provide the capability of expressing instantaneous forced expiratory flow rates as a function of volume (flow-volume curve); however, the flow-volume representation offers few advantages over the conventional volume-time plot (Fig. 6-1). Peak expiratory flow can be measured with a Wright peak flow meter or derived from the volume-time curve (maximum slope) or the flow-volume curve (peak flow). The validity of the measurements of forced expiratory volume and flow depends on the accuracy of the instrument and the full cooperation of the patient. In the physically exhausted patient suffering from a severe attack of asthma, it is often impossible to obtain reliable measurements of VC or forced expiratory flow (FEF).

(2) Measurement of **airway resistance** (R_{aw}) with a whole-body plethysmograph is occasionally useful in the evaluation of the response of an asthmatic patient to bronchodilator therapy when the FEV_1 does not change or appears to decrease paradoxically following a bronchodilator. Such "paradoxical" FEV_1 responses can be due to the constrictor effect of a single maximal inspiration or to dynamic airway compression of the more compliant "relaxed" airways during forced exhalation. These effects can be obviated by measurement of R_{aw} since the latter does not require deep inhalation or forced exhalation maneuvers, which can induce bronchoconstriction in some asthmatic patients. Airway resistance is elevated in asthma and decreases appreciably (usually > 35%) after bronchodilator therapy. **Partial expiratory flow-volume curves,** in which patients inhale submaximally before exhaling forcibly, are another means of avoiding such spirometer-induced bronchospasm when assessing responses of asthmatic patients to bronchodilator therapy.

(3) Measurement of the various subdivisions of lung volume **(RV, TLC, FRC)** is accomplished using an inert gas-dilution or N_2 washout technique or a whole-body plethysmograph, all of which are generally available only in specially equipped hospital laboratories.

c. **Indications for pulmonary function testing** are as follows: (1) confirming the diagnosis of asthma by documenting the presence of reversible airflow obstruction; (2) quantitating the severity of the obstruction and determining its reversibility in response to a bronchodilator; (3) following the course of a hospitalized patient with severe asthma or of an outpatient with chronic asthma who requires maintenance bronchodilator medication (particularly if corticosteroids are being used) to serve as a guide for changes in therapy; and (4) preoperative evaluation of risk for surgery. Simple measurements of FEV_1 and VC or of PEFR alone suffice as a guide for routine office management or for following the course of an asthmatic patient in the emergency room or hospital. A complete set of pulmonary function tests (including timed spirometry, lung volume measurements, and, at times, diffusing capacity determination) should be obtained only for diagnostic purposes or after the patient has been optimally treated. For patients with suspected asthma in remission in whom documentation of reversible obstructive airways disease is desired for diagnostic purposes, a methacholine inhalation challenge test (see **10**) can be very helpful.

9. **Arterial blood gases.** Arterial PO_2 (PaO_2) (see Appendix X for mean values, prediction equation, and hemoglobin dissociation curve) is often decreased, even in asymptomatic asthma, as a result of maldistribution of airflow in relation to pulmonary blood flow. At times, PaO_2 may be normal, but the alveolar-arterial oxygen difference [(A-a)DO_2] is abnormally widened.

a. To determine (A-a)DO_2, PaO_2 is calculated from the alveolar gas equation:

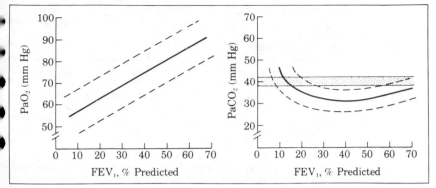

Fig. 6-4. Arterial PO_2 and PCO_2 values in asthma in relation to airflow obstruction of varying severity (indicated by percentage of predicted FEV_1). Shaded area represents normal range of $PaCO_2$ values. FEV_1 = forced expiratory volume in 1 second.

$$PAO_2 = PIO_2 - \frac{PaCO_2}{R},$$

where PIO_2 (inspired PO_2) = 150 mm Hg at sea level and R = 0.8. Therefore, if the arterial PCO_2 ($PaCO_2$) is low, PAO_2 may be normal or near-normal despite an abnormality in oxygenation as indicated by a widened $(A-a)DO_2$.

b. Acute attacks of asthma are accompanied by further impairment in oxygenation, as indicated by decreases in PaO_2 that are proportional to the severity of the obstruction of flow (Fig. 6-4). Conversely, acute attacks of asthma are often associated with **hyperventilation** (decreased $PaCO_2$), the magnitude of which is **inversely** proportional to the severity of the attack (Fig. 6-4). Therefore, mild attacks may result in considerable hyperventilation, and severe attacks may result in little or no hyperventilation or even **hypoventilation** ($PaCO_2 > 42$ mm Hg). Consequently, the presence of an elevated or even normal $PaCO_2$ in a dyspneic patient during an attack of asthma indicates a severe degree of obstruction and the need for aggressive therapy and frequent monitoring of arterial blood gases.

c. Arterial pH is usually normal or slightly **alkaline** during asthmatic attacks of mild to moderate severity due to the accompanying hypocapnia **(respiratory alkalosis)** with or without metabolic compensation through renal bicarbonate loss. However, in severe asthma ($FEV_1 < 15$–20% predicted), varying degrees of **acidemia** may occur as a result of **metabolic acidosis** (base excess < -2 mEq/liter) (due to lactic acid accumulation) with or without accompanying respiratory acidosis ($PaCO_2 > 42$ mm Hg) (due to alveolar hypoventilation). Metabolic (lactic) acidosis is probably secondary to (1) the markedly increased work of breathing associated with severe airflow obstruction and hyperinflation, and (2) tissue hypoxia due to reduced venous return (and reduced cardiac output) associated with hyperinflation and arterial hypoxemia.

d. **Arterial blood gases should be obtained in any patient who exhibits features of severe acute asthma** (marked dyspnea, relative resistance to bronchodilator drugs, tachypnea, tachycardia, signs of hyperinflation, use of accessory muscles of respiration, suprasternal retractions, and pulsus paradoxus), especially if there is any disturbance of consciousness. If significant hypoxemia ($PaO_2 < 60$ mm Hg) and/or a normal or elevated PCO_2 are present, vigorous therapy, including supplemental oxygen, is required, and arterial blood gases need to be monitored serially to ascertain the adequacy of arterial oxygenation, alveolar ventilation, and tissue perfusion.

10. Bronchial provocation

   a. The inhalation of the cholinergic agent methacholine (Provocholine) produces a reduction of airflow in most asthmatic patients, in most of those with a history of asthma, and in many of those with upper respiratory allergy without asthma. Less than 10% of normal persons have positive responses. False-positive responses may occur with a recent upper respiratory infection ($<$ 6 weeks), recent influenza vaccination, and heavy allergen or air pollution exposure. False-negative responses sometimes occur with concurrent bronchodilator therapy.

   (1) The test is done by first determining the FEV_1 and then comparing the FEV_1 2–3 minutes after inhalation of a control substance (normal saline) and various dilutions of methacholine (the reduction of FEV_1 after inhalation of the control substance should not be more than 10%).

   (2) A **positive** response to methacholine is defined as a reduction of FEV_1 of more than 20% below the postdiluent control. The test solutions are administered as a nebulized mist in one to five deep inhalations, beginning with a concentration of 0.075 mg/ml and doubling the concentration with successive challenges every 5 minutes until a positive result is observed. At the maximal concentration of 25 mg/ml, a **negative** response indicates a negative challenge test.

   (3) **Histamine** can be substituted for methacholine in bronchial provocation testing since the response is similar in most patients. The test is done in the same manner as with methacholine inhalation. The concentration of histamine begins at 0.03 mg/ml and is doubled with each challenge to a maximum of 10 mg/ml. A negative response at 10 mg/ml indicates a negative test.

   (4) **Other provocation tests** include exercise challenge; inhalation of cold, dry air with isocapnic hyperventilation; and hypotonic saline inhalation accompanied by the measurement of changes in airflow.

   b. When extrinsic allergens are suspected as possible provocative factors in asthmatic attacks on the basis of allergy skin testing or a radioallergosorbent test (RAST), but the clinical significance is not clear from the history, bronchial provocation testing with an allergen can sometimes help to determine the significance of that allergen. This test is difficult and time-consuming, and can precipitate an acute or delayed asthma attack. **Bronchial provocation with methacholine, histamine, or allergen should be done in a controlled setting by experienced personnel and only during a symptom-free interval (FEV_1 $\geq$ 75% of predicted).**

   (1) Administer the test material in the same manner as a methacholine challenge, preceded by measurement of FEV_1 and response to a diluent control.

   (2) Begin provocation with five inhalations of an allergen in a 1:1,000,000 dilution and then serial dilutions of 1:500,000; 1:100,000; 1:50,000; 1:10,000; 1:5000; 1:1000; 1:500; and 1:100; given at 10-minute intervals until a positive response is obtained. A reduction of FEV_1 of 20% or more lasting for 10–20 minutes after inhalation indicates a **positive** response. A **negative** response to a 1:100 dilution of allergen indicates a **negative** response.

   (3) Use only one allergen in a single day, and instruct the patient, if tolerated, to stop bronchodilator drugs, cromolyn sodium, and antihistamines for 24 hours prior to testing.

   (4) Delayed asthma attacks can occur (4–12 hours after bronchial provocation testing), even when the immediate response is negative.

Therefore, warn the patient, or if asthma is severe, observe the patient for at least 12 hours after testing.

III. **Complications**
   A. **Infection** can occur secondary to an acute or chronic asthmatic attack or can precede asthma symptoms and precipitate an attack. Respiratory infections commonly initiate wheezing in both childhood and adult asthma. Young children are particularly prone to the development of wheezing with "colds," which frequently is the early presentation of asthma. **Any child who has repeated chest colds and bronchitis should be suspected of having asthma.**
      1. **Viral respiratory infections** alone are the principal types implicated in provoking asthma attacks. Respiratory syncytial virus, parainfluenza, influenza, rhinovirus, and adenovirus are the most common and probably act by directly triggering the hyperactive airway of the asthmatic patient, although other mechanisms have been suggested, including virus-specific IgE antibody, virus-induced beta-adrenergic subsensitivity, and virus-enhanced mediator release.
      2. **Bacterial infections** are not usually involved in precipitating attacks, and mycoplasmal agents are of questionable importance.
      3. **Pneumonia** can occur secondary to an asthma attack, usually when attacks are persistent, with increased mucus accumulation and mucus plugging. Viral pneumonia is most common under the age of 5 years. *Mycoplasma* pneumonia is most common from 5–30 years, and bacterial pneumonia, especially pneumococcal, is most common after 30 years.
   B. **Atelectasis.** Lobar, segmental, or subsegmental atelectasis can occur in both acute and chronic asthma, usually secondary to bronchial obstruction with mucus plugs. Atelectasis should be suspected in the patient who has worsening or persistence of cough, wheezing, dyspnea, or fever following a course of therapy, especially when associated with the findings of localized, reduced breath sounds and dullness to percussion. Atelectasis of the right middle lobe is common and can go undetected in an asymptomatic patient. The diagnosis of atelectasis is substantiated by chest x-ray. Atelectasis is most common in young children and frequently recurs at the same site.
   C. **Pneumothorax and pneumomediastinum**
      1. **Pneumothorax** is an uncommon complication in acute asthma. Recurrence in the same patient suggests the presence of some other anatomic abnormality (e.g., pulmonary bleb or cyst, congenital lobar emphysema). Repeated or violent coughing or intermittent positive pressure breathing (IPPB) can precipitate pneumothorax. The latter should be suspected if there is a sudden development of pleuritic chest pain associated with dyspnea, tachypnea, and, occasionally, cough. Pneumothorax is confirmed by chest x-ray. A small pneumothorax ($<$ 25%), if unassociated with severe dyspnea or chest pain, may be allowed to resolve spontaneously with bed rest. Most patients with pneumothorax have a lung collapse greater than 25% and are best treated with closed thoracotomy and water-seal drainage with or without suction.
      2. **Pneumomediastinum** and **subcutaneous emphysema,** usually involving the neck and clavicular area, are more common than pneumothorax. They are usually asymptomatic and are detected as an incidental finding on chest x-ray or as soft-tissue swelling or a crunching sound on skin pressure about the neck and chest. A crunching sound on auscultation over the heart (Hamman's crunch) indicates mediastinal emphysema. Pneumomediastinum and subcutaneous emphysema can be precipitated by vigorous coughing or by the use of a positive pressure breathing apparatus. Pneumomediastinum can present with substernal pain and, in more severe cases, dyspnea, tachypnea, tachycardia, hypotension, and cyanosis, especially over the upper body. Most patients require no treatment, but in patients with severe disease (cardiovascular and respiratory compromise), needle aspiration or mediastinostomy is necessary.

Table 6-1. Differential diagnosis of asthma

Acute onset
  Respiratory infections
  Cardiac failure
  Aspiration
  Upper airway obstruction: hypertrophic tonsils and adenoids, foreign body, angio-
    edema, epiglottiditis, and laryngeal infections
  Hyperventilation
  Pneumothorax
  Pulmonary embolism
Chronic presentation
  Chronic obstructive lung disease
  Allergic bronchopulmonary aspergillosis and hypersensitivity pneumonitis
  Chronic upper respiratory obstruction: foreign body, hypertrophic tonsils and
    adenoids, laryngeal disease, subglottic stenosis, tracheomalacia, tracheal tumor,
    and vascular ring
  Central airway obstruction: bronchogenic carcinoma, sarcoidosis, vasculitis
  Factitious asthma
  Carcinoid syndrome
  Cystic fibrosis
  Alpha-1-antitrypsin deficiency

D. **Bronchiectasis** rarely occurs in asthma; when it does occur, it is usually associated with concomitant chronic bronchitis, persistent atelectasis, chronic infection, or allergic bronchopulmonary aspergillosis. Chronic cough, purulent sputum, and hemoptysis are frequent symptoms. Digital clubbing, which does not occur in uncomplicated asthma, is a suggestive physical finding. The diagnosis can sometimes be made by chest x-ray but usually requires tomography or computerized axial tomography and, in rare instances, bronchography.

E. **Bronchopulmonary aspergillosis** is an infestation by and hypersensitivity to the organism *Aspergillus fumigatus*. It occurs primarily in adult asthmatic patients (see Chap. 7).

F. **Cardiovascular complications.** Arrhythmias are the most common cardiovascular complication in asthma and vary from occasional premature ventricular contractions to severe or fatal ventricular arrhythmias. Arrhythmias are more common in asthmatic patients with underlying cardiac disease and are aggravated by hypoxemia and the excessive use of adrenergic drugs. Right heart strain can occur during an acute asthma attack, but right heart failure is rare except in the presence of prolonged severe hypoxemia and fluid overload. Pulmonary hypertension may occur during an acute asthma attack, but cor pulmonale is rare unless it is associated with chronic bronchitis, emphysema, or both.

Treatment is directed at relieving hypoxemia by oxygen administration and by the minimization of systemic adrenergic bronchodilator and theophylline therapy in the case of arrhythmias. In severe arrhythmias and right heart failure, digitalis (if the arrhythmia is not digitalis-related) and other antiarrhythmic agents (observing for complications of bronchospasm with beta-blocking agents and emphasizing calcium-channel blockers, e.g., verapamil) may be required.

G. **Status asthmaticus and respiratory failure.** See sec. VII.

IV. **Differential diagnosis.** It is important to differentiate conditions with an **acute onset** of respiratory symptoms from an acute asthma attack (Table 6-1). It is also necessary to differentiate conditions associated with **chronic** or **prolonged** episodic respiratory symptoms from chronic asthma.

A. **Acute onset**

1. **Respiratory infections,** especially bronchiolitis, bronchitis, croup, epiglottiditis, tonsillitis, and tonsillar abscess, can present with acute onset of

respiratory difficulty and wheezing. Bronchiolitis is more common in infancy; upper respiratory infection with obstruction is more common in childhood. The response to bronchodilator therapy and persistence or recurrence of wheezing usually distinguish asthma from these conditions.

2. **Left ventricular failure,** especially with pulmonary edema, can present with acute respiratory distress and wheezing. A concomitant history of cardiac disease, the findings of crackles or moist rales in the chest, and a third heart sound on auscultation will usually distinguish this condition from asthma.

3. **Aspiration** of a foreign body, with lodgment in a main stem, lobar, or segmental bronchus, can cause wheezing. A history and physical finding of unilateral wheezing will usually distinguish it from asthma. A chest x-ray may reveal a foreign body, segmental or lobar atelectasis, or unilateral hyperinflation. Bronchoscopy may be necessary to confirm the diagnosis and for treatment.

4. **Upper airway obstruction.** Patients with acute obstruction of the upper airway present with respiratory difficulty that is usually accentuated on inspiration. Common causes include hypertrophic tonsils and adenoids, aspirated foreign body, epiglottiditis, laryngeal infections, laryngeal dysfunction, and hysterical laryngospasm ("factitious asthma").

5. **Hyperventilation** is associated with rapid, shallow respirations and is usually accompanied by anxiety and peripheral numbness and tingling. Hyperventilation can also occur during an asthmatic attack. This condition is generally evident from the history and physical findings and is improved by reassurance and relaxation. Rebreathing from a bag is helpful, but not advised in patients during an acute asthma attack or patients with chronic obstructive lung disease in whom hypoxemia is suspected.

6. **Pneumothorax.** See sec. III.C.

7. **Pulmonary embolism** usually presents with tachypnea and dyspnea with or without cough, hemoptysis, and pleuritic chest pain, depending on the development of associated pulmonary infarction. There is often a history of predisposing factors (e.g., congestive heart failure, obesity, malignancy, thrombophlebitis, prolonged bed rest, oral contraceptives). The arterial PO_2 is characteristically, but not necessarily, low (≤ 60 mm Hg), but the alveolar-arterial oxygen gradient is almost always widened. The diagnosis may be supported by a ventilation-perfusion lung scan but often requires pulmonary angiography for definitive confirmation.

B. **Chronic presentation**

1. Clinically, **chronic obstructive pulmonary disease,** including chronic bronchitis, emphysema, and bronchiectasis, can mimic the findings of asthma. These conditions are distinguished by their relative lack of significant reversibility in response to bronchodilator therapy. Each of these conditions can coexist in asthmatic patients, and more detailed studies (pulmonary function testing and radiographic studies) may be necessary to determine their presence.

2. **Allergic bronchopulmonary aspergillosis and hypersensitivity pneumonitis.** See Chap. 7.

3. **Chronic upper respiratory obstruction** caused by a foreign body, hypertrophic tonsils and adenoids, laryngeal disease, or, less commonly, subglottic stenosis, tracheomalacia, tracheal tumor, and vascular ring presents with episodic or persistent respiratory difficulty, usually with inspiratory stridor.

4. **Carcinoid syndrome** can be associated with episodic wheezing similar to that of asthma. The diagnosis is confirmed by a history of paroxysmal flushing and diarrhea and the presence of increased 5-hydroxyindoleacetic acid in the urine.

5. **Cystic fibrosis** presents as a chronic obstructive pulmonary disease, usually in childhood, and is manifested by chronic cough, wheezing, and recurrent infections. Malabsorption, foul, bulky stools, and failure to thrive are

common. The diagnosis is confirmed by a sweat chloride concentration greater than 60 mEq/liter.

6. **Alpha-1-antitrypsin deficiency,** an inherited autosomal recessive disorder, is characterized by the onset of progressive emphysema, usually in young adulthood. Although homozygotes express the disease, emphysema can also develop in heterozygotes. The diagnosis is confirmed by measuring the serum alpha-1-antitrypsin level and by protease inhibitor phenotyping.

V. Therapeutic modalities

A. **Nonpharmacologic measures.** Drug therapy is the basis of treatment for symptomatic asthma. Nonpharmacologic measures are primarily for the prevention of symptoms or as adjuncts to drug therapy.

1. **Education.** The more patients understand asthma the better they can cope with its symptoms and comply with treatment. Instruction materials are available from a number of sources (e.g., the American Lung Association, the National Institute of Allergy and Infectious Disease, and the Asthma and Allergy Foundation of America).

2. **Avoidance** or minimization of exposure to known trigger factors is the most important aspect of prevention. The initial evaluation should attempt to determine all known exposures (e.g., diet, drugs, habits, hobbies, work, home, allergen exposure, emotional factors, climate, infections) (see Chap. 2). Decisions to relocate the home or change occupations should be made only after careful consideration of alternative measures.

Table 6-7 presents a complete list of inciting allergens or chemicals associated with various occupations. Environmental control measures are presented in Table 4-1.

3. **Immunotherapy** for appropriate allergens, determined by skin testing, RAST, or bronchial provocation, is helpful in the management of extrinsic asthma (see Chap. 4). **Immunotherapy does not preclude attempts at environmental control.**

4. **Relaxation and control of emotional factors,** especially at the onset of or during an acute attack, may help abort or relieve symptoms. To be effective, this requires education and practice during symptom-free periods. Since panic is a definite component of any attack and tends to increase the respiratory rate and aggravate bronchospasm, patients should be trained to relax their breathing.

a. The following instructions are helpful: Cease activity and relax. Take slow, deep breaths. Place one hand on the upper abdomen to determine expansion (diaphragmatic movement). Inhale through the nose, letting the abdominal area expand (instead of the upper chest). Slowly exhale through pursed lips (as though blowing out a candle), allowing the abdominal muscles to relax.

b. The following **positions** will enhance relaxation and abdominal breathing (whichever suits the patient):

(1) **Sitting in a chair**

(a) **First position.** Lean forward, resting the elbows on the knees.

(b) **Second position.** Lean forward over a table, resting the shoulders, arms, and head on a pillow placed on the table. When short of breath for a prolonged period, one can sleep in this position.

(2) **Standing**

(a) **First position.** Stand facing a wall, about 12–18 in. away, with the forearms resting against the wall. Rest the head on the forearms, and put one foot forward in a stepping position to relax abdominal muscles.

(b) **Second position.** Lean with the back against a wall, with the feet about 12 in. from the wall and the knees and trunk slightly bent.

c. The patient should be encouraged to practice relaxed breathing exercises frequently during symptom-free periods.

d. Other measures that are helpful in controlling anxiety and enhancing relaxation include transcendental meditation, autohypnosis, progressive relaxation training, and relaxation with biofeedback. Identification and control of ongoing stress factors are an important part of prevention. Psychiatric or psychological counseling may be necessary for patients with complicating emotional disorders.

5. **Fluid therapy** is important to prevent or treat dehydration and thereby reduce the viscosity of mucus and enhance expectoration. Instruct asthmatic patients to increase fluid intake even during symptom-free periods. Oral fluids should be increased at the start of symptoms and continued unless vomiting is aggravated. More severe attacks are usually associated with some degree of dehydration because of reduced fluid intake and increased fluid loss resulting from hyperventilation, sweating, and/or vomiting. In such instances, especially in unresponsive attacks and status asthmaticus, intravenous fluid therapy is indicated. Volumes and rates of fluid administration vary with the extent of dehydration; attention should be given to possible overload (i.e., pulmonary edema), especially during prolonged treatment.

6. **Postural drainage with chest percussion and vibration** is helpful in mobilizing and facilitating expectoration of mucus in patients with acute attacks of asthma complicated by atelectasis, mucus plugging, or pneumonia. These measures can also be useful in the chronic asthmatic patient with thick or copious sputum. The procedure is usually well tolerated in patients with moderate symptoms but may aggravate wheezing in more severe attacks. Patients often notice improvement about 30 minutes after these procedures, but if, instead, symptoms worsen, the procedures should be discontinued. Postural drainage is best accomplished after periods of recumbency (e.g., morning awakening) and may be repeated 2–3 times a day, depending on need. Postural drainage should be preceded by inhalation of a nebulized or pressurized bronchodilator.

   a. The patient is placed in various chest-dependent positions to permit gravity drainage of secretions. For 1–2 minutes, a therapist applies percussion with cupped hands over the chest area to be drained. The patient is encouraged to breathe slowly and deeply. In individual patients, particular positions are chosen or emphasized based on clinical or radiographic evidence of retained secretions. Figure 6-5 presents the various positions and areas of percussion to drain specific segments.

   b. These maneuvers are **contraindicated** in patients with hemoptysis, pneumothorax, or convulsions.

7. **Oxygen** is indicated for acute attacks in which hypoxemia is pronounced (documented clinically or by arterial blood gas analysis).

   a. Oxygen must be **fully humidified** and can be administered by nasal cannula, face mask, or Venturi mask. Small children who do not tolerate nasal cannulas or face masks may require tents; however, in tents, oxygen levels are more difficult to maintain and monitor.

   b. Administer oxygen at **low flow rates,** usually 2–4 liters/minute, trying to maintain the arterial PO_2 level between 70 and 100 mm Hg. Hypoventilation secondary to oxygen therapy may occur in hypercapnic patients, but this is more common in patients with chronic obstructive pulmonary disease than in others.

B. **Drug therapy**

   1. **Bronchodilators**

      a. **Adrenergic drugs** (see Chap. 4) act by directly stimulating the alpha- and beta-adrenergic receptors of the sympathetic nervous system. Alpha-adrenergic receptor stimulation leads primarily to vasoconstriction, uterine contraction, intestinal smooth-muscle relaxation and sphincter contraction, ureteral contraction, contraction of the spleen, and pupillary dilatation. There are two types of beta-adrenergic receptors: the **beta-1 receptor,** which, when stimulated, promotes cardiac contraction, acceleration of heart rate, relaxation of coronary artery and

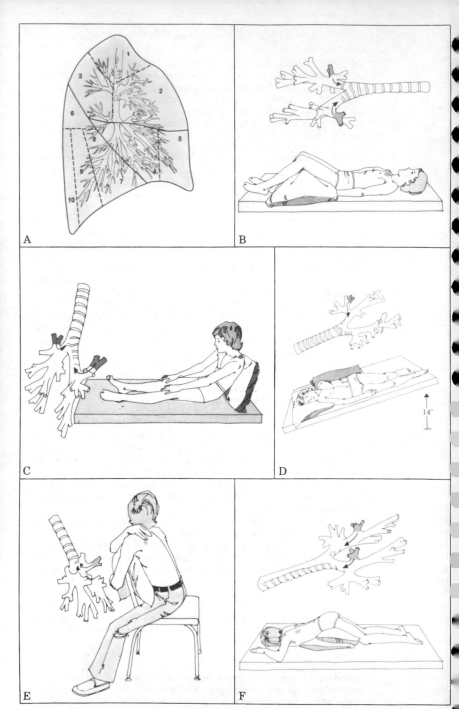

Fig. 6-5. Positions for postural drainage of various lung segments. **A.** Segments of the lung (right or left). Numerals refer to segments drained by various positions. **B.** Upper lobes, anterior segment 2, bed or drainage table flat. Patient lies flat on back with pillow under knees. (Clap between clavicle and nipple on each side of chest.) **C.** Upper lobes, apical segment 1, bed or drainage table flat. Patient leans back on pillow at a

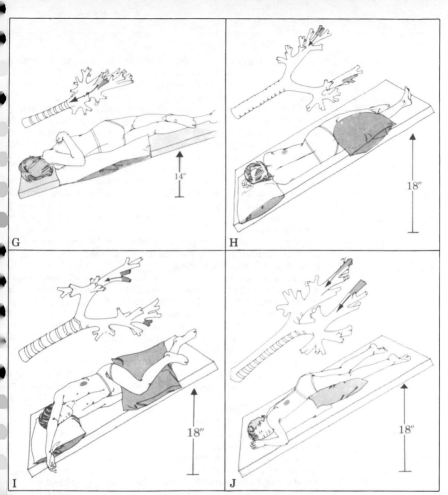

30-degree angle. (Clap over area between clavicle and top of scapula on each side.) **D.** Left upper lobe, lingular segment, superior 4, inferior 5, foot of table or bed elevated 14 in. or about 15 degrees. Patient lies head down on right side and rotates one-quarter turn backward. Pillow may be placed behind patient from shoulder to hip. Knees should be flexed. (Clap over left nipple area.) **E.** Upper lobes, posterior segment 3, bed or drainage table flat. Patient leans over folded pillow at a 30-degree angle. (Clap over upper back on each side of chest.) **F.** Lower lobes, superior segment 6, bed or table flat. Patient lies on abdomen with pillows under hips. (Clap over middle of back below tip of scapula on either side of spine.) **G.** Right middle lobe, lateral segment 4, medial segment 5, foot of table or bed elevated 14 in. or about 15 degrees. Patient lies head down on left side and rotates one-quarter turn backward. Pillow may be placed behind patient from shoulder to hip. Knees should be flexed. (Clap over right nipple area.) **H.** Lower lobes, lateral basal segment 9, foot of table or bed elevated 18 in. or 30 degrees. Patient lies on abdomen, then rotates one-quarter turn upward. Upper leg can be flexed over a pillow for support. (Clap over uppermost portion of lower ribs.) **I.** Lower lobes, anterior basal segment 8, foot of table or bed elevated 18 in. or 30 degrees. Patient lies on side, head down, pillow under knees. (Clap over lower ribs just beneath axilla.) **J.** Lower lobes, posterior basal segment 10, foot of table or bed elevated 18 in. or 30 degrees. Patient lies on abdomen, head down, with pillow under hips. Upper leg can be flexed over a pillow for support. (Clap over lower ribs close to spine on each side of chest.) (A–J adapted from B. C. Hilman. *The How and Why of Bronchial Drainage.* New York: Breon Laboratories, 1979.)

intestinal smooth muscle, and stimulation of lipolysis; and the **beta-2 receptor,** which, when activated, leads to relaxation of bronchial smooth muscle, skeletal muscle tremor, uterine relaxation, and promotion of glycogenolysis and glycolysis.

(1) Adrenergic drugs have varying effects on alpha, beta-1 and beta-2 receptors. Agents with predominant beta-2 and minimal beta-1 effects are most suited for the treatment of asthma. Adrenergic drugs are available in injectable, inhaled, and oral forms and are used both in the treatment of acute asthma symptoms and in ongoing maintenance therapy. They can be used alone or in conjunction with methylxanthines. Adrenergic drugs should be used **with caution** in patients with cardiovascular disease, especially cardiac arrhythmias. Maintenance therapy with any beta-adrenergic–stimulating agent may be associated with the development of some degree of subsensitivity. This condition is associated with a reduction in the number of available beta-adrenergic receptors. However, the extent to which subsensitivity develops in bronchial smooth muscle and its clinical significance are unclear.

(2) Intermittent positive pressure breathing (IPPB) or compressor-driven nebulizers as a means of delivering an aerosolized adrenergic bronchodilator are helpful in reversing an acute attack when oral bronchodilators alone are not successful. This modality can be used as an adjunct or an alternative to subcutaneous epinephrine in acute attacks and is also useful in the management of persistent attacks and in conjunction with chest physical therapy. Pressure-cycled machines (usual peak inspiratory pressures, 15–20 mm Hg) powered by compressed oxygen with air mixtures are used for nebulization of a bronchodilator (isoproterenol, isoetharine, metaproterenol, or albuterol) added with 1–3 ml of normal saline to a medication nebulizer. The treatment usually lasts about 5–10 minutes, and the patient is instructed by the therapist to take slow deep breaths with momentary rests. Care must be taken to sterilize and maintain equipment adequately.

(3) The regular use of compressor-driven nebulizers for delivery of an aerosolized bronchodilator in chronic asthma is generally not indicated except in patients who are unable to use simpler hand nebulizers (metered-dose inhalers) properly or fail to achieve relief of symptoms from the latter. Intermittent positive pressure breathing is **contraindicated** when pneumothorax is present, and it should be used with caution in patients with a history of pneumothorax.

(4) Available adrenergic agents include the following:

   (a) Epinephrine (Adrenalin) possesses alpha- and beta-adrenergic activity. It is most useful for immediate relief of an acute asthma attack, especially when oral medications are ineffective. A 1:1000 aqueous solution is injected subcutaneously in a dose of 0.2–0.5 ml (0.01 ml/kg in children). A response is usually noted within 15 minutes. The dose can be repeated at 20-minute intervals. Failure to respond after the **third injection** indicates impending status asthmaticus and need for additional therapy. The **side effects** of epinephrine include tachycardia, nausea, vomiting, headache, hypertension, chest pain, nervousness, tremor, and dizziness. Epinephrine should be used with caution in elderly patients and especially in patients with cardiovascular disease.

   Epinephrine is available in an aqueous suspension (1:200 dilution, Sus-Phrine), which has both immediate and sustained action for 6–8 hours (dosage is 0.1 ml–0.3 ml [0.005 ml/kg in children], given subcutaneously). In an acute attack, it is best to use epinephrine 1:1000 initially to determine the extent of reversibility and to use the suspension 20–30 minutes later for prolonged bronchodilatation. The suspension can be administered at 8-hour intervals. It has the same side effects as epinephrine.

(b) **Ephedrine,** a naturally occurring epinephrinelike compound, is used orally, in liquid or tablet form, frequently in combination with a methylxanthine. It is a less potent bronchodilator than epinephrine, but has the advantage of oral effectiveness. The usual dose is 25–50 mg (0.5–1.0 mg/kg in children) every 4–6 hours. The side effects are similar to those of epinephrine; specifically, it tends to cause nervousness, difficulty in sleeping, and tachycardia, especially in children. Because of these side effects ephedrine has generally been replaced by the more selective beta-2 agonists.

(c) **Ethylnorepinephrine** (Bronkephrine) is an effective bronchodilator with side effects similar to those of epinephrine. It is a short-acting, injectable, aqueous preparation. Indications for its use are similar to those for epinephrine. Dose ranges are 0.3–1.0 ml (0.02 ml/kg in children), given subcutaneously or intramuscularly. It can be repeated at 20-minute intervals as with epinephrine.

(d) **Isoproterenol,** a beta-1 and beta-2 stimulator, is a potent bronchodilator but causes marked cardiac stimulation and vasodilatation. It is relatively inactive orally and is usually administered by inhalation as an aerosol of a 1:100 or 1:200 aqueous solution added to a Venturi-type nebulizer driven by compressed gas or from hand nebulizers (metered-dose inhalers) pressurized with inert propellants (usually dichlorotetrafluoroethane and dichlorodifluoromethane). Inhalation of isoproterenol produces rapid bronchodilatation in seconds to minutes, with diminishing effects over 1–2 hours. In a progressively worsening attack, too-frequent use may fail to produce any significant or lasting bronchodilatation while at the same time exposing the patient to the danger of serious cardiac side effects, such as arrhythmias. In severe attacks with hypoxemia, isoproterenol must be used cautiously since it can further diminish ventilation-perfusion ratios because of its pulmonary vasodilating effect and thereby worsen hypoxemia. Abuse of inhaled bronchodilators is a common problem among asthmatic patients and should be avoided. Longer acting and more selective beta-2 agonists are generally used in place of isoproterenol.

(e) **Isoetharine** is a derivative of isoproterenol that is relatively selective for beta-2-adrenergic receptors and therefore has fewer cardiac side effects than isoproterenol. However, its duration of action is only slightly longer (about 2–3 hours) than that of isoproterenol. It is also administered primarily by inhalation in nebulized mist or metered-dose inhaler (0.34 mg/inhalation, one to two inhalations every 3–4 hours).

(f) **Metaproterenol** is a noncatecholamine isoproterenol derivative with a slower metabolism and, consequently, a longer duration of action (up to 5 hours). It is available both as an oral preparation (dosage, 10–20 mg [0.5 mg/kg in children] every 4–6 hours), as a metered-dose inhaler (0.65 mg/inhalation), one to three inhalations every 4–6 hours, and as a nebulizer solution (5% 0.2–0.3 ml [0.1–0.2 ml in children] in 2.5 ml sterile water or saline) every 4–6 hours. Although not as potent as isoproterenol, its longer duration of action and oral availability make it advantageous. Nervousness, tremor, and tachycardia are the most common side effects. The simultaneous use of oral metaproterenol and metaproterenol by inhalation in the usual recommended doses enhances its bronchodilator effect without appreciably increasing its side effects. (See Table 4-7 for pediatric dosage.)

(g) **Terbutaline** is similar to metaproterenol but has beta-2-adrenergic selectivity and an even longer duration of action. It is used orally (2.5–5.0 mg every 8 hours), by inhalation in a metered-dose inhaler (0.25 mg/inhalation, one to three inhalations every 4–6 hours), or by subcutaneous injection (0.25 mg of a 1 mg/ml solution; not recommended for children) with the same indications as for epinephrine. When injected subcutaneously, terbutaline has a bronchodilator effect equivalent to that of epinephrine, with a comparable duration of action. Unfortunately, it also has comparable cardiac side effects, so that it has only marginal advantages over subcutaneous epinephrine for treatment of an acute asthma attack. Oral terbutaline has a rapid onset of action (within 15–30 minutes), which persists for 6–8 hours. Terbutaline is not recommended for use in children under 12 years of age. Palpitations and nervousness are frequent, but the most common side effect is a nonintentional muscle tremor, which can occur in up to 50% of patients. The tremor frequently diminishes or disappears after regular use of terbutaline.

(h) **Albuterol** has beta-2-adrenergic selectivity similar to that of terbutaline, with a comparable time course of action. It is administered orally (2–4 mg every 6–8 hours) or by inhalation from a metered-dose inhaler (90 μg/inhalation), 2 inhalations every 4–6 hours or nebulizer solution 0.5% (2.5 mg) in adults every 4–6 hours. Its side effects are similar to those of terbutaline, with muscle tremors being the most annoying. (See Table 4-7 for pediatric dosage.)

(i) **Bitolterol** is a catecholamine, selective beta-2-adrenergic agent with a relatively long duration of action. It is administered by inhalation from a metered-dose inhaler (0.37 mg/inhalation, 1–3 inhalations every 8 hours).

(j) **Fenoterol*** is a selective beta-2-adrenergic agent with effects similar to those of terbutaline, albuterol, and bitolterol.

b. **Methylxanthines** produce bronchodilatation by blocking adenosine receptors (stimulation of which cause bronchoconstriction) and possibly by an effect on intracellular calcium. Since these compounds do not act on beta-adrenergic receptors, their action is additive to, or synergistic with, that of the adrenergic drugs.

(1) **Theophylline** is the prototype of this group of agents. In its anhydrous form it is an active bronchodilator whose effectiveness and side effects are directly proportional to serum theophylline concentrations (optimal effectiveness with relatively few side effects is achieved with serum concentrations between 8 and 20 μg/ml). Because of the log-linear relationship between bronchodilator effect and serum concentration, the benefit-risk ratio decreases when serum concentrations are above 15 μg/ml.

(a) **Common side effects** are nausea, vomiting, diarrhea, diuresis, headache, and nervousness. Less obvious side effects are difficulty sleeping, personality disturbances, and poor school or work performance.

(b) Although side effects can occur when serum levels are within the therapeutic range, they are more common when serum concentrations exceed 15–20 μg/ml (Table 6-2). Serum levels are dependent on the rate of hepatic metabolism of theophylline

*Not approved for use in the United States.

Table 6-2. Relationship between theophylline serum concentration and toxic effects

Serum theophylline concentration (μg/ml)*	Toxic effect
15–25	Abdominal cramps
	Agitation
	Diarrhea
	Gastrointestinal upset
	Headache
	Nausea
	Tremors
	Vomiting
25–35	Sinus tachycardia (> 120)
	Occasional premature ventricular contractions
Over 35	Frequent premature ventricular contractions
	Ventricular tachycardia
	Gastrointestinal bleeding
	Grand mal seizures

*These ranges are generalizations. Toxic effects have been observed at higher and lower serum concentrations.

which varies markedly among individuals (see Table 4-8). Children have a more rapid metabolic clearance (0.6–2.2 ml/kg/minute) than adults (0.37–1.57 ml/kg/minute). Clearance is significantly reduced (serum theophylline half-life prolonged) in patients with liver disease and heart failure. Clearance of theophylline is increased (serum half-life shortened) by tobacco or marijuana smoking. Certain drugs alter the metabolism of theophylline or are themselves affected by theophylline. Drugs and other factors affecting theophylline clearance are listed in Table 4-8. The selection of a proper dose of theophylline requires attention to factors affecting clearance (e.g., disease, smoking habits); the dose should be individually titrated in each patient by monitoring effectiveness, side effects, and serum theophylline levels. Dosing frequency of long-acting preparations (every 8–24 hours) can be determined by measuring peak and trough serum levels. Patients with slow metabolism can often be managed successfully with every 24 hour dosing, especially with some long-acting preparations (Uniphyl and Theo-24).

(c) The side effects of nausea or abdominal discomfort are useful end-dose titration points in most patients. However, in certain patients, more serious and **potentially fatal** side effects (cardiac arrhythmias or convulsions and coma) can occur without the early signs of toxicity. Therefore, serum levels should be monitored during dose titration in any patient who is on a high-dose regimen. Serum theophylline determinations using spectrophotometric, high-pressure liquid chromatography or the more rapid enzyme immunoassay techniques can be done in most reference and hospital laboratories. Rapid and accurate serum theophylline levels can be obtained by a monoclonal antibody technique available in self-contained kits (AccuLevel)* ideally suited for office determinations. Salivary theophylline concentration correlates somewhat with serum concentration, but ratios between the two vary over time and among individuals,

*Syntex Medical Diagnostics, Palo Alto, CA 94304.

reducing the usefulness of the salivary theophylline determination.

(d) Administration. Theophylline is administered orally, rectally, and intravenously. Oral administration in liquid (aqueous and hydroalcoholic) or uncoated tablet form results in rapid and complete absorption in the intestine, so that adequate serum levels are reached in 30–60 minutes (liquid and micronized tablet forms are most rapidly absorbed). Long-acting oral preparations in tablet or capsule form reach peak serum levels in 4–? hours and are particularly suited to continuous therapy. Rectal administration is slower and more erratic (liquids are more predictable than suppositories) and is a **less preferred route, especially in suppository form,** except when oral preparations are not tolerated. Theophylline solution is available for intravenous administration.

The usual beginning dose for most adults is 150–200 mg orally every 6 hours with short-acting preparations or 100–200 mg every 12 hours with long-acting preparations. In selecting a beginning dose, consideration must be given to the factors affecting clearance (see Table 4-8). The usual adult maintenance dose range will fall between 100 and 400 mg every 6 hours with short-acting preparations and 200–500 mg every 12 hours for long-acting preparations. Single-dose (24-hour) preparations are effective in a 200- to 1000-mg range, especially in adults but may require every 12 hour divided dosing in patients with more rapid clearance. Bioavailability and absorption vary among the various long-acting preparations available. Some preparations are affected by concurrent food ingestion either by retardation or by rapid absorption, and others are affected by simultaneous administration of antacids. Therefore, caution must be taken with consideration to serum theophylline levels when different preparations or generics are substituted. Children are best started at 16 mg/kg/24 hours (see Chap. 4 for dosing in infants) in divided doses every 6 hours for short-acting preparations and every 8–12 hours for long-acting preparations, but some may require doses above 24 mg/kg/24 hours. Patients who have rapid clearance require more frequent doses (every 4 hours for short-acting preparations and every 8–12 hours for long-acting preparations), to maintain a constant theophylline level. Dose titration can take several days to weeks. In difficult cases, dose changes should be made every 2–3 days, and then the serum theophylline level should be determined at the anticipated peak level (2 hours after the oral dose of a short-acting theophylline and 5 hours after the oral dose of a long-acting theophylline) until it reaches a steady state (i.e., same dose for ? days). See Table 4-9.

Rectal theophylline is administered in a dose range of 250–500 mg (7 mg/kg/12 hours in children) every 8 to 12 hours. Serum theophylline levels should be monitored closely with repeated use of rectal preparations because of irregular absorption. Intravenous theophylline solution* (1.6 mg/ml, which is equivalent to 2 mg/ml of aminophylline) is administered in repeated doses (3–5 mg/kg every 6 hours) or preferably by continuous infusion (0.6–1.0 mg/kg/hour in patients under 50 years of age without other disease; 0.4–0.6 mg/kg/hour in older patients; and 0.1–0.4 mg/kg/hour in those with cardiac or liver disease) after an initial intravenous loading dose (5 mg/kg in patients with no prior

*Travenol Laboratories, Inc., Garden Grove, CA 92647.

Table 6-3. Intravenous aminophylline (theophylline) dosage for patient population (current FDA recommendations)

Not currently receiving theophylline products:

Group	Loading dose[a,b]	Maintenance dose for next 12 hours[a,b]	Maintenance dose beyond 12 hours[a,b]
Children 6 mo–9 yr[c]	6 mg/kg (5)	1.2 mg/kg/hr (1.0)	1.0 mg/kg/hr (0.80)
Children 9–16 and young adult smokers	6 mg/kg (5)	1.0 mg/kg/hr (0.80)	0.8 mg/kg/hr (0.65)
Otherwise healthy nonsmoking adults	6 mg/kg (5)	0.7 mg/kg/hr (0.60)	0.5 mg/kg/hr (0.40)
Older patients and patients with cor pulmonale	6 mg/kg (5)	0.6 mg/kg/hr (0.5)	0.3 mg/kg/hr (0.24)
Patients with congestive heart failure, liver disease	6 mg/kg (5)	0.5 mg/kg/hr (0.4)	0.1–0.2 mg/kg/hr (0.08–0.16)

Currently receiving theophylline products:

1. Determine time, amount, and route of administration of last dose.
2. Determine the loading dose on the expectation that each 0.5 mg/kg (lean body weight) of theophylline (0.6 mg/kg aminophylline) will result in a 1 μg/ml increase in serum theophylline concentration. Defer the loading dose and calculate based on serum theophylline concentration if this can be obtained rapidly.
3. If rapid determination of serum theophylline concentration is unobtainable, there is sufficient respiratory distress, and there is no evidence of theophylline toxicity, give 3 mg/kg aminophylline IV as a loading dose.
4. Maintenance dosage is the same as for those not currently receiving theophylline products.

[a] Based on estimated lean (ideal) body weight.
[b] Equivalent anhydrous theophylline doses are indicated in parentheses.
[c] See Chap. 4 for theophylline dosing in infants.

theophylline; 2 mg/kg in patients who have received theophylline within the past 12–24 hours) (Table 6-3).

(2) **Aminophylline,** an ethylenediamine derivative of theophylline, is an effective bronchodilator when given orally, rectally, or intravenously. It has about 80% of the bioavailability of anhydrous theophylline (Table 6-4). It is metabolized to theophylline, and the indications for its use and its side effects are the same as for theophylline. Aminophylline is more water soluble than pure theophylline, although the newer microcrystalized preparations of anhydrous theophylline have enhanced solubility.

(a) The oral **dosage** should be about 20% higher than for oral theophylline preparations. Aminophylline is available in short-acting liquid and tablets and long-acting tablets. The usual rectal dose is 300 mg every 8 hours (children 5 mg/kg every 8 hours), with the same precautions as for rectal theophylline.

(b) The **major benefit** of aminophylline is its safety in intravenous administration. In persistent, severe attacks, it can be adminis-

Table 6-4. Bioavailability of methylxanthines

Preparation	Bioavailability (%)[a]
Theophylline anhydrous (theophylline base)	100
Theophylline monohydrate	91
Aminophylline anhydrous	84–86
Aminophylline hydrous	78–82
Dyphylline[b]	70
Oxytriphylline	62–66
Theophylline calcium salicylate	48–50
Theophylline sodium glycinate	45–47

[a]Dosage is calculated on percentage of bioavailability (effective theophylline) of each preparation.
[b]Bioavailability of dyphylline is variable; 70% is an estimate.

tered in repeated doses (4–6 mg/kg every 6 hours) or preferably by continuous intravenous infusion (0.7–1.2 mg/kg/hour in patients under 50 years of age without other disease; 0.5–0.7 mg/kg/hour in older patients, and 0.1–0.5 mg/kg/hour in those with cardiac or liver disease) after an initial intravenous loading dose (6 mg/kg in 50–100 ml 5% dextrose in water over 20–30 minutes in patients with no prior theophylline; 3 mg/kg in patients who have received theophylline within the past 12–24 hours) (see Table 6-3). A serum theophylline concentration should be obtained 1–2 hours after the loading dose and every 12–24 hours with a continuous aminophylline infusion, or 4–6 hours following a change in the maintenance infusion rate. Administration of an additional bolus dose should be followed in 1–2 hours by a serum theophylline determination.

(3) Oxytriphylline is a choline salt of theophylline that is metabolized to theophylline, with a bioavailability of 65% of anhydrous theophylline. It is administered orally in a liquid and a short-acting and long-acting tablet form. It is supposedly better absorbed and less irritating to the intestine than older preparations of pure theophylline and may therefore be useful in patients who cannot tolerate other theophylline preparations. The oral dosage should be 35–40% higher than for oral theophylline preparations.

(4) Dyphylline (dihydroxypropyltheophylline) is an alkylated derivative of theophylline. It is an effective bronchodilator with a varying bioavailability equivalent of 70% of anhydrous theophylline. **Dyphylline is not detected by the standard serum theophylline assay** (it can be measured by modified techniques). It is claimed to have fewer side effects than theophylline and is available in oral and intramuscular preparations. The usual starting dose for adults is 15 mg/kg, given orally every 6 hours (dosage in children has not been established).

The bronchodilator effects of theophylline derivatives and the adrenergic agents are mutually enhancing. Each has a different mode of action, and maintenance therapy with theophylline, unlike that with adrenergic drugs, is not associated with the development of tachyphylaxis. In some patients reduced doses of each in combination yield a similar improvement in FEV_1, with fewer side effects, to either administered alone in maximal dose. Therefore, this combination is especially useful in patients who canno tolerate higher doses of either drug because of side effects. Alternatively, optimal doses of theophylline, in combination with an inhaled beta-agonist administered by metered-dose inhaler every 4 to 8 hours around-the-clock as part of maintenance therapy, can achieve additive bronchodilatation without added side effects, since the inhaled route of administration of a beta-agonist minimizes systemic side effects.

   c. Anticholinergic agents are effective as bronchodilators because they reduce the cholinergic-induced tone and irritability of bronchial smooth muscle. They can be of benefit in the occasional patient who does not tolerate or is not responding to aerosolized adrenergic agents. They can also be more effective than beta-agonists in asthma provoked by psychogenic factors, inadvertent use of beta-adrenergic blocking drugs, or conditions with marked bronchorrhea. Anticholinergic agents for bronchodilatation include atropine sulfate (1–2 mg) delivered by a hand-bulb or compressor- or pressure-driven nebulizer (not FDA-approved for use by inhalation), and the poorly absorbed, quaternary ammonium derivative of atropine, ipratropium bromide (Atrovent*), which is available for delivery by a metered-dose inhaler (18 μg/inhalation), 1–2 inhalations 3–4 times/day. The concentration of atropine sulfate should be adjusted according to the method of delivery (e.g., 4–10 mg/ml by hand-bulb nebulizer or 0.4–1.0 mg/ml by compressor- or pressure-driven nebulizer). Compared with the newer, longer-acting beta-agonists, aerosolized anticholinergics have a slightly slower onset of action (within minutes), a much slower rise to peak action (60 minutes), and a similar duration of action (up to 4–6 hours). Side effects of atropine include dry mouth and occasional blurring of vision, urinary hesitancy, and palpitations. However, systemic side effects of ipatropium are negligible.

2. Cromolyn sodium is a disodium salt of chromone that appears to act by preventing the degranulation of mast cells, induced by antigen-antibody interaction, and the release of histamine, leukotrienes, and other mediators. It may have a nonspecific effect on bronchial hyperreactivity. **Cromolyn sodium has no bronchodilator activity.** Because the drug is poorly absorbed from the gastrointestinal tract, it is administered by inhalation as a micronized powder combined with lactose, as a nebulizer solution, or by metered-dose inhaler. (See Chap. 4.)

   a. Indications. Cromolyn sodium is used for prophylaxis only and is indicated primarily in the patient with chronic asthma that is not readily controlled by or as an alternative to bronchodilators, or to obviate or reduce the need for corticosteroids in chronic asthma. Cromolyn sodium also prevents bronchospasm in patients with bronchoconstriction induced by the inhalation of chemical dusts and vapors, in "late" allergic reactions possibly triggered by antigen-antibody complexes, and in exercise-induced asthma. Cromolyn sodium is **not** indicated for the treatment of an acute attack of asthma, since it can aggravate wheezing.

   b. Dosage. The usual starting and maintenance dose is 20 mg inhaled into the airways by a Spinhaler device or solution by power nebulizer 4 times/day, although the dose can be reduced with long-term use. Alternatively, cromolyn sodium may be administered by metered-dose inhaler (1600 μg, 4 times/day). Patients who experience bronchial or throat irritation or a mild bronchospastic reaction on inhaling the drug may benefit by pretreatment (10–20 minutes) with a pressure-nebulized bronchodilator (metered-dose inhaler) and by rinsing the mouth and throat with water after inhalation. A 4- to 8-week trial is desirable when initiating cromolyn sodium administration. If there is no change in the frequency or severity of asthmatic attacks, or if other medication cannot be reduced without an increase in symptoms, the drug should be

*Boehringer Ingelheim Pharmaceuticals, Ltd., Ridgefield, CT 06877.

discontinued. Cromolyn sodium can be effective in reducing allergen- or exercise-induced bronchospasm when administered 10–15 minutes, but not more than 60 minutes, before exposure.

   c. The most common **side effects** are bronchospasm, cough, nasal congestion, and pharyngeal irritation. Less common side effects include laryngeal edema, urticaria and dermatitis, nausea, hemoptysis, parotitis, and pulmonary infiltrates.

3. Corticosteroids are very effective in the treatment of asthma, especially in patients with chronic, intractable wheezing or status asthmaticus. The method of action is not fully known but may be related to a reversal of beta-adrenergic subsensitivity with restoration of adrenergic responsiveness and inhibition of phospholipase A_2, thus decreasing production of arachidonic acid metabolites (leukotrienes, thromboxanes, prostaglandins). Corticosteroids do not have any direct bronchodilator action, as is evident by their delayed onset of action (6–24 hours).

Hydrocortisone, the biologically active hormone, is produced by the adrenal cortex, while other forms of corticosteroids are converted in the liver to hydrocortisone. The relative dosages, properties, and side effects of the various corticosteroid preparations are reviewed in Chap. 4.

   a. Indications and dosage

      (1) Acute attacks. Corticosteroids are indicated in the acute attack that is unresponsive to bronchodilator therapy. They can be administered orally (prednisone, 40–80 mg/day; 1–2 mg/kg/day in children), usually for 3–4 days, and then discontinued (the dose should be tapered over 3–5 days if the initial course of therapy is over 5–7 days). In more severe attacks or in status asthmaticus, intravenous corticosteroid therapy is indicated (hypoxemia may improve more rapidly with early institution of corticosteroid therapy). The usual intravenous dosage recommendations vary from 200 mg of hydrocortisone sodium succinate (4–6 mg/kg in children) every 4–6 hours to 40–80 mg of methylprednisolone (1 mg/kg in children) every 6–8 hours. If improvement is not evident within 24 hours, the dose should be increased, maximum doses being as high as 250 mg of methylprednisolone every 6 hours in adults. With high-dose corticosteroid therapy, vital signs and fluid and electrolyte status must be followed closely.

      (2) Prolonged corticosteroid therapy is indicated in **chronic asthma** uncontrolled by standard therapy. Initial control should be attempted with metered-dose inhaled preparations that afford minimal systemic absorption (beclomethasone dipropionate, 50–200 μg, or triamcinolone acetonide, 100–400 μg 4 times/day, or flunisolide, 250–1000 μg 2 times/day). These preparations are often effective in chronic asthma in obviating or minimizing the need for systemic corticosteroids. It is frequently helpful to pretreat (by 10–20 minutes) with a beta-agonist by metered-dose inhaler and to rinse the mouth and throat after each dose to prevent oral and pharyngeal irritation.

   b. The most common **side effects** of inhaled corticosteroids are throat irritation, dysphonia, and oropharyngeal candidiasis, which are reversible with discontinuation or reduction in the dose of the drug. Candidiasis can be treated with nystatin suspension (400,000–600,000 units 3–4 times/day). The use of a spacer or aerosol chamber attachment to the metered-dose inhaler (provided with the triamcinolone preparation) substantially reduces oropharyngeal deposition and can prevent or minimize local side effects (see **4**). Beclomethasone, triamcinolone, and flunisolide are not significantly absorbed and do not appear to cause significant adrenal suppression in adults in recommended doses. Therefore when the patient is switched from a systemic corticosteroid, it must be tapered to prevent withdrawal symptoms. In long-term therapy the daily dose of corticosteroid inhalation may gradually be reduced after symptomatic improvement occurs.

c. **Alternate-day versus daily therapy.** When systemic corticosteroids are required, a single morning dose on alternate mornings will frequently control symptoms with less adrenal suppression than with daily therapy. In alternate-day therapy, short-acting preparations (i.e., prednisone, methylprednisolone) are used to minimize suppression of adrenal output. Longer-acting preparations (e.g., dexamethasone) will cause adrenal suppression even with alternate-day therapy. Alternate-day therapy with prednisone in doses greater than 20 mg (less in young children) can cause adrenal suppression. When daily therapy is required, the **minimal dose possible** is given, preferably as a single morning dose. With long-term corticosteroid therapy, tapering the dose is attempted very gradually (e.g., 1–5 mg prednisone every 1–4 weeks). Patients on long-term or recurrent corticosteroid therapy should be examined regularly to detect the early onset of secondary complications (see Chap. 4).

d. **Troleandomycin (TAO),** a macrolide antibiotic, can enhance the effectiveness of systemic corticosteroids in asthma when administered simultaneously.* This enhancement is specifically limited to methylprednisolone. Although the mechanism of enhancement is unclear, inhibition of elimination of methylprednisolone and elevation of serum levels occur 1 week after initiation of TAO. Increased cushingoid features seen with TAO-methylprednisolone therapy tend to disappear at low doses of each, and the clinical improvement of asthmatic symptoms appears to be greater than that achieved by increasing the corticosteroid dose alone. Table 6-5 gives a protocol for TAO-methylprednisolone therapy.

Troleandomycin has known liver toxicity with elevation of liver enzymes and jaundice. In doses as low as 500 mg daily, elevation of serum aspartate aminotransferase (AST) (serum glutamic-oxaloacetic transaminase [SGOT]) and serum alanine aminotransferase (ALT) (serum glutamic-pyruvic transaminase [SGPT]) may occur. Commonly (up to 50% of the time), patients receiving 1 gm of TAO daily for 2 weeks or more experience some liver enzyme elevation. **A persistent rise in serum AST (SGOT) or serum ALT (SGPT) necessitates tapering and occasionally discontinuation of the regimen.** Initial, mild enzyme elevations usually subside as the TAO-methylprednisolone doses are reduced.

Troleandomycin reduces theophylline elimination presumably by inhibiting demethylation of theophylline in the liver. Consequently, when TAO-methylprednisolone therapy is initiated, theophylline dosage must be reduced by 25–50% and then monitored by serum theophylline levels. Patients must be selected carefully for TAO-methylprednisolone therapy and limited to those who are chronic, severe, on optimal conventional asthma therapy, and who require high-dose corticosteroid therapy (> 15–20 mg of prednisone/day). The risks of such therapy must be fully explained to prospective patients or parents of children and weighed against the risks of continued high-dose corticosteroid therapy. An informed consent for the use of TAO-methylprednisolone therapy should be obtained.

Common side effects of TAO-methylprednisolone therapy include an initial increase in corticosteroid-related side effects (see Chap. 4), nausea, and abdominal cramping.

4. **Spacer devices** are chambers of varying sizes designed to adapt to the various metered-dose inhalers (MDIs) to enhance delivery of the inhaled

---

*Troleandomycin-methylprednisolone therapy for asthma is not currently approved by the FDA.

Table 6-5. Suggested protocol for the use of troleandomycin (TAO) in corticosteroid-dependent asthmatics

A. Initiation phase
  1. Select only severe, chronic, corticosteroid-dependent and -resistant asthmatics.
  2. Optimize conventional asthma therapy (medical and psychological).
B. Methylprednisolone trial phase
  1. Switch to methylprednisolone at corticosteroid equivalent dose that maintains maximal clinical status and pulmonary function.
  2. Attempt to reduce methylprednisolone.
  3. Add TAO only if there is:
    a. Absence of liver disease
    b. Absence of drug allergy to macrolide antibiotics
    c. No response to methylprednisolone
    d. Favorable response to methylprednisolone *but*
      (1) Methylprednisolone required daily in children and adolescents
      (2) Methylprednisolone required in doses greater than 12–16 mg daily in adults
      (3) Methylprednisolone required in frequent high-dose bursts
      (4) Adrenal suppression persists
      (5) Patient remains poorly functional
C. TAO trial phase
  1. Inform and educate the patient.
  2. Obtain baseline studies (spirometry, liver function tests, serum theophylline and cortisol levels, eye examination).
  3. Reduce theophylline dosage by 25–50% depending on baseline levels.
  4. Consider reducing high-dose daily methylprednisolone ($\geq$32 mg) by 25% both at initiation of TAO and again at the end of the first week if the patient is doing well.
  5. Begin TAO, 250 mg qd (or 3.5 mg/kg/day).
    a. Determine a serum theophylline level in 1 wk.
    b. Determine responsiveness to TAO at the end of 2 weeks by clinical well-being or spirometric improvement or both. Obtain liver function tests at this time.
      (1) If unfavorable, attempt an increased TAO dose (see 6).
      (2) If favorable, continue TAO and follow the tapering guide (see D).
  6. If the initial response is unfavorable, attempt an increased TAO dose.
    a. Week 1, TAO dose: 250 mg qid (or 14 mg/kg/day)
    b. Week 2, TAO dose: 250 mg tid (or 10 mg/kg/day)
    c. Determine weekly liver and pulmonary function tests and serum theophylline levels.
    d. Determine responsiveness to TAO at the end of 2 wk by clinical well-being or spirometric improvement, or both.
      (1) If unfavorable, discontinue TAO.
      (2) If favorable, continue TAO and follow the tapering guide.
D. TAO-methylprednisolone tapering phase (if favorable response at TAO dose of 250 mg/day progress to 4; if following the high dose TAO regimen, begin with 1).
  1. Week 3, TAO dose: 500 mg qd (or 7 mg/kg/day).
  2. Week 4, TAO dose: 250 mg qd in morning (or 3.5 mg/kg/day).
  3. Determine weekly liver enzymes, spirometry, and serum theophylline levels until TAO dose of 250 mg or less per day is reached.
  4. Reduce daily methylprednisolone dose by 4 mg weekly if possible (spirometry stable, patient asymptomatic) to 4 mg/day (more rapid tapering can be attempted on an individual basis).
  5. Switch to methylprednisolone, 16 mg qod.
  6. Then, in 1 to 2 wk, switch to TAO, 250 mg qod (administered on the same day as methylprednisolone).
  7. Taper methylprednisolone slowly by 2-mg qod decrements every 1–2 wk to 10 mg qod, then every 2–4 wk to lowest possible dose.
  8. May try cromolyn sodium when spirometry is maximal.
  9. Consider a trial of an inhaled corticosteroid when the lowest effective methylprednisolone dose is established.
  10. Obtain a morning serum cortisol level when doses of methylprednisolone, 16 mg qod (or less), and TAO, 250 mg qod, are reached.

Source: Adapted from R. S. Zeiger et al. Efficacy of troleandomycin in outpatients with severe corticosteroid-dependent asthma. *J. Allergy Clin. Immunol.* 66:438, 1980, and J. A. Wald et al. An improved protocol for the use of troleandomycin (TAO) in the treatment of steroid-requiring asthma. *J. Allergy Clin. Immunol.* 78:36, 1986.

medication and reduce oropharyngeal deposition. These devices allow for reduction of laminar flow of the aerosol, with sedimentation of larger droplets and more even distribution of medication on inhalation. They also reduce impaction of material on the soft palate and pharynx. The observed benefit of spacers does not warrant their routine use with MDIs; however, they may be helpful in patients with problems of coordination and in patients subject to irritation, especially those with a tendency to oropharyngeal candidiasis from inhaled corticosteroids. One-way valve spacers can be helpful in small children by allowing multiple breaths to inhale medication from an MDI. Commonly available spacers include InspirEase* and the one-way valve spacers Inhal-Aid* and Aerochamber.†

To achieve maximum effectiveness from an MDI, patients must be properly instructed and observed in their use. Instruct the patient to properly shake the inhaler. With the head tilted slightly back and the aperture of the MDI placed at, or 1 in. beyond, the open mouth and directed toward the posterior pharynx, have the patient take a deep, slow breath, actuating the MDI at the start of inhalation. Some patients may benefit from a sigh just prior to inhalation. At the end of inhalation the breath is held for 10 seconds before exhalation. When multiple inhalations are indicated, allow proper timing between inhalations (3–4 minutes for beta-adrenergic agonists, 1 minute for corticosteroids). Rinsing the mouth and throat on completion can reduce side effects and is most important with inhaled corticosteroids.

5. **Expectorants** enhance the removal of mucus from the bronchial passages. The only preparation with definite effectiveness is water, especially in the dehydrated patient.

   a. Maintenance or restoration of adequate **hydration** (12–16 eight-oz. glasses of liquid/day in adults) helps to prevent bronchial mucus from drying, thereby retarding the formation of mucus plugs and loosening those already formed. In patients with severe asthma and very thick secretions, inhalation of a large volume of a bland aerosolized fluid (e.g., 0.5N saline) from a large-volume nebulizer over 20–30 minutes 3–4 times/day helps to mobilize retained secretions. Since aerosol droplets are irritating to the airways and can provoke bronchospasm, such therapy should always be preceded or accompanied by inhalation using an aerosolized bronchodilator.

   b. If bronchospasm continues to develop, bland aerosol therapy is discontinued. Aerosolized fluid and bronchodilator therapy is best accompanied by postural drainage with chest percussion and vibration.

   c. The efficacy of **other expectorant preparations** is dependent on an adequate fluid intake, and their use in asthma is of questionable value.

      (1) **Glyceryl guaiacolate** (guaifenesin) is believed to act by stimulating the secretion of a more watery mucus and by reducing the surface tension of mucus. It is a relatively nontoxic preparation with few side effects and is compounded in many "cough" preparations. The usual dose is 200 mg (100 mg in children) every 4 to 6 hours, taken with increased amounts of fluid. Its efficacy in asthma is limited, and it does not replace bronchodilator therapy.

      (2) **Iodides** appear to reduce the viscosity of sputum in the presence of adequate fluid intake. Their efficacy is probably equivalent to that of glyceryl guaiacolate. Their effect is dose dependent, and they can be administered orally (saturated solution of potassium iodide, 10–15 drops in water 3 times/day or iodinated glycerol 30–60 mg 3–4 times/day) or intravenously (sodium iodide, 1–2 gm in 5% dextrose in water daily in adults). The intravenous route does not offer any greater advantage. The major limitation in the use of iodides is the common occurrence of **side effects,** including acneiform skin erup-

*Key Pharmaceuticals, Kenilworth, NJ 07033.
†Monaghan Company, Littleton, CO 80160.

tions (especially in adolescents) and other forms of dermatitis parotid and submandibular salivary gland inflammation, nausea, vomiting, anorexia, abdominal pain, and diarrhea. A metallic taste is common. Thyroid enlargement can occur and may be associated with hypothyroidism. Side effects are more common with potassium iodide than with iodinated glycerol. Because of the frequent side effects, iodides should not be used regularly, are generally contraindicated during pregnancy and for breast-feeding mothers, and are of limited value in the management of acute asthma.

   (3) N-acetylcysteine decreases the viscosity of sputum, presumably by splitting mucoproteins. Its effects are dose-dependent (1–10 ml of a 20% solution or 2–20 ml of a 10% solution delivered as an aerosol 1–4 times daily as needed in adults and children). N-acetylcysteine may be immediately followed by mucus accumulation; therefore treatments should be followed immediately by vigorous coughing and postural drainage. It is irritating to the tracheobronchial tree and commonly precipitates bronchospasm in patients with hyper-reactive airways; therefore, the preparation must always be used in conjunction with a bronchodilator (2–3 ml of a 10% solution of N acetylcysteine with 0.25–0.50 ml of 1% isoetharine or 0.30 ml of 5% metaproterenol). It must be discontinued if the bronchospastic effect cannot be prevented by concomitant bronchodilator therapy. Stomatitis can also occur as a side effect. Because of N-acetylcysteine's tendency to produce bronchospasm, it should be reserved for the asthmatic patient with thick, tenacious bronchial mucus that cannot be thinned and mobilized by other measures.

6. **Antihistamines** are of questionable benefit in the treatment of the acute symptoms of asthma. Some patients are benefited by the use of these preparations, probably by a reduction in coughing and the symptoms of upper respiratory tract allergy. It is permissible to use antihistamines for the control of upper respiratory allergy symptoms in conjunction with regular bronchodilator therapy in the management of acute asthma symptoms. Ketotifen, a drug closely related to cyproheptadine, has both antihistamine and bronchial relaxing properties. Although not available in the United States, it is widely used in Europe. Likewise, cetirizine, an experimental piperazine H_1 histamine antagonist, produces significant bronchodilation.

7. The routine use of **antibiotics** during acute and chronic asthma symptoms is unnecessary and is not associated with any enhanced response. Although asthma is often exacerbated by respiratory tract infection, such infection is most often viral and only infrequently of bacterial origin.

   a. The usual secondary bacterial infections occurring with asthma are sinusitis, bronchitis, and pneumonia. In acute bacterial sinusitis, the most common pathogens are *Haemophilus influenzae, Streptococcus pyogenes, Streptococcus pneumoniae,* and *Staphylococcus aureus.* On microscopic examination of gram-stained smears in acute bronchitis complicated by bacterial infection, expectorated sputum shows numerous neutrophils rather than eosinophils, as well as potential pathogens (most often *S. pneumoniae* and *H. influenzae*). Chronic sinusitis is usually associated with infection by anaerobic bacteria or *H. influenzae.* The appropriate antibiotic therapy for acute and chronic sinusitis is given in Chap. 5.

   b. The most common cause of pneumonia varies with the age of the patient. In patients under 5 years of age, many cases are viral and in these antibiotic therapy is therefore unnecessary. In patients between 5 and 30 years of age, viruses or mycoplasmas are the most common causes; mycoplasmal infection is appropriately treated with tetracycline or erythromycin. In patients beyond 30 years of age, *S. pneumoniae* is common and is treated with penicillin or a cephalosporin. In all cases of suspected pneumonia, gram-stained smear and culture of the sputum are essential for identifying the offending bacterial agent.

VI. **Approach to therapy.** The primary goal of treatment is to keep the patient as symptom-free as possible on a minimum of medication. The most important aspect of treatment is education about the disease and instruction in measures of avoiding or lessening attacks. These include avoidance of precipitating or aggravating factors, treatment of concomitant allergies or infections, and the modalities to control attacks previously outlined. Further treatment can be separated into the treatment of acute symptoms and the treatment of chronic symptoms. Exercise-induced asthma, the aspirin- and sulfite-sensitive asthmatic patient, asthma in pregnancy, and asthma with gastroesophageal reflux require special consideration.

A. **Onset of symptoms** of asthma can occur abruptly in an asymptomatic patient or be manifested in a symptomatic patient already on medication.

1. Initially, instruct the patient to rest, to try to relax, and to breathe slowly and deeply. Encourage the taking of oral fluids.

2. In a previously asymptomatic patient on no medication, one to three inhalations of a bronchodilator by metered-dose inhaler usually provides relief in a few minutes. Alternatively, give a rapid-acting oral theophylline preparation (preferably a micronized tablet or liquid) or an oral beta-2-adrenergic agonist (onset of action is slower, generally 30–60 minutes).

3. If symptoms persist or recur or if the patient has a history of prolonged attacks, begin **around-the-clock oral maintenance bronchodilator therapy** with oral theophylline or a beta-2-adrenergic agent or both.

   a. Start with a **long-acting** theophylline preparation (see sec. **V.B.1** for dosage) every 12 hours or, alternatively, a short-acting theophylline preparation every 6 hours (see Chap. 4 for dosing and preparations and Table 6-4 for bioavailability). If the dose is not tolerated, it is reduced and supplemented with an oral beta-2-adrenergic agonist, or an alternative theophylline preparation (e.g., oxytriphylline) can be tried. If theophylline is well tolerated but symptoms are not adequately controlled, **increase the dose** every 2–3 days, monitoring serum theophylline levels to obtain an optimal therapeutic response. If symptoms are still not satisfactorily controlled, or as an alternative to theophylline, give an **inhaled or oral beta-2-adrenergic agent** (see Table 4-7 for dosing and preparations). If side effects of the oral beta-2-adrenergic stimulant occur, **temporarily reduce** the dosage and increase as tolerance develops. If necessary, enhance the bronchodilator effect of the beta-2-adrenergic stimulant by using both routes of administration (oral and inhaled) in combination. One or two inhalations of the beta-2-adrenergic metered-dose inhaler can be used as needed in between regular maintenance doses. **A maximum of 16 inhalations/24 hours should not be exceeded.** Ipratropium bromide (Atrovent) can be given (one or two inhalations by metered-dose inhaler 3–4 times/day) as an alternative to beta-2-adrenergic agents, especially if the latter agents are poorly tolerated, or in addition to the other types of bronchodilators, if symptoms are not adequately controlled.

   b. The **duration** of treatment depends on patient response. It is best continued for at least 2–3 symptom-free days. The minimal amount of medication required to control symptoms is continued.

4. Institute **corticosteroid therapy** if the patient fails to respond to the preceding regimen, especially if there is a history of severe attacks or prior corticosteroid therapy. Begin with a "burst" (e.g., prednisone, 40–80 mg/day or 1–2 mg/kg/day), given orally in a single or divided dose for 3–4 days. A response usually occurs within 6–24 hours but can take up to 2–3 days. When the response is favorable, discontinue the corticosteroid without tapering, but continue oral bronchodilators for at least an additional 5–7 days before attempting dose reduction. If corticosteroids are used for over 5 days, taper the dose over the same number of days as high-dose therapy is given.

5. If the patient fails to respond to such a regimen of corticosteroids, **hospitalize** for more intensive management (see sec. **VII**).

B. Acute asthma attack. The patient with an acute attack of asthma not responding to the usual therapeutic measures should immediately consult a physician.

  1. Assess the **severity** of the attack and obtain **blood gases** if indicated. Employ measures of relaxed breathing and give reassurance.

  2. Administer **supplemental oxygen** if indicated (2–4 liters/minute), to maintain the PaO_2 above 60–65 mm Hg.

  3. Give **epinephrine** 1:1000, 0.2–0.3 ml (0.01 ml/kg in children) subcutaneously and repeat in 20–30 minutes as needed, with a maximum of 3 doses (see **5** as an alternative). The response is usually rapid and, if it is sustained, discharge the patient on an oral bronchodilator regimen with appropriate follow-up. (See **V.B.1.a.(1)** for precautions.)

  4. If rebound bronchospasm occurs or is suspected (by the history) give **Sus-Phrine** (0.1–0.3 ml; 0.005 ml/kg, 0.15 ml maximum in children) subcutaneously 30 minutes after the last epinephrine dose.

  5. If the patient fails to respond to epinephrine, or as an initial alternative to epinephrine, administer a **nebulized bronchodilator** (e.g., 0.25–0.50 ml of 1% isoetharine or 0.20–0.30 ml of 5% metaproterenol or 0.5 ml of 0.5% albuterol in 1–3 ml normal saline) by nebulizer or positive pressure.

  6. As an alternative measure or as the next step, administer an intravenous infusion of **fluids** and **aminophylline** (loading dose of 6 mg/kg over 20–30 minutes [see Table 6-3]). Use a lower dose of aminophylline if the patient is already receiving maintenance oral theophylline. Continue to infuse aminophylline in a maintenance dose of 0.5 mg/kg/hour (0.2–1.2 mg/kg/hour), depending on factors affecting metabolic clearance (see Table 4-8), and monitor the serum theophylline level. Intravenous theophylline can be used in place of aminophylline (see Table 6-3). If the patient has a history of prior corticosteroid therapy or is on a maintenance corticosteroid regimen, begin an oral "burst" regimen as described in **A.4** (alternatively, give an intravenous infusion of hydrocortisone, 5 mg/kg, or methylprednisolone, 1–2 mg/kg, followed by an oral "burst" regimen). If the patient responds, continue a brief oral regimen of corticosteroids along with oral bronchodilators, and arrange for an appropriate follow-up.

  7. If the patient fails to respond to this regimen, hospitalize for the treatment of status asthmaticus.

C. Chronic asthma. The chronic asthmatic patient is one who has continuing or daily symptoms or requires regular medication to remain symptom-free. In such a patient, stress nonpharmacologic measures, and investigate possible aggravating environmental or psychological factors.

  1. Theophylline. Initially, give an oral theophylline preparation in a dosage to maintain a therapeutic serum level (8–20 µg/ml). Administer as a long-acting preparation every 8–12 hours. Patients in whom nocturnal or early-morning breakthrough symptoms develop should take a long-acting preparation, especially at bedtime. Monitor side effects and adjust the dose accordingly.

  2. Adrenergic drugs. If oral theophylline alone does not control symptoms or adequate doses are not tolerated, add or substitute a beta-2-adrenergic agonist, either orally or by inhalation or both (preparation, dosage, and frequency are described in Table 4-7). If intolerable side effects occur, attempt treatment with a low dose of one or both preparations in combination (theophylline and beta-2 agonist).

    Corticosteroid therapy is usually indicated for the chronic asthmatic patient who remains symptomatic despite the preceding regimen or who cannot tolerate bronchodilator medication (see under **4**).

  3. Cromolyn sodium can be tried in any chronic asthmatic patient, as an alternative to chronic bronchodilator therapy, especially one with an extrinsic component who does not tolerate bronchodilator therapy well, who is receiving maintenance corticosteroid therapy, or in whom corticosteroid therapy is anticipated. Attempt a 4- to 8-week trial with cromolyn sodium by Spinhaler, metered-dose inhaler, or nebulized solution 4 times/day. Before and during the trial period, have the patient keep an accurate symptom and medication record. If cromolyn sodium is found to be effective (reduced symptoms or need for other medication or both), continue treatment indefinitely, with regular attempts to reduce the dosage in the well patient (i.e., dropping 1 dose/day every 1–2 weeks). Some patients respond well with a twice-daily dosing, especially in combination with an inhaled beta-agonist.

4. **Corticosteroids**

   a. **Inhaled corticosteroids.** In the patient on a continuous systemic corticosteroid regimen, or if such a regimen is anticipated, attempt a trial of corticosteroid inhalation by metered-dose inhaler for a 4-week period (see sec. **V.B.3** for preparations and dosage). Reduce the inhaled corticosteroid gradually if symptoms are adequately controlled. Also use inhaled corticosteroids in conjunction with oral corticosteroids to reduce the systemic dosage. When inhalation causes airway irritation or bronchospasm, or when bronchial obstruction interferes with peripheral penetration of the inhaled corticosteroid, have the patient, 10–20 minutes before each dose, pretreat with one to three inhalations of a beta-2 agonist by metered-dose inhaler. Each actuation of the corticosteroid inhaler should be drawn deeply into the chest and the breath held for 10–15 seconds. Multiple inhalations should be spaced 1 minute apart. The mouth and throat should be rinsed with water after each inhalation.

   b. **Systemic corticosteroids.** If symptoms are not controlled by the foregoing measures, give systemic corticosteroids. If the patient has acute symptoms, give an initial "burst" of prednisone (see **A.4**), and then taper to the lowest dose necessary to control symptoms. Usually, a 3- to 4-day burst of prednisone will suffice. Follow by reduction to a dose of 20 mg/day (0.5 mg/kg/day in children) and then taper by 2.5–5.0 mg every 1–2 days to the lowest dose that controls symptoms.

   c. To minimize the side effects of continuous daily corticosteroids, attempt **alternate-day therapy,** beginning either by tapering the alternate daily dose until no medication is given on the alternate day, or by doubling the daily dose and giving every other day. If symptoms are not controlled on the off-corticosteroid day, resume daily therapy. Give daily and alternate-day corticosteroids as a single morning dose on arising. Administer antacids 20–30 minutes after the oral corticosteroid dose if gastric irritation occurs or there is a history of peptic ulcer disease. Restrict salt intake and provide a potassium supplement if necessary, especially in patients receiving diuretic therapy. If acute symptoms occur during daily or alternate-day therapy with corticosteroids, triple the single dose and give daily in a divided dose for 2–3 days. Then attempt to return to the previous regimen as tolerated. Make regular attempts to reduce the dose gradually in symptom-free patients and observe the patient closely for the usual complications of corticosteroid therapy (see Chap. 4).

   The use of corticosteroids should not take the place of usual bronchodilator or cromolyn sodium therapy.

   d. In chronic, severe asthmatics requiring high-dose corticosteroid therapy, a trial of troleandomycin-methylprednisolone can be considered (see sec. **V.B.3.d**).

5. Encourage the patient with chronic asthma to maintain a good fluid intake. Although the regular use of expectorants is of limited value, it may help some patients with thick, tenacious sputum or copious secretions. Also, postural drainage, especially in the morning and at bedtime, can be helpful in these patients.

6. In the patient with **severe obstruction,** the regular use of intermittent positive pressure breathing or continuous pump-driven nebulizers for delivery of aerosolized bronchodilator medication occasionally produces greater

relief of bronchospasm than do pressurized hand nebulizers. Possibly, this is because the longer duration of aerosol administration using the former devices leads to more effective topical delivery of the bronchodilator to the tracheobronchial tree in these patients.

   7. Use **antibiotics** only for secondary bacterial infections (see sec. **V.B.7**).

D. Exercise-induced asthma. Most patients with asthma and many patients with allergic rhinitis experience bronchial obstruction, indicated by a significant fall in FEV_1 after 5–10 minutes of sustained exercise. In some patients, exertion is the only factor that precipitates the asthma. Exercise-induced wheezing tends to be more pronounced in severe asthma, both extrinsic and intrinsic.

   1. The occurrence and degree of exercise-induced bronchospasm depend on the **type of exercise.** Vigorous running is the most likely to induce wheezing; jogging and bicycling are less likely to do so, while swimming is usually best tolerated. Exercise-induced asthma typically begins 5–10 minutes after cessation of activity, usually lessens with rest, but can persist for over an hour or lead to a severe asthma attack. Repeating the exercise in less than 2 hours can lead to increased tolerance.

   2. The **cause** of exercise-induced asthma appears to be related to respiratory heat loss with cooling of the airways during the hyperpnea of exercise, although the mechanism coupling airway cooling with bronchospasm is not defined. Evidence also exists that mediator release is involved.

   3. The **treatment** of exercise-induced asthma is directed toward the type and duration of exercise and pretreatment with medication. Select the exercise or activity best tolerated by the patient. Instruct the patient to take moments of rest between brief bursts of activity. If the patient continues to have symptoms, pretreat with medication. Initially, instruct the patient to take his or her regular oral bronchodilator (theophylline, adrenergic drug, or both) 1–2 hours before the activity. Alternatively, use a beta-2 agonist by metered-dose inhaler 15–20 minutes prior to exercise. Inhaled adrenergic agonists are the most effective therapy for exercise-induced asthma. Pretreatment with **cromolyn sodium,** 20 mg by Spinhaler or 1600 µg by metered-dose inhaler, alone or in conjunction with the preceding inhalation of an adrenergic agonist, 15–60 minutes before exercise can protect against exercise-induced bronchospasm in some patients and is useful in patients who experience side effects with other medications. Anticholinergic agents, ipratropium bromide (Atrovent) (1–2 inhalations by metered-dose inhaler), or atropine sulfate (1–2 mg inhaled through a hand-bulb nebulizer [see sec. **V.B.1.c**]) can be helpful in some patients when inhaled 15–30 minutes prior to exercise.

E. Aspirin-sensitive asthma. A subgroup of asthmatic patients exhibits marked sensitivity to aspirin (acetylsalicylic acid), often associated with vasomotor rhinosinusitis and nasal polyposis. These patients are characteristically nonallergic adults with a long history of vasomotor rhinitis and subsequent development of asthma and reactions to aspirin.

   1. The **typical reaction** usually begins in minutes (up to 24 hours) after ingestion of aspirin and consists of watery rhinorrhea, vascular flushing, and dyspnea or wheezing. The asthmatic reactions are often **very severe;** some patients can experience urticaria, angioedema, or shock. The mechanism is not understood, but is probably related to cyclooxygenase inhibition with reduction in the synthesis of bronchodilating prostaglandins (which in some asthmatic persons may play an important homeostatic role) or to the shunting of arachidonic acid metabolism in the direction of lipoxygenase products, including leukotrienes.

   2. **Do not challenge these patients with aspirin.** The primary treatment is avoidance of aspirin and aspirin-containing preparations. Other chemically unrelated preparations that can cause the same reaction in these patients include indomethacin and other nonsteroidal anti-inflammatory drugs, mefenamic acid, antipyrine, aminopyrine, and tartrazine (see Table 12-10 and Appendix XII). Other salicylates and acetaminophen generally do not

produce these reactions. The symptoms are treated by the standard modalities previously discussed, but since the precipitated asthma attacks are frequently severe, hospitalization and corticosteroid therapy are often necessary. Manage anaphylactic reactions as presented in Chap. 10.

3. Some asthmatic persons, including children, who do not have the preceding syndrome have bronchospasm associated with the use of aspirin. Aspirin should be avoided in these patients. **Educate patients to all sources of these substances, especially proprietary medications,** and instruct patients with severe reactions to carry identification of their sensitivity (see **F**).

F. **Sulfite-sensitive asthma.** Sulfiting agents can provoke asthmatic reactions in some patients. These chemicals, which include potassium metabisulfite, potassium bisulfite, sodium metabisulfite, sodium bisulfite, sodium sulfite, and sulfur dioxide, are added to many foods and medicines as antioxidants and preservatives to inhibit enzymatic and microbial browning and spoilage. **Potassium metabisulfite** is the most common of the sulfiting agents to induce asthmatic reactions. Reactions to these agents may occur in 5% of asthmatics, but most commonly occur in a subset of chronic, severe, corticosteroid-dependent adult asthmatics who may be either atopic or nonatopic. Cross-reactivity with other food additives and aspirin does not occur. Reactions vary from mild to severe but often present with immediate, severe to life-threatening bronchospasm and may be associated with other anaphylaxis-like symptoms.

The mechanism of provocation of bronchospasm by sulfiting agents is unknown. Direct mast cell degranulation, effects on arachidonic acid metabolism, and cholinergic stimulation by released sulfur dioxide are proposed. Specific IgE antibodies to sulfites have been demonstrated.

Diagnosis can usually be made by the clinical presentation of chest tightness, wheezing, and dyspnea, often with erythematous flushing of the chest and face occurring immediately after ingestion of a sulfite-containing food (e.g., salad, wine, shrimp), usually in a restaurant. Specific reactions to sulfiting agents in medications, including inhalant bronchodilating solutions, and to sulfur dioxide in smog are undefined but are proposed mechanisms of refractoriness in some asthmatics. The clinical presentation is sufficient to make a presumptive diagnosis. Confirmation can be established by oral and inhalation challenge. This challenge should be attempted only in a hospital or clinic setting by physicians experienced in the procedure.

Treatment of sulfite sensitivity consists of proper patient education in recognizing and avoiding those substances containing sulfiting agents. Appendix XII presents common substances containing sulfiting agents. Sulfitest* paper test strips are available for testing suspected foods for the presence of sulfites. False-negative results are common, and certain foods, depending on color, acidity, or presence of other chemicals, cannot be tested. Thus the test is not an absolute indication of the presence or absence of sulfites. Current FDA regulations prohibit the use of sulfiting agents on raw fruits and vegetables (excluding potatoes), packaged foods are required to be labeled if sulfites are present at 10 parts/million or more, and prescription drugs are to be labeled if sulfites are present in the final form. Treatment of asthmatic reactions follows the usual guidelines and depends on severity. Because of possible inadvertent exposure, patients with a history of severe reactions to sulfiting agents are encouraged to carry a source of epinephrine (ANA-Kit,† EpiPen*) and identification of their sensitivity (e.g., Medic Alert‡ badge) when exposure risk is increased, as in dining out.

G. **Asthma and pregnancy**
   1. **Physiologic changes**
      a. **Respiratory changes.** Maternal minute ventilation increases, and functional residual capacity decreases. Forced expiratory flow rates, in-

---

*Center Laboratories, Inc., Port Washington, NY 11050
† Hollister-Stier Laboratories, Spokane, WA 99220
‡ Medic Alert Foundation, Turlock, CA 95380

spiratory capacity, diffusing capacity, and oxygen consumption remain the same. A drop in PaO_2 occurs from maternal to fetal blood.
   b. **Hormonal changes** include an increase in chorionic gonadotropin and in plasma cortisol and a small increase in cyclic AMP. These changes may reduce the effects of histamine release. Further, serum IgE levels tend to decrease in pregnancy.
   c. **Clinical changes.** Asthma improves in one-third of pregnant asthmatic patients, while one-third remain unchanged, and one-third worsen. Severe asthma tends to worsen during pregnancy. Some patients experience worsening asthma in the postpartum period. There is a suggestion of a slightly increased incidence of prematurity and spontaneous abortions in pregnant asthmatic women compared with nonasthmatic pregnant women.
   2. The **management** of asthma during pregnancy is similar to that in the nonpregnant asthmatic woman. However, strict control must be placed on environmental irritants, and known allergens must be avoided. Standard pharmacologic agents are not contraindicated in pregnancy but must be used with knowledge of their current categorization for use in pregnancy (see Table 6-6) and attention given to the risk-to-benefit ratio. The rationale for use of these agents and the concept of the risk-to-benefit ratio must be discussed with each patient.
      a. Continue immunotherapy or initiate cautiously when indicated (see Chap. 4), and treat respiratory infections appropriately. Instruct the patients in breathing exercises, and encourage them to practice these exercises. Use postural drainage with modified positions when indicated. Avoid hydroxyzine and iodides, and employ local anesthesia during delivery if possible.
      b. Treat the symptoms of asthma with a **theophylline** or a **beta-2-adrenergic agonist** preparation in the usual dosage or both in combination. **Cromolyn sodium** can be used for prophylaxis. Give **corticosteroids,** either by inhalation or systemically, when indicated (sparingly and in moderate doses if possible). Newborns of mothers treated with high-dose corticosteroid therapy should be observed for adrenal insufficiency.
H. **Asthma and gastroesophageal reflux.** Regurgitation and aspiration of gastrointestinal contents can trigger wheezing in the asthmatic patient. Gastroesophageal reflux should be considered in any asthmatic patient with gas, heartburn, or other peptic symptoms, a hiatal hernia or esophageal dysfunction, recurrent pneumonia, or recurrent infiltrates on chest x-ray. Gastroesophageal reflux can occur without symptoms and should be considered in the chronic asthmatic patient unresponsive to therapy.
   1. **Diagnosis.** A barium esophogram is often not adequate to identify gastroesophageal reflux. Determination of lower esophageal sphincter pressure and, preferably, the demonstration of a fall in the pH of the lower esophageal contents with recumbency (acid reflux test) are indicated for evaluation.
   2. **Treatment.** When gastroesophageal reflux is demonstrated or suspected, place the patient on an antireflux regimen consisting of a bland diet, no eating for 2 hours before bedtime, antacid therapy, and elevation of the head of the bed (15–20 cm). Addition of ranitidine or metocolpramide can be helpful. Continue this regimen if effective. Selected patients may require surgical repair of gastroesophageal abnormalities.
   Theophylline and beta-adrenergic agonists relax the smooth muscles of the lower esophageal sphincter. This may affect gastroesophageal reflux in some patients.
I. **Occupational asthma.** Exposure to agents in the workplace can induce the onset of asthma in 5% of workers. Such exposure can also aggravate or reactivate asthmatic symptoms in previously diagnosed atopic and nonatopic patients. Provocation can result from known allergens or from a variety of materials that enhance bronchial responsiveness.
   The presentation of occupational asthma is variable, but typically a worker

Table 6-6. Pregnancy risk categories of pharmacologic agents used in asthma

Drug[a]	Risk category[b]
Adrenergic agents	
Epinephrine	C
Ephedrine	NC[c]
Ethylnorepinephrine	C
Isoproterenol	NC
Isoetharine	NC
Metaproterenol	C
Terbutaline	B
Albuterol	C
Bitolterol	C
Theophylline	C
Aminophylline	NC
Oxytriphylline	NC
Dyphylline	C
Ipratropium bromide (Atrovent)	B
Cromolyn sodium	B
Inhaled corticosteroids	
Beclomethasone	NC[d]
Triamcinolone	D
Flunisolide	C
Systemic corticosteroids (e.g., prednisone, methylprednisolone)	NC

[a]Category is the same for all routes of administration for each drug.
[b]Risk categories determined by the FDA include: A, no risk in well-controlled studies; B, no adequate human studies and either some risk or no risk in animal studies; C, no adequate human studies and some risk in animal studies or no adequate human and animal studies available; D, drugs shown to be associated with birth defects but are acceptable for use when the need outweighs the risk; X, birth defects exist and the risk clearly outweighs the benefit.
[c]NC indicates a noncategorized drug; in such drugs, use is acceptable but the risk must be weighed against the need for use.
[d]For beclomethasone, category NC refers to use in asthma; use for nasal inhalation is category C.

complains of coughing, wheezing, and chest tightness occurring at work, with improvement on weekends and vacations. Some workers have immediate symptoms on arrival at the workplace **(within 1 hour).** Others may not become symptomatic for 4–12 hours after exposure, or they may present with a **dual response**—immediate symptoms on arrival at work that are often mild, resolving in 1–4 hours, and the recurrence of more severe, late symptoms occurring toward the end of the work day (see sec. **I.B.5**). Some workers develop chronic symptoms that do not remit during prolonged absence from work or persist indefinitely. Workers who develop a chronic cough or have associated rhinitis and recurrent colds should be suspected of early onset of work-induced asthma. Over 100 work-related materials are known to cause or provoke asthma. The Occupational Safety and Health Administration (OSHA) establishes exposure limits for all industrial materials. Threshold limits are based on exposure levels affecting normal individuals. Thus, individuals with hyperresponsive airways are often provoked in occupationally safe environments. Sulfur dioxide gas, a common industrial agent, causes airway aggravation in normal individuals at levels above 5 parts/million (ppm). Workers with mild asthma may react at levels less than 0.5 ppm. Some of the more common industrial agents include isocyanates, anhydrides, and wood dusts. **Toluene diisocyanate (TDI),** a polymerizing catalyst used in the production of paints and polyurethane products, may produce cellular damage to the airway lining, leading to prolonged sensitivity. Serum IgE reactive to TDI can be demonstrated in some patients, although an immediate hypersensitivity reaction is unclear. **Trimellitic** and **phthalic anhydrides** are used in the production of paints and plastics and produce reactions similar to TDI. **Plicatic acid** in western red cedar dust produces a chemical irritation of the airways and, with chronic exposure, symptoms may persist for several years following elimination. Table 6-7 lists the common causes of occupational asthma and correlates the type of occupation where exposure for each is likely.

1. **Diagnosis** of work-related asthma is usually evident from the history and physical examination. Early diagnosis is important in preventing long-term morbidity. Reactivity can be documented by pre- and post-shift spirometry, or the worker can be instructed to record expiratory peak flow responses hourly through the work day with a portable peak flowmeter. If a specific substance is suspected, the diagnosis can be confirmed by bronchial provocation testing (see sec. **II.C.10**). This testing should be performed in a hospital or clinic setting by physicians experienced in the procedure, with particular attention to late reactions occurring up to 12 hours after provocation.

2. **Treatment** of occupational asthma is directed to avoidance of the offending agent. This often requires job retraining. Attention must be given to the chronic and progressive course produced by many of these agents, especially with prolonged exposure. Symptomatic therapy follows standard guidelines, but is not recommended as a substitute for avoidance. Immediate reactions are usually blocked by pretreatment with bronchodilators or cromolyn sodium; late reactions are less affected by these agents and respond best to corticosteroids.

VII. **Status asthmaticus and ventilatory failure**

A. **Definition.** Status asthmaticus is severe asthma unresponsive to the usual methods of treatment, including bronchodilator medication, subcutaneous epinephrine, and intravenous aminophylline. Status asthmaticus is associated with a 1–3% mortality; it should be treated, therefore, as a life-threatening medical emergency.

B. **Precipitating factors** are the same as those that may provoke any attack of asthma and include exposure to an allergen or primary irritant, viral respiratory tract infection, change in ambient temperature or humidity, an emotional crisis, gastric acid aspiration, or poor compliance in taking prescribed medication. Often, there may be no obvious initiating factor.

C. **Clinical features**

1. The following **historic features** strongly suggest that a patient is approaching status asthmaticus:

   a. **Change in the pattern of symptoms,** including increasing frequency and severity of attacks of dyspnea and wheezing, progressive exertional intolerance, and cough that has become productive of scantier amounts of tenacious sputum, which may be discolored.

   b. **Refractoriness to bronchodilator drugs** that, despite more frequent use and even abuse, result in a lesser magnitude and duration of effect.

   c. **Personality changes,** including increasing anxiety and irritability and, at times, panic.

   d. **History of recent and frequent repeated episodes of severe asthma** treated either in the emergency room and/or hospital with only short-lived benefit.

2. **Physical findings** include the following:

   a. An **anxious patient** with tachypnea and obviously labored breathing interfering with speech.

   b. **Suprasternal retractions,** use of accessory muscles of respiration (especially the sternocleidomastoids), and signs of hyperinflation (low diaphragms, decreased lateral excursions of the chest, hyperresonance).

Table 6-7. Common causes of occupational asthma

Material	Occupation at risk
Chemical	
Isocyanates	
Toluene diisocyanate (TDI)	Polyurethane workers, insulators, laminators
Diphenylmethane diisocyanate	Laminators, polyurethane foam workers
Hexamethylene diisocyanate	Painters, plastics workers
Naphthalene diisocyanate	Chemists, rubber workers
Anhydrides	
Trimellitic anhydride	Chemical workers
Phthalic anhydride	Painters, plastics workers
Hexahydrophthalic anhydride	Epoxy resins workers
Tetrachlorophthalic anhydride	Epoxy resins workers
Polyvinyl chloride vapor	Meat wrappers
Formaldehyde	Laboratory workers, embalmers, insulators, textile workers
Dimethylethanolamine	Paint sprayers
Ethylenediamine	Rubber workers, photographic processors
Persulfate salts	Chemical workers, beauticians
Ethylene oxide	Medical sterilizers
Pyrethrin	Fumigators
Ammonium thioglycolate	Beauticians
Monoethanolamine	Beauticians
Hexamethylenamine	Beauticians
Wood dusts	
Western red cedar	Woodworkers
Cedar of Lebanon	Woodworkers
Mahogany	Woodworkers
California redwood	Woodworkers
Oak	Woodworkers
Iroko	Woodworkers
Boxwood	Woodworkers
Cocabolla	Woodworkers
Zebrawood	Woodworkers
Mansonia	Woodworkers
Mulberry	Woodworkers
Metals	
Chromic acid	Chrome platers, welders
Potassium chromate and dichromate	Chrome workers, cement workers
Platinum salts	Platinum refiners
Chloroplatinic acid	Platinum refiners, chemists
Nickel sulfate	Nickel platers, welders
Nickel carboxyl	Chemical workers, nickel platers, welders
Vanadium	Boiler cleaners, turbine cleaners
Dyes	
Anthraquinone	Fabric dyers
Carmine	Cosmetics and dye workers
Paraphenyl diamine	Fur dyers
Hexafix brilliant yellow	Dye manufacturers
Drimaren brilliant blue	Dye manufacturers
Cibachrome brilliant scarlet	Dye manufacturers
Henna extract	Beauticians

Table 6-7 (*continued*)

Material	Occupation at risk
Fluxes	
Colophony (soft-core solder)	Solderers, electronics workers
Aminoethylethanolamine	Aluminum solderers
Drugs	
Benzyl penicillin	Pharmaceutical workers
Ampicillin	Pharmaceutical workers
Sulfathiazole	Pharmaceutical workers
Tetracycline	Pharmaceutical workers
Psyllium	Pharmaceutical workers
Methyldopa	Pharmaceutical workers
Albuterol	Pharmaceutical workers
Piperazine dihydrochloride	Pharmaceutical workers
Chloramine T	Pharmaceutical and laboratory workers
Organophosphates	Farm workers, pesticide formulators, fumigators
Enzymes	
Pancreatic extracts	Pharmaceutical workers
Bacillus subtilis	Detergent manufacturers
Papain	Food processors
Trypsin	Plastics and rubber workers
Flaviastase	Pharmaceutical workers
Bromelain	Food processors
Pectinase	Food processors
Animals	
Domestic animals (hair, dander)	Farmers, veterinarians, meat processors
Birds	Poultry breeders, bird fanciers
Mice, guinea pigs (dander, urine)	Laboratory workers
Fish (glue)	Bookbinders, postal workers
Silkworms	Silk sericulturers
Insects, mites	Grain mill and storage workers, bakers
Plants	
Wheat	Farmers, grain handlers
Buckwheat	Bakers
Grain dust	Farmers, grain handlers, bakers
Rye flour	Bakers
Hops	Brewers
Tamarind seeds	Millers, spice processors
Castor beans	Farmers, castor bean workers
Coffee beans	Farmers, coffee bean workers
Wool	Textile workers
Tobacco dust	Cigarette manufacturers
Tea	Food processors
Cotton, flax, hemp	Textile workers
Vegetable gums	
Acacia	Printers
Tragacanth	Printers, food processors
Karaya	Food processors
Arabic	Printers

     c. **Diminished breath sounds,** expiratory prolongation, and wheezes heard on both inspiration and expiration. When obstruction is very severe, however, there is little air movement and flow rates are too low to generate a wheeze, so that wheezing can be absent ("silent chest").

     d. **Paradoxical pulse** ($>$ 10 mm Hg decrease in systolic blood pressure during inspiration). Suprasternal retractions and pulsus paradoxus are frequently present ($\sim$50%) when the FEV_1 is less than 1.0 liter in adults but are rarely present when the FEV_1 is greater than 1.25 liters.

     e. Evidence of **increased sympathoadrenal activity,** including tachycardia, increase in systolic blood pressure, and diaphoresis.

3. Differential diagnostic considerations include:

     a. **Upper airway obstruction,** e.g., acute epiglottitis, laryngeal edema, tumor or paralysis, acute laryngotracheobronchitis, tracheal stenosis, tracheomalacia, tracheal tumor, foreign body, and extrinsic compression of the trachea. In extrathoracic upper airway obstruction, a characteristic inspiratory stridor is generally heard localized to the upper airway.

     b. **Congestive heart failure** ("cardiac asthma"). Diagnostic features include a history of heart disease and paroxysmal nocturnal and exertional dyspnea, physical findings of cardiomegaly, a third heart sound, and inspiratory rales; and radiographic evidence of interstitial or alveolar edema, distended upper lobe pulmonary veins, Kerly "B" lines, and absence of hyperinflation.

     c. **Pulmonary embolism** can present with the sudden onset of wheezing ($\sim$4% of cases). It is suggested by the presence of predisposing factors (e.g., congestive heart failure, carcinoma, thrombophlebitis), a history of previous pulmonary embolism, symptoms of pleuritic pain with or without hemoptysis, signs of congestive heart failure, a pleural friction rub or pulmonary consolidation, and characteristic chest radiographic findings (e.g., localized area of oligemia, elevated hemidiaphragm).

     d. **Recurrent aspiration** of foreign material is suspected in the patient with alcoholism, seizure disorder, or difficulty swallowing and with radiographic evidence of atelectasis.

     e. **Carcinoid syndrome** is associated with wheezing in 20–30% of cases. It is generally readily differentiated from asthma by the characteristic features of paroxysmal flushing, watery diarrhea, and abdominal pain.

4. Laboratory tests that are indicated include:

     a. **Measurement of FEV_1 and VC or PEFR** before and after treatment with a bronchodilator administered either subcutaneously or as an aerosol via a pressure-powered nebulizer or intermittent positive pressure breathing (IPPB). Patients with severe asthma generally have an FEV_1 less than 15–30% of predicted, a VC less than 30–50% of predicted, and a PEFR less than 100 liters/minute in adults. Those with both severe obstruction initially ($FEV_1 < 0.7$ liter; PEFR $<$ 100 liters/minute) and only small increases in FEV_1 or PEFR after bronchodilator therapy ($<$ 0.3 liter or $<$ 60 liters/minute, respectively), have a strong likelihood of relapse and usually require hospitalization. Adult patients with severe acute asthma should be treated to achieve an FEV_1 greater than 2.1 liters or a PEFR greater than 300 liters/minute before discharge.

     b. **Arterial blood gases.** During severe asthma the PaO_2 can be decreased below 60 mm Hg, whereas the $PaCO_2$ is often normal (38–42 mm Hg) or slightly low but can be elevated (alveolar hypoventilation) when obstruction is very severe. In contrast, during mild to moderate asthma, PaO_2 is usually only modestly reduced, and $PaCO_2$ is frequently low (respiratory alkalosis). In severe asthma, arterial pH can be normal or slightly alkaline due to mild respiratory alkalosis; however, acidemia is not uncommon due to metabolic acidosis (base excess < -2 mEq/liter) or respiratory acidosis ($PaCO_2 > 42$ mm Hg) or both. Both metabolic acidosis and respiratory acidosis are more common in children with severe asthma than in corresponding adults. Metabolic acidosis accompanying status asthmaticus reflects lactic acid accumulation secondary (1) to the markedly increased work of breathing and (2) to diminished venous return, cardiac output, and tissue perfusion presumably due to the effects of marked hyperinflation. During less severe attacks, a mild hyperchloremic, non-anion-gap metabolic acidosis is common, due to renal loss of bicarbonate in compensation for a preceding period of hyperventilation and respiratory alkalosis. Respiratory acidosis occurs when $PaCO_2$ increases due to very severe obstruction, fatigue of the respiratory muscles, and/or sedative-induced respiratory center depression resulting in alveolar hypoventilation.

Frequent arterial blood gas determinations are recommended in status asthmaticus to detect the rise in PCO_2 to or above normal levels that signals the imminence of respiratory failure. A PCO_2 of 50–60 mm Hg that does not fall below 50 mm Hg in the first 8 hours of treatment or a PCO_2 greater than 60 mm Hg on admission are indications for intubation and mechanical ventilation (each case must be individualized and PCO_2 levels used as guidelines). Repeated measurements of PEFR or FEV_1 can aid, or may substitute for arterial blood gases, in the detection of emerging respiratory acidosis. Hypercapnia rarely develops unless the PEFR is less than 130 liters/minute; also, a rise in PEFR (even if initially < 130 liters/minute) is not associated with the development of hypercapnia in patients who are eucapnic initially.

c. **Chest x-ray.** The chest roentgenogram usually demonstrates only marked hyperinflation, sometimes with transient densities due to mucus plugging causing subsegmental atelectasis. The major value of the chest x-ray is to evaluate the possibility of a pulmonary complication of severe asthma (e.g., pneumothorax, pneumomediastinum, or segmental or lobar atelectasis), to exclude an acute bronchopneumonia that may have precipitated the asthmatic attack, and to suggest other disorders (e.g., pulmonary embolism with infarction and congestive heart failure).

d. **Complete blood count and differential.** The white blood count is increased in about 50% of cases (this increase can result from previously administered epinephrine or corticosteroids), averaging approximately 15,000/mm³; higher counts are found in the presence of infection, or dehydration. Marked eosinophilia (1000–1500 eosinophils/mm³) suggests an allergic cause of the asthmatic exacerbation, whereas an infectious etiology of the worsening of asthma results in only a modest eosinophilia. In patients already receiving therapy, corticosteroid responsiveness is usually associated with an eosinophil count less than 50–100/mm³, whereas the unresponsive state is characterized by a high eosinophil count, indicating the need for more corticosteroids.

e. **Theophylline serum concentrations** should be determined in patients on maintenance treatment with oral theophylline to ascertain compliance and to serve as a guide to further theophylline therapy.

f. **Sputum examination.** Before therapy, sputum is generally thick, opalescent, and adhesive with many threadlike mucinous strands. Microscopic examination should be performed initially on an unstained, unfixed wet preparation. The presence of many eosinophils in the wet sputum preparation militates against an infectious episode. On the other hand, the presence of many polymorphonuclear leukocytes suggests an infectious etiology and indicates the need for a gram-stained smear and culture of the sputum to identify bacterial pathogens. Only about 5% of asthmatic attacks in adults are associated with bacterial respiratory infection.

g. **A 12-lead electrocardiogram** should be obtained, especially in the older asthmatic patient. Pulmonary hypertension in severe asthma often causes a shift of the mean electrical axis to the right and can lead to right ventricular predominance and a right bundle branch block pattern. Use of large doses of beta-adrenergic agonists and theophylline drugs can lead to supraventricular and ventricular arrhythmias, particularly when hypoxemia and acid-base disturbances are present. Myocardial ischemia or infarction can also complicate status asthmaticus in the older patient.

5. **Indications of impending respiratory failure** requiring aggressive, intensive, in-hospital therapy include:

    a. Disturbance of consciousness.

    b. Obvious physical exhaustion.

    c. "Silent" chest.

    d. A $PaCO_2$ greater than 45 mm Hg.

    e. Central cyanosis.

    f. An FEV_1 less than or equal to 0.6 liter or a PEFR less than 60 liters/minute without response to bronchodilator therapy.

    g. Pneumothorax or pneumomediastinum.

D. **Treatment.** The patient with status asthmaticus must be treated aggressively, preferably in an intensive-care unit staffed by a team of medical and paramedical personnel who are knowledgeable and experienced in the care of severe respiratory disorders. Arterial blood gases should be obtained periodically and at least once daily as long as the patient remains unresponsive or poorly responsive to bronchodilator therapy. The electrocardiogram should be monitored continuously in severe and unstable patients and in patients with cardiac disease, as long as theophylline is being administered by continuous intravenous infusion. Treatment should include the following measures:

1. **Continuous low-flow oxygen** via nasal prongs or Venturi mask to maintain PaO_2 over 60 mm Hg.

2. **Nebulized 0.5% isoproterenol,** 0.25–0.50 ml, 1% **isoetharine,** 0.25–0.50 ml, 5% **metaproterenol,** 0.20–0.30 ml, or 0.5% albuterol, 0.5 ml in 1–3 ml of normal saline by a pressure-driven jet-nebulizer or intermittent positive pressure breathing with supplemental oxygen every 1–3 hours as needed initially. Alternatively, or if nebulized bronchodilator therapy is not initially effective, epinephrine (1:1000), 0.3 ml, or terbutaline, 0.25 mg subcutaneously, repeated once, if necessary, after 15–20 minutes. In patients with severe airflow obstruction ($FEV_1 \leq 35\%$ predicted), the bronchodilator response to a nebulized beta-agonist alone is significantly greater than that to subcutaneous epinephrine alone. It may be worthwhile to administer beta-adrenergic agonists by mouth (terbutaline, 2.5–5.0 mg every 8 hours, or albuterol, 2–4 mg every 8 hours, or metaproterenol, 10–20 mg every 6 hours) as well as by the inhaled route (as indicated above) to achieve an additive bronchodilator effect, particularly on smaller airways to which the aerosolized drug has only limited access. See Table 4-7 for pediatric dosage.

3. **Intravenous aminophylline or theophylline** administered as a loading dose followed by a continuous infusion via a peripheral vein (never a central vein) using the dosing guidelines already described (see sec. **V.B.1.b** and Table 6-3). Rapid relief of dyspnea can occur within 15 minutes after a loading dose of aminophylline but is often delayed for hours if a maintenance infusion is given without a loading dose. Theophylline blood concentration should be measured:

    a. Prior to the loading dose in patients who have received theophylline within the previous 12–24 hours.

    b. One to two hours after administration of a loading dose to ascertain whether the expected increase in theophylline serum concentration (2 μg/ml for each 1 mg/kg of loading dose) has occurred after saturation of the volume of theophylline distribution. If the theophylline serum level is still not in the therapeutic range (8–20 μg/ml), an additional partial loading dose (e.g., one-half the initial loading dose) is required.

    c. Every 12–24 hours during maintenance therapy to ascertain that the serum level remains in the therapeutic range (8–20 μg/ml).

    d. Four to six hours after a change in maintenance infusion rate, then every 12–24 hours.

e. **At the first sign of toxicity.** The relationship between theophylline serum concentration and toxic effects is shown in Table 6-2. Although gastrointestinal symptoms are usually the first manifestation of toxicity (often at levels < 20 μg/ml), serious cardiac arrhythmias (usually at levels between 20 and 40 μg/ml) and grand mal seizures (generally at levels > 40 μg/ml but occasionally at lower serum levels) can occur without any prior evidence of toxic effects. Arrhythmias can lead to hypotension and cardiac arrest, and theophylline-induced convulsions are fatal in about 50% of instances in adult patients (less in children, although morbidity is significant). Consequently, careful monitoring of serum theophylline concentration in patients receiving infusions of aminophylline or theophylline is mandatory. Blood must be drawn from a vein far enough from the infusion site to avoid falsely high serum theophylline levels.

4. **Corticosteroids.** Prompt use of corticosteroids in the emergency treatment of severe asthma can help terminate attacks, decrease morbidity, and reduce the need for hospitalization. Corticosteroids are indicated if there is no sustained improvement or less than the desired improvement after 1–3 hours of vigorous therapy as outlined in sec **VII.D.1–3**, or if the patient had already received corticosteroid therapy within the previous month or had been on long-term corticosteroid therapy (> 2 weeks) within the previous year. Corticosteroids should be given in moderate to high doses. Dosage recommendations for hydrocortisone vary from 200 mg intravenously 4 times/day in adults only to as much as 4–6 mg/kg every 4–6 hours; the dosage of methylprednisolone varies from 60–250 mg (1–2 mg/kg in children) every 6 hours. If significant improvement is not evident with initial dosing within 24 hours, the dose should be increased—for example, by progressively doubling the dose every 24 hours within the dose ranges indicated above.

5. **Hydration.** Dehydration (5% average deficit in total body water) is common in acute asthma and can contribute to the increase in tenacity of the bronchial secretions. Dehydration should be corrected with 5% glucose and 0.25–0.50 normal saline intravenously over 6–12 hours, followed by maintenance of hydration with oral and intravenous fluids. Intake and output should be monitored to avoid overhydration, and parenteral fluids should be administered cautiously to patients with cardiac disease.

6. **Antibiotics,** if examination of the gram-stained sputum reveals evidence of bacterial bronchopulmonary infection (see sec. **V.B.7**).

7. **Sodium bicarbonate** intravenously if severe acidemia (pH ≤ 7.20) is present and is not reversed promptly by other measures to reduce airflow obstruction and thereby improve ventilation and decrease the work of breathing. Acidemia reduces the responsiveness of beta-adrenergic receptors to stimulation by endogenous and exogenous catecholamines. If sodium bicarbonate is administered, only enough should be given to correct the metabolic component by one-half (or less), because full correction of the metabolic acidosis may lead to alkalemia when improved lung function corrects the overproduction of lactic acid and the lactic acid already accumulated is rapidly metabolized by the liver. The potentially harmful effects of alkalemia (which rapidly replaces acidemia) include cardiac arrhythmias, hypotension, and depression of central ventilatory drive. Administration of bicarbonate in the amount of **0.3 × body weight (in kg) × base excess (in mEq/liter)** can be expected to return an abnormal pH approximately halfway to the normal value of 7.40, assuming there is no change in respiratory acid-base status.

8. **Bronchial hygiene measures,** including controlled cough encouragement, chest physical therapy, and, at times, large-volume aerosol therapy, if tolerated. The technique of controlled cough increases cough effectiveness and conserves energy. After less than a full inspiration, the patient is instructed to cough in staccato fashion with only moderate effort down to low-lung volumes to milk secretions toward the mouth while avoiding dynamic air-

way compression, induction of bronchospasm, and exhaustive and wasteful expenditure of energy. In selected patients who have difficulty raising secretions, **postural drainage** with chest percussion and vibration may help mobilize and facilitate expectoration of mucus, provided these techniques do not induce additional bronchospasm. In asthmatics with very thick secretions, inhalation of large volumes of a warm, bland aerosolized liquid (e.g., 0.5 N saline) over 20–30 minutes several times a day may help mobilize retained secretions (see sec. **V.B.5**). However, since the aerosol droplets may irritate the airways and induce reflex bronchospasm, such therapy should be preceded or accompanied by the administration of a nebulized bronchodilator and, if appreciable bronchospasm still develops, aerosol therapy should be discontinued. Because of the greater tendency for the smaller particles generated by ultrasonic nebulizers to induce bronchoconstriction, treatment with these nebulizers is often not tolerated.

9. **Continuation of in-hospital treatment.** Dose and frequency of all drugs should be adjusted according to the patient's clinical course, which should be monitored closely. Ancillary measures for evaluating progress include periodic determinations of arterial blood gases (particularly if the $PaCO_2$ was initially > 40 mm Hg and the PaO_2 was < 60 mm Hg), measurement of FEV_1 (using a portable spirometer), or peak expiratory flow rate (using a Wright peak flowmeter) before and after treatment with an aerosol bronchodilator, and daily total blood eosinophil counts to ascertain the adequacy of the corticosteroid dose (the corticosteroid dose should be increased if the total eosinophil count has not fallen below $50/\mu l$ within 24 hours). Lack of an acute or sustained improvement in flow rates in response to bronchodilator aerosol therapy indicates the need for continued high-dose corticosteroids, frequent beta-agonist nebulizer treatments, and intravenous aminophylline or theophylline.

10. **Sedation should be avoided in most cases, especially if the $PaCO_2$ is normal or elevated,** to prevent respiratory center depression and resultant hypoventilation and respiratory acidosis. Occasionally, however, severe anxiety and the central nervous system side effects of drug therapy require very cautious administration of a tranquilizing agent such as diazepam (2–5 mg 4 times/day), alprazolam (0.25–0.50 mg 3 times/day) or hydroxyzine (25 mg 3 times/day). These are adult doses.

11. **Treatment of ventilatory failure.** Intubation and mechanical ventilation are rarely necessary in the management of status asthmaticus, provided conventional measures are vigorously applied and corticosteroids are used when indicated. Despite all these measures, however, a few patients develop progressive ventilatory failure ($PaCO_2$ > 50–60 mm Hg) associated with moderately severe acidemia (pH < 7.25) due to combined respiratory and metabolic acidosis. The acidemia may result in mental obtundation that impairs the patient's ability to cooperate with therapeutic measures such as aerosolized bronchodilator treatments and controlled cough with expectoration of obstructing mucous secretions. In addition, patients may be so exhausted as a result of the markedly increased work of breathing that their respiratory muscles fatigue, resulting in further ventilatory failure and acidosis. Under these circumstances, intubation with a cuffed endotracheal tube is required so that the work of breathing may be assumed by a mechanical ventilator and effective ventilation provided to return the PCO_2 and pH gradually toward normal. Adequate arterial oxygenation (PaO_2 > 65 mm Hg) is maintained by providing sufficient supplemental oxygen (inspired oxygen concentration generally ≤ 40%). Young children with severe asthma may be more likely than adults to require assisted or controlled ventilation since their airways are smaller and are therefore more readily occluded to the extent of causing severe hypoventilation

   a. **A continuous intravenous infusion of isoproterenol** is an alternative to tracheal intubation and mechanical ventilation in patients with ventilatory failure resulting from status asthmaticus.

(1) A dilution of 0.1 μg/kg/minute is begun using a syringe pump to ensure a constant infusion (0.5 mg isoproterenol in 50 ml of fluid gives 10 μg/ml). Increase the dose stepwise at 10- to 15-minute intervals in increments of 0.1 μg/kg/minute until the heart rate (with continuous electrocardiographic monitoring) approaches 200 beats/minute, an arrhythmia develops, or a satisfactory clinical response and improvement in arterial blood gases are observed.

(2) Every 15–30 minutes, monitor **PaO$_2$ and PaCO$_2$**, obtained from an indwelling arterial catheter, while dose changes are made. Similarly, monitor the blood pressure continuously through the arterial catheter.

(3) During the intravenous infusion of isoproterenol, discontinue all adrenergic aerosols and continue intravenous aminophylline and corticosteroid therapy (infused through a separate intravenous line). The simultaneous intravenous administration of **aminophylline** and **isoproterenol** should be done **cautiously**, with close attention to serum theophylline levels, since aminophylline may accentuate the side effects of adrenergic drugs.

(4) Progressive ventilatory failure necessitates **intubation** and **mechanical ventilation.**

(5) When an adequate clinical response is obtained (PaCO$_2$ consistently < 45 mm Hg), generally after 24–48 hours of a usual maintenance dose of 0.25–0.75 μg/kg/minute (up to 3.5 μg/kg/minute in some children), reduce the isoproterenol dose by 0.1 μg/kg/minute at hourly intervals. Serial PaCO$_2$ tensions are obtained with dose changes; if the PaCO$_2$ increases by 5 mm Hg, raise the concentration to the next higher dose.

(6) Both experience with and evidence for the efficacy of intravenous isoproterenol are greater in children; adolescents and adults have a greater incidence of arrhythmias and myocardial toxicity. **Intravenous isoproterenol should generally be limited to use in children and should not be used in patients with a history of heart disease.** More selective beta-2-adrenergic agonists are currently being employed intravenously or by continuous nebulization on an investigational basis. These agents appear to have less toxicity than isoproterenol.

b. Intubation and mechanical ventilation are associated with numerous potential complications, including barotrauma (subcutaneous emphysema, pneumothorax, tension pneumothorax) secondary to the high inspiratory pressures usually required, atelectasis due to intubation of the right main bronchus, endotracheal tube malfunction (e.g., cuff leak causing hypoventilation or gastric distention), ventilator malfunction, ineffective ventilation, nosocomial pneumonia, mucus plugging, post-extubation subglottic stenosis, and sepsis. Consequently, these procedures should be carried out by an experienced and knowledgeable medical team in an intensive care setting.

(1) An indwelling arterial catheter should be inserted and maintained for continuous monitoring of blood pressure and for arterial blood samples.

(2) Very frequently, asthmatics who are intubated and mechanically ventilated need to be narcotized with intravenous morphine (and sometimes paralyzed with a curariform agent), at least initially, to allow ventilation to be completely controlled. This practice is necessary to prevent discoordination between the ventilator and the patient's spontaneous breathing efforts, which, if uncorrected, could lead to ineffective ventilation and more severe respiratory acidosis.

(a) Morphine sulfate is administered intravenously in a dose of 3–5 mg (0.1–0.2 mg/kg in children) initially over 4–5 minutes while systemic blood pressure is monitored; if necessary, additional doses of morphine are given at 5- to 10-minute intervals until the patient is adequately narcotized.

(b) If hypotension develops, the effect of morphine can be reversed with **naloxone hydrochloride** administered intravenously in a dose of 0.1–0.2 mg (0.01 mg/kg in children) at 2–3-minute intervals as required for reversal of hypotension.

(c) If ventilation cannot be controlled adequately with morphine alone, paralysis of voluntary respiratory muscle activity can be achieved by administering **pancuronium bromide** intravenously in an initial dose of 0.04 mg/kg and repeated in 4–5 minutes if adequate paralysis has not occurred.

(d) Continuous sedation with diazepam (2–5 mg every 4–6 hours) or lorazepam (1–2 mg every two hours) relaxes the patient and may prevent violent muscular efforts. Repeat doses of morphine (1–2 mg/hour) or pancuronium (or both) can be given if discoordination between the ventilator and the patient recurs. These are adult doses.

(e) If effective ventilation of the intubated patient is not achieved despite narcotization and paralysis, **cautious intravenous isoproterenol** can sometimes produce dramatic benefit (see **a**).

c. Volume-limited ventilators are generally preferable to pressure-limited machines to ensure an adequate tidal volume is delivered to the patient.

(1) Ventilators should be adjusted initially to deliver a tidal volume of 10 ml/kg body weight at a rate of 10–12 breaths/minute (increase frequency in infants and children; see Appendix I.B for nomogram to determine breathing rate). The inspiratory flow rate must be adjusted to allow the desired tidal volume to be delivered in the time allowed for inspiration while avoiding excessively high peak inspiratory pressures due to turbulence generated by high flow rates in the presence of a high inspiratory resistance. Occasionally, slower controlled rates are required to allow adequate time both for delivery of the desired tidal volume and for adequate exhalation through the markedly obstructed airways to prevent progressive air trapping ("auto-PEEP"). On the other hand, lowering the tidal volume while slightly increasing the respiratory rate is sometimes indicated to reduce excessively high peak inspiratory pressures.

(2) One hundred percent oxygen should be given before and immediately after intubation and initiation of mechanical ventilation.

(3) Arterial blood gases should be obtained within 30 minutes of initiation of mechanical ventilation or any ventilator adjustments. Changes in the ventilator settings should be made to provide a gradual reduction in the degree of hypercapnia (5–10 mm Hg/hour) and maintenance of a PaO_2 greater than or equal to 60 mm Hg.

(4) Overly rapid correction of PCO_2 must be assiduously avoided to prevent the development of alkalemia due to unmasking of a partially compensatory metabolic alkalosis as respiratory acidosis is corrected.

d. While the patient is being mechanically ventilated, all other therapeutic measures must be pursued with undiminished vigor.

(1) Catheter endotracheal suctioning should be carried out aseptically, expeditiously, with minimal trauma to the tracheobronchial mucosa, and as frequently as needed to eliminate excessive airway secretions.

(2) As a supplement to the water vapor contained in the humidified gas delivered by the ventilator, additional water may need to be added to the airways in the form of heated or ultrasonically generated mist to loosen viscid secretions that are difficult to mobilize. Avoid this therapy if bronchospasm is worsened.

(3) If viscid secretions are extensively plugging the tracheobronchial tree and cannot be loosened by aggressive bronchial hygiene measures, 10% **N-acetylcysteine** (2–3 ml) inhaled as an aerosol every 3–4 hours together with an aerosolized bronchodilator can be tried followed by endotracheal suctioning and chest physical therapy. Although *N*-acetylcysteine can produce effective lysis of mucoid secretions, it is very irritating to the respiratory tract and often cannot be tolerated because of its bronchospastic effect.

(4) An occasional patient with severe asthma fails to respond to bronchodilators, corticosteroids, and bronchial hygiene measures and remains ventilator-dependent due to severe obstruction from secretions that cannot be mobilized effectively. In such patients, consideration can be given to bronchial lavage via bronchoscopy under general anesthesia to remove endobronchial casts. **This procedure is potentially hazardous and not always effective, and therefore should be regarded as a measure of last resort.**

e. **After adequate ventilation is restored, patients should be weaned off the ventilator and extubated as quickly as possible.** Intubation interferes with effective cough (which is dependent on an intact glottic mechanism) and therefore with elimination of bronchial secretions, the major contributing cause of the severe airway obstruction and hypoventilation initially.

(1) Criteria for weaning from mechanical ventilatory assistance include the following:

(a) Vital capacity over 1000 cc (15 cc/kg in children).

(b) Provision of adequate arterial oxygenation by an inspired oxygen concentration of 40% or less.

(c) Ratio of dead space ventilation to total ventilation (V_D/V_T) less than 60%.

(d) Peak inspiratory ventilator pressure less than 25 cm H_2O.

(e) Minute ventilation less than 10 liters/minute (1.5 times the predicted normal minute ventilation in children*).

(f) Ability of the patient to achieve a minute ventilation of 20 liters/minute off the ventilator (3 times the predicted normal ventilation in children*).

(2) Prior to extubation, thoroughly lavage and suction the trachea. Muscle paralysis can be reversed by giving 0.6–1.2 mg of atropine sulfate (0.02 mg/kg in children) and 0.5–2.0 mg of neostigmine methylsulfate (0.07 mg/kg in children) together intravenously—use separate syringes and inject neostigmine slowly. To ensure adequate spontaneous ventilation prior to extubation, administer humidified oxygen at 5–10 liters/minute through a T-piece adapter attached to the endotracheal tube. The endotracheal tube can usually be removed within 6–12 hours.

3. **Weaning problems** can result from psychological dependence on the ventilator or acquired weakness of the respiratory musculature following a prolonged period of mechanical ventilation. Psychological dependence can often be inferred from a combination of patients' attitudes toward weaning attempts and arterial blood gases during weaning trials. Respiratory muscle weakness is often difficult to separate from severe obstructive lung disease with inadequate pulmonary reserve as a cause of weaning failure. These problems can often be resolved by the use of intermittent mandatory ventilation (IMV), which allows patients to breathe spontaneously while, at periodic intervals, their lungs are inflated by the mechanical ventilator. By breathing on their own while assisted in part by the ventilator, patients

---

*Estimation of minute ventilation in children is tidal volume (approximately 10 cc/kg of body weight) times the respiratory rate in breaths/minute (18–30 in children, 30–50 in infants). Nomogram for determination of minute ventilation is shown in Appendix I.B.

gain more confidence in their own ability to breathe and also have the opportunity to retrain their respiratory muscles, which may then gradually resume normal function.

E. After-crisis care

1. Depending on the patient's progress as assessed by reduction in symptoms and signs and sustained improvement in FEV_1 or PEFR, the frequency of aerosolized bronchodilator treatment is gradually reduced from every 1–2 hours to every 4–6 hours while oral beta-agonist drugs are continued.

2. Intravenous corticosteroids should be tapered daily, if possible, by progressive halving of the dose until a dose of approximately 40 mg of methylprednisolone or the equivalent is reached; then oral corticosteroid therapy with prednisone or methylprednisolone can be substituted, with more gradual tapering subsequently.

3. Intravenous aminophylline or theophylline is converted to oral therapy by discontinuing the infusion 3 hours before the first maintenance oral dose is administered. For most individuals, 0.80 times the total daily intravenous dose of aminophylline (or an equivalent dose of intravenous theophylline) can be divided into two equal parts given as an oral sustained-release theophylline preparation at 12-hour intervals. Children have a shorter theophylline half-life than adults, and sustained-release preparations may need to be given every 8–12 hours (see sec. **V.B.1.b.(1)**). During maintenance oral therapy, blood samples obtained at the time of suspected peak blood theophylline level (approximately 5 hours after administration of a 12-hour sustained-release preparation) as well as a trough level obtained prior to the next dose are helpful to ensure that the level is always within the therapeutic range and below toxic concentrations. Serum theophylline levels are obtained every 2–3 days during stabilization of oral therapy as a guide to therapeutic dose adjustment.

4. Because symptoms and signs of asthma can disappear when significant airflow obstruction is still present (i.e., when FEV_1 and $FEF_{25-75\%}$ are reduced by as much as 50% and 70%, respectively, below normal values; see Fig. 6-2), it is important to **continue intensive therapy** until maximal improvement has been achieved, as assessed by objective tests of lung function, if recurrence of severe asthma is to be prevented.

5. Advantage should be taken of hospitalization by reinforcing patient education regarding the disease and its treatment. **Arrangements for adequate follow-up care are essential to prevent recurrences of life-threatening asthma.**

Selected Readings

Fanta, C. H., Rossing, T. H., and McFadden, E. R. Treatment of acute asthma. *Am. J. Med.* 80:5, 1986.

Fiel, S. B., et al. Efficacy of short-term corticosteroid therapy in outpatient treatment of acute bronchial asthma. *Am. J. Med.* 75:259, 1983.

Goldstein, R. A. (ed.). Advances in the diagnosis and treatment of asthma. *Chest* 87:1S–113S, 1985.

Littenberg, B., and Gluck, E. H. A controlled trial of methylprednisolone in the emergency treatment of acute asthma. *N. Engl. J. Med.* 314:150, 1986.

Rebuck, A. S., and Read, J. Assessment and management of severe asthma. *Am. J. Med.* 51:788, 1971.

Sheffer, A. L., and Rachelefsky, G. S. (eds.). Asthma '84: Pharmacologic update. *J. Allergy Clin. Immunol.* 76:249, 1985.

Weiss, E. B., Segal, M. S., and Stein, M. (eds.). Bronchial Asthma: Mechanisms and Therapeutics (2nd ed.). Boston: Little, Brown, 1985.

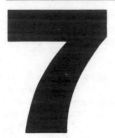

Immunologic Diseases of the Lung

Henry Gong, Jr.

The lung is an important and vulnerable target in immunologic diseases. Not only does the lung participate in systemic immunopathologic processes, it also is capable of initiating local immune reactions that may be beneficial or adverse to the host. Excluding asthma, primary and secondary immunologic lung diseases are discussed in this chapter according to their presentation, pathologic features, diagnostic criteria, differential diagnosis, treatment, and prognosis. The various entities are often different clinically, but are either known or proposed to have immunologic mechanisms. These entities include hypersensitivity pneumonitis, allergic bronchopulmonary aspergillosis, pulmonary infiltrates with eosinophilia, Goodpasture's syndrome, idiopathic pulmonary hemosiderosis, Wegener's granulomatosis, sarcoidosis, and diffuse interstitial fibrosis of the lung.

Hypersensitivity Pneumonitis

Hypersensitivity pneumonitis (or extrinsic allergic alveolitis) is a common and well studied immunologically mediated lung disease. It consists of a group of diffuse interstitial or alveolar-filling (or both) granulomatous diseases resulting from inhalation of organic dusts and subsequent immunopathologic reactions localized in the lung (without systemic involvement). Since hypersensitivity pneumonitis develops in only 5–15% of the exposed population, and the majority of patients are nonatopic and nonsmokers, other factors determine how a person will respond to inhalation of organic dust. An atopic person will respond with production of reaginic (IgE) antibodies, whereas a nonallergic person is likely to produce precipitating (IgG) antibodies. The antigenic materials are usually of animal or vegetable origin and must be less than 5 μ in diameter to penetrate to the alveoli. Acute or chronic exposures and intensity of exposure are critical but unpredictable factors. Evidence also suggests a genetic predisposition to the development of hypersensitivity pneumonitis. In general, there are no age, sex, or significant geographic predilections.

I. **Causative antigens.** The antigens listed in Table 7-1 are recognized as capable of sensitizing susceptible persons and subsequently causing hypersensitivity pneumonitis. This is only a partial list, and new sources from occupational exposure, homes, and hobbies are reported annually. Despite this long, expanding list, these conditions have striking similarities in their clinical, x-ray, and pathologic features.

II. **Clinical features**

    A. **Acute hypersensitivity pneumonitis** occurs when exposure is heavy but intermittent.

        1. **Symptoms and signs.** Acute symptoms, including fever, chills, dyspnea, chest tightness, and dry cough, appear 4–6 hours after each exposure and remit when the causative agent is avoided. This is considered a late, or Arthus (type III), immune reaction (see Chap. 1). Only a few rhonchi or rales are noted on physical examination of the chest.

        2. **Blood tests.** Peripheral neutrophilia (without eosinophilia) and increased IgG levels are commonly seen in the acute form. Serum IgE levels are usually within normal limits.

        3. **X-ray findings.** X-ray abnormalities will typically develop with repeated

Table 7-1. Principal causes of hypersensitivity pneumonitis

Clinical condition	Source of antigen	Antigen
Farmer's lung	Moldy hay	*Micropolyspora faeni, Thermoactinomyces vulgaris*
Bird fancier's or breeder's lung	Pigeon, parakeet, parrot, turkey, chicken, etc.	Sera, protein, and droppings
Bagassosis	Pressed sugar cane (bagasse)	*Thermoactinomyces sacchari*
Suberosis	Cork dust	?
Malt worker's lung	Barley	*Aspergillus* sp.
Maple bark disease	Maple bark	*Cryptostroma corticale*
Sequoiosis	Redwood sawdust	*Graphium* sp., *Pullularia* sp.
Woodworker's lung	Oak, cedar dusts, pine, spruce pulp	Wood dust, *Alternaria* sp.
Humidifier lung	Contaminated home humidifier and air conditioning ducts	*Thermoactinomyces* sp.
Mushroom worker's lung	Compost	*Micropolyspora faeni Thermoactinomyces vulgaris*
Paprika slicer's lung	Paprika	*Mucor stolonifer*
Cheese washer's lung	Moldy cheese	*Penicillium casei*
Miller's lung	Wheat weevils	*Sitophilus granarius*
Furrier's lung	Animal hairs	?
Chemical worker's lung	Polyurethane products, meat wrapping	Toluene diisocyanate (TDI), methylene diisocyanate (MDI), phthalic anhydride, vinyl chloride

antigen exposure and usually parallel the severity of the clinical symptoms. Bilateral, finely granular or nodular mottling is characteristic and is due to alveolar inflammation (alveolitis).

   4. **Physiologic tests.** Pulmonary function tests show hypoxemia and a restrictive ventilatory pattern, with reduced vital capacity, total lung capacity, diffusing capacity, and static compliance. Airway obstruction is not typical unless the patient is a smoker or is atopic.

B. **Acute hypersensitivity pneumonitis in asthmatic patients.** Approximately 10% of patients with hypersensitivity pneumonitis have atopy and asthma or asthmatic bronchitis. A two-stage reaction develops in these patients if they are exposed to organic dust. The immediate asthmatic, or type I, immune reaction will be manifested by dyspnea, wheezing, and an obstructive ventilatory pattern. This reaction subsides and is followed in 4–6 hours by a type III immune reaction.

C. **Chronic hypersensitivity pneumonitis** occurs when exposure is mild but more continuous (e.g., from a single parakeet).

   1. **Symptoms and signs.** Progressive dyspnea, decreased exercise tolerance, productive cough, and weight loss develop insidiously. Acute episodes of chills and fever are less likely. Wheezing, cyanosis, clubbing, and cor pulmonale develop as pulmonary inflammation and fibrosis progress.

   2. **X-ray findings.** The diffuse nodular pattern characteristic of the acute and

subacute stages is replaced by a medium-to-coarse reticular pattern, loss of lung volume, a honeycomb pattern, and compensatory overinflation (emphysema) of less involved lung zones. These changes are typical of diffuse interstitial fibrosis of any origin, and such findings usually indicate an irreversible stage.

   3. **Physiologic testing.** Pulmonary function tests show severe restrictive disease, with variable airway obstruction and air trapping.
III. **Immunologic features**
   A. **Serum precipitins.** The characteristic immunologic feature of hypersensitivity pneumonitis is the presence of precipitating (usually IgG) antibody to the offending antigen. Serum antibodies or precipitins are readily and reproducibly demonstrated by the Ouchterlony double-gel diffusion technique. However, the presence of serum precipitins against an antigen present in a patient's environment is not prima facie evidence that it is the causal antigen in hypersensitivity pneumonitis. Although the **positive precipitin test** is clinically helpful, it actually indicates prior exposure and sensitization, not necessarily with clinical sequelae. Precipitins are observed in 90% of patients with active farmer's lung, but the percentage of detectable antibodies falls as time passes. Serum precipitins without clinical pneumonitis may develop in up to 50% of asymptomatic patients. Conversely, there are rare patients with clinical disease and no demonstrable antibodies. Antibodies may be demonstrated by more sensitive techniques such as immunoelectrophoresis and immunofluorescence. The correct antigen must be used to detect antibodies, but many causative antigens have not been identified. In addition, commercial gel diffusion kits are available, but extracts prepared by individual investigators give substantially more positive precipitin reactions than do the commercial kits. Thus, a negative precipitin test in the face of convincing clinical evidence does not exclude the diagnosis, whereas a positive test without appropriate clinical findings does not establish it.
   B. **Skin testing.** Commercial antigens* are now available for skin testing for many of the conditions listed in Table 7-1. The important exceptions are extracts of thermophilic actinomycetes, which act as nonspecific irritants. When protein antigens such as pigeon serum are used, skin testing will generally result in a dual response consisting of an immediate wheal and flare (type I immune reaction) and a late response (type III immune reaction) at 3–8 hours, which subsides in 24–48 hours.
   Although the immediate intracutaneous reaction is due to IgE antibody in atopic persons, a short-term sensitizing IgG antibody may be responsible in nonatopic persons. Positive late reactions closely correlate with both clinical disease and presence of precipitins.
   C. **T cell involvement.** Since a type III immune reaction alone cannot adequately explain the pathogenesis of hypersensitivity pneumonitis, a combination of types III and IV (and also type I in atopic persons) is probably involved. Circulating T cells sensitized to antigen (e.g., pigeon proteins) are capable of in vitro lymphocyte transformation and production of macrophage inhibition factors. Bronchoalveolar lavages in patients with hypersensitivity pneumonitis have shown increased lymphocyte numbers, increased percentage of T cells, increased subset of suppressor T cells (T8), and elevated IgG and IgM levels as compared with the findings in peripheral blood. The finding that bronchoalveolar lymphocytes (T cells) can proliferate when exposed to antigens in vitro and induce macrophage-migration inhibition strongly suggests that pulmonary as well as systemic cell-mediated immunity occurs in hypersensitivity pneumonitis.
IV. The **pathologic features** of all forms of hypersensitivity pneumonitis are similar and nonspecific unless one is fortunate enough to identify fungus (e.g., maple bark disease), vegetable fibers (bagassosis), or cork dust (suberosis) within lesions. The histologic reflection of precipitating antigen-antibody complexes and activation of the complement cascade in lung tissue is best demonstrated in early hypersensitivity pneumonitis. This pathologic reaction consists of acute vasculitis of alveolar

*Hollister-Stier Laboratories, Spokane, WA 99220

capillaries, fibrin thrombi, and influx of neutrophils, eosinophils, and mononuclear cells. The acute alveolar damage is associated with bronchiolitis (25–100% of cases) and later with noncaseating granulomas (similar to those in sarcoidosis) and significant interstitial pneumonitis with mononuclear cells. Over the course of several months the lesions become nonspecific as the granulomas disappear and interstitial fibrosis and obliterative bronchiolitis predominate, resulting eventually in emphysema and a honeycomb lung. Antigen (*Micropolyspora faeni*), antibody (IgG, IgA, and IgM), and complement (C3) have been found in the lung tissue of some patients.

V. Diagnostic approach

A. Specific etiologic approach

1. **A high index of suspicion** is based on a detailed environmental history. Although patients often associate recurrent exposures with symptoms in the acute form of hypersensitivity pneumonitis, the chronic form is much more difficult to identify.

2. Positive or consistent **chest x-rays**; adenopathy and pleural effusions are not typical.

3. Compatible **pulmonary function tests,** serum precipitins, and skin tests.

4. **Trial of avoidance and controlled reexposure** to the suspected antigen or environment. Deliberate repetition of natural exposure to the suspected antigenic environmental source (e.g., barn, factory) and observing the clinical response (by physical examinations, chest x-rays, and spirometry before and after exposure) constitute simple, relatively safe diagnostic procedures.

B. An allergen inhalation challenge test.
In instances in which the specific diagnosis remains in doubt because the relevance of a particular exposure is questionable, allergen inhalation or bronchial challenge tests can be useful in establishing a definitive diagnosis. Various dusts or liquids in the home or work area can be collected and cultured and extracts prepared from these for gel diffusion or inhalation challenge studies in order to identify the responsible antigen.

1. Positive reactions to aerosolized extracts of the appropriate antigen will produce symptoms and signs of hypersensitivity pneumonitis as immediate, late, or dual reactions. Within minutes, measurable bronchospasm (without associated fever or leukocytosis) develops in susceptible persons and subsides spontaneously in 1–3 hours. Late reactions occur 4–6 hours after inhalation and show primarily systemic symptoms, a restrictive ventilatory defect, and leukocytosis. Pretreatment with beta-adrenergic bronchodilators and cromolyn sodium will block or inhibit the immediate response, while corticosteroids will inhibit the late reaction. The late reaction alone is more commonly present than a dual reaction. Almost all patients with either late or dual reactions have serum precipitins to the appropriate antigen.

2. Bronchial challenge tests must utilize **purified extracts** to be diagnostically helpful. The patient can become severely ill during the procedure and require hospitalization and parenteral corticosteroids. Thus, this procedure should **not** be performed routinely but only in laboratories experienced in its administration.

C. Differential diagnosis.
Both the acute and chronic forms of hypersensitivity pneumonitis may be confused with recurrent pneumonias, drug-induced lung disease, allergic bronchopulmonary aspergillosis, sarcoidosis, and collagen vascular diseases. The long list of interstitial lung diseases that may mimic hypersensitivity pneumonitis is summarized in Table 7-3. Farmers are exposed to multiple respiratory antigens, and only a careful history can distinguish the diagnosis of farmer's lung, grain dust asthma, silo-filler's disease, and pulmonary mycotoxicosis. Although the historic and physical findings can usually differentiate and limit the possibilities, open lung biopsy is justified in puzzling cases or in patients without an environmental history.

VI. Treatment

A. General treatment measures

1. **Avoidance.** If possible, avoiding the offending antigen is the most important treatment of hypersensitivity pneumonitis, especially in the acute

form. Masks or dust filters, alteration of ventilatory or air-conditioning systems, education of the patient, and even changing occupations are other preventive or therapeutic measures.

2. **Bronchodilators** and cromolyn sodium usually alleviate or prevent acute asthmatic symptoms.

3. **Hyposensitization** is **not** useful or advisable because of the potential danger that parenteral injection of an antigen might increase the levels of precipitins and set the stage for a severe reaction on reexposure to the airborne allergen.

B. **Corticosteroid therapy** is indicated when the offending antigen cannot be avoided or when symptoms are severe or prolonged. Corticosteroids hasten the resolution of symptoms and physiologic abnormalities and possibly prevent tissue damage from the inflammatory reaction. The response to **prednisone,** 60 mg/day for a week, with tapering to 20 mg/day over 2 weeks and then weekly 5 mg decrements, is often dramatic, with the chest x-ray and spirometric findings (except diffusing capacity) rapidly returning to normal. The initial pediatric dose of prednisone is 2 mg/kg/day in this disease and in other severe respiratory diseases (requiring pharmacologic anti-inflammatory therapy) described subsequently in this chapter. Whether or not prednisone is administered, patients should be followed periodically by chest x-rays and spirometry. The chronic form of the disease is unfortunately less easy to treat, and a short trial of corticosteroids should be given empirically with the assumption that part of the interstitial disease is potentially reversible. The use of inhaled corticosteroids is of questionable value.

VII. The **prognosis** is excellent, provided the antigen is avoided and/or corticosteroid therapy is instituted before irreparable tissue damage (fibrosis) occurs. In the patient with acute disease, avoidance of the offending antigen will result in a return to normal pulmonary function. However, in chronic disease, pulmonary fibrosis and advanced respiratory failure often exist when these patients first present for treatment.

Allergic Bronchopulmonary Aspergillosis

Allergic bronchopulmonary aspergillosis is immunologically classified as both an immediate hypersensitivity and immune complex disease. It is caused by *Aspergillus fumigatus* and is characteristically associated with asthma and proximal bronchiectasis. Allergic bronchopulmonary aspergillosis occurs most frequently in atopic patients, and a history of asthma is always obtained. The incidence is relatively high in the United Kingdom and low in the United States, but the geographic differences in the incidence of the disorder may be due in part to lack of recognition. In the majority of patients, the diagnosis is made after the age of 20 years.

I. **Clinical presentation**

A. **Clinical features**

1. **Symptoms and signs.** Patients present typically with episodes of fever, wheezing, productive cough, minimal hemoptysis, shortness of breath, leukocytosis, and sputum and blood eosinophilia, particularly during the winter months. Patients usually expectorate brownish plugs or flecks and occasionally, bronchial casts. The casts contain the causative fungus, which is seen on microscopic examination and by culture (67% of the time). A single sputum culture growing *Aspergillus* is not diagnostic because the organism is ubiquitous and is a possible contaminant. Repeatedly positive sputum cultures, however, are suspicious.

2. **X-ray findings.** Chest x-rays frequently show transient or fixed pulmonary infiltrates resulting from proximal saccular bronchiectasis. Upper lobe fibrosis occurs in patients with chronic disease.

3. **Physiologic tests.** The presence of mucus plugging (mucus impaction syndrome) and airway damage is commonly, but not always, associated with

evidence of reversible airway obstruction and lowered diffusing capacity on pulmonary function testing. A restrictive ventilatory pattern may occur with pulmonary fibrosis and may not reverse with corticosteroid therapy.

B. Immunologic features. Skin tests positive for *Aspergillus* show both an immediate wheal-and-flare reaction (type I) and a late erythema and edema or Arthus reaction (type III). Serum precipitins to the fungus and markedly elevated serum IgE levels (> 1000 units/ml) are common findings.

C. Pathologic features. The pathogenesis of allergic bronchopulmonary aspergillosis is not known. Although thick, tenacious mucus plugs with fungal elements fill the affected bronchi, the organism does not invade the bronchial wall or lung parenchyma. The bronchial-wall damage is associated with intense infiltration by eosinophils and mononuclear cells and the presence of granulomas (bronchocentric granulomatosis in some patients).

II. Diagnostic approach

A. Specific etiologic approach. The diagnosis is certain if the following conditions (usually present in over 90% of patients) are present:

1. **Episodic bronchial obstruction (asthma).**
2. **Peripheral blood eosinophilia.**
3. **Transient or fixed pulmonary infiltrates.**
4. **Proximal bronchiectasis.** Obtain computerized tomography or, in selected patients, bronchograms of suspicious areas on the chest x-ray. Proximal bronchiectasis with distal bronchial tapering is absolutely confirmatory but not essential because the bronchi may be normal or minimally altered early in the course of the disease.
5. **Immediate skin reactivity** to *Aspergillus* antigen on prick or intradermal testing. Patients with a history of recurrent asthma and pulmonary infiltrates should be evaluated initially with skin tests for *Aspergillus*. If both prick and intradermal tests are negative, and assuming the *Aspergillus* antigen is reliable, it is very unlikely that allergic bronchopulmonary aspergillosis is the cause of the symptoms.
6. **Precipitating antibodies** against *Aspergillus* antigen.
7. **Elevated serum IgE** by radioimmunoassay. Patients with positive skin tests should have confirmatory serum precipitin and IgE (total and antigen-specific) levels evaluated since they reflect disease activity.

B. Differential diagnosis. Patients with allergic bronchopulmonary aspergillosis frequently have had prior diagnosis of intractable asthma, chronic bronchitis, recurrent pneumonia, tuberculosis, or bronchiectasis due to other causes. However, it is possible for some of these entities to coexist with the fungal hypersensitivity. Allergic bronchopulmonary aspergillosis may be confused with other conditions exhibiting pulmonary infiltrates with eosinophilia (Table 7-2).

III. Treatment

A. General treatment. Bronchodilators and antibiotics (if bacterial infection is suspected) will improve the asthmatic component of the disease, especially during acute exacerbations. Flexible fiber-optic or rigid bronchoscopy can effectively clear secretions and mucus plugs in difficult cases. Hyposensitization with *Aspergillus* extracts is **not** recommended because it may accentuate local and asthmatic reactions.

B. Corticosteroids. Oral **prednisone** (0.5 mg/kg/day, or 20–40 mg/day) is currently the treatment of choice, although its mechanism of action is not known. Symptoms, expectorated plugs, positive cultures, and infiltrates seen on x-ray resolve or decrease in frequency rapidly (in days to weeks) with daily prednisone therapy.

1. Although the responses of precipitins and total serum IgG to corticosteroid therapy are variable, total serum IgE levels fall significantly with remission and are of benefit in monitoring and predicting disease activity.
2. A 2- to 3-month course of prednisone therapy with subsequent tapering and monitoring (by history, chest x-rays, and serum IgE levels) will suffice in most patients. However, in some patients, the disease may be exacerbated

Table 7-2. Eosinophilic syndromes with pulmonary involvement

Syndrome	Etiology	Symptoms	Physical findings	Blood eosinophilia	Chest x-ray	Other features	Treatment	Prognosis
Simple pulmonary eosinophilia (Löffler's syndrome)	Drugs, parasites	None or minimal	None or minimal	10–30%	Transient peripheral infiltrates		None; self-limited	Excellent
Prolonged pulmonary eosinophilia (chronic eosinophilic pneumonia)	? Drugs, parasites; fungal and bacterial infections in some patients	Severe cough, dyspnea, fever; wheezing in two-thirds of patients	Wheezing	20–40% in two-thirds of patients	Dense, recurring peripheral infiltrates	Females; asthma with onset	Corticosteroids	Good with prolonged therapy
Tropical (filarial) eosinophilia	Microfilariae	Dry cough, wheezing, dyspnea, fever	None or wheezing; adenopathy	> 20–50%	Diffuse nodular infiltrates	High levels of filarial antibodies and IgE; residence in tropics	Diethylcarbamazine	Good
Pulmonary eosinophilia with asthma (allergic bronchopulmonary aspergillosis)	Atopic host with aspergillus	Wheezing, productive cough, fever	Wheezing	10–20%	Migratory, recurrent infiltrates, occasional bronchiectasis	High IgE levels; positive precipitins and skin tests	Corticosteroids	Good; possible recurrence
Pulmonary eosinophilia with polyarteritis nodosa and variants	?	Fever, chest pain, cough, hemoptysis; extrapulmonary multisystem involvement	Nonspecific and variable	> 20% in 20–30% of patients	Variable	Vasculitis in medium-sized arteries	Corticosteroids, cyclophosphamide	Poor

after corticosteroids are discontinued, and, after repeated courses, they may require prednisone therapy indefinitely (e.g., at least 10 mg/day).

3. The efficacy of alternate-day corticosteroids or inhaled corticosteroids is limited since asymptomatic pulmonary infiltrates can continue to develop during either kind of therapy.

IV. Prognosis. Pulmonary infiltrates and further lung destruction continue to develop in untreated patients. Irreversible bronchiectasis, pulmonary fibrosis, recurrent pneumonias, and, eventually, respiratory failure result. On the other hand, effective treatment with corticosteroids is associated with significantly fewer recurrences of pulmonary infiltrates and less bronchial damage. Fungal invasion or extension in patients on long-term corticosteroid therapy has not been documented.

Pulmonary Infiltrates with Eosinophilia

Pulmonary infiltrates with eosinophilia (PIE) is a generic term applied to a group of eosinophilic (blood or tissue or both) syndromes with pulmonary involvement. In this section, simple and prolonged pulmonary eosinophilia, tropical eosinophilia, and polyarteritis nodosa will be discussed. Allergic bronchopulmonary aspergillosis, another member of this spectrum of diseases, is discussed separately. Although the commonly used classification of PIE (see Table 7-2) is somewhat arbitrary, the scheme will continue to serve as a useful clinicopathologic approach until the immunologic roles of eosinophils and eosinophilia are better characterized.

I. Simple pulmonary eosinophilia (Löffler's syndrome)

A. Clinical presentation

1. **Clinical features.** Patients are usually asymptomatic or have minimal constitutional symptoms. They have blood eosinophilia and transient, migratory infiltrates on serial chest x-rays. Radiographic changes are patchy, homogeneous, peripheral (pleura based), and either unilateral or bilateral. The syndrome probably represents an allergic response to several causative or associated agents: *Ascaris, Strongyloides,* para-aminosalicylic acid, sulfonamides, chlorpropamide, nitrofurantoin, and chemicals such as nickel carbonyl. Idiopathic cases are also reported.

2. **Pathologic features.** Light and electron microscopy of lung tissue show interstitial eosinophilic pneumonia without necrosis or vasculitis.

B. Diagnostic approach. Because of the lack of absolute criteria, the diagnosis of simple pulmonary eosinophilia is based on a **retrospective** clinical impression. A mildly symptomatic patient with blood eosinophilia, transient pulmonary infiltrates, and spontaneous resolution of these findings within a month meets the strict criteria for the diagnosis. Stools should be examined for parasites. Some cases of simple pulmonary eosinophilia possibly develop into the prolonged variety of PIE.

Since increasing numbers of diagnostic studies have documented specific causes of simple pulmonary eosinophilia (and other eosinophilic syndromes), the use of the term has become limited.

C. Treatment. Because the symptoms are minimal and improvement is spontaneous, medication is usually not necessary. However, there may be recurrences if the susceptible patient is reexposed to the same or other offending agents. Corticosteroids or antihelminthic drugs can be given for severe systemic reactions.

D. The **prognosis** is excellent, and there is no evidence of permanent damage to the lung parenchyma if the offending agent is withdrawn or treated.

II. Prolonged pulmonary eosinophilia (chronic eosinophilic pneumonia)

A. Clinical presentation

1. **Clinical features.** Patients with this syndrome have moderate to severe symptoms (fever, sweats, weight loss, cough, dyspnea, and wheezing in the majority) that persist over a month. A variety of agents or conditions (parasites, fungi, bacteria, hypersensitivity pneumonitis, drug allergies) cause prolonged pulmonary eosinophilia. Patients with chronic eosinophilic pneu-

monia present with chronic, severe symptoms, chest x-ray changes, blood eosinophilia, and a restrictive ventilatory pattern (with decreased diffusing capacity and hypoxemia). The outcome is potentially fatal unless the patient is vigorously treated with corticosteroids. Asthma may occur for the first time during the typical presentation of chronic eosinophilic pneumonia and persist in the years following. Although a history of atopy is present in one-third of the patients, the etiology of chronic eosinophilic pneumonia remains unknown.

   2. Pathologic features. The alveoli and interstitium of the lung are characteristically filled with eosinophils and mononuclear cells. There may be occasional granuloma formation in "eosinophilic abscesses" and, rarely, microangiitis.

B. Diagnostic approach
   1. Criteria. The typical patient with chronic eosinophilic pneumonia presents with the preceding clinical features and, most important, with a chest x-ray appearance that is diagnostic; in fact, the diagnosis can be made by the astute radiologist in 75% of cases. Progressive dense infiltrates without lobar or segmental distribution are seen opposed peripherally to the pleura. The appearance is that of a photographic negative or reversal of the shadows commonly seen in pulmonary edema. The opacities disappear and then recur in exactly the same locations. Blood eosinophilia is confirmatory, but its absence (in one-third of cases) does not exclude the diagnosis. Lung biopsy is unnecessary to confirm the diagnosis unless there is a reasonable doubt, e.g., when peripheral eosinophilia or the characteristic radiographic pattern is lacking.

   2. Differential diagnosis. The clinician may initially suspect polyarteritis nodosa, vasculitis, recurrent viral or bacterial pneumonia, tuberculosis, allergic bronchopulmonary aspergillosis, or sarcoidosis.

C. Treatment. Corticosteroid therapy causes a dramatic and complete clinical recovery and clearing of the chest x-ray within a few days, as well as histologic resolution of the eosinophilic infiltration. Although the symptoms vary from patient to patient, all patients should receive prednisone (60 mg/day initially, 1–2 mg/kg in children), with gradual tapering and maintenance on an individual basis. The optimal duration of corticosteroid therapy is not known and must be individualized; it may be necessary indefinitely in difficult cases. Empirical reduction or omission of therapy frequently causes exacerbation of symptoms and chest infiltrates. The therapeutic benefit of inhaled corticosteroids in this disease is not known. Bronchodilators will be helpful if a bronchospastic component is present. Supplemental oxygen is necessary during acute episodes.

D. The **prognosis** is excellent with corticosteroid therapy, although recurrences are frequent if the dosage is reduced or if the therapy is discontinued prematurely.

III. Tropical eosinophilia
A. Clinical presentation
   1. Clinical features
      a. Symptoms and signs. Infected persons in the tropics (or any area where human filariasis is transmitted and importable) have an insidious onset consisting of dry cough, dyspnea, nocturnal wheezing, malaise, anorexia, weight loss, and low-grade fever. The patients are usually males (4:1 sex ratio) in their third and fourth decade. Coarse rales, rhonchi, and wheezing are heard during symptomatic episodes. Moderate lymphadenopathy and hepatomegaly are common in children but not in adults. The eosinophil count is extremely high ($> 3000/mm^3$), and the eosinophilia persists for weeks.

      b. X-ray findings. Chest x-rays are almost always abnormal during episodes and show increased bronchovascular markings and diffuse 1- to 3-mm nodules or mottled opacities, without hilar adenopathy or pleural effusions.

      c. Physiologic tests. Pulmonary function evaluation shows a restrictive ventilatory pattern and diffusion impairment, particularly in long-standing disease. Airway obstruction can be seen in 25–30% of patients.

2. **Pathologic features**

   a. **Lungs.** The pulmonary lesions are related to the duration of illness and are distinctly different from those of asthma. Patients with a short history of symptoms show an alveolar and interstitial infiltration by histiocytes. This picture then evolves into an eosinophilic bronchopneumonia and eosinophilic abscesses. Radiographically apparent nodules are found histologically to be interstitial granulomatous reactions surrounding degenerated microfilariae or necrotic centers. These nodules may progress to predominantly histiocytic, granulomatous changes with increasing parenchymal fibrosis.

   b. **Lymph nodes.** Infected peripheral lymph nodes show microfilariae and a foreign-body, granulomatous response with a prominence of eosinophils.

B. **Diagnostic approach**

   1. **Specific etiologic approach.** Establishing the diagnosis of tropical pulmonary eosinophilia is difficult because the adult host apparently sequesters the parasite in the pulmonary parenchyma, and there is no microfilaremia in either day or night blood samples. The diagnosis must be based on the clinical presentation, history of prolonged (usually months) residence in an endemic area, hypereosinophilia, markedly elevated IgE levels (over 1000 units/ml), and high titers of antifilarial antibodies. Lung biopsy is not necessary to find microfilariae. Enlarged lymph nodes are more likely to yield microfilariae from tissue specimens. Marked improvement in 7–10 days with therapy (diethylcarbamazine) is another diagnostic criterion.

   2. **Differential diagnosis.** Few, if any, of the other eosinophilic lung diseases exhibit this x-ray pattern. Diseases with both pulmonary and systemic manifestations include polyarteritis nodosa and other vasculitides, drug allergies, hypereosinophilic syndrome (associated with leukemia, fibroplastic endocarditis, or collagen vascular diseases), and parasitic infections such as *Ascaris, Strongyloides, Ancylostoma,* and *Toxocara canis.*

C. **Treatment.** Diethylcarbamazine (5 mg/kg/day) will produce marked clinical improvement in the vast majority of patients after 7–10 days of therapy. Patients with chronic symptoms respond variably. Patients who improve may relapse and then respond again to another course of treatment.

IV. **Polyarteritis nodosa**

A. **Clinical presentation**

   1. **Clinical features.** Lung involvement in polyarteritis nodosa is uncommon; a combination of eosinophilia and pulmonary infiltration occurs in 10% of patients. Up to 30% of patients have peripheral eosinophilia during life, and 25% have pulmonary involvement at autopsy. Patients usually present after their third decade of life. The clinical manifestations of the disease are varied and occur singly or in combination over a short or long course.

      a. **Symptoms and signs.** Patients have a sudden onset of intractable wheezing, especially associated with systemic involvement, e.g., fever, hypertension, renal failure, congestive heart failure, abdominal pains, peripheral neuritis, myalgias, and generalized weakness. Dry cough, hemoptysis, and pleuritic chest pain are common with lung involvement.

      b. **X-ray findings.** The abnormal chest x-ray most commonly shows transient patchy infiltrates, consolidations, and nodules that rarely cavitate.

      c. **Laboratory findings.** Nonspecific laboratory findings include anemia, leukocytosis, eosinophilia, elevated erythrocyte sedimentation rate and serum IgE, cryoglobulinemia, hypocomplementemia, and decreased renal function.

   2. **Pathologic features**

      a. **Histologic features.** Diffuse and focal inflammation of medium-sized arteries of any organ may be involved. Thrombosis, infarction, or hemorrhage in vital organs accounts for the majority of presenting complaints. The lesions are segmental, and this can be diagnostically confusing on tissue biopsy. The affected lung tissue is characterized by vasculitis of the arterioles or by both vasculitis and granuloma formation. Eosinophils, when present, accumulate in a pattern similar to that in prolonged pulmonary eosinophilia. Hypersensitivity angiitis and allergic granulomatosis (of Churg and Strauss) are variants or separate entities, although unequivocal differentiation on clinical or histopathologic criteria is very difficult.

    b. Pathogenesis. The cause of polyarteritis nodosa is unknown. It has been described in association with serous otitis media, drug abuse, hepatitis B antigenemia, penicillin, sulfonamides, equine serum sickness, preceding respiratory infections, and even allergic hyposensitization (the latter for presumptive extrinsic bronchial asthma). Some patients have asthma several years before the first recognized manifestation of polyarteritis nodosa.

B. Diagnostic approach

    1. Criteria. Although the presenting symptoms and chest x-ray appearance are similar to the findings in prolonged pulmonary eosinophilia, the presence of multisystem involvement is indicative of polyarteritis nodosa with lung involvement. Two or more organ systems are involved in over 80% of the patients.

        a. Biopsy. The diagnosis of polyarteritis nodosa requires confirmation of arterial vasculitis, and biopsy of an affected organ (skin, muscle, kidney, testes, or liver) is necessary.

        b. Angiography of the kidney or other abdominal viscera is a useful screening procedure. Many clinicians regard angiographic findings of multiple aneurysms as diagnostic, but it should be emphasized that sufficient angiographic data have not been compiled in other collagen vascular diseases and vasculitides.

    2. Differential diagnosis. Without tissue confirmation, the differential diagnosis of this multisystem disease includes the collagen vascular diseases, hypersensitivity angiitis, allergic granulomatosis, Wegener's granulomatosis, and, when eosinophilia is present, the other pulmonary eosinophilic syndromes (see Table 7-2).

C. Treatment. The treatment of polyarteritis nodosa has been unsatisfactory. Corticosteroids may provide symptomatic improvement, but there is conflicting evidence as to their long-term benefit and effect on survival. Initial therapy for polyarteritis nodosa should be high-dose corticosteroids (prednisone, 1–2 mg/kg/day), with subsequent monitoring of the clinical and laboratory response. If the response to corticosteroids is poor, cyclophosphamide (1–2 mg/kg/day) or azathioprine (1–2 mg/kg/day) can be tried.

D. The **prognosis** in patients with polyarteritis nodosa is generally poor despite therapy. The estimated 5-year survival is 50–60%, and most deaths occur within the first 3 months after the initial diagnosis. Patients with multiorgan involvement (particularly with hypertension and renal disease) tend to have a more fulminant course than those with more limited organ involvement. The major causes of death are hemorrhage, rupture of viscera, renal or respiratory failure, and sepsis coincident with immunosuppressive therapy.

Goodpasture's Syndrome

Goodpasture's syndrome is one of the first diagnostic possibilities raised when the clinician is confronted with pulmonary hemorrhage associated with nephritis. Its immunopathologic nature is underscored by its more accurate alternative term, **anti–basement-membrane antibody-induced glomerulonephritis and pulmonary hemorrhage.** Although Goodpasture originally described the syndrome as a sequela of influenza, and it is now accepted as due to an antigen-antibody reaction (type II), its actual cause and the predisposing factors remain unclear. This disease typically affects young adult males (usually during the second decade of life), with occasional familial occurrence. Less than 20% of reported cases of Goodpasture's syndrome involve women.

I. Clinical presentation

A. Clinical features

1. **Symptoms and signs.** Patients invariably present with mild or frank hemoptysis days or months prior to clinical manifestations of renal disease. Other symptoms include dyspnea (57%), fatigue (51%), cough (41%), fever (22%), and, eventually, hematuria (90%). Symptoms attributed to a viral syndrome are found in 20% of patients. Physical findings include pallor (51%), mild hypertension (13%), retinal hemorrhages and exudates (11%), edema (25%), and rales or wheezes (37%). Skin purpura is rare.

2. **Blood and urine findings.** Iron deficiency anemia is present in 98% of patients. Other laboratory findings include leukocytosis (50% incidence), proteinuria (88%), red and white blood cell casts (> 70%), granular casts (56%), and progressive azotemia (71%). The urinalysis is initially normal in 10% of patients.

3. **X-ray findings.** The chest x-ray will initially show widespread bilateral patchy airspace consolidation that simulates pulmonary edema in 90% of cases. Serial x-rays show either progressive acinar consolidation during continued pulmonary hemorrhage or a reticular pattern whose distribution matches that of the airspace process (or both). The chest x-ray findings may return to normal in days after the acute episode.

   Progressive interstitial fibrosis results from repeated hemorrhage and increasing hemosiderin deposition within the lung interstitium. Hilar adenopathy can occur during acute episodes, but pleural effusions are rare.

4. **Physiologic tests.** Pulmonary function tests commonly reveal a predominantly restrictive ventilatory pattern with or without arterial hypoxemia at rest. Diffusing capacity for carbon monoxide is absolutely decreased, but the ratio of gas transfer to alveolar volume is increased over 50% of the predicted value, suggesting pulmonary hemorrhage.

B. Immunologic features.
Antistreptolysin O titers and blood coagulation tests and collagen vascular serologic tests are normal or negative. However, serum anti-glomerular-basement-membrane (GBM) antibody is invariably positive by radioimmunoassay, and titers correlate with pulmonary hemorrhage.

C. Pathologic features

1. The **lungs** are the only site of hemorrhage and reveal extensive intraalveolar hemorrhage during an acute episode. Light microscopy will reveal hemosiderin-laden macrophages, intact alveolar and endothelial cells, and a component of interstitial fibrosis in patients with chronic disease. In contrast to collagen vascular diseases affecting the lung, vasculitis and pulmonary arteritis are minimal or absent in Goodpasture's syndrome. However, electron microscopy shows vascular damage with wide endothelial gaps and occasionally fragmented basement membrane. Immunofluorescence microscopy shows diagnostic linear deposits of IgG and, often, complement bound to the basement membranes of alveoli.

2. **Kidneys.** Renal biopsy shows acute glomerulonephritis that progresses to interstitial inflammation and glomerular fibrosis without vasculitis. Electron microscopy reveals endothelial cell proliferation and swelling, increased basement membrane materials, and fibrin deposition beneath the capillary endothelium. Immunofluorescence findings are similar to those found in the lung.

II. Diagnostic approach

A. Specific etiologic approach

1. Goodpasture's syndrome can be diagnosed by satisfying the following criteria: **pulmonary hemorrhage,** which may be recurrent; iron deficiency

anemia; **glomerulonephritis;** serum anti-GBM **antibodies;** and positive **immunofluorescence** for IgG in a linear pattern along glomerular or alveolar basement membranes or both.

2. **Radioimmunoassay** of anti-GBM antibody is an excellent, complementary diagnostic test that is reliable and sensitive, with a very low incidence of false-positive reactions. The assay may not be readily available in some areas, but can be performed in a matter of days in reference laboratories equipped for the technique.

3. The diagnosis of Goodpasture's syndrome is best confirmed by **renal biopsy** with **ultrastructural** and **immunofluorescence analyses,** particularly if clinical glomerulonephritis is present and thus must be differentiated from other causes. Renal biopsy should be performed with the first manifestations of kidney involvement to determine the extent and severity of damage, as well as to establish an early diagnosis. Renal changes by light microscopy may be nonspecific and do not exclude Goodpasture's syndrome unless immunofluorescence studies and electron microscopy are also done. Transbronchial lung biopsy will be helpful only if sufficient alveoli are obtained, and it cannot be performed as easily and serially for accurate follow-up as can percutaneous renal biopsies.

B. The **differential diagnosis** includes idiopathic pulmonary hemosiderosis, uremic pneumonitis, acute (poststreptococcal) glomerulonephritis, pneumococcal or viral pneumonia with nephritis, polyarteritis nodosa, Wegener's granulomatosis, and systemic lupus erythematosus (see Chap. 14). Many of these diseases may carry a more favorable prognosis than Goodpasture's syndrome, and they must be systemically evaluated to distinguish their clinical, pathologic, and immunologic features. Several cases of pulmonary-renal disease similar to Goodpasture's syndrome but without anti-GBM antibodies have been reported and presumably involve other immunopathologic mechanisms.

III. Treatment

A. **General measures.** Blood transfusions, oral iron therapy, careful maintenance of fluid and electrolyte balance, supplemental oxygenation, intubation and mechanical ventilation, and peritoneal dialysis or hemodialysis are often necessary for emergency stabilization in individual cases.

B. **Immunosuppressive therapy.** The current treatment of choice consists of early plasmapheresis to remove circulating anti-GBM antibody and prednisone (1 mg/kg/day) and cyclophosphamide (1–2 mg/kg/day) to suppress further anti-GBM antibody production. Pulmonary hemorrhage usually stops promptly, but recurrences require repeat plasmaphereses. Plasmaphereses should be continued until circulating anti-GBM antibody is no longer detectable and renal function has stabilized. Chest radiographs and pulmonary function usually return to normal in days to weeks, whereas renal function either improves or progresses to endstage disease depending on the presenting severity of renal damage. Corticosteroid therapy alone may temporarily ameliorate the pulmonary hemorrhage but not the glomerulonephritis. Bilateral nephrectomy is no longer necessary.

IV. Prognosis.
Early studies indicated a rapidly fatal course, with death resulting from pulmonary hemorrhage or asphyxia in 50% of patients, and from uremia in the other 50%. The mean duration of survival for 90% of patients after the appearance of the first symptom was 4–6 months. However, recent data suggest that the clinical course and the likelihood of survival are better than previously considered due to early plasmapheresis and long-term maintenance with prednisone and cyclophosphamide. Although many patients develop chronic renal failure despite therapy, recovery can follow even prolonged anuria.

Idiopathic Pulmonary Hemosiderosis

Idiopathic pulmonary hemosiderosis is a rare syndrome of unknown etiology and pathogenesis and consists of pulmonary hemorrhage (hemoptysis) and anemia without renal abnormalities or discernible immunologic defects. Idiopathic pulmonary hemosiderosis occurs most commonly in children below the age of 16 years. There is no sex predominance. However, there have been several reports of the disease occurring in adults over 40 years of age.

I. **Clinical presentation**

    A. Clinical features. The onset of idiopathic pulmonary hemosiderosis can be insidious with a prolonged course or can be characterized by recurrent acute episodes of hemoptysis. Clinical myocarditis, positive cold agglutinins, increased serum IgA, and enlarged liver, spleen, and lymph nodes can occasionally ($<$ 20%) occur. Although renal abnormalities and serum anti-GBM antibodies are lacking, the rest of the clinical presentation is similar to that of Goodpasture's syndrome. Iron deficiency anemia invariably results from sequestration of blood and iron in the lungs.

    B. Pathologic features. The light-microscopic appearance of the lung in Goodpasture's syndrome and idiopathic pulmonary hemosiderosis is similar and can be differentiated only by electron microscopy and immunofluorescence studies. Elastic-fiber fragmentation, focal ruptures of the basement membrane, hydropic changes in pneumocytes, and collagen deposition within the basement membrane are present in idiopathic hemosiderosis. The inability to detect immunoglobulin, complement, or albumin in the lung or kidney is consistent with idiopathic pulmonary hemosiderosis.

II. **Diagnostic approach**

    A. Specific etiologic approach. The diagnosis is often one of exclusion. The combination of a compatible clinical history, tissue pathology, and exclusion of other causes of pulmonary hemorrhage is necessary for diagnosis. The most direct and productive diagnostic procedure is open lung biopsy, with subsequent iron stains, electron microscopy, and immunofluorescence studies. The lack of renal and serologic abnormalities excludes Goodpasture's syndrome and makes renal biopsy unnecessary. If renal abnormalities occur in a patient with suspected idiopathic pulmonary hemosiderosis, a renal biopsy is necessary for proper immunologic diagnosis as well as for evaluation of the severity and extent of renal damage.

    B. The **differential diagnosis** is similar to that in Goodpasture's syndrome, but without a renal component. Idiopathic pulmonary hemosiderosis occasionally may be associated with collagen vascular diseases such as rheumatoid arthritis or systemic lupus erythematosus.

III. **Treatment.** Significant anemia can be treated with blood transfusions and/or iron replacement. Corticosteroids (prednisone, 1 mg/kg/day) have been administered, with variable benefit. Cyclophosphamide and azathioprine have been successful during acute episodes. Because of the association of pulmonary hemosiderosis with cow's milk sensitivity (in the presence or absence of serum milk precipitins), a trial off cow's milk products (see Appendix XII) is warranted.

IV. The **prognosis** is difficult to determine. The average survival from diagnosis to death was 2.5 months in one series, but instances of survival for as long as 20 years are not uncommon. The disease has a variable course, with spontaneous remissions and exacerbations. Pulmonary fibrosis is a common sequela.

Wegener's Granulomatosis

Although Wegener's granulomatosis is a relatively infrequent disease of undetermined immunologic origin, it must be considered in the differential diagnosis of aseptic multisystem illnesses involving necrotizing granulomas and vasculitis. Controversy now exists regarding the relationship of **classic,** or **generalized,** Wegener's granulomatosis (involving the upper airways, lung, and kidneys), **limited** Wegener's granulomatosis (involving the upper airways and lung or the lung alone), and **midline granuloma** (involving the upper airways alone). The three entities may constitute a continuum or spectrum of the same disease process, with the manifestations influenced by the tempo of organ involvement and intervening treatment. Generalized Wegener's granulomatosis can occur at any age, but it commonly affects patients in the fourth and fifth decades of life—men slightly more often than women.

I. **Clinical presentation**
   A. **Clinical features**
      1. **Symptoms and signs**
         a. **General.** Wegener's granulomatosis can involve virtually any organ system with vasculitis or granuloma, or both as seen in one series: upper airways (93% of patients); eyes or middle ear (40%); lungs (100%); heart (29%); nervous system (24%); skin (48%); and joints (57%). Fever, with weakness and weight loss, may be due in part to the primary necrotizing process, but is primarily due to secondary infection (usually *Staphylococcus aureus*) of the sinuses in up to one-third of the patients.
         b. **Respiratory.** The classic complaints are referable to the upper respiratory tract (rhinorrhea, paranasal sinus pain and drainage, nasal mucosal ulcerations, and otitis media with hearing loss). Chest symptoms (cough, purulent sputum production, hemoptysis, pleuritic chest pain) are usually associated with upper airway symptoms and occasionally precede them.
         c. **Renal findings.** Although renal manifestations occur in the majority of patients (> 80%) at some time in the course of the disease and constitute the hallmark of generalized Wegener's granulomatosis, they are rarely the presenting feature. Renal involvement is manifested by proteinuria, hematuria, and erythrocyte casts, with or without functional impairment initially.
      2. **X-ray findings.** The chest x-ray patterns of Wegener's granulomatosis take many forms and are often fleeting and asymptomatic. Typically, there are multiple, usually bilateral, sharply circumscribed nodules of varying size that change or disappear rapidly. Cavitation occurs eventually in one-third to one-half of the patients and leaves shaggy, thick walls that gradually become thin and resolve with therapy. Acute airspace infiltrates are common and occur with or without the discrete nodules. Uncommonly, small pleural effusions and hilar and mediastinal lymphadenopathy are seen.
   B. **Immunologic features.** Anemia, leukocytosis, hyperglobulinemia (particularly IgA and IgE), and elevated erythrocyte sedimentation rate are characteristically observed prior to therapy. Peripheral eosinophilia, cryoglobulins, antinuclear antibody, and L. E. cell phenomena are not usually present. Serum complement levels are normal or slightly elevated. Anergy is not a feature of untreated Wegener's granulomatosis.
   C. **Pathologic features**
      1. **Lungs.** Pulmonary involvement is characterized by necrotizing granulomas, situated near the bronchi but usually independent of the vasculitic lesions. The granulomas are composed of a largely mononuclear infiltration and multinucleated giant cells of either the foreign body or Langhans' type. Immunoglobulin and complement deposits of the coarse, granular type have been reported.
      2. **Kidney.** Renal biopsies show necrotizing vasculitis that results in thrombosis and infarction. A variable focal and segmental glomerulonephritis can be found in biopsy specimens even from patients without clinical evidence of renal involvement. Electron microscopy reveals subepithelial deposits of immune complexes that are coarse and granular and stain for IgG and complement.

II. **Diagnostic approach**
   A. **Criteria.** No clinical or pathologic features are absolutely diagnostic of Wegener's granulomatosis. However, the clinicopathologic triad of (1) necrotizing granulomatous, small-vessel vasculitis involving the upper and lower respiratory tracts, (2) focal glomerulonephritis, and (3) vasculitis disseminated to a greater or lesser degree should enable one to make or exclude the diagnosis of

generalized Wegener's granulomatosis with considerable certainty in most instances.

The definitive diagnosis thus requires the documentation of granulomas and vasculitis. These can be confirmed in biopsies from the upper and lower respiratory tract (in midline granuloma or limited Wegener's granulomatosis) or the kidney (in generalized Wegener's granulomatosis).

B. Specific etiologic approach

   1. Lung biopsy. Lung lesions are a sine qua non of limited and generalized Wegener's granulomatosis, and the diagnosis should probably not be made unless there is pulmonary involvement.

   2. Renal biopsy is usually the procedure of choice in **generalized** Wegener's granulomatosis. Although the focal glomerulonephritis is not specific for or pathognomonic of Wegener's granulomatosis, its presence in association with upper and lower respiratory tract lesions is virtually diagnostic. The renal biopsy is also important to assess the extent of renal involvement accurately, particularly in patients who may have clinically limited Wegener's granulomatosis or who are in the early stages of the disease process.

   3. Nasopharyngeal biopsy. Since nasopharyngeal symptoms are often the initial symptoms in over 90% of patients, nasopharyngeal biopsies may be diagnostic in approximately 60% of patients and show necrotizing granulomas with or without vasculitis.

C. Differential diagnosis. Wegener's granulomatosis must be differentiated from diseases with vasculitis, granulomas, glomerulonephritis, or all three. Polyarteritis nodosa, hypersensitivity angiitis, polymorphic reticulosis, lymphomatoid granulomatosis, the vasculitis of collagen vascular disease, Goodpasture's syndrome, infectious granulomatous diseases, and neoplastic diseases are the most important to consider.

III. Treatment

A. Specific treatment

   1. Cytotoxic agents. The efficacy of cytotoxic drugs in treating generalized Wegener's granulomatosis, and especially the renal lesion, is now convincing. Oral cyclophosphamide (1–2 mg/kg/day) for 2 weeks is the initial recommended regimen. If a favorable clinical response is not seen, the daily dosage is adjusted in increments of 25 mg for 2-week periods until a definite clinical response is seen or until serious toxicity results. The criteria for clinical response are a decrease in respiratory symptoms and signs, remission of peripheral manifestations of vasculitis, and, more significantly, arrest of renal deterioration and improvement in renal function. Therapy can be tapered and stopped 1 year after all traces of disease activity disappear. Therapy should be continued for a longer period if the disease persists or resolves slowly.

   2. Corticosteroids. Although corticosteroids may rapidly decrease inflammatory reactions and improve symptoms, they have serious side effects with long-term use and cease to be beneficial by themselves when the disease progresses to significant pulmonary and renal involvement. Short courses of oral prednisone (1 mg/kg/day) should be used, in addition to cytotoxic drugs, to control constitutional symptoms or severe inflammatory or vasculitic flares.

Prednisone (1 mg/kg/day) alone may be sufficient to control localized lesions of midline granuloma and limited Wegener's granulomatosis. Patients with extensive midline granuloma who fail to respond to corticosteroids should be treated with high-dose, deep local irradiation. Cyclophosphamide should be added to ongoing prednisone therapy for resistant midline granulomas and limited Wegener's granulomatosis. There are no firm guidelines for determining the duration of therapy in these patients.

   3. Surgery. Cicatricial and destructive residua in the nose and tracheobronchial tree may require surgical management despite effective immunosuppressive therapy.

IV. Prognosis

A. The prognosis in untreated **generalized** Wegener's granulomatosis is extremely poor, with an average life span of 5 months after onset and a mortality of 93% in 2 years. In 80% of patients the cause of death is renal failure, while the remaining patients die of respiratory insufficiency. Cyclophosphamide has produced favorable results in up to 90% of patients.

B. Patients with **limited** Wegener's granulomatosis have a more favorable prognosis and longer survival than those with the generalized form. Some patients have spontaneous remission of pulmonary lesions and require no therapy for years. Death, if it occurs, is usually within the first 6 months after onset and is due to progressive lung involvement.

C. Untreated **midline granuloma** is characterized as a relentless, destructive disorder with a progressive downhill course lasting from 1–3 years after onset.

Sarcoidosis

Sarcoidosis is a systemic granulomatous disease of unknown origin, involving multiple organs with variable frequency and intensity, but invariably the lung. Sarcoidosis has a high incidence in certain populations (e.g., American black females, Puerto Ricans in New York City, Scandinavians) and age groups (third to fourth decade of life). The incidence in the United States ranges from 30–60/100,000, but is over 10 times more common in blacks than in whites and causes more disability than pulmonary tuberculosis. Although there is no patient-to-patient transmission, sarcoidosis has occurred in families, suggesting a constitutional susceptibility or a common exogenous etiologic mechanism.

I. Clinical presentation

A. Clinical features

1. **Symptoms and signs**

   a. **General.** Approximately 50% of patients have symptoms at the time of diagnosis. Constitutional symptoms (fever, weight loss, fatigue, malaise) frequently develop insidiously and indicate multisystem involvement. Persistent daily fevers (to 39° C) may be associated with tuberculosis, hepatic inflammation, and/or with the acute onset of erythema nodosum (the latter is more common in young Scandinavian women).

   b. **Pulmonary.** Respiratory symptoms occur in over 95% of patients and include shortness of breath, dry cough, occasionally blood-streaked sputum, and substernal chest discomfort, usually attributable to excessive coughing. The physical findings are variable (depending on the stage) and nonspecific, consisting of tachypnea, restricted diaphragmatic excursion, crackling rales (diffuse or basilar), and, sometimes wheezing (indicating localized endobronchial involvement).

   c. **Extrapulmonary sarcoidosis** is common and must be evaluated. Adenopathy (80%), splenomegaly (75%), hepatomegaly (50%), skin lesions (30%), uveitis (25%), arthritis (10%), arrhythmias (5%), and peripheral nerve involvement (5%) are seen early or years after the initial presentation. Salivary gland enlargement (6%) can occur, with facial nerve palsy, fever, and uveitis. All patients suspected of having sarcoidosis should have a careful slit-lamp examination to rule out uveitis.

2. **Blood and urine findings.** Mild anemia with leukopenia (30%), eosinophilia (30%), and elevated erythrocyte sedimentation rate (> 70%) may be found in active disease. Serum alkaline phosphatase is elevated in 30–45% of patients, as are serum globulins (50%). The serum albumin is characteristically reduced. Hypercalciuria occurs in 30% of patients with chronic sarcoidosis and hypercalcemia in less than 15%, but nephrocalcinosis, nephrolithiasis, and metastatic calcification are rarely seen.

3. **X-ray findings.** In as many as 88% of patients, the chest x-ray changes in pulmonary sarcoidosis consist of symmetric bilateral hilar adenopathy with or without parenchymal involvement. Approximately 25% of patients pre-

sent with diffuse, symmetric reticulonodular x-ray changes. Pulmonary fibrosis with coarse scarring and emphysema is seen in 20% of patients who have parenchymal changes for over 2 years. Right paratracheal adenopathy is a common but not a pathognomonic feature of sarcoidosis. Gallium-67 radionuclide studies may show abnormal uptake in the lungs, lymph nodes, and salivary glands.

4. **Physiologic tests.** Pulmonary function tests commonly show a restrictive ventilatory pattern with a decrease in vital capacity, total lung capacity, diffusing capacity, and static compliance. Airway disease is rare unless the patient is a smoker, or has endobronchial involvement, or both. A widened alveolar-to-arterial oxygen gradient (hypoxemia) is associated with hypocapnia.

B. **Immunologic features.** Anergy to a battery of skin tests (e.g., tuberculin, coccidioidin, *Trichophyton*, mumps) is characteristic of patients with sarcoidosis and is seen in over two-thirds of these patients. Although the depression of delayed hypersensitivity (type IV reaction) may vary with the duration and activity of sarcoidosis, the patient with a positive tuberculin skin test must be evaluated for active disease. Defective cell-mediated immunity is seen in vitro by the poor responses of lymphocytes to mitogens, decreased circulating T cell percentages and inhibition of leukocyte migration by sarcoid tissue suspension (Kveim antigen).

The lungs show ample evidence of increased immune activity (alveolitis) in patients with active sarcoidosis. Bronchoalveolar lavage data indicate increased lymphocyte numbers, increased proportion of T cells, increased helper (T4) lymphocytes, and secretion of interleukin-2, a glycoprotein that stimulates proliferation of T cells. Polyclonal increase in immunoglobulins, particularly IgG, and enhanced B cell function are present in lung lymphocytes.

C. **Pathologic features.** The most characteristic pathologic feature of established sarcoidosis is the presence of noncaseating granulomas composed of epithelioid and multinucleated giant cells. Asteroid or Schaumann's bodies are frequently seen, and some central fibrinoid necrosis may occur. A peripheral inflammatory reaction is absent. The granulomas transform into nonspecific fibrotic hyaline scars or resolve completely over time. These findings occur in multiple organs, and deposits are scattered throughout the lung interstitium and bronchial walls even when the chest x-ray appears normal. Typical noncaseating granulomas are seen in the skin biopsy specimens from sarcoid patients whose Kveim tests are positive. In the Kveim test a sarcoid spleen suspension is injected intradermally 4–6 weeks prior to skin biopsy. This diagnostic test is not used commonly, however, because of its lack of antigen standardization, specificity, and availability.

II. **Diagnostic approach**

A. **Criteria.** The diagnosis requires three primary criteria:
1. A compatible clinical and radiographic presentation.
2. Histologic evidence of noncaseating granuloma from a tissue biopsy.
3. A careful exclusion of other disease processes, especially infectious diseases.
The diagnosis of sarcoidosis is still presumptive even with these criteria, and prudent longitudinal follow-up is required. Although gallium-67 lung scans and bronchoalveolar lavage are useful to stage the activity of the immune process and in research protocols, they are currently not diagnostic by themselves.

B. **Biopsy sites.** In asymptomatic, young patients with bilateral hilar adenopathy alone, biopsy of any suspicious skin lesion or palpable lymph node should be done. If there are no extrapulmonary lesions available for biopsy and corticosteroids are not administered, the histologic diagnosis may be postponed and the patient observed.
1. Active or recently symptomatic (< 2 years) pulmonary disease can yield a positive biopsy from scalene nodes (80% yield), other palpable nodes or hilar nodes (80–90%), lung (> 90%), skin (30%), bronchus (30–60%), and conjunctiva (25%). Liver biopsy yields noncaseating granulomas in 70% of patients (especially if serum alkaline phosphatase is increased), but the hepatic

histologic picture is nonspecific and may not reflect the intrapulmonary disease process.

2. **Mediastinoscopy** is helpful in histologic diagnosis if hilar adenopathy is present, but this procedure requires general anesthesia and is invasive.

3. If there is clinical uncertainty about the significance of biopsy results from the skin or lymph nodes (e.g., due to foreign-body reactions or infectious complications), and if there are diffuse pulmonary changes, a **transbronchial biopsy** using a fiberoptic bronchoscope is the procedure of choice. It is a safe procedure with a 70–100% yield.

4. An **open lung biopsy** will give virtually a 100% diagnostic yield if previous techniques are unsuccessful.

C. **Angiotensin-converting enzyme** measurement is a potentially useful diagnostic serologic test since serum elevations occur in 83% of patients with active sarcoidosis (particularly those with both hilar adenopathy and lung infiltrates). The epithelioid cells in the sarcoid granulomas of lymph nodes may be the source of the elevated serum enzyme level. The specificity of the test is now controversial in that some patients with Gaucher's disease, tuberculosis, lymphoma, or leprosy also have elevated angiotensin-converting enzyme levels. Thus, while the test may be performed rapidly in a reference laboratory, only significantly high levels are helpful (and one must still fulfill the three primary diagnostic criteria for sarcoidosis), and normal activity does not rule out the disease. The assay assumes more clinical importance when a patient is unwilling to have a diagnostic biopsy.

D. **Differential diagnosis.** It is important to emphasize that noncaseating granulomas are **nonspecific** and are seen in tuberculosis, fungal infections, lymphoma, foreign-body responses, berylliosis, hypersensitivity pneumonitis, and lymph nodes draining malignant tumors. These possibilities cannot be excluded in the absence of further investigation. The clinical similarity and occasional coexistence of the other diseases previously mentioned make the accurate diagnosis of sarcoidosis extremely important, especially since corticosteroids may be administered.

III. **Treatment**

A. **General measures.** Ocular sarcoidosis generally responds to topical corticosteroids. Skin lesions frequently respond to intralesional injections of corticosteroids, or low-dose systemic corticosteroids. Isoniazid (300 mg/day; 10 mg/kg/day in children) should be administered prophylactically for at least 1 year in patients treated with systemic corticosteroids whose tuberculin tests are positive.

B. **Corticosteroids.** According to the American Thoracic Society, indications for treatment are progressive respiratory impairment or symptoms, ocular disease, clinical myocardial disease, central nervous system involvement, cutaneous lesions, and persistent hypercalcemia or hypercalciuria with renal insufficiency.

1. Oral corticosteroids (prednisone, 40–60 mg/day [1–2 mg/kg/day in children], in divided doses) should be given for 4–6 months and then gradually tapered to maintenance doses of 10–20 mg daily, if possible. Therapy should be continued for another 6–12 months, or as long as there is disease activity, with periodic attempts to reduce the dosage or discontinue the drug.

2. Since interruption or premature discontinuation of therapy often precipitates exacerbations, **alternate-day** prednisone (e.g., 40 mg every other day) with 10-mg decrements every 3 months may be an effective maintenance regimen.

3. If there is physiologic or clinical deterioration, the corticosteroid dose should be doubled and given on a daily basis. Unresponsiveness to high doses suggests irreversible changes.

4. Despite the strong impression that corticosteroids produce symptomatic improvement, objective criteria (complete pulmonary function tests [including diffusing capacity], chest roentgenograms, and angiotensin-converting enzyme levels) should be monitored before and during corticosteroid therapy to document therapeutic efficacy.

IV. **Prognosis.** Approximately one-third of patients have spontaneous clinical and physiologic resolution within months to 2 years. In another one-third the condition resolves, with some residual symptoms and radiologic or physiologic abnormalities. The remaining one-third have severe disability, usually involving the lungs or eyes. The prognosis is poorer in blacks, in those with an intermittent course and frequent relapses, and in those with systemic manifestations (skin, bone, eyes, salivary glands, and hepatosplenomegaly). Mortality in sarcoidosis is up to 10%, with most patients dying of cor pulmonale secondary to chronic pulmonary fibrosis and some dying suddenly from a cardiac arrhythmia.

Diffuse Interstitial Fibrosis of the Lung

Diffuse interstitial fibrosis is a convenient term to encompass a large group of pulmonary diseases characterized histologically by an interstitial inflammatory response (alveolitis) and thickening of the alveolar walls, with a strong tendency to fibrosis. Since this term encompasses more than 100 individual disease entities, multiple terms (e.g., **Hamman-Rich syndrome, idiopathic pulmonary fibrosis, cryptogenic** or **diffuse fibrosing alveolitis**), as well as etiologic, immunologic, and histopathologic classifications, have been devised. No cause is found in more than 50% of patients after intensive investigation. The following discussion is primarily limited to the large group in which the major clinical and pathologic abnormalities are confined to the lung.

Diffuse interstitial fibrosis now represents 15–20% of the noninfectious disorders of the lung. All age groups are affected, but the disease occurs most often in those between the ages of 30 and 70 years. Although there is no sex or race predilection, familial forms are transmitted by a simple mendelian autosomal dominant characteristic.

I. **Clinical presentation**

A. **Clinical features.** The clinical presentation of diffuse interstitial fibrosis is varied, reflecting diverse causes, environmental factors (e.g., smoking), genetic background, and rate of disease progression.

1. **Symptoms and signs.** Insidious and progressive breathlessness, initially during exercise, is present in all patients. Over 80% of patients have a nonproductive cough, and fewer than 50% complain of systemic or constitutional symptoms. Purulent sputum indicates possible intercurrent bacterial infection. Tachypnea, clubbing, bibasilar dry crackles ("Velcro" rales), and evidence of cor pulmonale and pulmonary hypertension are often found, depending on the extent and chronicity of the disease process.

2. **X-ray findings.** Initially, the chest x-ray reveals a nonspecific, bilateral, fine reticular or nodular pattern or a combination of both, predominantly in the lung bases. Serial chest x-rays show progressive coarse reticulation, 3- to 10-mm thin-walled cysts (honeycomb lung), and loss of lung volume. The chest x-ray in early diffuse interstitial fibrosis correlates roughly with disease activity (alveolitis), but there is less reliable correlation with physiologic and morphologic variables in midcourse. Gallium-67 lung scans may help stage alveolitis but are nonspecific, and a negative scan does not exclude disease.

3. **Physiologic tests.** Pulmonary function studies invariably reveal a restrictive ventilatory defect, with reduction in vital capacity, total lung capacity, diffusing capacity, static compliance, resting arterial oxygenation (hypoxemia), and carbon dioxide tension. The latter is due to hyperventilation induced by intrapulmonary stretch-receptor stimulation. Although the forced expiratory volume in 1 second (FEV_1) and airway resistance are normal, sophisticated physiologic tests show small-airway narrowing in over 50% of nonsmokers with morphologically documented pulmonary fibrosis, thus supporting the concept that ventilation-perfusion imbalances cause resting hypoxemia in this disease process. The most useful physiologic tests to stage and follow the fibrotic process are determinations of

volume-pressure curves (compliance) and arterial oxygen tensions during exercise.

B. Immunologic features. Excluding diffuse interstitial fibrosis associated with systemic disease or other known causes, the idiopathic lung process is definitely associated with abnormalities of the immune system.

1. Over 90% of patients have elevated erythrocyte sedimentation rates during active disease. Antinuclear antibodies, rheumatoid factors, cryoimmunoglobulins, and hyperglobulinemia (IgG, IgM, and IgA) are present in over 30% of patients, but no antibodies specific to the lung have been identified. High levels of circulating immune complexes as determined by the Raji-cell assay strongly correlate with intrapulmonary deposition of immune complexes in patients with predominantly cellular lung disease.

2. Immunofluorescence studies of lung biopsy tissue generally show granular deposits of IgG and usually complement (C3) in alveolar walls and capillaries.

3. Bronchoalveolar lavages in patients with active alveolitis reveal increased percentages of polymorphonuclear leukocytes and significant elevation of IgG as compared with controls.

These data suggest that immune complex deposition may cause lung injury which then elicits the nonspecific production of rheumatoid and antinuclear antibodies. However, not all forms of diffuse interstitial fibrosis have an apparent immunologic basis.

C. Pathologic features. Diffuse interstitial fibrosis is a reparative reaction to a variety of lung-injuring agents and is modified by the host's defense mechanisms. Two major patterns of lung reaction, desquamative interstitial pneumonia and usual interstitial pneumonia, are considered to represent early and later stages of diffuse interstitial fibrosis, respectively. Actually, both histologic patterns can appear in the same patient at the same time, and they probably represent the same disease process at different stages of evolution.

1. **Desquamative interstitial pneumonia (DIP).** The desquamative histologic pattern shows intraalveolar spaces uniformly filled with macrophages and granular pneumocytes (type II alveolar cells), with minimal alveolar-wall thickening and interstitial inflammatory cell infiltration.

2. **Usual interstitial pneumonia (UIP).** The other end of this spectrum of reactive changes is the mural pattern (corresponding to UIP), in which the predominant findings are thickening and lymphocytic and monocytic infiltration of alveolar walls. Intraalveolar exudate is sparse or absent. If the process advances, alveolar obliteration results in the formation of cystic spaces (honeycomb lung), cholesterol-ester clefts (associated with pulmonary hypertension), generalized smooth-muscle proliferation, atypical epithelial metaplasia (with possible development of lung carcinoma), and pulmonary arteriolar fibrointimal thickening and obliteration. Arteritis, granulomas, and evidence of minerals are absent in the lungs of patients with the idiopathic disease.

II. Diagnostic approach

A. Specific etiologic approach. Diffuse interstitial fibrosis can be diagnosed with a high degree of accuracy on clinical and laboratory grounds. Since the injured lung responds to many diseases with similar clinical and histologic changes, determination of the etiology and pathogenesis is difficult unless there is historic or physical evidence of infection, exposure to a toxin, multisystem involvement (e.g., collagen vascular disease), and so forth. A definite diagnosis of diffuse interstitial fibrosis and possibly determination of its cause can be made only by histologic examination and culture of tissue obtained by **lung biopsy.** Lung biopsy is clearly indicated when the disease is progressive and other methods fail to establish a diagnosis. Although transbronchial biopsy using the fiber-optic bronchoscope can be performed initially, open-lung biopsy provides the more optimal and representative tissue specimen for histologic, microbiologic, and mineral analyses. At least two lung sites (including a less diseased area) should be biopsied, since histologic activity can vary from one area to

Table 7-3. Principal causes of diffuse interstitial fibrosis

Infections	Malignancy
Tuberculosis	Bronchioloalveolar carcinoma
Fungi	Lymphangitic carcinomatosis
Viruses	Leukemia
Pneumoconioses	Pulmonary edema
Silicosis	Left ventricular failure
Asbestosis	Mitral stenosis
Coal worker's pneumoconiosis	Adult respiratory distress syndrome
Berylliosis	Collagen vascular diseases
Inhaled gases	Rheumatoid arthritis
Nitrogen dioxide	Scleroderma
Sulfur dioxide	Polymyositis
High oxygen concentrations	Systemic lupus erythematosus
Hypersensitivity pneumonitis	Diseases of unknown origin
Chronic aspiration	Sarcoidosis
Drugs	Eosinophilic granuloma
Busulfan	Goodpasture's syndrome
Nitrofurantoin	Pulmonary alveolar proteinosis
Bleomycin	Desquamative interstitial pneumonia
Chest irradiation	Usual interstitial pneumonia or idiopathic diffuse interstitial fibrosis

another in the same biopsy specimen and since changes of end-stage pulmonary fibroses are nonspecific.

All tissue must be examined for arteritis, granulomas, minerals, and infection. Unfortunately, in spite of vigorous diagnostic efforts, the cause frequently remains unknown. However, the possible decision to administer potentially dangerous drugs (e.g., corticosteroids) carries with it an obligation not only to eliminate a mistaken diagnosis but also to assess the degree of irreversible fibrosis as a guide to possible therapeutic benefits.

B. Differential diagnosis. The many diseases that should be considered are listed in Table 7-3. Many of these diseases are serious, and management and prognosis will be influenced by the specific diagnosis. Every effort should be made to identify treatable diseases such as tuberculosis and other infections, collagen vascular diseases, and hypersensitivity pneumonitis.

III. Treatment

A. General measures. Supportive therapy consists of prompt treatment of respiratory tract infections, supplemental oxygen, and treatment of cor pulmonale.

B. Corticosteroids. Besides avoidance of the causal agent (if known), the only currently effective treatment is a therapeutic trial of systemic corticosteroids, used in much the same fashion as used in sarcoidosis. Patients with significant respiratory symptoms or clinical deterioration should receive prednisone in an initial dose of 60 mg daily (1–2 mg/kg/day in children) for at least 30–60 days. These patients must be carefully followed with serial pulmonary function tests, chest x-rays, and possibly gallium lung scans and circulating immune complex determinations. Maintenance prednisone therapy (0.5 mg/kg/day), with or without other agents, may be continued for 1 year, but clear guidelines are not available.

1. Patients who respond to corticosteroids usually have a preponderance of a DIP pattern, or have been treated early in the course of the disease, or both.

2. Patients with predominantly irreversible mural fibrosis rarely respond to corticosteroids, but their disease often progresses slowly. Corticosteroid therapy can be attempted empirically in individual patients with UIP. The results with azathioprine (3 mg/kg/day) or cyclophosphamide (2 mg/kg/day) have been generally disappointing, but large controlled studies are not available.

IV. Prognosis. Although Hamman and Rich originally described patients presenting with a rapidly fatal course of 1–6 months' duration, the majority of cases subsequently reported indicate that the course of idiopathic diffuse interstitial fibrosis is more variable and frequently chronic and slowly progressive, particularly in DIP. Recent studies have shown a mortality in DIP of 28% and a mean survival of 12 years, as compared with 66% and 6 years in UIP. Without treatment, 22% with DIP but none with UIP improved. With corticosteroid therapy, 62% with DIP and only 12% with UIP improved; the disease worsened in 27% with DIP and 69% with UIP. The relatively good prognosis in treated (and untreated) DIP probably reflects its reversible, cellular nature (alveolitis) and response to early treatment. Neither the extent of chest x-ray abnormalities nor the presence of circulating rheumatoid and antinuclear factors influences subsequent survival.

The main causes of death are respiratory failure, cor pulmonale, infection, and lung carcinoma. Spontaneous pneumothorax is relatively uncommon.

Selected Readings

Hypersensitivity Pneumonitis

Fink, J. N. Hypersensitivity pneumonitis. *J. Allergy Clin. Immunol.* 74:1, 1984

Leatherman, J. W., et al. Lung T-cells in hypersensitivity pneumonitis. *Ann. Intern. Med.* 100:390, 1984.

Pepys, J. *Hypersensitivity Diseases of the Lungs Due to Fungi and Organic Dusts.* Basel: Karger, 1969.

Roberts, R. C., and Moore, V. L. Immunopathogenesis of hypersensitivity pneumonitis. *Am. Rev. Respir. Dis.* 116:1075, 1977.

Slavin, R. G. Hypersensitivity diseases of the lung. *Adv. Asthma Allergy Pulm. Dis.* 5:25, 1978.

Allergic Bronchopulmonary Aspergillosis

Greenberger, P. A. Allergic bronchopulmonary aspergillosis. *J. Allergy Clin. Immunol.* 74:645, 1984.

McCarthy, D. S., and Pepys, J. Allergic bronchopulmonary aspergillosis. *Clin. Allergy* 1:261 and 415, 1971.

Rosenberg, M., et al. Clinical and immunological criteria for the diagnosis of allergic bronchopulmonary aspergillosis. *Ann. Intern. Med.* 86:405, 1977.

Rosenberg, M., et al. The assessment of immunologic and clinical changes occurring during corticosteroid therapy for allergic bronchopulmonary aspergillosis. *Am. J. Med.* 64:599, 1978.

Pulmonary Infiltrates with Eosinophilia

Citro, L. A., Gordon, M. E., and Miller, W. T. Eosinophilic lung disease (Or how to slice P.I.E.). *Am. J. Roentgenol.* 117:787, 1973.

Fauci, A. S. Vasculitis. *J. Allergy Clin. Immunol.* 72:211, 1983.

Neva, F. A., and Ottesen, E. A. Tropical (filarial) eosinophilia. *N. Engl. J. Med.* 298:1129, 1978.

Ottesen, E. A. Eosinophilia and the Lung. In. C. H., Kirkpatrick and H. Y. Reynolds (eds.), *Immunologic and Infectious Reactions in the Lung.* New York: Dekker, 1976.

Pearson, D. J., and Rosenow, E. C. Chronic eosinophilic pneumonia (Carrington's). A follow-up study. *Mayo Clin. Proc.* 53:73, 1978.

Sack, M., Cassidy, J. T., and Bole, G. G. Prognostic factors in polyarteritis. *J. Rheumatol.* 2:411, 1975.

Goodpasture's Syndrome

Lockwood, C. M., et al. Immunosuppression and plasma-exchange in the treatment of Goodpasture's syndrome. *Lancet* 1:711, 1976.

Proskey, A. J., et al. Goodpasture's syndrome. A report of five cases and review of the literature. *Am. J. Med.* 48:162, 1970.

Thomas, H. M., and Irwin, R. S. Classification of diffuse intrapulmonary hemorrhage. *Chest* 68:483, 1975.

Wilson, C. B., and Dixon, F. J. Anti-glomerular basement membrane antibody-induced glomerulonephritis. *Kidney Int.* 3:74, 1973.

Idiopathic Pulmonary Hemosiderosis

Boat, T. F., et al. Hypersensitivity to cow's milk in young children with pulmonary hemosiderosis and cor pulmonale secondary to nasopharyngeal obstruction. *J. Pediatr.* 87:23, 1975.

Byrd, R. B., and Gracey, D. R. Immunosuppressive treatment of idiopathic pulmonary hemosiderosis. *J.A.M.A.* 226:458, 1973.

Donald, K. J., Edwards, R. L., and McEvoy, J. D. S. Alveolar capillary basement membrane lesions in Goodpasture's syndrome and idiopathic pulmonary hemosiderosis. *Am. J. Med.* 59:642, 1975.

Soergel, K. H., and Sommers, S. C. Idiopathic pulmonary hemosiderosis and related syndromes. *Am. J. Med.* 32:499, 1962.

Wegener's Granulomatosis

DeRemee, R. A., et al. Wegener's granulomatosis. Anatomic correlates, a proposed classification. *Mayo Clin. Proc.* 51:777, 1976.

Fauci, A. S., et al. Wegener's granulomatosis: Prospective clinical and therapeutic experience with 85 patients for 21 years. *Ann. Intern. Med.* 98:76, 1983.

Schechter, S. L., Bole, G. G., and Walker, S. E. Midline granuloma and Wegener's granulomatosis: Clinical and therapeutic considerations. *J. Rheumatol.* 3:241, 1976.

Sarcoidosis

Ceuppens, J. L. et al. Alveolar T-cell subsets in pulmonary sarcoidosis: Correlation with disease activity and effect of steroid treatment. *Am. Rev. Respir. Dis.* 129:563, 1984.

Daniele, R. P., et al. Bronchoalveolar lavage: Role in the pathogenesis, diagnosis, and management of interstitial lung disease. *Ann. Intern. Med.* 102:93, 1985.

Hunninghake, G. W., et al. Maintenance of granuloma formation in pulmonary sarcoidosis by T-lymphocytes within the lung. *N. Engl. J. Med.* 302:594, 1980.

Johns, C. J., et al. Extended experience in the long-term corticosteroid treatment of pulmonary sarcoidosis. *Ann. N.Y. Acad. Sci.* 278:722, 1976.

Keough, B. A., et al. The alveolitis of pulmonary sarcoidosis: Evaluation of natural history and alveolitis-dependent changes in lung function. *Am. Rev. Respir. Dis.* 128:256, 1983.

Kirks, D. R., McCormick, V. D., and Greenspan, R. H. Pulmonary sarcoidosis. Roentgenologic analysis of 150 patients. *Am. J. Roentgenol.* 117:777, 1973.

Lawrence, E. C., et al. Serial changes in markers of disease activity with corticosteroid treatment in sarcoidosis. *Am. J. Med.* 74:747, 1983.

Mitchell, D. N., and Scadding, J. G. Sarcoidosis. *Am. Rev. Respir. Dis.* 110:774, 1974.

Sharma, O. P. *Sarcoidosis: Clinical Management.* London: Butterworths, 1984.

Diffuse Interstitial Fibrosis of the Lung

Carrington, C. B., et al. Natural history and treated course of usual and desquamative interstitial pneumonia. *N. Engl. J. Med.* 298:801, 1978.

Crystal, R. G., et al. Interstitial lung disease: Current concepts of pathogenesis, staging and therapy. *Am. J. Med.* 70:542, 1981.

Crystal, R. G., et al. Interstitial lung diseases of unknown cause: Disorders characterized by chronic inflammation of the lower respiratory tract. *N. Engl. J. Med.* 310:154, 235, 1984.

Kunstling, T. R., Goodwin, R. A., Jr., and Des Prez, R. M. Diffuse interstitial pulmonary fibrosis (cryptogenic fibrosing alveolitis). *South. Med. J.* 69:479, 1976.

Reynolds, H. Y., et al. Analysis of cellular and protein content of broncho-alveolar fluid from patients with idiopathic pulmonary fibrosis and chronic hypersensitivity pneumonitis. *J. Clin. Invest.* 59:165, 1977.

Wall, C. P., et al. Comparison of transbronchial and open biopsies in chronic infiltrative lung disease. *Am. Rev. Respir. Dis.* 123:280, 1981.

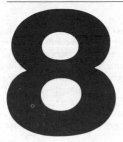

Allergic Diseases of the Skin

Anne W. Lucky,
Glenn J. Lawlor, Jr., and
Thomas J. Fischer

Atopic Dermatitis

Atopic dermatitis is the cutaneous component of a group of immediate hypersensitivity disorders that also include allergic rhinoconjunctivitis and asthma. Unlike allergic rhinoconjunctivitis and asthma, the exact relationship of atopic dermatitis to IgE sensitization and mediator release is unclear. Atopic dermatitis can occur in all age groups, alone or associated with the other atopic disorders. A family history of atopy is common. The incidence of atopic dermatitis is highest in infants and children, occurring in 1–3% of infants in the first 2 years of life. Of childhood eczema, 60% occurs before the age of 1 year and 90% before the age of 5 years. Distinction by appearance from other inflammatory dermatoses (e.g., seborrheic dermatitis) can be difficult. The diagnosis is usually based on the clinical course and the presence of other atopic findings.

I. **Pathophysiologic features.** Although the cause(s) of atopic dermatitis and its relationship to other atopic disorders are not completely known, certain features are characteristic.

   A. **Immunologic findings.** Of persons with atopic dermatitis, especially with coexisting allergic respiratory symptoms, 80% have significant elevations of serum IgE and significant peripheral eosinophilia. The serum level of IgE generally does not parallel the degree of dermatitis, although in a specific patient it can reflect the severity and return to normal levels during prolonged inactive phases of the dermatitis. Also, the relationship of disease activity with exposure to specific allergens (identified by skin testing or the radioallergosorbent test [RAST]) is inconsistent.

   A reduction of **cell-mediated immunity** in atopic dermatitis is suggested by increased susceptibility to cutaneous infections with *Staphylococcus,* herpes simplex, vaccinia, common warts, and molluscum contagiosum. There is a reduced incidence of allergic contact dermatitis, decreased contact sensitization to dinitrochlorobenzene, and often negative delayed hypersensitivity to intradermal antigens. However, in vitro T-cell function is more often normal. Abnormal T-cell subpopulations with decreased numbers of suppressor cells (T8) and an increased ratio of helper (T4) to suppressor (T8) cells has been documented. Whether this abnormal ratio is primary or secondary is unclear.

   B. **Neurogenic and vascular features**

      1. **Pruritus and hyperirritability** of the skin are the most consistent features of atopic dermatitis and seem to be related to excessive amounts of histamine. Disease activity can be directly correlated with exposure to irritants and trauma (heat, sweating, dryness, harsh fabrics, scratching). Indeed, lesions are characteristically secondary to the trauma of scratching and tend to appear in areas of increased sweating and hypervascularity.

      2. Altered cutaneous vascular responses to **catecholamines** and other neurogenic mediators are also characteristic features of atopic dermatitis. The most evident of these reactions are **white dermatographism** and **delayed blanching** of the skin following stroking. Normal skin reacts to stroking by

producing immediate erythema, with gradual fading. In persons with atopic dermatitis, immediate redness is followed in 15–30 seconds by pallor (secondary to edema rather than vasoconstriction), which persists for 1–3 minutes. With injection of methacholine, the typical flare is replaced by pallor lasting up to 30 minutes. Reduction in cutaneous blood flow with reduced skin temperature (i.e., fingers and toes) occurs, although increased blood flow and skin temperature are characteristic in active areas.

  3. Abnormally low leukocyte **cyclic adenosine monophosphate** levels may be due to increased levels of its degrading enzyme, phosphodiesterase.

C. Excessive dryness of the skin, a common feature that can be of primary or secondary importance, may be related to alterations in sweating, lipid content, and sebaceous-gland activity in the skin.

D. Histopathologic findings fall into three categories: (1) **acute** dermatitis characterized by epidermal spongiosis and mixed lymphohistiocytic dermal infiltrate (not eosinophils); (2) **chronic** dermatitis **(lichen simplex chronicus),** which is characterized by thickening of the epidermis (acanthosis), changes in the uppermost layers of collagen, and proliferation of nerve endings; and (3) **subacute** dermatitis, which falls in between acute and chronic.

II. **Clinical course.** Atopic dermatitis presents as a chronic, relapsing inflammation of the skin. **Itching** is the primary symptom. Active lesions, generalized or limited to small single patches, are characterized by erythema that can progress to edema, excoriations, weeping, bleeding, and secondary infections. Chronically involved areas of the skin become thickened (lichenified), with fissuring, scaling, and hyperpigmentation. The **pattern of distribution, age of onset,** and **prognosis** allow classification of atopic dermatitis into three clinical stages.

A. **Infantile eczema** affects children from approximately 2 months to 2 years of age. Lesions have a predilection for the face (especially the cheeks), the scalp, the neck, the trunk, and **extensor** surfaces of the extremities. Infants older than 18 months tend to have more generalized involvement. Infantile eczema can resolve or abate in intensity by 3 years of age, persist through childhood, or recur in the prepubertal period.

B. **Childhood eczema,** more chronic and persistent than infantile eczema, can begin from 2–12 years of age or can be an extension of the infantile form. Lesions tend to be more localized, lichenified, and less exudative, with characteristic involvement of the flexor surfaces of the extremities, especially the antecubital and popliteal fossae, neck, wrists, and ankles. **Dennie's lines,** deep single or multiple transverse furrows of the lower eyelids, are frequently seen in this stage (although they are nonspecific for atopic dermatitis).

C. **Adolescent and adult eczema** begins between the ages of 12 and 20 years, or it can be an extension of the childhood form. Lesions are mainly lichenified and primarily on flexor surfaces of the extremities. The most troublesome form of dermatitis involves the hands. Single, persistent, thickened pruritic plaques of lichen simplex chronicus may occur. Facial involvement also occurs, with the production of dried, lichenified plaques in the periorbital and perioral areas. There tends to be a characteristic facial pallor. Adult-onset atopic dermatitis tends to be chronic.

D. Associated cutaneous findings that occur more frequently in atopic dermatitis than expected in the general population are:

  1. Dennie-Morgan folds, or "atopic pleats," are extra creases beneath the lower eyelids.
  2. Atopic "shiners" or dark rings are found infraorbitally.
  3. Hyperlinearity with increased number and prominence of skin markings is prominent on the palms and soles.
  4. Pityriasis alba is seen as irregular patches of finely scaling hypopigmentation on the cheeks, upper trunk, arms, and legs. It represents mild dermatitis.
  5. Keratosis pilaris results from keratotic perifollicular plugs, usually on the

extensor surfaces of the upper arms and thighs. In children, keratosis pilaris commonly occurs on the cheeks and is often mistaken for acne.

E. The **prognosis** in atopic dermatitis is dependent on the severity and age of onset. Significant improvement occurs in most infantile and childhood forms, so that 50–75% are symptom-free by adulthood. Patients with severe infantile atopic dermatitis have a more prolonged course, are susceptible to the development of allergic rhinitis and asthma, and often progress to the more localized adult type, which is usually persistent.

III. Differential diagnosis. The age of the patient can help to differentiate atopic dermatitis from other cutaneous diseases.

A. Infantile eczema

1. **Seborrheic dermatitis** presents between 3 weeks and 3 months of life. It characteristically affects the scalp and the flexural areas, such as the diaper area, the neck, and the axillae, which may be spared in infantile atopic dermatitis. At times, it can be indistinguishable from atopic dermatitis.

2. **Diaper dermatitis**, either irritant or secondary to *Candida* infection, is characterized by its specific perineal localization or involvement of skin folds.

3. **Other rare forms** of dermatitis include erythroderma desquamativum (Leiner's disease), immunodeficiency disorders, dermatitis exfoliativa neonatorum (Ritter's disease), histiocytosis (Letterer-Siwe disease), and metabolic disorders (e.g., phenylketonuria, histidinemia, gluten-sensitive enteropathy, acrodermatitis enteropathica, essential fatty acid deficiency, and biotin-dependent carboxylase deficiencies).

B. Childhood eczema

1. **Contact dermatitis** to various chemical agents occurs in childhood. Foot dermatitis is frequently difficult to distinguish since atopic dermatitis presents similarly with eczematoid pruritic plaques. A correlative atopic history and the use of patch testing can help to differentiate these disorders.

2. **Tinea infections,** especially tinea pedis, can resemble atopic dermatitis. A potassium hydroxide slide preparation or fungal culture of material from the vesicular and scaling lesion is diagnostic. Tinea pedis is rare prepubertally.

3. **Pityriasis rosea** appears as pale, erythematous, papulosquamous lesions, typically on the torso, and often with a herald patch. The lack of pruritus in some cases and its self-limited nature are distinguishing features.

4. **Scabies** is often confused with acute flares of atopic dermatitis and should be considered in all pruritic papular eruptions.

C. Adult eczema

1. **Psoriasis** is usually distinguished by its well-defined scaly plaques and by extensor and axial involvement. Pruritus is rarer than in atopic dermatitis.

2. **Pyoderma** can usually be distinguished by the clinical course; pruritus is a less common feature in pyoderma than in atopic dermatitis.

3. **Dyshidrotic eczema** manifests as pruritic vesicles of the palms and soles, aggravated by hyperhidrosis.

IV. Laboratory features. The diagnosis of atopic dermatitis is usually made by history and clinical presentation. Laboratory studies may be helpful in atypical presentations.

A. Eosinophilia on peripheral blood smear, a common occurrence, can correlate with the degree and activity of atopic dermatitis. Elevated neutrophil counts suggest secondary infection.

B. Serum IgE levels are elevated in 80% of patients with atopic dermatitis, especially if allergic respiratory symptoms coexist.

C. Allergy skin testing can reveal positive reactions in a majority of patients with atopic dermatitis. Positive reactions to foods are common, especially in infants and young children. **The role of incriminated antigens is often unclear, and challenge or elimination may not alter the clinical course** (see Chap. 2).

D. The **radioallergosorbent test (RAST)** has similar sensitivity as scratch or prick allergy skin tests (see Chap. 2). It can be useful in patients who have generalized dermatitis that precludes skin testing.

   E. Skin biopsy findings show a variety of changes, depending on the clinical stage
      (see sec. **I.D**).
V. Complications
   A. Secondary infection is increased by frequent rubbing and scratching, which
      breaks down the protective barrier of the skin.
      1. Secondary bacterial infection, the most common complication, is usually
         caused by *Staphylococcus aureus*. This organism colonizes atopic skin more
         commonly than the skin of normal individuals. Staphylococcal infections
         usually remain superficial in atopic dermatitis and are manifested by ex-
         udate, crusting, or erythema. Dermatitis tends not to improve in the pres-
         ence of bacterial infection. Rarely, other bacteria may be cultured. Second-
         ary bacterial infections are treated with systemic antibiotics.
      2. Viral infections
         a. Eczema herpeticum (Kaposi's varicelliform eruption) is a generalized
            vesiculopustular infection caused by herpes simplex virus. It occurs
            maximally in areas of active atopic dermatitis, but can also involve
            normal skin, and usually lasts from 1–2 weeks. A Tzanck smear (scrap-
            ings obtained from the base of a vesicle, smeared on a microscope slide,
            and stained with Giemsa or Wright's stain) identifies multinucleated
            giant cells produced by viral transformation of epidermal cells. Viral
            culture can distinguish herpes simplex from varicella-zoster. Electron
            micrographs of the blister can help differentiate herpes simplex virus
            (round spheres) from the brick-shaped virions of vaccinia. Treatment is
            symptomatic unless severe complications occur; systemic antiviral
            agents (e.g., acyclovir) are indicated for treatment.
         b. Eczema vaccinatum results from exposure to the attenuated vaccinia
            virus (smallpox vaccine). The lesions can occur anywhere on the skin
            and begin a few days after exposure either by vaccination or by contact
            with a vaccinated person. The administration of vaccinia immune globu-
            lin is most efficiently used as a prophylactic measure. Symptomatic
            treatment is also indicated.
         c. Molluscum contagiosum appears to be more common in atopic individ-
            uals. This pox virus causes firm, white, often umbilicated papules 1–6
            mm in size. Lesions have a central core or "molluscum body," which is
            composed of virally transformed epidermal cells with cytoplasmic inclu-
            sions. Lesions may resolve in 1 or 2 years, but because of pruritus,
            secondary infection, and spread, treatment is recommended. Des-
            quamating agents, acids, cryotherapy, or incision and curettage of indi-
            vidual lesions can all be used.
         d. Warts, both common warts on glabrous skin (verruca vulgaris) and
            plantar warts, may be persistent in patients with atopic dermatitis.
      3. Yeast and fungal infections (e.g., *Candida* and *Trichophyton*) can develop
         in areas of active dermatitis, especially in the moist areas of the skin folds
         and feet. These infections usually respond to topical, fungicidal prepara-
         tions.
   B. Cataracts (posterior or anterior lenticular opacities) occur in up to 5% of pa-
      tients with atopic dermatitis, usually adolescents or adults. **Keratoconus** (a
      conical protrusion of the cornea) occurs less commonly.
VI. Treatment
   A. General measures. Because atopic dermatitis is chronic, with exacerbations
      and remissions, therapy **must** be tailored according to the needs of the individ-
      ual patient. Atopic skin is more sensitive to a variety of local factors, and many
      stimuli are perceived as "itch." Exacerbating factors include rough textures
      such as wool, a dry cool environment, excessive sweating, and occlusion with
      synthetic fabrics. Diet plays a role in atopic dermatitis in less than 20% of
      patients; some patients may benefit from avoiding foods suspected of aggravat-
      ing symptoms. Four major factors need to be considered in therapy (see Table
      8-1):

Table 8-1. Guidelines in treating atopic dermatitis

I. Reduce itching and scratching
   A. Avoid local irritants (e.g., wool or fur garments); soft cotton fabrics are preferable. Wash clothing and bed sheets in a mild detergent (e.g., Ivory Flakes, Dreft) and rinse well. Avoid starch and fabric softeners.
   B. Keep fingernails short; use mittens or socks on hands of small children.
   C. Keep affected areas covered.
   D. Keep ambient temperature at 68–72°; humidify dry heat in winter.
   E. Avoid animals, dust, sprays, and perfumes.
   F. Use oral antihistamines as directed.
II. Keep skin moisturized
   A. Daily baths (not showers) will hydrate skin. Use mild neutral soaps. Avoid deodorant and perfumed soaps. Immediately apply topical corticosteroids to affected areas and emollients to entire **wet** skin surface to keep skin moist.
   B. Use topical skin moisturizers 2–4 times/day or as needed.
   C. Remember that occlusion with ointments is greater than with creams or lotions (in that order). Ointments provide better lubrication but are not always acceptable to patients.
   D. Bath oils and oilated oatmeal products (e.g., ½–1 cup of corn starch, oatmeal, or Aveeno to tepid bathwater) may be soothing.
III. Prevent inflammation
   A. Use topical corticosteroids on affected skin.
   B. Use of systemic corticosteroids is indicated in rare cases in adults.
   C. Use coal tar as a helpful adjunct.
IV. Treat infection (use systemic antibiotics to eliminate *Staphylococcus aureus* whenever necessary).

---

1. **Itch.** Patients should avoid local irritants and try to suppress pruritus with adequate doses of systemic antihistamines. Pruritus is worse in times of stress and in the evening and at bedtime.
2. **Dryness.** Dry skin itches. Although there are two seemingly contradictory approaches to therapy, both approaches are popular: (a) avoidance of water and use of nonsoap washes, or (b) good hydration of the skin with application of emollients. Both may be used interchangeably.
3. **Inflammation.** Edema, erythema, and infiltrated papules and plaques respond to anti-inflammatory measures such as topical corticosteroids and tar.
4. **Infection.** Systemic antibiotics are necessary to successfully eliminate superinfection, usually due to *S. aureus*.
   B. **Specific treatments**
   1. **Antihistamines** are used to control pruritus (see Table 4-5 for a list of preparations and dosages). These agents are administered orally as needed 3–4 times/day. A bedtime dose is most helpful, especially in small children who scratch during sleep. Hydroxyzine (Atarax or Vistaril), 10–100 mg/dose (2–5 mg/kg/day in children), diphenhydramine (Benadryl), 25–50 mg/dose (5 mg/kg/day in children), and cyproheptadine (Periactin), 2–4 mg/dose, are particularly useful agents. Newer nonsedating drugs such as terfenidine (Seldane), 60 mg twice a day in patients over age 12 years, are useful in patients made drowsy by standard H_1 antihistamines.
   2. **Emollients** (moisturizers) (Table 8-2). Effective use of emollients are the mainstay of therapy for atopic dermatitis. In general, ointments more than creams, and creams more than lotions, provide lasting protection from dryness and itching, but heavy occlusion may not be tolerated by all patients. Emollients are more effective if applied while the skin is wet. Daily baths (rather than showers) for 20 minutes to hydrate the skin, followed immediately by application of a thick emollient before the skin is allowed to

Table 8-2. Topical emollients

Preparation	Form of emollient			Contents of emollient			
	Ointment	Cream	Lotion	Lanolin	Urea	Parabens	Petrolatum
Acid mantle		+					
Almay Deep Mist Moisturizing Cream		+					
Almay Deep Mist Moisturizing Lotion			+			+	+
Aquacare, Aquacare HP		+	+	+	+	+	+
Aquaglycolic			+	+		+	+
Aquaphor	+						
Carmol 10	+				+		
Carmol 20					+		
Complex 15		+	+		+		
Curel		+	+	+		+	+
Eucerin		+	+	+		+	+
Keri			+			+	
Lac-Hydrin*			+			+	
LactiCare			+		+		

Lubriderm

Moisturel

Neutraderm

Neutrogena Facial Moisturizer

Neutrogena Norwegian Formula

Nivea Cream

Nivea Lotion

Purpose

RV Cream

RV Lotion

Sarna

Shepard's

Tritle's

Ultra Mide 25

Vaseline (Petrolatum)

Vaseline Derm Formula

Vaseline Intensive Care

Wondra

*Prescription item.

dry, is the preferred treatment for dry atopic skin. Addition of oilated oatmeal (Aveeno) or bath oils are useful in some patients. Some patients may become sensitized to lanolin or parabens (a preservative) in some emollients or in the vehicle bases of corticosteroid creams.

3. **Corticosteroids**

   a. Topical corticosteroids, used initially to control active dermatitis, are available as fluorinated and nonfluorinated products. In general, the fluorinated group has greater anti-inflammatory capabilities but more side effects than the nonfluorinated group. (Table 8-3 lists available topical corticosteroids and their relative potencies based on vasoconstrictor activity.) Some nonfluorinated corticosteroids are quite potent and have the same potential for side effects as the fluorinated group. These preparations are available in a wide variety of vehicles, the type of vehicle affecting spreadability, absorption, occlusiveness, and drying. Some vehicles may have components that irritate the skin or to which cutaneous allergy is present.

      (1) Ointments, creams, lotions, and gels are more occlusive and less drying, in that order. The greasy feel of ointments is cosmetically unacceptable to some patients. Lotions are most useful in the scalp. The most occlusive ointment vehicles provide greater penetration of corticosteroids. Occlusive dressings such as plastic wrap increase penetration. If occlusion is to be used, instruct the patient to apply topical creams and then cover the area with a commercial plastic wrap. Occlusion therapy should be limited to 5–7 days. All topical corticosteroid preparations can be applied 2–4 times/day to active areas and should **not** be used widespread as emollients. Emollients may be applied over topical corticosteroids.

      (2) Potent fluorinated corticosteroids are used to control acute, severe lesions, while nonfluorinated preparations are used for milder acute lesions, for maintenance therapy, and for sensitive areas such as the face, neck, and groin. Potent corticosteroids (group I) are rarely indicated in children, especially in infancy and during the pubertal growth spurt, and 1% or 2.5% hydrocortisone suffices for most clinical situations. It should be noted that several topical corticosteroids are available in preparations that span the potency range (i.e., 0.025, 0.1, and 0.5% triamcinolone), and thus concentration as well as name should be considered before prescribing.

      (3) Percutaneous absorption occurs, and systemic side effects of corticosteroids can become a problem with topical preparations used in large amounts over weeping surfaces. Adrenal suppression can occur in adults if more than 50 gm/week (10 gm/week in children) of a group I topical corticosteroid is applied (see Table 8-3). The most common local side effects of topical therapy include skin atrophy, telangiectasia, folliculitis, and acne (Table 8-4). These conditions can be prevented by cautious use of the potent preparations, especially in areas of enhanced absorption (i.e., face, neck, and groin). In general, the smallest amount of the lowest potency corticosteroid used as little as possible to control symptoms is safest.

   b. **Intralesional corticosteroids.** Local intradermal injections of corticosteroids are occasionally used to treat recalcitrant localized plaques of lichen simplex chronicus. Triamcinolone acetonide or triamcinolone hexacetonide suspensions, in dilutions of 2.5–10.0 mg/ml (up to 0.5 mg/ sq. in. of affected skin), are injected intralesionally through a 30-gauge needle. Injections of up to 10 mg total can be safely repeated every 4–6 weeks. Because this method increases systemic and local side effects, maintenance of controlled lesions should be accomplished with topical preparations.

   c. **Systemic corticosteroids.** If the dermatitis is extensive or not responsive to topical treatment, systemic corticosteroids can be administered

Table 8-3. Topical corticosteroid preparations[a]

	Group I (High potency)
0.05%	Betamethasone dipropionate[b] (Diprosone, Diprolene)
0.1%	Amcinonide[b] (Cyclocort)
0.25%	Desoximetasone[b] (Topicort)
0.5%	Triamcinolone acetonide[b]
0.2%	Fluocinolone acetonide[b] (Synalar HP)
0.05%	Diflorasone diacetate[b] (Florone, Maxiflor)
0.1%	Halcinonide[b] (Halog)
0.05%	Fluocinonide[b] (Lidex, Topsyn)
0.05%	Clobetasole propinate[b] (Temovate)

	Group II (Intermediate potency)
0.2%	Hydrocortisone valerate (Westcort)
0.025%	Betamethasone benzoate[b] (Uticort, Benisone)
0.025%	Flurandrenolide[b] (Cordran)
0.1%	Betamethasone valerate[b] (Valisone)
0.05%	Desonide (Tridesilon)
0.025%	Halcinonide[b] (Halog)
0.05%	Desoximetasone[b] (Topicort L.P.)
0.05%	Flurandrenolide[b] (Cordran)
0.1%	Triamcinolone acetonide[b]
0.025%	Fluocinolone acetonide[b]

	Group III (Low potency)
0.1%	Fluocinolone acetonide[b] (Synalar, Fluonid)
0.01%	Betamethasone valerate[b] (Valisone)
0.025%	Fluorometholone[b] (Oxylone)
0.025%	Triamcinolone acetonide[b] (Aristocort, Kenalog, Triacet)
0.1%	Clocortolone pivalate[b] (Cloderm)
0.03%	Flumethasone pivalate[b] (Locorten)

	Group IV (Lowest potency)
0.25–2.5%	Hydrocortisone
0.25%	Methylprednisolone acetate (Medrol)
0.04%	Dexamethasone[b] (Hexadrol)
0.1%	Dexamethasone[b] (Decaderm)
1.0%	Methylprednisolone acetate (Medrol)
0.5%	Prednisolone (Meti-Derm)
0.2%	Betamethasone[b] (Celestone)

[a]Grouped according to potency as determined by vasoconstrictor activity. Topical side effects are directly related to potency.
[b]Fluorinated corticosteroids.
Source: Adapted from D. B. Robertson and H. I. Maibach. Topical corticosteroids. *Int. J. Dermatol.* 21:59, 1982.

Table 8-4. Side effects of topical corticosteroids*

Burning	Hypopigmentation
Itching	Perioral dermatitis
Irritation	Allergic contact dermatitis
Dryness	Maceration of the skin
Telangiectasia	Secondary infection
Folliculitis	Skin atrophy
Hypertrichosis	Striae
Acneiform eruptions	Miliaria

*Side effects are enhanced under occlusive dressings.

(see Table 4-12). Besides the usual corticosteroid side effects, rebound flares of atopic dermatitis often occur after systemic therapy.

   (1) Oral administration is preferable. Prednisone can be started in a dose of 40–60 mg/day in adults and tapered by 5–10 mg every 2 or 3 days when stable (not recommended for children). Topical corticosteroids are used for maintenance. Therapy for more than 10–14 days carries the potential for adrenal suppression.

   (2) Intramuscular injections of corticosteroids can be used as an alternative to oral administration in selected cases. Table 4-12 lists preparations and doses.

4. **Coal tar.** For chronic, recalcitrant lichenified plaques, various tar preparations act as anti-inflammatory agents and can significantly decrease the use of topical corticosteroids. Most over-the-counter preparations (e.g., Estar Gel, Phototar) are gels and may burn or irritate the skin. A mild crude coal tar, liquor carbonis detergans (LCD), can be compounded in 2–5% strengths in a variety of vehicles such as petrolatum or Aquaphor.

5. **Open wet dressings.** When patients with atopic dermatitis have an acute flare with generalized erythema, edema, heat loss, fluid loss, and desquamation of foul-smelling keratin (acute erythroderma), or when localized areas become superinfected with exudative, crusting, weeping surfaces, the application of open wet dressings is indicated. A thin cotton material (i.e., sheet or pillowcase) soaked in lukewarm tap water or in aluminum acetate solution (Burow's solution; mix 1–2 commercially available packets or tablets [Domeboro] to 1 pint of water [1:40 to 1:20 dilution]) and applied to the affected area will lessen erythema, edema, itching, and pain. The dressings should be applied for 15 minutes every 3–4 hours.

6. **Antibiotics.** Systemic antibiotics are essential when dermatitis becomes infected. *S. aureus* is the usual organism. Erythromycin is the first choice, but resistance may occur in some communities. Dicloxacillin, cloxacillin, amoxicillin with clavulanic acid (Augmentin), or a cephalosporin can also be used. Topical antibiotics may accelerate emergence of resistant strains.

7. **Immunotherapy** (hyposensitization) is usually **not** helpful for atopic dermatitis. Immunotherapy can be given to patients with atopic dermatitis for their coexisting respiratory allergies.

8. **Ultraviolet B light.** In some recalcitrant cases, ultraviolet B light treatments are useful.

Contact Dermatitis

Contact dermatitis is a cutaneous inflammation caused by exposure to external agents. There are four basic types: **irritant, allergic, phototoxic,** and **photoallergic. Irritant dermatitis** results from contact with a substance that chemically or physically damages the skin on a nonimmunologic basis. **Allergic contact dermatitis** occurs as a result of a substance contacting the skin and causing a specific alteration in its immunologic reactivity on the basis of a type IV hypersensitivity reaction (see Chap. 1). The term **contact dermatitis** is often used synonymously with **allergic contact dermatitis**. **Phototoxic contact dermatitis** resembles the irritant type but requires sun and a chemical in combination to damage the epidermis. **Photoallergic contact dermatitis** is similar to allergic contact dermatitis but requires light exposure in addition to allergen contact to produce immunologic reactivity in the skin. Contact dermatitis is widespread, affecting 3–4% of the adult population and accounting for 10% or more of the patients treated by dermatologists. The incidence varies widely by country because of different degrees of industrialization and thus different chemical exposures.

I. **Irritant dermatitis** often occurs after the first exposure to a strong irritant (e.g., battery acid); this reaction does not require a presensitization phase. It can also result from repeated exposures to milder irritants over an extended time (e.g., detergents or home cleaning solutions).

   A. **Clinical presentation.** The first stage of irritant dermatitis is usually dryness, lasting from days to months or even years. The second stage, characterized by vesiculation, fissuring, and/or cracking, is often difficult to differentiate from true allergic contact dermatitis, even by skin biopsy.

   Irritant reactions are enhanced by occlusion and vary with each individual and according to the specific irritant. The hands and lower arms are the most common locations for irritant dermatitis because of their repeated exposure. Dryness (e.g., caused by excessive water immersion) predisposes the skin to irritant reactions. Similarly, patients with inflammatory dermatoses (e.g., atopic dermatitis) have easily irritated skin. The same irritant can cause different degrees of eruption on different areas of the skin.

   B. The **diagnosis** of irritant dermatitis is based on clinical judgment (e.g., location of the reaction and type of chemical) and appropriate negative patch tests results that exclude allergic dermatitis. Examine every patch test critically, looking for an irritant response. A sharply demarcated reaction resembling a chemical burn suggests an irritant response; a progressively spreading eczematous reaction or erythema and vesiculation suggest allergic contact dermatitis. Other patch test phenomena suggesting irritant responses include the production of pustules and the presence of multiple positive reactions, especially to the more irritating materials such as nickel and formalin, which indicate hyperirritable skin prone to false-positive reactions.

   C. **Treatment.** First, the source of irritation must be identified and removed. This alone often suffices. The inflammatory component is treated in the same manner as for other dermatitides (see sec. II and Atopic Dermatitis, sec. VI). Application of a hydrophilic cream (see Table 8-2) or petrolatum is soothing and protective. Apply compresses for weeping lesions and topical corticosteroids for more stubborn cases. Administer antibiotics systemically for secondary infection and oral antihistamines for pruritus.

II. **Allergic contact dermatitis,** which results from a delayed hypersensitivity (type IV) reaction to the contacting substance, requires a sensitization period of 10–14 days. Sensitization occurs when lymphocytes, altered by exposure to the antigenic component of the contact sensitizer, are disseminated throughout the body, producing sensitivity of the entire skin. This alteration of lymphocytes takes place in the regional lymph nodes that drain the area of initial contact. For sensitization to simple chemicals, the chemical (hapten) must combine with skin protein to form the actual sensitizer reactive in the lymph nodes. Passive transfer is demonstrable with lymphocytes from a sensitive person but not with serum.

   The onset and intensity of contact sensitivity are dependent on a number of factors, including variable sensitivity to sensitization among individuals, easier sensitization of young or middle-aged adults as compared with children or elderly persons, and the capacity of a contactant as a sensitizer. The risk of sensitization increases by increasing the concentration of material on the skin, increasing the skin area exposed to the chemical, applying to inflamed skin, occluding the skin site (i.e., dressings, clothing) exposed to the sensitizer, and repeated exposure. Generally, contact sensitivity remains for life. Persons who are atopic are less likely to develop allergic contact dermatitis.

A. Pathologic features. The histologic changes in contact dermatitis are the same as those produced by fungal infections, atopic dermatitis, infectious eczematous dermatitis, or nummular dermatitis. Consequently, microscopic examination of a skin biopsy specimen is not diagnostic unless fungal hyphae are demonstrated or disorders with a characteristic histologic picture are identified (e.g., lichen planus or discoid lupus erythematosus).

  1. Acute contact dermatitis produces microscopic changes before gross alterations are usually evident. Vasodilatation and perivascular infiltrates in the dermis are typically seen within 3 hours after application of the sensitizer to the skin of sensitized persons. The changes in the dermis at 6 hours are more evident, with mononuclear cells infiltrating into the epidermis, where intracellular edema (spongiosis) is present in the uppermost layers. If the reaction proceeds, the intracellular edema becomes more marked within 12–24 hours and can actually form intraepidermal vesicles. As the mononuclear cell infiltrate extends throughout the epidermis, from the basal cell layer to the stratum corneum, thickening of the epidermal layer (acanthosis) appears, and the perivascular infiltrates become more evident. Intracellular edema disappears after 2 days but the intraepidermal vesicles and acanthosis persist, and parakeratosis (retention of the nuclei in the stratum corneum) develops.

  2. Chronic contact dermatitis is characterized histologically by the nonspecific changes of acanthosis, hyperkeratosis, and a variable inflammatory cell infiltrate.

B. Etiologic agents. The list of materials causing contact dermatitis is constantly increasing as people are exposed to a variety of new chemical substances. Antimicrobial agents, dyes, formaldehyde-containing resins, cosmetics and perfumes, rubber products, metals such as nickel and chromium, plants, and topical medications are the most common causes of contact dermatitis. A list of the common allergic contact sensitizers is given in Table 8-5.

Cross-sensitization can exist when allergic contact dermatitis is produced by one sensitizer but subsequently evoked by secondary exposure to chemically related substances. Multiple sensitization to different substances can also occur when products containing multiple sensitizers are used.

C. Clinical presentation and diagnosis

  1. History. To make an accurate diagnosis, a thorough, detailed history is

Table 8-5. Common allergic contact sensitizers

Substance* and percent concentration for patch testing	Area or source of contact	Comment
PLANTS		
1. *Rhus*		
Poison ivy	United States, except Southwest	
Poison oak	Pacific coast	
Poison sumac	Damp swampy areas, especially east of Mississippi	
Oak-leaf poison ivy	Southeastern United States	
2. Compositae Chrysanthemum, daisy, ragweed, artichoke	Ubiquitous	Cross-reacts with turpentine, balsam of Peru, and benzoin

Table 8-5. (continued)

Substance* and percent concentration for patch testing	Area or source of contact	Comment
PLANTS (cont.)		
3. Liliaceae Tulip, hyacinth, asparagus, garlic, onion	Ubiquitous	
4. Amaryllidaceae Daffodil, narcissus	Ubiquitous	
5. Umbelliferae Carrots, celery	Ubiquitous	
6. Cannabinaceae Nettles, hops	Ubiquitous	
7. Rutaceae Orange, lemon, grapefruit	Ubiquitous	
8. Lichen Various species	Ubiquitous	
9. Primula Primrose	Great Britain	
METALS AND METAL SALTS		
1. Nickel sulfate (2.5%)	Jewelry, watches, clasps, hairpins, garter belts, earrings, stainless steel wire, some dyes	
2. Potassium dichromate (0.5%)	Leather, bleaches, yellow paint, tanning agents, photographic materials	
3. Mercury bichloride (0.1%)	Disinfectants, silk, wire, batteries, skin lighteners, thermometers	
4. Cobalt sulfate and chloride (2%)	Tattoos, clays, adhesives, hair dyes, hematinics	
5. Ferric chloride (2%)	Monsel's solution, styptic	Rare sensitizer
6. Gold chloride (2%)	Photographic materials	
7. Copper sulfate (5%)	Insecticides, food processing, dyes, coins	
8. Silver nitrate (2%)	Caustic pencils, hair dyes	Use open patch test to avoid irritation
9. Aluminum chloride (2%)	Antiperspirants, antiseptics	
10. Sodium arsenate (10%)	Hair tonics, insecticides, arsenical soaps	
RUBBER CHEMICALS	Clothing, adhesive tape, latex cements, glues, gums, resins	
1. Mercapto compounds (1%) Mercaptobenzothiazole Dibenzothiazoldisulfide	Rubber vulcanizers and accelerators, cements	Most common rubber sensitizer
2. Thiuram compounds (1%)	Rubber vulcanizer, rubber gloves	

Table 8-5. (continued)

Substance* and percent concentration for patch testing	Area or source of contact	Comment
RUBBER CHEMICALS (cont.)		
Tetramethyl-thiuram disulfide		
Tetramethyl-thiuram monosulfide		
3. Naphthyl compounds (1%)	Rubber antioxidant	
4. Paraphenylenediamines (1%)	Vulcanizer for industrial black rubber	
5. Carba compounds (3%)	Rubber accelerator	
OTHER CHEMICALS AND MEDICAMENTS		
1. Coal tar (5%)	Adhesives, insecticides, wood preservatives, resins, dyes, topical medicaments	
2. Ethylenediamine (1%)	Topical medicaments, tincture of Merthiolate	Possible eruption with oral or parenteral aminophylline
3. Formalin (2%)	Disinfectants, toothpaste, antiperspirants, permanent wave solutions, soaps, fingernail hardeners	
4. Ammoniated mercuric chloride (1%)	Topical medicaments, bleaching creams	Cross-reacts with organic and inorganic mercury compounds (not Merthiolate).
5. Neomycin sulfate (20%)	Topical antibiotic	
6. Thimerosal (0.1%)	Merthiolate, preservatives in medications	
7. Turpentine (10%)	Solvents, thinners, dry cleaners, varnishes, adhesives, cleaning fluids	
8. Wool wax alcohols (30%)	Ointments, creams, bath oils, cosmetics	Fraction of lanolin
9. Lanolin (100%)	Ointments, creams, cosmetics, bath oils	Purified wool fat
10. Acrylic monomer (10%)	Artificial fingernails, dentures, Lucite, plastics, Plexiglas, resins	All acrylic monomers cross-react.
11. Balsam of Peru (25%)	Perfumes, topical medicaments, rectal suppositories, cosmetics, hair tonics, flavoring, oil paint	Cross-reacts with vanilla, cinnamon, benzoic acid, benzyl alcohol, clove.
12. Benzyl alcohol (5%)	Essential oils, food flavoring, perfumes, local anesthetics, antiseptics	
13. Benzocaine (5%)	Local anesthetics, lozenges, suppositories, denture adhesives, sunburn medicaments	Cross-reacts with procaine, tetracaine, butacaine, sulfonamides, azo dyes.

Table 8-5. (continued)

Substance* and percent concentration for patch testing	Area or source of contact	Comment
OTHER CHEMICALS AND MEDICAMENTS (cont.)		
14. Other caine derivatives	Local anesthetics	
Amethocaine, procaine, dibucaine		Strong sensitizers
Mepivacaine, lidocaine		Weak sensitizers
15. Diaminodiphenylmethane (0.5%)	Epoxy hardener, anticorrosives, insecticides	Cross-reacts with paraphenylenediamine.
16. Dichlorophen (0.5%)	Fungicide, cosmetics, soaps	Photopatch tests may be necessary.
17. Epoxy resins (1%)	Adhesives, protective coatings, paints	All epoxy resins cross-react.
18. Nitrofurazone (0.2%)	Furacin and other topical antibacterial agents	
19. Hexachlorophene (0.5%)	Antiseptic in soaps and cosmetics	Photopatch test may be necessary.
20. Parabens (3% each) Ethylparaben, methylparaben, propylparaben, butylparaben, and benzylparaben	Cosmetics, preservative in medicaments, topical corticosteroid creams and ointments, sunscreens, lipstick, hair lotions	
21. Tripelennamine	Antihistamine in creams, ointments, nasal sprays	
22. Paratertiary butylphenol (2%)	Adhesives, resins, duplicating paper, rubber	
23. Triethylenetetramine (0.5%)	Epoxy hardener	Same exposure as epoxy resins
24. Iodochlorohydroxyquinoline	Vioform and other antibacterial topical medicaments	
25. Quaternary ammonium compounds (1:1000 aqueous solution)	Topical disinfectants in tape, gauze, creams, lotions	
26. Colophony (20%)	Rosins to increase friction (i.e., athletes)	
27. Wood tars (12%)	Perfumes, cosmetics, topical medicaments	
28. Hydroxycitronellal (4%)	Oil of turpentine, perfumes, cosmetics, food flavorings	
29. Parachloro-m-xylenol (1%)	Antiseptic in cosmetics and topical medicaments	
30. Quaternium (2%)	Preservative in cosmetics	
31. Imidazolidinyl urea (2%)	Preservative in cosmetics	
32. Captan (1%)	Agricultural fungicide, bacteriostatic agent in soaps and cosmetics	

*When multiple substances are listed under the same numbered heading, they are cross-reactive.

mandatory, not only during the initial evaluation but also on repeated visits. Special inquiries should be directed to the following areas:

   a. Obtain information on **previous** skin problems. Topical therapy of an existing dermatitis can produce a new allergic contact dermatitis.

   b. A **family history** of skin disease suggests endogenous dermatitides, such as atopic dermatitis, seborrheic dermatitis, or psoriasis.

   c. Specifically inquire about materials that commonly cause contact dermatitis. **Cross-sensitizing materials should also be noted.** The patient may consider these materials as harmless and unimportant unless specifically questioned about them (see Table 8-5).

      (1) Cosmetics are a frequent cause, and a cause not limited to women. They commonly include deodorants, hair dressings, hair dyes, perfumes, after-shave lotions, hand creams, face creams, bath oils, and body lotions.

      (2) Drugs, including prescription drugs and over-the-counter preparations, are common sensitizers when used topically or given parenterally. Common topical preparations causing sensitization include neomycin, ethylenediamine, topical anesthetics, thimerosal, mercury, lanolin, and preservatives (e.g., parachlorometaxylenol, dichlorophen, and parabens).

      (3) Hobbies are a frequent source of contactants. Inquire as to the use of paints, solvents, and synthetic glues, especially the epoxy glues.

      (4) Occupational exposures commonly include formaldehyde, solvents, nickel, epoxy and other glues, cement, oils and greases, and rubber products. Rubber products, in particular, contain accelerators, antioxidants, and other materials that can produce "rubber contact dermatitis." **Specifically inquire about the use of rubber gloves.**

      (5) Plants provide sensitizing substances, with poison ivy and poison oak the most common offenders in North America. The possibility of plant contact through pets, clothing, or smoke from burning plants should be explored.

      (6) Metals, particularly nickel or chromium, are common sensitizers. Nickel sensitivity is common in women because of jewelry exposure, especially with ear piercing. Small amounts of chromates are found in most forms of cement, and chrome salts are employed in tanning, dying, and printing; thus, chrome sensitivity is primarily an industrial problem.

2. A careful **physical examination** in patients with suspected contact dermatitis is essential to help exclude systemic disorders mimicking contact dermatitis or coexisting with it. Determination of the distribution of the dermatitis often suggests a possible cause. Approximately one-half of contact dermatitis reactions are located on the hands (the percentage is higher for occupational contact dermatitis, in which up to 90% of patients have hand involvement). The rashes are usually on the dorsal aspect of the hands unless the contact is caused by solid objects, e.g., nickel-plated objects that can cause dermatitis in the palm. In hand dermatitis, note the materials encountered at work and exposure to topical drugs, lubricants and hand lotions, metal jewelry, plants, and rubber gloves. Other common associations between contactants in relation to body site are noted in Table 8-6.

3. Patch testing is used to discover and confirm the cause of an allergic contact dermatitis. Chemical substances are applied to an area of skin in an attempt to reproduce the allergic contact dermatitis seen clinically.

   a. Indications. If a material is obviously causing an allergic contact dermatitis, patch testing is not indicated for that patient. Eczematous dermatitides from various causes, however, can clinically mimic allergic contact dermatitis and make diagnosis based solely on history or gross morphology difficult. Indications for patch testing include the following:

      (1) To prove a clinically diagnosed case of contact dermatitis.

Table 8-6. Suspected sources of contact sensitizers for specific body areas

Area	Suspected source
Hands	Jewelry, plants, cosmetics, topical medicaments, rubber, metals (most cases are irritant)
Arms	Wood dust, metals, plants, textiles, dyes (otherwise same as hands, with later onset)
Face and head	Topical medicaments, cosmetics (usually involve hands as well), sunscreens, nail preparations
Lips and perioral	Lipstick, toothpaste, denture preparations, nail polish, metals, citrus, mangoes; fluorinated topical corticosteroids are common irritants
Eyelids	Contactants from fingertips, plants, cosmetics and eye makeup, metals, topical medicaments
Forehead	Hair preparations
Ears	Metals and jewelry, topical medicaments, acrylic hearing aids and earphones, ear plugs (resins), hair preparations
Scalp	Hair preparations (e.g., sprays, wave sets, dyes, tonics), topical medicaments
Axillae	Antiperspirants, topical medicaments, textiles, dyes
Trunk	Topical medicaments, sunscreens, cosmetics, buttons, zippers, leather, rubber, plastics, plants
Genitalia	Antiseptics, topical fungicidals and antibacterials, rubber, wood dust in clothing, perfumes
Perianal	Topical anesthetics, antiseptics, and antibiotics, dyes, textiles, perfumes, suppositories (balsam of Peru and mercury)
Thighs and lower legs	Wood dust in clothing, textiles, dyes, topical medicaments, rubber, metals, and contents of pockets
Feet	Shoes, leather, rubber, shoe polish, dyes, powders, topical medicaments, plants, stockings, textiles

    (2) To determine the actual sensitizers among many clinically suspected materials.
    (3) To detect relevant but clinically unsuspected contact sensitizers, especially in puzzling clinical cases.
    (4) To determine which materials a patient can safely tolerate, especially the highly sensitive patient.
  b. Contraindications. Patch testing is contraindicated in acute, widespread dermatitis. Testing in these circumstances can worsen the dermatitis or evoke nonspecific test reactions at the patch test site. Delay patch testing for approximately 1 month until such widespread dermatitis has cleared.
  c. Patch testing methods. The classic **closed patch test** consists of applying the test substance to a piece of cloth or soft paper that is placed on the skin, covered with an impermeable material, affixed with tape, and removed after 48 hours. At this time, the characteristics of the underlying skin are examined. To standardize the patch test, the International Contact Dermatitis Research Group* has established guidelines to help standardize critical factors such as skin test site, size and material of the patch, and occlusiveness of the patch. The test substances **must be nonirritating** and diluted in a preferred diluent (usually white pet-

* Address: c/o The Journal of Contact Dermatitis, Post Box 2148, 35 Norre Sogade, DK-1016, Copenhagen K, Denmark

rolatum). The International Contact Dermatitis Research Group has published lists for recommended patch test concentrations for common contact allergens. **Carefully follow these recommendations.** Information about technique and availability or the proper concentration of the material in question can be obtained from the contact dermatitis research groups.* The following **guidelines** should be used in patch testing procedures:

(1) The preferred test site is the midportion of the upper back or, alternatively, the upper outer arm. The skin used for testing must be completely normal, because even trace amounts of dermatitis make a site unsuitable. If no areas are free of dermatitis, testing should be deferred.

(2) Mark test sites using four rows of tests, two rows spaced evenly apart on each side of the midline on the back. Mark the test sites with a felt-tipped, waterproof marking pen. The patient should remain in a neutral, relaxed position during testing to avoid stretching or wrinkling of the skin.

(3) The basic patch test unit, the AL-Test (manufactured in Sweden and available through Hollister-Stier Laboratories), consists of round disks of cellulose affixed to polyethylene-coated aluminum paper. Place a small amount of the agent to be tested on the fabric portion of the patch. A consistent amount of the material must be applied. The standard patch test materials are usually provided in syringes, tubes, or other dispensers so designed that the proper amount of the patch test material in a petrolatum base is delivered if one squeezes out a strip of material corresponding in length to the diameter of the disk (1 cm).

(4) When testing multiple substances, record the results on a standardized printed form (Table 8-7) to avoid confusion. Recording of the results can be simplified by labeling the locations of the test materials in vertical rows and then numbering the position within each row, starting from the top.

(5) Correct application of the patch test is critical to obtain an occlusive patch. (Also check to see that the test patches correspond and are exactly oriented to the marked sites.) If the patches will not adhere for the full length of time, use nonallergenic, reinforcing tape (e.g., Blenderm or Dermacil).

(6) Instruct the patient to avoid wetting the patch test, to remove promptly any test patch that produces severe itching or discomfort, and at 48 hours to remove all test patches before returning for the patch test reading (**at least 1–2 hours before the visit**).

(7) Patch test interpretation is made at a minimum of 1–2 hours after removal of the test substance (actually, a period of 4–24 hours is more desirable). **Delayed patch test readings** 2–3 days after **removal** of the test substance are essential because with certain substances, notably formalin and neomycin, a test can be negative or weakly reactive on the initial reading yet produce a strong, eczematous reaction at the later time. These initial weak reactions can progress to an infiltrated eczematous patch, suggesting that the initially weak reaction probably represented the early stage of a true allergic response.

d. Patch test interpretation. Skin test response is graded using criteria established by the International Contact Dermatitis Research Group: 1+ represents strong erythema and infiltration; 2+ indicates vesicles;

---

*Address: c/o The American Academy of Dermatology, 820 Davis Street, Evanston, IL 60201, and c/o The Journal of Contact Dermatitis, Post Box 2148, 35 Norre Sogade, DK-1016, Copenhagen K, Denmark. Standard commercial patch testing materials are not currently available because of FDA requirements.

Table 8-7. Standardized patch test form

Substance* and percent concentration	Reaction				
	24 hours	48 hours	72 hours	Delayed reading	Remarks
1. Caine mix 1%					
2. Paraben mix 15%					
3. Nickel sulfate 2.5%					
4. Potassium dichromate 0.5%					
5. Ethylenediamine 1%					
6. Parachloro-m-xylenol 1%					
7. Ammoniated mercuric chloride 1%					
8. Neomycin sulfate 20%					
9. Wool wax alcohol 30%					
10. Lanolin 100%					
11. Mercapto mix 1%					
12. Mercaptobenzothiazole 1%					
13. Thiuram mix 1%					
14. Naphthyl mix 1%					
15. Paraphenylenediamine mix 1%					
16. Carba mix 3%					
17. Acrylic monomer 10%					
18. Balsam of Peru 25%					
19. Benzyl alcohol 5%					
20. Hydroxycitronellal 4%					
21. Paratertiary butyl phenol 2%					
22. Epoxy resin 1%					
23. Imidazolidinyl urea 2%					
24. Captan 1%					
25. Quaternium 2%					
26. Other					
27. Control (petrolatum)					

Key: 1+ = strong erythema and infiltration; 2+ = vesiculation; 3+ = severe reaction with blistering; IR = irritant reaction.
*Substances included on the form are those recommended by the North American Contact Dermatitis Group. Substances are in petrolatum except for quaternium and imidazolidinyl urea, which are in water.

and 3+ indicates an extremely severe blistering reaction. **Distinguish irritant responses from allergic contact dermatitis.** Primary irritant reactions are characterized by a reaction in a few minutes or within an hour. The reaction tends to fade rapidly after the patch is removed and usually stays within the perimeter of the patch (whereas an allergic reaction tends to extend beyond the perimeter of the patch).

To ensure accuracy in patch testing methods, be aware of known causes for false-positive and false-negative patch test reactions.

(1) **False-positive patch tests** can result from excessively high concentrations of test material, hyperirritable skin, bacterial infection under a patch test site, or a combination of each.

(2) **False-negative patch tests** can result from the following:
   (a) Inadequate penetration of the allergen at the test site.
   (b) Inadequate concentration of the allergen.
   (c) Failure to do delayed skin test readings 2–3 days after patch removal.
   (d) Lack of an adequately occlusive patch.
   (e) Failure to reproduce conditions such as sweating or friction.
   (f) Failure to use photopatch testing in relevant situations when photo contact materials are suspected, i.e., by material or sun exposure.
   (g) Failure to observe test sites at 30 minutes after application in cases of suspected contact urticaria.

e. **Complications of patch testing.** Although complications are relatively uncommon, the following can occur:

(1) Patch testing can produce a marked **flare** of the original contact dermatitis, often noticeable within 6 hours in highly sensitive patients. If a sufficiently severe exacerbation occurs, a 2- to 3-day course of systemic corticosteroids (e.g., prednisone) can effectively control these reactions.

(2) **Marked** localized patch test reactions occasionally occur and can be controlled with topical corticosteroids or, if severe, by administration of systemic corticosteroids for 2–3 days.

(3) Rare **systemic** reactions can occur within minutes of placing the test substance. Awareness of this reaction is mandatory to be able to treat life-threatening anaphylaxis (see Chap. 10).

(4) Patch testing can lead to sensitization of the patient to the **test materials.** When standardized concentrations of allergen are employed, this complication is infrequent. Using environmental agents whose sensitization potential or safe concentrations are undetermined is a greater hazard.

f. There are no simple rules for patch testing with uncommon materials that the patient with contact dermatitis may bring to the physician for testing. However, general guidelines include the following:

(1) Most items intended for direct, undiluted application to the skin can usually be patch tested as such, with the exception of cosmetics containing a volatile and irritating solvent (e.g., nail polish or mascara) or any aerosol preparation. Allow these materials to evaporate on the patch for 10–15 minutes before application to the skin (perfumes, however, should be tested wet and not be allowed to evaporate).

(2) **Fabrics** and **clothing** can be tested by placing the suspected material on the skin and covering with an occlusive, nonirritating tape.

(3) **Soaps** and **detergents** must be diluted to avoid irritant reactions. Because of the dilution effect, the final concentration of many sensitizers in soap (e.g., perfumes, antimicrobials, or other additives) is often below the threshold level for detection.

(4) **Solid objects** are difficult to test since they can produce friction

artifacts. Powders or scrapings of these solid materials may yield more reliable results but still can be very irritating.

D. Differential diagnosis. Allergic contact dermatitis can resemble atopic eczema, nummular eczema, psoriasis, seborrheic dermatitis, or eruptions from orally or parenterally administered medications. Allergic contact dermatitis can also be mistaken for cellulitis, herpetic infection, or fungal infection such as tinea corporis or tinea pedis. The rashes seen in lupus erythematosus, erythema multiforme, dermatomyositis, viral exanthems, or pityriasis rosea generally differ from contact dermatitis by their symmetrical and usually noneczematoid appearance. Contact dermatitis often preferentially affects select areas of the body; e.g., shoe contact dermatitis is usually seen in the dorsa of the toes and feet, with relative sparing of the interdigital webs (as seen with infection) or sparing of the plantar surface (as seen with psoriasis). Similarly, psoriasis often affects the palm and volar aspects of the arm in contradistinction to contact involvement of the dorsa of the hands.

E. Complications. In acute contact dermatitis, complications include disability and discomfort, secondary infection, and sensitization to topically applied treatments. Chronic contact dermatitis can lead to psychological complications and economic loss to the patient who is unable to work or who must change jobs.

F. Treatment

1. **Prevention.** Avoidance of the offending material is the primary treatment for contact dermatitis. This approach can be simple (e.g., avoidance of poison ivy and poison oak) or difficult (e.g., the rubber-sensitive patient with multiple chances of exposure). It is imperative to find the offender, indicate cross-sensitizing materials, and, if possible, advise substitutes for other necessary materials (e.g., use of mineral spirits instead of turpentine; plastic gloves instead of rubber gloves; acrylic resin synthetic tapes instead of tapes with rubber adhesive; and stainless steel studs or wire in place of nickel ear studs).

2. **Therapy of active dermatitis**

   a. **Compresses.** Use aluminum acetate solution or cool water as drying compresses for vesiculation and oozing (see Atopic Dermatitis, sec. **VI.B.5**). **Avoid calamine lotion** to prevent accumulation of residue on the skin. Warn the patient to avoid topical antihistamines or anesthetics because of their sensitizing potential.

   b. **Corticosteroids**

      (1) **Systemic corticosteroids** are the primary mode of therapy for the acute stage of severe contact dermatitis. They are given in a tapering regimen, usually for 7–14 days, as needed. Use short-acting preparations (prednisone) as a divided or single morning dose, following the usual precautions (see Chap. 4). The usual starting dose of prednisone is 60–100 mg/day for adults (1–2 mg/kg/day for children).

      (2) **Topical corticosteroids** (see Table 8-3) are applied in **mild** contact dermatitis or in the later resolving stages of severe dermatitis. Because of inadequate penetration in severe, acutely edematous, blistering skin, avoid topical agents until systemic corticosteroids have taken effect. Fluorinated topical corticosteroids are more potent than hydrocortisone and should not be used on the face, to avoid acneiform eruptions, or in the skin-fold areas, to avoid skin atrophy (see Atopic Dermatitis, sec. **VI.B.3**). Topical corticosteroids can be applied 3–4 times/day or more during the acute phase of a mild contact dermatitis. Occlusion with a plastic film for about 6 hours a day increases penetration of the topical corticosteroid and accelerates healing. However, limit occlusive therapy to periods of 5–7 days.

   c. Orally administered **antihistamines** are used adjunctively to corticosteroids to help relieve pruritus. Hydroxyzine, 25–100 mg 4 times/day for adults (2–5 mg/kg/day for children), is particularly helpful.

Table 8-8. Common photoallergic contact sensitizers

Substance	Occurrence
Salicylanilides	Antiseptics in soaps, detergents, cosmetics
Sulfonamides	Topical antibiotics
Paraminobenzoic acid	Sunscreening agents
Digalloyl trioleate	Sunscreening agents
Bithionol	Antiseptic soaps, cosmetics
Hexachlorophene	Antiseptic soaps, cosmetics
Dichlorophen	Antiseptic soaps, cosmetics
Phenothiazines	Medicaments, insecticides
Quinine	Hair tonics
Dyes	Lipsticks, chemicals, stains
Eosin	
Fluorescein	
Rose bengal	
Acridine	
Methylene blue	
Chlorsalicylamide	Fungicide

    d. Hyposensitization has been attempted for allergic contact dermatitis, but its efficacy is uncertain. Consequently, this form of therapy is not generally accepted or used.

  G. Prognosis. Fortunately for most patients, the prognosis is excellent if the contactant is removed and appropriate therapy is quickly instituted.

III. Phototoxic and photoallergic contact dermatitis consist of reactions similar to irritant dermatitis and allergic contact dermatitis except that they require the addition of ultraviolet light either from the sun or from an artificial source. In **phototoxic contact dermatitis,** phototoxic substances cause an irritant reaction after initial exposure if the substance is strong enough or the light exposure long enough. Phototoxic substances include such drugs as sulfonamides, griseofulvin, and chlorothiazide, and some dyes. **Photoallergic contact dermatitis** is an immunologic reaction that occurs in a small number of people who become sensitized to the combination of an allergen and ultraviolet light. Cross-reactions can occur. Common substances included in this group are salicylanilides, sulfonamides, dichlorophen, and some sunscreens (Table 8-8).

  A. The **diagnosis** of photoallergic contact dermatitis is made by photopatch testing, which requires the application of the allergen plus a suitable light source. The following are guidelines for the test.

    1. Perform the test in duplicate, placing exposed phototests on the upper outer arm and the nonexposed, control sets on the back.

    2. After 48 hours, expose the phototest on the arm to the noontime sunlight or a hot quartz lamp using ultraviolet wavelengths. The simplest method is to use ordinary daylight. Generally, 10 minutes of light exposure in the summer or 60 minutes during the winter is required in most climates, with intermediate amounts required in the spring and fall. Without sunlight, exposure of the test site for 1 hour to an overcast sky at noon for 3 successive days will often suffice.

    3. Read all tests 24 hours later, i.e., 1 day after exposure to light. Be sure to include a delayed reading 48 hours later. Interpret as for closed patch testing.

  B. The **treatment** for phototoxic and photoallergic contact dermatitis is the same as outlined for the other dermatitides. Avoidance of any sensitizing material is critical. Occasionally, a material (e.g., declomycin) can produce persistent symptoms ("persistent light reactor") despite discontinuation of the sensitizer. In such patients, the use of a cinnamate, benzophenone-type sunscreen (TiScreen or SolBar PF15) applied 2 or 3 times/day to exposed areas can help ameliorate the symptoms. The frequency of application is increased when the patient is swimming or involved in physical activity with increased perspiration.

Selected Readings

Fisher, A. *Contact Dermatitis* (3rd ed.). Philadelphia: Lea & Febiger, 1986.

Fitzpatrick, T. B., et al. *Dermatology in General Medicine.* New York: McGraw-Hill, 1979.

Hanifin, J. M. Basic and clinical aspects of atopic dermatitis. *Ann. Allergy* 52:386, 1984.

Lucky, A. W. Principles of the use of glucocorticosteroids in the growing child. *Pediatr. Dermatol.* 1:226, 1984.

Moschella, S. L., Pillsbury, D. M., and Hurley, H. J. *Dermatology* (2nd ed.). Philadelphia: Saunders, 1985.

Rasmussen, J. E. Recent developments in the management of patients with atopic dermatitis. *J. Allergy Clin. Immunol.* 74:771, 1984.

Rook, A., et al. (eds.). *Textbook of Dermatology* (4th ed.). London: Blackwell, 1986.

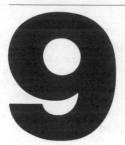

Urticaria and Angioedema

Stanley M. Fineman

Urticaria (hives) is a well-demarcated skin reaction characterized by erythematous or blanched cutaneous elevations of the upper corium of the dermis, usually associated with pruritus. **Angioedema** is a similar lesion but mainly involves the deeper subcutaneous tissues and is usually not associated with pruritus. Although angioedema commonly occurs in association with urticaria, it occurs alone in about 10% of cases.

Vascular permeability is the most important factor in the pathophysiology of urticarial lesions. Histopathologic examination of urticarial lesions reveals dilatation and engorgement of minute cutaneous blood vessels, dilated lymphatics, and a minimal perivascular infiltrate that may predominantly contain eosinophils. The "triple response" of Lewis is basic to the understanding of these findings: initial redness, due to dilatation of capillaries; secondary flare, produced by arteriolar dilatation mediated by nerve axon reflexes; and, finally, the wheal, caused by extravasation of fluid with increased vascular permeability.

Urticaria is a common problem, affecting 10–20% of the population during their life. **Acute urticaria,** defined as lasting less than 6 weeks, is more common in children and young adults. It is frequently a self-limited disorder caused by an allergic reaction or infection. **Chronic urticaria,** persisting more than 6 weeks, is more common in middle-aged women. The cause of chronic urticaria is not found in approximately 80–90% of patients.

I. **Classification and etiologic factors.** See Table 9-1.
   A. **Immunologic.** Urticaria and angioedema are considered to be of immunologic origin if specific antigens, antibodies, or sensitized cells have been identified.
      1. The **anaphylactic, or type I, hypersensitivity reaction** (see Chap. 2) is the most common immunologic mechanism producing acute urticaria. Homocytotropic antibodies, especially IgE antibodies to specific allergens, sensitize cutaneous mast cells. Subsequent challenge by the appropriate allergen produces release of chemical mediators, especially histamine, and causes the cutaneous phenomena of urticaria or angioedema or both. These cutaneous responses may occur either as a manifestation of systemic anaphylaxis or as the only symptom of immediate hypersensitivity. Homocytotropic or reaginic antibodies can be passively transferred from the serum of sensitized persons to an unafflicted recipient (Prausnitz-Küstner reaction). The most common antigens causing hives through the anaphylactic mechanism include foods, especially fish, nuts, eggs, and cow's milk; drugs, especially penicillin and sulfonamides; stinging insects; and animal dander or saliva.
      2. **Type II hypersensitivity reactions,** initiated by cytotoxic antibodies, are responsible for the urticaria that accompanies transfusion reactions. IgG and IgM antibodies react with isoantigens on donor erythrocytes, resulting in the subsequent activation of the complement cascade and production of biologically active chemical mediators, especially C3a and C5a anaphylatoxins.
      3. **Type III hypersensitivity reactions** are triggered by antigen-antibody complexes acting as toxic immune complexes that activate the complement pathway and cause mediator release. Serum sickness is a type III hypersen-

Table 9-1. Classification of urticaria

Immunologic	Pressure
Anaphylactic (type I)	Vibratory
Cytotoxic (type II)	Aquagenic
Immune complex (type III)	Miscellaneous
Anaphylactoid	Papular urticaria
Hereditary angioedema	Urticaria pigmentosa
Chemical mediator–releasing	Systemic mastocytosis
agents	Infection
Aspirin sensitivity	Cutaneous vasculitis and collagen
Physical	vascular diseases
Dermatographia	Malignancy
Cold	Endocrine
Heat	Psychogenic
Cholinergic	Amyloidosis with deafness
Solar	Idiopathic

Table 9-2. Agents commonly causing histamine release

X-ray contrast material

Opiates: codeine, morphine

Anti-infective agents: chlortetracycline, polymyxin, quinine

Muscle relaxants: curare, d-tubocurarine

Vasoactive drugs: atropine, amphetamine, hydralazine

Miscellaneous: bile salts, thiamine, dextran, deferoxamine

Foods: egg white, strawberries, citrus fruits, tomatoes, lobster

sitivity reaction induced by antigen-antibody complexes and manifested as urticaria, arthralgias, and fever. Immune complex–mediated urticaria and IgE-mediated urticaria may be simultaneously operative.

B. Anaphylactoid. The mechanisms of urticaria and angioedema in anaphylactoid reactions can involve certain immunologic or biochemical pathways but without involvement of known specific antigens or antibodies.

1. Hereditary angioedema is a clinical syndrome characterized by recurrent attacks of painful angioedema involving the skin and mucosa of the upper respiratory and gastrointestinal tracts. The lesions are not urticarial or pruritic and last for 2–4 days, affecting mainly the limbs, trunk, and neck. Death from laryngeal edema may occur in as many as 26% of affected persons. Many factors can initiate an attack, including minor trauma, emotional upset, infections, and exposure to sudden temperature changes.

Hereditary angioedema is an autosomal-dominant, genetically determined deficiency or malfunction of the C1-esterase inhibitor, the inhibitor of the first component of the complement system. Without this inhibitor the complement cascade is activated, with the generation of a kininlike fragment (C kinin) and the release of other pharmacologically active chemical mediators that produce angioedema.

2. Histamine liberators. Certain drugs, foods, and chemicals have been shown to cause urticaria by direct degranulation of mast cells, with subsequent histamine release (Table 9-2). These substances produce local wheal and flare reactions when injected intradermally and produce local or generalized histamine release in some patients following systemic administration. The mechanisms responsible involve other immunologic pathways, including hapten or complement-dependent reactions.

3. **Aspirin** acts not only as a primary cause of urticaria, but it also frequently exacerbates hives secondary to other causes. Persons with aspirin hypersensitivity may have urticaria or angioedema following the ingestion of tartrazine, other azo dyes, benzoic acid derivatives, or other nonsteroidal antiinflammatory drugs. The urticarial response by these agents may relate to their effect on arachidonic acid metabolism and the subsequent release of various chemical mediators.

C. **Physical.** Urticaria and angioedema of the physical category can be elicited by various physical or environmental factors.

1. **Dermatographia** ("writing on the skin"), the most common type of physical urticaria, has been reported in 5–20% of the general population, but may occur with greater frequency in association with chronic urticaria. Minor trauma, especially firm stroking of the skin, will initiate the local hives (peaking in about 10 minutes and clearing rapidly) in this condition. Although the exact mechanism of dermatographia is not understood, IgE may mediate this reaction in certain patients.

2. **Cold urticaria** can occur in either familial or acquired forms.
   a. The **familial** cold urticaria is a rare autosomal-dominant condition, usually manifested by nonpruritic, burning, erythematous papules that may have a delayed presentation—30 minutes to 4 hours—after cold exposure. Fever, arthralgias, chills, headaches, myalgias, and leukocytosis are present.
   b. The more common acquired, **idiopathic** cold urticaria occurs more often in adults, although any age group or sex can be affected. Cold exposure results in localized or generalized urticaria or angioedema within a few minutes, especially in the body area exposed to the cold. The lesions are often maximal after rewarming. There is evidence of associated mast cell degranulation and increases in plasma histamine levels. In certain patients this urticarial response can be passively transferred with serum.
   c. Cold urticaria also presents as a symptom associated with other underlying diseases characterized by the presence of abnormal proteins that have cold-dependent properties. These diseases include syphilitic paroxysmal cold hemoglobinuria, cryofibrinogenemia and cryoglobulinemia, and cold-agglutinin disease.

3. **Cholinergic urticaria** (generalized heat urticaria) is characterized by a generalized pruritic eruption with multiple wheals 1–3 mm in diameter with surrounding erythematous flares. It occurs immediately or within minutes following heat exposure, emotional stress, or vigorous exercise. The mechanism of cholinergic urticaria probably involves the release of histamine mediated by acetycholine from cholinergic sympathetic nerve fibers. The cholinergic urticarial response has been passively transferred with serum. In certain patients, systemic cold challenge produces a response clinically identical to cholinergic urticaria. This condition is termed **cold-induced cholinergic urticaria.**

4. **Direct contact with heat** (localized heat urticaria) also causes immediate or delayed urticarial reactions. The pathophysiologic mechanism of this rare form of heat urticaria, separate and distinct from cholinergic urticaria, is unknown and not subject to passive transfer.

5. **Solar urticaria** is an uncommon disorder in which exposure to light causes pruritic, erythematous wheals within minutes after exposure. The lesions are confined to exposed skin areas and usually subside within 2 hours. Although it is more common in adults, it can occur at any age. Solar urticaria is classified into six types, depending on the wavelength of light that elicits the reaction and the ability to transfer the phenomenon passively with serum.
   a. Types I and IV are associated with wavelengths of 2800–3200 Å and 4000–5000 Å respectively. Both types have been passively transferred with serum.

    b. Types II, III, and V are induced by wavelengths of 3200–4000 Å, 4000–5000 Å, and 2800–5000 Å respectively, and cannot be passively transferred with serum.

    c. Type VI is a metabolic disorder (erythropoietic protoporphyria) in which protoporphyrin IX is a photosensitizer at a wavelength of 4000 Å.

  6. Pressure urticaria and angioedema can be differentiated into immediate and delayed types. Immediate pressure urticaria is rare and has been seen in patients with hypereosinophilic syndrome. Pressure or rubbing of the skin may elicit the urticarial response within a few minutes. Delayed pressure urticaria is more common and is characterized by deep, painful edematous wheals that usually occur 4–6 hours (although they can occur within minutes) after the application of pressure to the skin. The lesions may persist for 2–24 hours and may or may not be pruritic. Constitutional symptoms such as malaise, fever, chills, and headache can occur during attacks.

  7. Vibratory angioedema is a rare autosomal-dominant, genetically transmitted disorder characterized by erythema and edema following the application of vibratory stimuli to the skin. The manifestations usually appear in infancy and persist through adulthood, although the severity decreases with age. The pathophysiologic mechanism is unknown, and passive transfer with serum has not been successful.

  8. Aquagenic urticaria has been described in a few patients following contact with water, regardless of its temperature. The lesions occur shortly after contact and consist of small, pruritic papules that resemble cholinergic urticaria.

D. Miscellaneous. In some clinical situations, urticaria and angioedema are not readily classified in any of the previous categories.

  1. Papular urticaria presents as crops of small, pruritic papules and wheals on exposed areas of the body (especially on the lower extremities in children). It is usually caused by bites of insects such as mosquitoes, bedbugs, or fleas. The lesions result from a biphasic reaction to either saliva or mouth parts left in the skin following the insect bite. The immediate wheal may be due to type I hypersensitivity; the delayed component may be a type IV reaction.

  2. Urticaria pigmentosa is an uncommon, usually localized disorder characterized by dermal infiltrations of mast cells. The skin lesions appear as areas of increased pigmentation that become urticated following mild stroking (Darier's sign). Urticaria pigmentosa is usually a mild, localized disorder in children and frequently disappears at puberty.

  3. Systemic mastocytosis is similar to urticaria pigmentosa. It is a more serious and rare disorder, characterized by accumulations of mast cells in the dermis, bone marrow, and gastrointestinal tract. Symptoms consist of flushing, headaches, and hypotension secondary to histamine release.

  4. Infections are frequently associated with urticaria. Although certain parasitic infestations are commonly accompanied by hives, urticaria also occurs with viral infections such as upper respiratory infections (especially in children), infectious mononucleosis, and hepatitis (usually in the preicteric stage). Bacterial infections are rarely associated with urticaria.

  5. Urticaria with underlying systemic diseases may occur.

    a. Collagen vascular diseases. Urticaria occurs in 10% of patients with systemic lupus erythematosus with or without cryoglobulinemia and is also seen in rheumatoid arthritis and Sjögren's syndrome.

    b. Malignancies, particularly carcinoma of the colon, rectum, or lung and lymphoma, can present with urticarial lesions. Patients with malignancy and associated angioedema have been reported with acquired C1-esterase inhibitor deficiency. In this condition, C1 depletion is more pronounced than C4, C2, or C3 depletion, which distinguishes it from the hereditary disorder.

    c. Endocrine hormone imbalance, such as in hyperthyroidism, pregnancy, and menopause, can present with urticaria.

    d. Urticaria is associated with the symptom complex consisting of **amyloidosis, nerve deafness, and limb pain** (Muckle-Wells syndrome).

    e. Rare patients have been reported to be deficient in the C3b inactivator and present with urticaria.

    f. Rare patients present with hypereosinophilia and recurrent attacks of massive angioedema, urticaria, fever, and marked, acute weight gain. Prednisone produces prompt and dramatic improvement.

6. Exercise can induce urticaria and angioedema, often associated with bronchospasm. Hypotension and syncope can occur in some patients (exercise-induced anaphylaxis), commonly associated when exercise is preceded by ingestion of specific foods.

7. Psychogenic factors can exacerbate existing urticaria due to other causes. Whether or not psychological influences alone can be the primary cause is unknown.

8. Idiopathic urticaria and angioedema occur in clinical conditions in which no cause can be determined. Although chronic urticaria and angioedema are common problems, their cause remains unknown in about 80–90% of cases. Generally these patients are not atopic and have normal IgE levels, erythrocyte sedimentation rates, and white blood cell counts. No systemic disease is evident. Skin biopsy reveals perivascular cuffing consisting predominantly of lymphocytes with some monocytes, mast cells, and, occasionally, eosinophils. Immunofluorescence studies of immunoglobulin and complement deposition are negative.

II. Diagnostic approach

A. General approach. A systemic approach to the evaluation of the patient with urticaria or angioedema begins with a thorough history and careful physical examination. If the cause is not readily elicited from the history and physical examination, specific etiologic factors are usually not detected. Occasionally, the question "What do you think is causing your hives?" yields the answer.

    1. Specific inquiry is directed to the following:

        a. Foods or inhaled aromas.

        b. Drugs, especially antibiotics, aspirin, vitamins, medications containing tartrazine, birth control pills, cold tablets, and topical preparations.

        c. Food additives, e.g., benzoic acid derivatives and azo dyes.

        d. Inhalants or contactants, e.g., animal dander or saliva, pollens.

        e. Occupation or hobbies.

        f. Recent infection.

        g. Stress and anxiety.

    2. Laboratory procedures usually can be limited to general screening tests (Table 9-3). Further studies are rarely revealing unless the cause is suspected.

B. Specific etiologic approach. When the history or physical examination suggests a specific cause, specific diagnostic tests are useful (Table 9-3). In most cases of acute urticaria, an abbreviated evaluation directed toward the suggested origin is adequate. Patients with chronic urticaria or atypical manifestations may need a more extensive evaluation, depending on the nature and severity of the problem.

    1. Atopic sensitivity

        a. On the basis of the history, avoidance of the suspected inhalant or drug or a strict elimination diet (including avoidance of food additives) should be initiated. The patient should keep a daily symptom diary.

        b. To confirm a causal relationship to a certain food, a controlled, double-blind **challenge** should be performed. This challenge should not be done if anaphylaxis was produced in the past by the suspected food.

        c. Prick or scratch tests to foods or prick, scratch, and intradermal skin tests to selected inhalant or drug allergens may help to confirm allergic sensitivity. A control test must be done to assess the presence of dermatographia. (RAST tests can also be used, especially when dermatographia occurs.)

Table 9-3. Diagnostic tests for urticaria and angioedema

Condition suspected	Test*
Atopic: food or drug (inhalant or contactant) sensitivity	Elimination of offending agent Daily symptom diary Skin tests or radioallergosorbent tests of suspected antigens Challenge with suspected foods Total serum IgE determination Eosinophil count
Cutaneous vasculitis or systemic collagen vascular disease	Immunoglobulin analysis Antinuclear antibody Rheumatoid factor Cryoglobulins, cryofibrinogens Complete complement profile C1q binding assay Skin biopsy with immunofluorescence
Hereditary angioedema	C4, C2 Total hemolytic complement (CH_{50}) C1-esterase inhibitor (immunochemical and functional assays)

Physical urticaria
  Dermatographia
  Cold
	
	Firm stroke on skin with tongue blade
	Ice cube test
	Cryoglobulins, cryofibrinogens
	VDRL test

Cholinergic urticaria	Exercise challenge Methacholine skin test
Solar urticaria	Exposure to various wavelengths of light Protoporphyrin and coproporphyrin determinations
Pressure urticaria and angioedema	Application of pressure with weights for 10 minutes
Vibratory angioedema	Vibratory stimulation of skin for 4 minutes
Aquagenic urticaria	Tap-water challenge at various temperatures
Infections	Appropriate cultures and x-rays Stool for ova and parasites Hepatitis B antigen and antibody
Urticaria pigmentosa	Test for dermatographia Skin biopsy
Malignancy with angioedema	Total hemolytic complement (CH_{50}) C$\bar{1}$ C$\bar{1}$-esterase inhibitor
C3b inactivator deficiency	C3, factor B, C3b inactivator determinations
Idiopathic urticaria	Skin biopsy with immunofluorescence (for exclusion of vasculitis)

*The general screening consists of a complete blood count, urinalysis, and erythrocyte sedimentation rate determination.

    d. Serum IgE and **blood eosinophil counts** may be elevated in patients with inhalant or contact urticaria, particularly involving pollen or animal dander sensitivity.

2. Cutaneous vasculitis and collagen vascular disease. When a collagen vascular disease or vasculitis is suspected clinically, the following determinations are indicated:

    a. Quantitative **immunoglobulin** analysis (IgG, IgA, IgM, IgE).

    b. Quantitative **complement** assays

        (1) C3, C4 (initial test).

        (2) Complete complement profile, including classic and alternative pathway analysis (immunochemical and functional assays).

    c. Antinuclear antibody, rheumatoid factor.

    d. Skin biopsy with immunofluorescence studies.

    e. Cryoglobulins, cryofibrinogens.

3. Hereditary angioedema

    a. A history of recurrent attacks of swelling, often following trauma, starting in childhood, and a positive family history (negative in up to 20% of patients) suggests hereditary angioedema.

    b. The level of C4 is diminished during asymptomatic periods and is usually undetectable during an attack. This determination is a readily available screen for hereditary angioedema.

    c. The level of C2 is usually normal during asymptomatic periods, but diminished during attacks. It serves to confirm the C4 decrease.

    d. Total hemolytic complement (CH_{50}) may be reduced.

    e. C1-esterase inhibitor assay is the most specific laboratory confirmation for hereditary angioedema. Most patients demonstrate a significant reduction in the serum concentration of this protein, although in approximately 15% of patients, a normal or elevated C1-esterase inhibitor level is detected using immunochemical techniques. In such patients, a **functional assay** is required to demonstrate the abnormal activity.

4. Physical urticaria

    a. In dermatographia, a firm stroke of the skin with a fingernail or wooden stick elicits a linear wheal that reaches peak intensity in about 10 minutes and spontaneously subsides within 20 minutes. A delayed variant occurs in which the initial wheal subsides within 20–30 minutes, recurs 3–8 hours later at the same site, and persists for 24–48 hours.

    b. The **ice cube test** confirms the diagnosis of **cold urticaria.** An ice cube is applied to the volar surface of the forearm for 5–10 minutes. The area is rewarmed, and characteristic wheals appear within 5–20 minutes. Occasionally, application of ice does not reproduce the lesions, but exposure to a cold environment (e.g., 4°C room) will.

    c. Exercising the patient to provoke perspiration (e.g., chair stepping, treadmill, or riding a stationary bicycle) is a readily available method of producing cholinergic urticaria under the usual clinical conditions. A **methacholine chloride (Mecholyl) skin test** will also produce the lesions of cholinergic urticaria. The intradermal injection of 0.05 ml of 0.02% methacholine chloride or of 0.002% carbamylcholine chloride (carbachol) produces a localized wheal with surrounding erythema and many small satellite wheals within 20 minutes. A skin test may not be positive during the refractory period immediately following an attack of cholinergic urticaria.

    d. A monochromatic light source using varying wavelengths accurately tests for **solar urticaria.** The skin should initially be exposed for 1–2 minutes. If the results are negative, a longer exposure may be needed. A fluorescent light emits a broad spectrum of wavelengths and can be used as a simple screening test. Filters should be employed to define the light spectrum that elicits the urticaria.

    e. Pressure urticaria usually occurs in areas where tight clothes, elastic bands, or straps are worn. A 7- to 14-kg weight (suspended by stockinette) hung around the arms or shoulders for 10 minutes may elicit this urticarial phenomenon.

  f. **Vibratory angloedema** may be elicited by applying an electric mixer, vibrator, or laboratory vortex to the skin for 4 minutes.

  g. **Aquagenic urticaria** is elicited in patients in whom wheals develop after contact with water and in whom tests for the other forms of physical urticaria are negative.

5. **Urticaria pigmentosa** is diagnosed by a positive test for dermatographia (Darier's sign), with confirmation by skin biopsy.

6. The diagnosis of **chronic idiopathic urticaria** is usually one of exclusion after the preceding evaluation is negative. Although frequently unnecessary, a skin biopsy with negative immunofluorescence supports the diagnosis.

III. **Treatment**
  A. **General treatment measures**
    1. **Elimination procedures.** The optimal treatment for urticaria and angioedema is identification and removal of the cause. This is especially true for urticaria secondary to certain drugs, foods, or animals. Avoidance of aspirin, benzoates, tartrazine, and other azo dyes by all patients with urticaria, regardless of its cause, may be beneficial. Avoidance of agents enhancing histamine release, especially foods, and caution regarding physical and emotional factors (e.g., temperature changes, pressure, exercise, topical irritants, anxiety, and tension) that increase peripheral circulation or enhance pruritus are also helpful.

    2. **Antihistamines** are usually effective in the control of urticaria and can be of benefit in angioedema, particularly if administered soon after the onset of symptoms. Because of individual variations in response to different antihistamines, therapeutic trials of drugs from several classes (see Table 4-5), with gradual increases in dosage in excess of the usual dose, may be necessary to control symptoms. In general, if one antihistamine fails to improve the urticaria or produces uncomfortable side effects, a drug from a different pharmacologic class should be used.

      a. **Hydroxyzine** is the drug of choice for the treatment of urticaria because of its prolonged effect in inhibiting wheal-and-flare skin reactions and more effective suppression of histamine-induced pruritus in comparison with the effect of antihistamines of other classes. The usual starting dose is 25 mg 4 times/day, increasing by 25-mg increments/dose as needed. The limiting side effect is drowsiness, which is frequently overcome with a few days of therapy. Total daily doses of 400 mg or more may be required for control of symptoms. The usual starting dose for children is 2 mg/kg/24 hours in 4 divided doses.

      b. **Cyproheptadine,** 4–8 mg (2–4 mg in children) 4 times/day, and **diphenhydramine,** 25–100 mg 4 times/day (5 mg/kg/day in children), are common substitutes for hydroxyzine.

      c. **Cimetidine,** an H_2 histamine receptor inhibitor, may be helpful, particularly when used in combination with an H_1 antihistamine such as hydroxyzine. The usual starting adult dose of cimetidine is 300 mg 4 times/day.

      d. **Terfenadine,** a nonsedating H_1 antihistamine, can be helpful especially in patients made drowsy by other H_1 antihistamines. The usual dose is 60 mg every 12 hours, but higher doses may be required. Astemizole (not currently FDA-approved) is a long-acting H_1 antagonist with few sedative side effects. It has been shown to be helpful in the treatment of chronic urticaria (10 mg 1–2 times/day).

      e. **Doxepin,** a tricyclic antidepressant with H_1 and H_2 antihistamine properties, can be effective in selected patients with chronic urticaria in an adult dose of 10–50 mg 3 times/day or as a single bedtime dose starting with the lower dose and gradually raising every few days as needed and tolerated.

3. Adrenergic drugs

a. In patients with severe, acute urticaria, especially with associated angioedema, give **subcutaneous epinephrine** (in children, 0.01 ml/kg of 1:1000 aqueous epinephrine; in adults, 0.2–0.3 ml). This can be repeated in 20–30 minutes or every 2–3 hours over short periods (24–36 hours) for recurrent symptoms (use cautiously in patients with cardiovascular disease).

b. **Sus-Phrine,** a longer-acting aqueous suspension of epinephrine, is useful for symptoms that recur rapidly. In adults, 0.1–0.3 ml subcutaneously, or for children, 0.005 ml/kg (maximal dose is 0.15 ml), can be used every 4–6 hours.

c. **Ephedrine sulfate,** widely used prior to the discovery of antihistamines, can be tried in conjunction with an antihistamine in either severe acute or chronic refractory urticaria. The usual dose for adults is 25–50 mg every 4 hours; for children, 3 mg/kg/24 hours divided into 4 doses.

d. Newer adrenergic agents (e.g., terbutaline, 2.5–5.0 mg 3 times/day, or albuterol, 2–4 mg 3–4 times/day) may be helpful in combination with an H_1 antihistamine, particularly in exercise-induced urticaria or angioedema or when drowsiness limits the use of antihistamines (see Table 4-7).

4. Corticosteroids effectively control urticaria and angioedema when given in pharmacologic dosages. In acute or chronic urticaria unresponsive to other treatment, a course of prednisone usually controls symptoms. A starting dose of 2 mg/kg/day is usually adequate, tapering as tolerated. The use of long-term corticosteroid therapy should be limited to patients whose symptoms are uncontrolled by other modalities and to the lowest daily or alternate-day dose possible, with the usual consideration of side effects (see Chap. 4).

B. Treatment regimen for specific disorders

1. Hereditary angioedema

a. Various regimens for long-term and short-term prophylaxis and for acute attacks have been used, including subcutaneous epinephrine, fresh-frozen plasma, androgens, antifibrinolytic agents (epsilon-aminocaproic acid and tranexamic acid), and corticosteroids. More recently, infusions of partially purified C1-esterase inhibitor, the functional deficient protein in these patients, has reproducibly terminated attacks within minutes to hours. However, this material is still investigational and not available for distribution.

b. During the **acute attack** (especially if mild), supportive treatment with mild analgesics and intravenous fluids may suffice. Although epinephrine, antihistamines, and corticosteroids have been used, only epinephrine appears to offer a modest degree of improvement. If pain is severe, limited early use of narcotics is indicated, although the distinct possibility of narcotic addiction must be constantly kept in mind. If laryngeal edema compromises respiratory function, endotracheal intubation by skilled operators should be performed. Tracheostomy should be performed if endotracheal intubation fails. Although fresh-frozen plasma has been used, some patients appear to worsen after the infusion. Infusion of partially purified C1-esterase inhibitor, an investigational agent, will also terminate these attacks.

c. For short-term preventive treatment when an attack is anticipated (e.g., dental surgery), fresh-frozen plasma (2 units, adult dose) given 1 day prior to the procedure may be beneficial.

d. For long-term prevention and treatment, androgen and androgen derivatives are superior to the antifibrinolytic agents such as epsilon aminocaproic acid (Amicar) and tranexamic acid (tranexamic acid has been removed from distribution because of animal toxicity studies). Danazol (200 mg 3 times/day), an attenuated androgen, appears to act by correcting the underlying biochemical abnormality, i.e., increasing the concentration of C1-esterase inhibitor and C4. In some patients, the initial dosage of Danazol can be reduced to as little as 15 mg every other day. Stanazolol, a newer anabolic steroid, is also effective in reducing symptomatology at low doses (2–4 mg/day). The dose is gradually reduced, and many patients can be maintained on 1–2 mg daily or every other day. All the androgens can produce similar side effects, which should be monitored. Their use in children and adolescents (who have not attained full growth stature) and during pregnancy is contraindicated.

2. Solar urticaria

   a. Sunlight should be avoided, especially around sand or snow. Patients should remain indoors between 10 A.M. and 4 P.M., particularly during the summer months. Opaque clothing should be worn, and topical sunscreens should be applied to the remaining exposed areas. Ultraviolet light of shorter wavelengths is effectively blocked by *p*-aminobenzoic acid–(PABA) based sunscreens; (PABA-free sunscreens [e.g., TiScreen, SolBar PF 15] can be used in patients sensitive to this substance). Sunscreening agents with a protective factor of 15 or greater should be used. Zinc oxide and titanium dioxide block all wavelengths, but unfortunately are less cosmetically appealing.

   b. Antihistamines such as hydroxyzine or diphenhydramine, with or without cyproheptadine, can be useful in solar urticaria, especially IgE-mediated types I and IV.

   c. Type VI solar urticaria, a metabolic disorder due to protoporphyrin IX, has been treated with oral beta carotene.

3. Cold urticaria

   a. A partial refractory state develops after cold exposure. In some patients, **desensitization** by gradually increasing exposure to cold water will reduce cold sensitivity. However, management of all forms of cold urticaria includes precautions to avoid cold exposure, especially when swimming or boating in cold water. Systemic exposure in these situations can produce severe hypotension and the risk of drowning.

   b. The antihistamine **cyproheptadine** will provide relief at a dose of 4–8 mg 3–4 times daily in adults. After administration, the ice cube test may become negative.

   c. **Epinephrine** is indicated for severe symptoms following generalized exposure (e.g., swimming), including instruction in self-administration.

4. Cholinergic urticaria

   a. **Limitation of exposure** to precipitating factors (e.g., overheating or pressure on the skin) is helpful in reducing the frequency of attacks.

   b. Rapid **cooling** once an attack is threatened may prevent a major attack.

   c. **Antihistamines** will reduce the tendency to urtication. **Hydroxyzine** is the current antihistamine of choice for cholinergic urticaria. For cold-induced cholinergic urticaria, cyproheptadine should be added to hydroxyzine for optimal control.

   d. A **refractory period** exists for a few hours to 24 hours after an attack. The use of an antihistamine may be combined with an attempt to induce an attack artificially (e.g., with a hot bath), producing a refractory period for a special event (e.g., a social engagement).

5. Pressure urticaria

   a. **Immediate pressure urticaria** is treated with antihistamines and control of any underlying disorder.

   b. **Delayed pressure-induced urticaria** or **angioedema** may at times respond to antihistamines, although symptom control often requires corticosteroids. The decision to use corticosteroids must be based on the severity of the disease, the amount of disability it produces, and the dose of corticosteroid required. Some patients have had improvement following use of nonsteroidal anti-inflammatory drugs.

6. Urticaria pigmentosa
   a. Antihistamines help to reduce the intense pruritus.
   b. Inadvertent trauma (e.g., tight-fitting clothes) to the lesions should be carefully avoided.
7. Chronic idiopathic urticaria often becomes a difficult treatment problem because of its chronicity and the lack of an identifiable cause. Treatment involves the general measures previously outlined.

IV. The **prognosis** depends on the underlying cause. Acute urticaria is self-limiting. Allergic or physical urticaria is limited by avoidance of the offending agent. In many cases the condition is transient, and future exposure is uneventful. In urticaria associated with systemic disease, the prognosis depends on control of the underlying condition.

Chronic urticaria is commonly a benign disorder, but the prognosis is variable. Most cases are idiopathic, and over half of these persist for periods longer than 6 months, often for years. Recurrences are common at variable periods of time up to 10 years or more.

Except for hereditary angioedema and cold urticaria with generalized exposure, urticaria is rarely associated with significant morbidity or mortality.

Selected Readings

Champion, R. H., et al. Urticaria and angioedema: A review of 554 patients. *Br. J. Dermatol.* 81:588, 1969.

Frank, M. M. Hereditary Angioedema. In L. M. Lichtenstein and A. S. Fauci (eds.), *Current Therapy in Allergy, Immunology, and Rheumatology (1985–1986)*. Philadelphia: Decker, 1985.

Gleich, G. J., et al. Episodic angioedema associated with eosinophilia. *N. Engl. J. Med.* 10:1621, 1984.

Harvey, R. P., Wees, H., and Shoket, A. L. A controlled trial in therapy of chronic urticaria. *J. Allergy Clin. Immunol.* 68:262, 1981.

Kaplan, A. P. Urticaria and Angioedema. In E. Middleton, C. E. Reed, E. F. Ellis (eds.), *Allergy—Principles and Practice* (2nd ed.). St. Louis: Mosby, 1983.

Matthews, K. P. Management of urticaria and angioedema. *J. Allergy Clin. Immunol.* 72:1, 1983.

10

Anaphylaxis

Glenn J. Lawlor, Jr., and
Howard M. Rosenblatt

Anaphylaxis is the clinical response to an immediate (type I) immunologic reaction between a specific antigen and a tissue-fixing (homocytotropic) antibody. The reaction is usually mediated by IgE antibody and occurs in three steps: (1) Antigen attaches to the IgE antibody fixed to the surface membrane of mast cells and basophils, causing cross-linking of these surface (sensitizing) antibodies, thus activating these target cells. (2) Activated mast cells and basophils release various mediators. (3) The effects of mediator release cause vascular changes, activation of platelets, eosinophils, and neutrophils, and activation of the coagulation cascade (see Chap. 2).

Anaphylactoid (anaphylaxis-like) **reactions** are clinically similar to anaphylaxis. They are not, however, mediated by antigen-antibody interaction, but result from substances that act directly either on the mast cells, causing the release of mediators, or on the tissues (e.g., anaphylotoxins of the complement cascade—C3a, C5a, etc.). Table 10-1 presents a classification of anaphylaxis and anaphylactoid reactions.

I. The **pathophysiology** of anaphylaxis is best defined by the physiologic effects of the primary and secondary mediators on the target organs (cardiovascular system, respiratory tract, gastrointestinal tract, and skin).

   A. **Histamine** promotes increased vascular permeability and vascular smooth-muscle relaxation, which lead to the following:
      1. Constriction of bronchial smooth muscle.
      2. Edema of the airways and larynx.
      3. Stimulation of smooth muscle in the gastrointestinal tract, causing tenesmus, vomiting, and diarrhea.
      4. Breakdown of cutaneous vascular integrity, resulting in flushing, urticaria, and angioedema.
      5. Vasodilation with reduction of circulating blood volume and progressive fall in blood pressure leading to shock.

   B. **Leukotrienes** act by altering bronchial smooth-muscle tone and enhancing the effects of histamine on its target organs.

   C. Basophil **kallikrein** generates **kinins,** which alter vascular permeability and blood pressure.

   D. **Platelet-activating factor** (PAF) enhances the release of **histamine** and **serotonin** from platelets. These substances affect smooth-muscle tone and vascular permeability.

   E. **Eosinophil chemotactic factors of anaphylaxis** (ECF-A) recruit eosinophils to areas of activity, and these cells release secondary mediators that may limit the effects of the primary mediators.

   F. **Prostaglandins** released from the metabolism of arachidonic acid from cell membrane phospholipids can affect smooth-muscle tone and vascular permeability.

II. **Etiology.** Several groups of agents cause anaphylactic reactions. The frequency of anaphylactic reactions to some agents is higher in persons with atopic disease (e.g., specific protein allergens). In some individuals, antigen exposure must be followed up to 3 hours by exercise to induce anaphylaxis. The two most common agents leading to serious anaphylactic reactions are drugs and insect stings. The frequency

Table 10-1. Classification of anaphylactic and anaphylactoid reactions

Anaphylactic reactions (type I immunologic reactions)
    IgE
    IgG homocytotropic antibody
    IgE associated with exercise
Anaphylactoid reactions
    Direct mediator release
        Drugs
        Foods
        Physical (e.g., exercise, cold)
        Mastocytosis
    Immune complex aggregation
        Reactions to gamma globulin
        IgG anti-IgA reactions
    Cytotoxic antibody transfusion reactions
        Red blood cells
        White blood cells
    Possibly prostaglandin-induced (aspirin and other drugs)
    Idiopathic

Source: Adapted from and reproduced with permission from *Current Views in Allergy and Immunology:* Lieberman, Phil: "Anaphylaxis and Anaphylactoid Reactions," Vol. IV, Program 1, January 1980, slides #6, #13, and #16, Copyrighted by Current Views in Allergy and Immunology, Inc., Atlanta, GA.

of reaction to these agents is not generally increased in atopic persons, and the family history is usually unrelated. A list of the more common etiologic agents is presented in Table 10-2.

III. Clinical findings
A. Types of reactions
1. **Local reactions** consist of urticaria and angioedema at the site of antigen exposure, or angioedema of the bowel after ingestion of certain foods. These local reactions can be severe but are rarely fatal.
2. **Systemic reactions** occur in the following target organs: respiratory tract, cardiovascular system, gastrointestinal tract, and skin. They usually occur within 30 minutes of exposure to the offending agent.
B. The **major signs and symptoms** of anaphylactic reactions, along with the proposed chemical mediators, are presented in Table 10-3.
1. **Mild systemic reactions.** The first symptoms of mild systemic reactions are a peripheral tingling and warm sensation, frequently accompanied by a fullness in the mouth and throat. Nasal congestion and periorbital swelling can accompany these initial symptoms. Itching of the skin and mucous membranes, tearing of the eyes, and sneezing can also occur. The onset is variable but usually occurs within the first 2 hours of exposure. The duration depends on treatment, but symptoms often last for 1 or 2 days and may be prolonged in chronic cases.
2. **Moderate systemic reactions** include any of the signs and symptoms of mild reactions plus bronchospasm and/or edema of the airways or larynx, with dyspnea, cough, and wheezing. Angioedema, generalized urticaria, nausea, and vomiting can occur. Flushing is a common symptom, and patients frequently complain of generalized pruritus, warmth, and anxiety. The onset and duration are like those in mild reactions.
3. The onset of **severe systemic reactions** is usually abrupt, with the signs and symptoms described in **1** and **2,** and progresses rapidly within minutes (and sometimes without preliminary symptoms) to intense bronchospasm and laryngeal edema, with hoarseness, stridor, severe dyspnea, cyanosis, and, rarely, respiratory arrest. Gastrointestinal edema and hypermotility cause dysphagia, intense abdominal cramping, diarrhea, and vomiting. Uri-

Table 10-2. Common causative agents of anaphylaxis and anaphylactoid reactions

Antibiotics
  Penicillin*
  Ampicillin
  Cephalosporins
  Bacitracin
  Neomycin
  Polymixin B
  Dimethylchlortetracy-
    cline
  Tetracycline
  Chloramphenicol
  Kanamycin
  Streptomycin
  Vancomycin
  Amphotericin B
  Sulfonamides
Arachidonic acid mod-
    ulators
  Acetylsalicylic acid*
  Other nonsteroidal anti-
    inflammatory drugs
  Tartrazine (possibly)
  Benzoates (presumed)
Allergen extracts*
  Ragweed
  Grass
  Molds
  Epidermals
Horse serum
  Tetanus antitoxin
  Diphtheria antitoxin
  Antilymphocyte globulin
  Rabies antitoxin
  Venom antitoxin

Hormones
  Insulin
  Pituitary extract
  ACTH
  Synthetic ACTH
  Vasopressin (Pitressin)
  Parathyroid extract
  Estradiol
Diagnostic agents
  Radiopaque dyes*
  Sulfobromophthalein
    (Bromsulphthalein)
  Benzylpenicilloyl-polyly-
    sine (Pre-Pen)
Polysaccharides
  Dextran
  Acacia
Venoms and saliva
  Hymenoptera*
  Deerfly
  Snake venom
  Fire ant
  Triatoma
Enzymes
  Trypsin
  Chymotrypsin
  Penicillinase
  Asparaginase
  Chymopapain
Blood products*
  Whole blood
  Gamma globulin
  Cryoprecipitate
Local anesthetics
  Tetracaine
  Hexylcaine
  Lidocaine
  Procaine

Foods
  Egg white
  Milk
  Shellfish*
  Sesame seed
  Soy bean
  Garbanzo bean
  Walnut
  Brazil nut
  Cashew
  Potato
  Buckwheat
  Cottonseed
  Halibut
  Salmon
  Cod
  Mango
  Beet
  Chocolate
  Chamomile tea
  Orange
  Tangerine
  Mustard
  Peanut*
Miscellaneous drugs
  Thiopental (Pentothal)
  Arginine
  Opiates
  d-Tubocurarine
  Mechlorethamine
  Vitamins
  Heparin

*Most frequent causative agents.
Source: Reproduced with minor changes from G. J. Donsky and R. P. Orange. Anaphylaxis. In E. Middleton, Jr., C. E. Reed, and E. F. Ellis (eds.), *Allergy: Principles and Practice,* 1978, St. Louis, The C.V. Mosby Co. With permission.

nary urgency, uterine cramping, and generalized seizures, either from central nervous system stimulation or hypoxia, can occur. Cardiovascular collapse leads to hypotension, cardiac arrhythmias, shock, and coma.

The sequence of events leading to **respiratory failure** and **cardiovascular collapse** is often very rapid and can be the first objective signs of anaphylaxis. The severity of the reaction relates directly to the rapidity of onset. Most fatal reactions occur in persons over 20 years of age. The most common cause of death in children is laryngeal edema; death in adults more commonly occurs from a combination of hypoxia, laryngeal edema, and cardiac arrhythmias.

Recurrence of acute symptoms can occur from 2–24 hours after the initial onset despite stabilization.

C. **Laboratory findings.** The diagnosis of anaphylaxis is clinical, but the following

Table 10-3. Clinical aspects of anaphylaxis by target organ and mediator

System	Symptoms and signs	Mediator
General (prodromal)	Malaise, weakness, sense of illness	
Dermal	Hives, erythema	Histamine
Mucosal	Periorbital edema, nasal congestion and pruritus, angioedema or flushing, and/or pallor, cyanosis	Histamine
Respiratory	Sneezing, rhinorrhea, dyspnea	Histamine
Upper airway	Laryngeal edema, hoarseness, tongue and pharyngeal edema, stridor	Histamine
Lower airway	Dyspnea, acute emphysema, air trapping (asthma, bronchospasm, bronchorrhea)	Histamine, leukotrienes, platelet-activating factor
Gastrointestinal	Increased peristalsis, vomiting, dysphagia, nausea, abdominal cramps, diarrhea (occasionally with blood)	Unknown
Cardiovascular	Tachycardia, palpitations, hypotension (cardiac arrest), coronary insufficiency with ST-T wave changes on ECG	Unknown
Central nervous system	Anxiety, seizures	Unknown

Source: Adapted from L. Goldfrank and A. Mayer. Anaphylaxis: The IVP emergency. *Hosp. Physician* 14:31, 1978. With permission.

laboratory findings help in unusual cases or in ongoing management:

1. A **complete blood count** may show an elevated hematocrit secondary to hemoconcentration, but usually there is no acute abnormality.
2. **Blood chemistries.** If myocardial damage has occurred, elevations of serum aspartate aminotransferase (AST) (glutamic-oxaloacetic transaminase [SGOT]), creatine phosphokinase (CPK), and lactic dehydrogenase (LDH) enzymes can be present. Elevated levels of serum tryptase, a neutral protease, selectively released from human mast cells have been demonstrated by immunoassay to correlate with histamine release and may indicate anaphylaxis or mastocytosis.
3. **Chest x-ray.** With bronchial involvement, the chest x-ray shows hyperinflation with or without areas of atelectasis. In some cases, pulmonary edema is evident.
4. **Electrocardiogram.** Unless myocardial infarction has occurred, ECG changes are usually transient and can include S-T wave depression, bundle branch block, atrial fibrillation, and various ventricular arrhythmias.

IV. **Differential diagnosis**

A. **Mild reactions.** When mild local or generalized reactions occur, the differential diagnosis includes the causes of urticaria and angioedema (see Chap. 9) or forms of extensive contact dermatitis (see Chap. 8).

B. **Severe reactions.** Consider all causes of respiratory distress, cardiovascular collapse, and unconsciousness. Table 10-4 presents characteristic features of the most common conditions confused with anaphylaxis. These conditions include:

1. **Vasovagal reactions and syncopal attacks** often occur with injections. The pulse is slow, and cyanosis usually does not occur. Although the blood pressure is low, it is usually easily detectable and generally higher than in anaphylaxis. **Pallor and diaphoresis are common features.**

Table 10-4. Differential diagnosis of anaphylaxis by clinical features

Condition	Anaphylaxis	Anaphylactoid reaction	Insulin reaction	Myocardial infarction	Vasovagal reaction
Pallor	+	+	+	+	+
Diaphoresis	±	±	+	+	+
Altered consciousness	+	+	+	±	+
Urticaria, angioedema	±	±	−	−	−
Dyspnea	+	+	−	+	±
Wheezing	±	±	−	±	−
Hyperinflation	+	+	−	−	−
Stridor	+	+	−	−	−
Hoarseness	+	+	−	−	−
Tachycardia	+	+	+	+	−
Hypotension	+	+	±	±	+
Arrhythmias	±	±	±	+	−
ECG and enzyme abnormality	±	±	−	+	−
Hypoglycemia	−	−	+	−	−

Key: + = usually present; ± = may be present; − = usually absent.

2. **Myocardial infarction.** The predominant symptom in myocardial infarction is chest pain, with or without radiation. Respiratory difficulty, developing more slowly, results from a restrictive abnormality without air trapping or other evidence of bronchial obstruction. There is no upper airway edema or obstruction.

3. **Insulin reactions** are characterized by weakness, pallor, diaphoresis, and unconsciousness. Airway obstruction and respiratory distress do not occur; the blood pressure is usually only moderately depressed.

4. In **hysterical reactions,** there is usually no objective evidence of respiratory distress, hypotension, or cyanosis. Paresthesias are more common than pruritus. Syncope can occur, but unconsciousness is momentary. Rapid assessment of vital signs and neurologic status will differentiate this condition from anaphylaxis.

Certain patients, especially those with recurrent episodes of anaphylaxis, may knowingly induce episodes with covert administration of an antigen (e.g., a drug such as penicillin or a food such as peanuts) and seek medical attention. Likewise, certain patients may knowingly simulate anaphylactic attacks. Recognition of such individuals is important, and appropriate psychiatric evaluation and treatment should be obtained.

V. **Treatment** of the patient with anaphylaxis depends on the severity of the reaction. Table 10-5 lists the equipment and medications that should be available to manage anaphylaxis properly. **Rapid action is of utmost importance.** The following approach is taken to counteract the effects of mediator release, support vital functions, and prevent further release of mediators:

A. **Evaluate quickly** airway patency and cardiac and respiratory status. If the patient has suffered cardiopulmonary arrest, institute basic cardiopulmonary resuscitation **immediately.** If shock is impending, place the patient in a recumbent position and elevate the legs.

B. **Epinephrine** (Adrenalin) in an aqueous solution of 1:1000 dilution (0.30–0.50 ml; 0.01 ml/kg in children) is administered subcutaneously in the upper extremity or thigh. If anaphylaxis has resulted from an injection or sting, provided the

---

Table 10-5. Equipment and medication for the office management of anaphylaxi?

Equipment
  Stethoscope and sphygmomanometer
  Tourniquets, syringes, hypodermic needles, and large-bore needles (14-gauge)
  Equipment for administering oxygen by mask
  Oral airway and equipment for endotracheal intubation
  Equipment and fluids for continuous intravenous infusion
Medication
  Aqueous epinephrine hydrochloride, 1:1000
  Diphenhydramine for intravenous injection
  Aminophylline for intravenous injection
  Corticosteroids for intravenous injection
  Vasopressor (e.g., levarterenol bitartrate or dopamine hydrochloride)

---

sting is not on the head, neck, hands, or feet, give a second injection of epinephrine (1:1000, 0.1–0.3 ml) in the injection or sting site to reduce antigen absorption. The initial epinephrine dose can be repeated at 15- to 20-minute intervals as needed. With **shock** or **vascular collapse** evident or impending, dilute epinephrine (1:1000) 0.1 ml in 10 ml of normal saline (1:100,000 dilution) and give 10 ml intravenously over 5–10 minutes. After initial dosing, if indicated, a continuous intravenous infusion of epinephrine (1 mg of a 1:1000 dilution in 250 ml of D5W [4 µg/ml]) can be given. Start the infusion rate at 1 µg/minute and increase to a maximum of 4 µg/minute as needed and tolerated under precise monitoring. In children, begin the infusion rate at 0.1 µg/kg/minute and increase by 0.1 µg/kg/minute increments to a maximum of 1.5 µg/kg/minute as needed and tolerated.* Epinephrine can be associated with significant morbidity in elderly patients or in those with underlying cardiovascular or cerebrovascular disease thus, each patient must be treated individually considering the risk to benefit.

C. **Tourniquet.** If the reaction is due to an injection or sting on an extremity, place a tourniquet proximal to the site of the injection. The tourniquet should be released for 1–2 minutes every 10 minutes.

D. **Oxygen** should be given to patients with cyanosis, significant dyspnea, or wheezing. Moderate-flow to high-flow oxygen (5–10 liters/minute) can be delivered by mask or nasal catheter (determine the presence of preexisting chronic obstructive pulmonary disease).

E. **Diphenhydramine** (Benadryl) can be administered intravenously (slowly over 5–10 minutes), intramuscularly, or orally (1–2 mg/kg) up to 50 mg as a single dose, depending on the severity of the reaction. **This drug is not a substitute for epinephrine.** Continue orally every 6 hours for 48 hours to prevent recurrence of the reaction, especially for urticaria and angioedema. Other antihistamin can be substituted for continued oral therapy. Although not proven to be of benefit for anaphylaxis, H_2 antihistamine blockers (e.g., cimetidine) can be added (see Chap. 4).

If the patient does not respond to the preceding measures, remains hypotensive, or has persistent respiratory difficulty, hospitalization in an intensive care unit i. necessary. Under these circumstances proceed with:

F. **Intravenous fluids,** administered through the largest-gauge line available at a rate necessary to maintain the systolic blood pressure at or above 100 mm Hg in adults and 50 mm Hg in children. Glucose (5%) in one-half normal saline is maintained at a rate of 2000–3000 ml/sq m body surface area/24 hours. See Appendix I for estimation of body surface area. In adults, 500–2000 ml of fluid in the first hour of therapy is appropriate. Children can receive an initial volume up to 30 ml/kg in the first hour, which can be repeated as necessary to

---

*R. D. White. Cardiovascular pharmacology: Part 1. In K. M. McIntyre, and A. J. Lewi. (eds.), *Textbook of Advanced Cardiac Life Support.* Dallas: American Heart Association, 1981, P. VIII–4.

maintain an acceptable blood pressure. Volume expanders such as normal saline or a colloidal solution should be administered if hypotension persists.

G. Aminophylline. If bronchospasm persists, give aminophylline intravenously, 4–7 mg/kg diluted in at least an equal volume of intravenous fluid, over 15–20 minutes. Depending on the degree of bronchospasm, continue as either a continuous intravenous infusion at a rate of 0.2–1.2 mg/kg/hour or 4–5 mg/kg intravenously over 20–30 minutes every 6 hours. Monitor serum theophylline levels (see Chaps. 4 and 6).

H. Vasopressors
   1. If intravenous fluids alone cannot maintain blood pressure, administer **levarterenol bitartrate** (Levophed), an alpha- and beta-adrenergic stimulant, intravenously. To 1000 ml of intravenous fluid (5% glucose in water or saline), add 4–8 mg (4–8 ml) and titrate the rate to maintain an adequate blood pressure (maximal rate, 2 ml/minute). In children, use 1 mg (1 ml) in 250 ml of intravenous fluid at a rate of 0.5 ml/minute. Levarterenol may produce tissue sloughing with subcutaneous infiltration.
   2. **Dopamine hydrochloride** (Intropin) is primarily a beta-adrenergic stimulant and can be used alternatively. It is administered as a continuous intravenous infusion at a rate of 0.3–1.2 mg/kg/hour (200 mg in 500 ml of 5% glucose in water or saline, which yields a dilution of 0.4 mg/ml). Begin the infusion at 0.3 mg/kg/hour, and titrate the dose to maintain blood pressure. Dopamine is preferable to levarterenol in patients with cardiac failure.

I. Intubation and tracheostomy are necessary if upper airway obstruction secondary to edema is so severe that the patient cannot maintain adequate ventilation. **Do not delay this procedure if it is indicated.** Tracheostomy is best performed in an operating room by a trained surgeon.

J. Corticosteroids are not helpful in the acute management of anaphylaxis, but in moderate or severe reactions they should be started early to prevent protracted or recurrent symptoms. Initially, give 7–10 mg/kg of hydrocortisone intravenously, followed by 5 mg/kg every 6 hours by a bolus infusion. An equivalent dose of other corticosteroid preparations can be used intravenously, intramuscularly, or orally (see Table 4-12). Treatment can usually be discontinued after 48–72 hours.

K. After the patient's condition has been stabilized, **maintain supportive therapy** with fluids and drugs as long as it is needed to support vital signs and functions. Depending on the severity of the reaction, this support can extend from a few hours to several days. Because of the potential of recurrences of acute symptoms several hours after the initial onset, patients with mild reactions must be so warned, and patients with more severe reactions must be observed for the first 12–24 hours. Most fatalities occur within the first 30 minutes. Recovery is usually complete unless myocardial infarction or central nervous system damage has occurred. Generally, subsequent challenges with the same antigen lead to more severe and more rapid reactions.

VI. Prevention is the most important aspect of the management of anaphylaxis (Table 10-6).
   A. A **careful history** of previous reactions to suspected antigens is **mandatory** before administering any medication (especially parenterally). Attempts to identify specific allergens should utilize immediate-type hypersensitivity skin tests or radioallergosorbent testing when available (see Chap. 2).
   B. The use of antibotics and other medications should be limited to specific **indications,** and **oral administration** is preferable to the parenteral route when possible.
   C. Skin testing or **conjunctival testing** with various vaccines and antivenoms derived from animal serum is mandatory before administration of therapeutic doses. A history of drug sensitivity should preclude the use of such drugs except in special circumstances (see Chap. 12).
   D. Identification information* should be worn at all times by patients who have had previous anaphylactic reactions.

*Medic Alert Foundation, P.O. Box 1009, Turlock, CA 95380.

Table 10-6. Prevention of anaphylaxis

1. Take a thorough drug allergy history.
2. Give drugs orally rather than parenterally when possible.
3. Have patients wait in office 30 minutes after drug administration.
4. Check all drugs for proper labeling.
5. Predisposed patients should carry warning identification.
6. Predisposed patients should be taught self-injection of epinephrine.
7. When antiserum is essential, use human serum preparations.
8. Give skin tests when appropriate.
9. The following drugs require special preventive protocols (Chap. 12):
   Radiographic contrast material
     Pretreatment
   Local anesthetics
     Skin testing
     Incremental challenge testing
   Blood and blood products in IgA-deficient patients
     Washed red blood cells
     Autotransfusion
     IgA-deficient blood used

Source: Adapted from and reproduced with permission from *Current Views in Allergy and Immunology:* Lieberman, Phil: "Anaphylaxis and Anaphylactoid Reactions," Vol. IV, Program 1, January 1980, slides #6, #13, and #16, Copyrighted by Current Views in Allergy and Immunology, Inc., Atlanta, GA.

Selected Readings

Perkin, R. M., and Anas, N. G. Mechanisms and management of anaphylactic shock not responding to traditional therapy. *Ann. Allergy* 54:202, 1985.

Peters, S. P. Systemic anaphylaxis. In L. M. Lichtenstein and A. S. Fauci (eds.), *Current Therapy in Allergy, Immunology, and Rheumatology, 1985–1986.* St. Louis: Mosby, 1985. P. 75.

Sheffer, A. Anaphylaxis. *J. Allergy Clin. Immunol.* 75:227, 1985.

Wasserman, S. I. Anaphylaxis. In E. Middleton, Jr., C. E. Reed, and E. F. Ellis. *Allergy: Principles and Practice* (2nd ed.). St Louis: Mosby, 1983. P. 689.

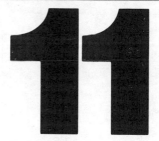

Insect Allergy

Thomas J. Fischer
and Glenn J. Lawlor, Jr.

Insect stings or bites can cause local or systemic reactions, ranging from mild to fatal responses, in susceptible persons. Because of the rapid onset of systemic reactions, they are true allergic emergencies. Insect sting allergy (Hymenoptera sensitivity) can occur in persons with no history of atopic disease and accounts for at least 30 deaths a year in the United States. The frequency increases in the summer months and with outdoor exposure.

Clinical Reactions

I. **Local reactions.** The response in a normal person to toxic sting or bite products consists of sharp, localized pain followed in minutes by a small reddened area at the site of the sting or bite. This reaction ususally resolves in 24 hours, although it can enlarge and become indurated, especially in a dependent portion of the body. Antivenom IgE antibodies can be found in patients with large local reactions that may precede an anaphylactic reaction on a subsequent sting.

Secondary infection can also complicate and prolong this immediate local reaction. **Any degree of swelling constitutes a local reaction provided it is continuous with the sting area.**

II. **Toxic systemic reactions.** Generalized reactions consisting of gastrointestinal symptoms, headache, vertigo, syncope, convulsions, or fever can occur following an episode of multiple stings. These reactions are not truly allergic, but result from histaminelike substances in the venom.

III. **Systemic allergic reactions**

    A. **Immediate** or **anaphylactic** reactions result from the interaction of IgE antibody with one or more constituents of the insect venom. These reactions are classified as mild, non-life-threatening reactions or severe systemic reactions. **Mild reactions** consist of disturbances beyond the sting site, usually itching and urticaria. **Severe systemic reactions** may consist of airway involvement (dyspnea, wheezing, chest tightness, hoarseness, fullness in the throat), hypotension manifested by disorientation, loss of consciousness, incontinence, nausea, vomiting, and abdominal pain. These severe reactions usually occur within 1 hour after the sting.

    B. **Delayed systemic reactions** occur from 2 hours to 3 weeks following the sting. They can take the form of serum sickness (fever, arthralgia, lymphadenopathy, urticaria, angioedema, or purpura); neurologic reactions such as peripheral neuritis, hemiplegia, or encephalopathy; or allergic vasculitis and coagulation defects.

    C. Systemic reactions are almost always caused by stinging insects of the order Hymenoptera. These insects include honeybees and bumblebees, wasps, hornets, yellow jackets, and fire ants. The individual characteristics of these insects are listed in Table 11-1. Biting insects (e.g., fleas, mosquitoes) rarely cause generalized reactions.

Table 11-1. Characteristics of common stinging insects (Hymenoptera)

Insect type	Appearance	Habitats	Sting characteristics	Venom constituents
Honeybee	Hairy bodies with yellow and black markings	Domestic hives, hollow trees or caves (rural and suburban)	Barbed stinger; only insect to leave stinger; stings only if provoked	Hyaluronidase, phospholipase A, histamine, lecithinase; smooth muscle contractor
Wasp	Hairless body with narrow waist, black or brown markings	Trees, shrubs, eaves of houses (rural and suburban scavenger)	Often contaminated	Histamine, serotonin, hyaluronidase, lecithinase
Hornet	Short waist, truncated body, with sparse hair, dark band under eyes	Oval and pear-shaped nests in trees and above ground (rural scavenger)	Often contaminated	Histamine, serotinin, kinins, acetylcholine
Yellow jacket	Similar to hornet, with yellow markings but without dark band under eyes	Nests in ground and walls (rural scavenger)	Often contaminated, aggressive	Histamine, serotonin, kinins
Imported fire ant	Appearance of domestic ants but with well-developed posterior stinging apparatus	Nests in ground, primarily in Gulf Coast states (scavenger)	Bites and stings; produces pustule for 3–8 days, with pain and burning	Cytotoxic and hemolytic alkaloids

Source: Drawings of honeybee, wasp, hornet, and yellow jacket from *Insect Allergy*, copyright 1978 by Hollister-Stier Laboratories, Spokane, WA. Drawing of fire ant from P. Anaphylaxis—Prenatal emergency. *Derm. Allergy* 3:45–19. With permission.

Diagnosis of Hymenoptera Sensitivity

I. **History.** A thorough account of the sting and subsequent reactions, including identification of the insect, presence or absence of the remaining stinger (see Table 11-1), and nature of the allergic reaction (generalized or localized), is a critical determinant for accurate diagnosis and appropriate therapy.

II. **Skin tests**
  A. Defer skin testing for 2–3 weeks following an allergic reaction to a bee sting. This delay allows for elimination of false-negative skin tests as seen during the refractory period following a systemic reaction.
  B. **Venom testing.** The development and commercial availability of specific venoms have allowed improved diagnostic accuracy over whole-body extracts. However, the degree of sensitivity to venom skin tests **will not** absolutely predict whether or not anaphylaxis will occur on a subsequent sting. Furthermore, there is a very narrow range between diagnostic and irritant concentrations of the venom. In approximately 95% of patients, clearly positive or negative skin tests are obtained at the recommended dilutions (up to 1.0 μg/ml). In the remaining patients, the results are equivocal.
    1. **Available venoms** include honeybee, yellow jacket, yellow hornet, white-faced hornet, and wasp. A mixed vespid preparation (equal amounts of yellow jacket, yellow hornet, and white-faced hornet) is available for treatment but not diagnostic purposes. These preparations are freeze-dried proteins (Pharmalgen,* Albay†) that must be reconstituted with a special diluent containing 0.9% sodium chloride, 0.03% normal serum albumin, and 0.4% phenol. This albumin solution has a protective effect on venom protein activity by reducing the absorption of venom protein to the glass surface of the vial. Observe the manufacturer's instructions concerning storage of the freeze-dried preparations, special diluents, and all venom dilutions **(do not freeze).** Observe the **current storage times** before expiration as noted in the product information insert.
    2. Using appropriate dilutions of the five single venom preparations, perform skin tests on patients with a **relevant** sting history (i.e., evidence of systemic reactions). Start skin testing with a preliminary scratch or prick test, using a venom concentration of 0.01 μg/ml of Pharmalgen venom protein or 1.0 μg/ml of Albay venom protein.‡ The preferred location for testing is usually the flexor surface of the forearm. Use aseptic technique and a separate, sterilized syringe and needle for each extract and each patient.
    3. Include a **negative control test** with diluent alone in both epicutaneous (prick or scratch) and intradermal tests. A positive control test using histamine base (0.1% for epicutaneous, 0.01% for intradermal) should be done initially to assure skin reactivity.
    4. An **exquisitely sensitive** patient can react to the scratch or prick test. For these patients, start the remaining intradermal tests at 0.0001 μg/ml.
    5. For patients with negative scratch tests, start individual testing at a concentration of 0.001 μg/ml, using injection volumes of 0.05 ml and reading the skin test 15 minutes after injection. If no reactions occur, continue intradermal testing with 10-fold increments in the concentration (0.01–0.1–1.0 μg/ml) until a clearly positive response has been obtained or until a concentration of 1 μg/ml has been tested (whichever comes first).
    6. **Interpretation** of skin response is based on wheal and erythema size and the presence of pseudopodia. Table 11-2 summarizes the recommended guidelines for skin test interpretation using Pharmalgen or Albay venom. Reactions at 1 + or greater at a concentration of 1 μg/ml or less of venom indi-

*ALK America, Inc., 132 Research Drive, Milford, CT 06460
†Hollister-Stier Laboratories, P.O. Box 3145 TA, Spokane, WA 99220
‡Manufacturers' recommendations.

Table 11-2. Interpretation of venom skin test responses

| Grade | Mean diameters (cm) | |
	Wheal	Erythema
0	<0.5	<0.5
±	0.5–1.0	0.5–1.0
1+	0.5–1.0	1.1–2.0
2+	0.5–1.0	2.1–3.0
3+	1.0–1.5; pseudopodia	3.1–4.0
4+	>1.5; many pseudopodia	>4.0

cates the patient is venom-sensitive (the 1+ reaction must be greater than that of the diluent control).

C. Skin tests with **whole-body extracts** of stinging insects **do not** differentiate sensitive from normal persons. Before venom proteins were available, they were used to determine safe starting concentrations for immunotherapy.

III. **Radioallergosorbent test (RAST).** Venom-specific IgE antibodies, demonstrable by in vitro RAST testing, can be found in sensitive persons. They can also be seen in patients with large local reactions who may be at risk of subsequent systemic reactions. The major advantage of RAST testing is lack of in vivo exposure of venom to extremely sensitive persons. Furthermore, because the inherent irritant qualities of the venom constituents limit the useful upper concentration of venom for skin testing to approximately 1.0 µg/ml, a patient with a suspicious clinical history and equivocal skin tests may also benefit from the RAST technique to further clarify sensitivity. Because of the cost, time delay, and the 15–20 percent frequency of negative responses in the presence of positive skin tests, it is not routinely used as a screening test.

IV. **Leukocyte histamine release** correlates with clinical anaphylactic sensitivity and is helpful in patients with equivocal skin test results. As a general diagnostic procedure, this technique is elaborate, available only on a research basis, and limited by the fact that the cells of 15% of insect-allergic persons will not release histamine even on challenge with anti-IgE globulin.

Treatment of Insect Allergy

I. **Management of acute reactions**
   A. Treatment of immediate systemic reactions is the same as for anaphylaxis from other causes (see Chap. 10).
   B. Treat local reactions with careful cleansing and application of ice to the sting site. If the stinger of a honeybee remains, flick it away with a blade or a fingernail to prevent further injection of venom.
   C. If secondary infection occurs, use **antibiotic** treatment.
   D. **Diphenhydramine** (Benadryl), 5 mg/kg/day (150 mg/day in adults) in 3–4 divided doses, can help relieve local itching and burning.
   E. Application of a topical corticosteroid cream or ointment to reduce local inflammation secondary to the venom components can be helpful.

II. **Prophylaxis**
   A. Instruct patients with a history of large local or generalized reactions about the characteristics of stinging insects and the measures necessary to decrease the risk of being stung (Table 11-3).
   B. Patients with a history of systemic reactions should carry and understand the use of an emergency kit for treating anaphylaxis. Barring a cardiac history, all patients unprotected by venom immunotherapy should immediately administer epinephrine after a sting whether or not a reaction is appreciated. In patients

Table 11-3. Patient information to limit the risk of insect stings

1. The risk increases in summer.
2. Exercise caution when doing yard work, handling garbage, picnicking, boating, camping or other outdoor activity.
3. Always wear shoes outdoors.
4. Avoid loose fitting clothing that may entrap insects. Insects are attracted to **bright** colors and floral patterns. Wear **light-colored** clothing; **white, green, tan,** and **khaki** are the least attractive.
5. Avoid scented perfumes, lotions, soaps, colognes, or hair preparations.
6. Look for insects in vehicles prior to driving, and keep vehicle windows closed.
7. Avoid rapid or jerking movement around insects. Most insects will not sting unless provoked.
8. All nests or hives in the vicinity of the home should be removed by a professional exterminator and **not** by the insect-sensitive patient.
9. Insect repellents should **not** be depended on for protection. Immunotherapy does **not** lessen the need for other measures of prevention.
10. Wear an identification tag or bracelet at all times.
11. Have an emergency kit available at all times, especially if at greater risk. Instruct family members and companions in its use.
12. Seek medical attention immediately after emergency treatment is given.

protected by venom immunotherapy, use epinephrine only for clear-cut reactions. A commercially available kit (ANA Kit*) contains: (1) a preloaded syringe with epinephrine 1:1000 dilution (sealed in nitrogen to avoid oxidation) to deliver 2 full doses of 0.3 ml each (0.01 ml/kg in children) subcutaneously; (2) an antihistamine tablet for immediate oral ingestion (e.g., chlorpheniramine, 4 mg); (3) a disposable alcohol sponge; and (4) a tourniquet to apply proximal to a sting on an extremity.

For the anxious or younger patient, the Epi-Pen† and the Epi-Pen Jr.† offer the advantage of an automatic, spring-loaded, self-injector that obviates the need for patients to give themselves injections. The Epi-Pen delivers 0.3 mg of epinephrine; the Epi-Pen Jr. delivers 0.15 mg of epinephrine.

1. Observe **expiration dates** on kits and replace as needed.
2. **Identification tags** or bracelets should be worn by patients with a history of systemic reactions.‡

C. **Venom immunotherapy**
1. **Indications.** The introduction of venom extracts has represented a major advance in the treatment of Hymenoptera-sensitive persons. At the present time, several classes of patients are considered as possible candidates.
   a. Adults and children with severe systemic reactions (airway involvement or hypotension) and a positive skin test are routinely treated.
   b. Adults with mild, non-life-threatening reactions (erythema or urticaria) and a positive venom skin test are routinely treated. Because children may require immunotherapy for six to eight decades (the long-term side effects of immunotherapy are not yet known) and because many children will naturally lose their sensitivity, the current recommendation leans toward avoiding therapy in most of these instances.
   c. Patients with a history of systemic reaction but negative venom skin tests are not candidates for venom immunotherapy because there is no indication which venom to use for treatment.
   d. Patients with a history of a large local reaction with a positive venom skin test can be at risk of subsequent systemic reactions. At the present

*ANA Kit, Hollister-Stier Laboratories, Spokane, WA 99220.
†Epi-Pen, Center Laboratories, Inc., Port Washington, NY 11050.
‡Medic Alert Foundation, Turlock, CA 95380.

time, however, the exact risk is unknown, and such patients are not routine candidates for venom immunotherapy.

e. Patients with a history of a large local reaction but a negative venom skin test are not candidates for venom immunotherapy.

f. Patients without a history of a systemic or local reaction but with a positive venom skin test are not suitable candidates for venom immunotherapy.

g. Patients previously treated with whole-body extracts require a complete reevaluation (e.g., history, skin tests) before starting venom immunotherapy.

h. In pregnant patients, the benefit-risk ratio of treatment must be carefully evaluated, especially in patients to be treated initially during pregnancy.

2. Contraindications. Injections are contraindicated in patients with bleeding disorders. Use cautiously in patients with immunologic diseases.

3. Immunotherapy regimen. The regimen currently recommended consists of a series of increasing doses of venom up to a maintenance dose of 100 µg/ml of venom protein (consult manufacturer's instruction insert regarding reconstitution, expiration, precautions, and dosage schedules). The usual progression occurs over a 15-week period, a shorter period ("rush") than routinely used with other allergens. A small percentage of patients are not able to tolerate this rapid progression due to large local or systemic reactions. These patients may take a full year to reach maintenance.

Table 11-4 is a representative treatment schedule using the Pharmalgen single venom preparation. Table 11-5 is a representative treatment schedule using the Albay single venom preparation. If a patient requires more than one venom preparation, the number of injections per visit is increased to include additional venom proteins. Each separate venom preparation should be given by separate injections. The mixed vespid preparation can be substituted for individual vespid preparations if the patient is allergic to all three of the venoms: yellow jacket, yellow hornet, and white-faced hornet. The treatment schedules are individualized to include a more dilute starting dose and smaller increments between doses in progressing to a maintenance dose of 100 µg, especially in extremely sensitive patients (those with a positive intradermal skin test response at a concentration of 0.001 µg/ml or less or those experiencing a systemic reaction to any venom skin test concentration).

Some experienced practitioners recommend decreasing the frequency of the maintenance dose to an interval of every 6 weeks (if tolerated) after the first 12 months of therapy.

4. Adverse reactions to venom immunotherapy include severe anaphylactic reactions or reactions limited to soreness and swelling at the injection site. The incidence of side effects is high, with one-half of treated patients having one or more local reactions and 1 in 6 adult patients having a systemic reaction at some time during their therapy. In children, both local and systemic reactions are much less common. Delayed reactions, such as serum sickness, also occur up to 48 hours after injection. Because of the high incidence of immediate systemic reactions, only physicians familiar with treating anaphylaxis should employ venom immunotherapy (see Chap. 10).

5. Length of therapy. The exact duration of treatment after reaching the monthly maintenance dose is not absolutely known. Current evidence suggests that treatment should be continued for several years (2–5 years), if not indefinitely, because sensitive patients appear protected even though their condition is not cured. Some experienced practitioners recommend that venom skin testing be repeated at 2-year intervals to assess loss of sensitivity. In patients whose skin tests become negative and who also have a negative RAST, it may be possible to consider discontinuation of venom therapy. However, conclusive data to support this approach are not currently available.

Table 11-4. Representative treatment schedule using Pharmalgen single venom preparation[a,b]

Week	Day	Number of doses per day at ½-hour intervals	Concentration of venom to be used (μg/ml)	Volume for subcutaneous injection (ml)	Amount of venom injected (μg protein)
1	1	1	0.01	0.1	0.001
		2	0.1	0.1	0.01
		3	1.0	0.1	0.1
2	8	1	1.0	0.1	0.1
		2	1.0	0.5	0.5
		3	10	0.1	1.0
3	15	1	10	0.1	1
		2	10	0.5	5
		3	10	1.0	10
4	22	1	100	0.1	10
		2	100	0.2	20
5	29	1	100	0.2	20
		2	100	0.3	30
6	36	1	100	0.3	30
		2	100	0.3	30
7	43	1	100	0.4	40
		2	100	0.4	40
8	50	1	100	0.5	50
		2	100	0.5	50
9	57	1	100	1.0	100
10	64	1	100	1.0	100
12	78	1	100	1.0	100
15	99	1	100	1.0	100
Monthly[c]		1	100	1.0	100

[a] The following *conditions for proceeding to next dose* must be observed: (1) If a single dose results in more than a moderate local reaction (> 5.0-cm wheal) within one-half hour, an additional dose should not be given during that visit. Repeat the same dose at the next visit(s) until tolerated. (2) If a systemic manifestation of sensitivity occurs during or following a visit, or a single dose results in an excessive local reaction (wheal > 10 cm) within one-half hour, do not administer an additional dose during the visit, and reduce the total dosage for the next visit to half the total resulting in the reaction. (3) Delayed (24–48 hours) local reactions < 10 cm do not require a dose adjustment. For delayed local reactions > 10 cm, hold dose at previous level.
[b] For the mixed vespid preparation, the total venom protein concentration and the total amount of venom protein injected will be triple the amounts shown, with no changes in injection volumes.
[c] If a patient on maintenance therapy is stung and has any systemic manifestation of sensitivity, the maintenance dosage should be increased to 200 μg for the relevant venom, using increments no greater than 50 μg.
Source: Pharmalgen Venom Extract Treatment Schedule. Courtesy of Pharmacia Diagnostics, Inc., Piscataway, NJ.

Table 11-5. Representative treatment schedule using Albay single venom preparation[a,b]

Week number	Concentration of venom to be used (µg/ml)	Volume for subcutaneous injection (ml)	Amount of venom injected (µg protein)
1	1	0.05	0.05
2	1	0.10	0.1
3	1	0.20	0.2
4	1	0.40	0.4
5	10	0.05	0.5
6	10	0.10	1
7	10	0.20	2
8	10	0.40	4
9	100	0.05	5
10	100	0.10	10
11	100	0.20	20
12	100	0.40	40
13	100	0.60	60
14	100	0.80	80
15	100	1.00	100
16	100	1.00	100
18	100	1.00	100
21	100	1.00	100
Monthly	100	1.00	100

[a] Precaution regarding progression is similar to that in Table 11-4.
[b] Multiple venom sensitivities are treated with individual single venom preparations given simultaneously at separate sites. Patients with such sensitivities have an increased risk of systemic reactions.
Source: Albay Hymenoptera Treatment Schedule. Courtesy of Hollister-Stier Laboratories, Spokane, WA.

6. IgG antibody to venom therapy can be measured by a number of techniques (see Appendix V). This IgG antibody response is associated with clinical protection if certain minimal IgG levels arbitrarily set by the laboratory are met (e.g., at the Johns Hopkins University Dermatology, Allergy, and Clinical Immunology laboratory, IgG venom antibody levels lower than 3.0 µg/ml have been associated with an increased risk of systemic sting reactions). IgG levels can be monitored every 6–12 months for patients on maintenance dosage. If the titers are below those considered to be protective, increase the venom dosage or decrease the interval between injections.
Although there is decided merit in determining venom-specific IgG antibody levels for research purposes, most experienced practitioners suggest this determination is of questionable value in clinical practice. They suggest, in addition to immunologic factors, there may be physiologic, psychologic, and biochemical factors that determine the patient's clinical response to insect stings.

Biting Insects

Insect (e.g., fleas, mosquitoes) bites are best prevented by avoidance, extermination, and use of repellents. Diet and vitamin B therapy are of no proved value. Similarly, immunotherapy or injection of extracts of biting insects does not reduce the risk of bites or the reaction to bites.

Systemic anaphylactic reactions can occur from the bites of insects of the *Triatoma* genus (kissing bugs). *Triatoma protracta* and *Triatoma rubida* are the species most commonly involved. Characteristically these insects are early morning feeders, and bites usually occur on exposed areas (e.g., arms, face) while the individual is sleeping. *Triatoma* occur in warm climates, especially in the Southwestern and Southeastern United States, Texas, and the Gulf states. Rodents are a common vector. Typical bite reactions appear as local inflammation and urtication lasting for several days. Anaphylaxis is rare, usually occurring in individuals with repeated bites, and reactions can be immediate and life-threatening. The antigen or antigens appear to be species-specific and are contained in the saliva of the insect. Specific IgE antibody to insect salivary gland protein has been demonstrated in sensitive individuals by the RAST technique.

Treatment is directed to the acute reaction and to prophylaxis as with Hymenoptera sensitivity. Immunotherapy has been attempted with some success using *Triatoma* salivary gland extract.

Selected Readings

Reisman, R. E. Insect Allergy. In E. Middleton, Jr., C. Reed, and E. F. Ellis (eds.), *Allergy: Principles and Practice* (2nd ed.). St. Louis: Mosby, 1983. P. 1361.

Rohr, A. S., Marshall, N. A., and Saxon, A. Successful immunotheraphy for *Triatoma protracta*–induced anaphylaxis. *J. Allergy Clin. Immunol.* 73:369, 1984.

Schuberth, K. C. Insect Sting Allergy in Children. In L. M. Lichtenstein and A. S. Fauci (eds.), *Current Therapy in Allergy, Immunology, and Rheumatology, 1985–1986.* St. Louis: Mosby, 1985.

Smith, P. L., et al. Physiologic manifestations of human anaphylaxis. *J. Clin. Invest.* 66:1072, 1980.

Yuninger, J. W. Insect Sting Allergy in Adults. In L. M. Lichtenstein and A. S. Fauci (eds.), *Current Therapy in Allergy, Immunology, and Rheumatology, 1985–1986.* St. Louis: Mosby, 1985.

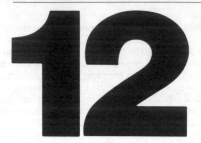

Drug Allergy

Michael H. Mellon,
Michael Schatz,
and Roy Patterson

Adverse reactions to drug therapy are a major consideration in clinical medicine. The first recognition of this problem came early in this century, when serum sickness was attributed to horse serum. Prior to the introduction of sulfonamides in the late 1930s, estimates of the incidence of adverse drug reactions approximated 0.5–1.5% of all patients. Currently, 15–30% of all hospitalized patients experience an adverse drug reaction that is an unintended or undesired consequence of drug therapy.

Classification of Adverse Drug Reactions

I. **Non-drug-related reactions**
  A. **Psychogenic reactions,** such as vasovagal reactions to injections, can be manifested as anxiety, nausea, lethargy, or syncope.
  B. **Coincidental symptoms,** caused by the disease under treatment, can be mistakenly attributed to a drug concurrently used, e.g., viral exanthemata in children treated with antibiotics.
II. **Drug-related reactions**
  A. **Adverse reactions occurring in nonsusceptible patients**
    1. **Overdosage** refers to toxic pharmacologic effects of a drug that are directly related to the systemic or local concentration of the drug in the body (e.g., respiratory depression with sedatives).
    2. **Side effects** are due to therapeutically undesirable but unavoidable pharmacologic actions of a drug occurring with normal drug dosages; side effects constitute the most frequent adverse drug reaction (e.g., tachycardia with epinephrine injection).
    3. **Secondary effects** are events only indirectly related to the primary pharmacologic action of the drug (e.g., the release of microbial antigens and endotoxins after antibiotic treatment, such as the Jarisch-Herxheimer reaction seen in certain cases of syphilis treated with penicillin).
    4. **Drug interactions** can alter the normal physiology of the host and change the response to one or a number of drugs (e.g., enzyme induction by one drug causing altered metabolism of another drug).
  B. **Adverse reactions occurring in susceptible patients**
    1. **Intolerance** is the production of a characteristic pharmacologic effect by small dosages of a drug in certain persons.
    2. **Idiosyncrasy** is a qualitatively abnormal response to a drug that is different from its pharmacologic effects. It occurs only in susceptible patients and does not involve an immune mechanism (although it can resemble an immunologic reaction clinically). Primaquine-induced hemolytic anemia in patients deficient in glucose 6-phosphate dehydrogenase is an example.
    3. **Allergy or hypersensitivity** to drugs occurs in selected patients in whom drug exposure results in the production of specific antibodies or sensitized lymphocytes (or both) directed against the drug or its metabolites. Only reactions mediated by immune mechanisms should be classified as allergic.

The **general features** of allergic drug reactions include the following:

a. Drug allergies occur in a small percentage of the population receiving the drug and can occur at low dosages of the drug.

b. Usually, there has been no reaction on initial exposure to the drug. (However, patients may be exposed without their knowledge, e.g., penicillin in beef.)

c. A latent period often occurs during which the drug is taken with no adverse effect.

d. Clinical manifestations of allergic drug reactions do not resemble known pharmacologic actions of the drug or the disease being treated.

e. Symptoms recur on readministration of the drug.

f. Symptoms usually subside within 3–5 days of discontinuation of the drug.

g. Penicillins and sulfonamides (including sulfonamide antibiotics, sulfonylurea hypoglycemics, thiazide diuretics, and carbonic anhydrase inhibitors) are the drugs most commonly associated with allergic drug reactions.

Clinical Manifestations of Allergic Drug Reactions

I. **Immunologic classification.** The clinical manifestations of drug reactions can be classified on the basis of the operative immunologic mechanism(s). The Gell and Coombs' classification of reactions (see Chap. 1) forms the basis of a useful immunologic classification of drug reactions that may have important clinical, diagnostic, and therapeutic implications (Table 12-1).

A. **Type I reactions**

1. Anaphylaxis, urticaria, and angioedema can result from immediate-type hypersensitivity to drugs. Bronchospasm occurs as part of the syndrome of anaphylaxis or following inhaled drugs (such as pituitary snuff). Immediate-type reactions generally occur within 30 minutes after drug administration. Although most drugs have been associated with anaphylaxis, penicillin remains the most common drug-induced cause of anaphylaxis today.

2. Reactions **resembling anaphylaxis** (but probably nonimmunologic in origin) are associated with several drugs, including contrast media, polymyxins, aspirin, and local anesthetics. Intravenous polymyxins, contrast media, and possibly aspirin may cause direct (nonimmunologic) mediator release. Opiates such as codeine and morphine also cause direct mediator release. However, except in drug abusers, the usual clinical manifestations of histamine release due to opiates are limited to a cutaneous wheal at an injection site.

B. **Type II reactions**

1. **Hematologic reactions.** The best examples of cytotoxic antibody-mediated drug reactions are the drug-induced Coombs'-positive hemolytic anemias (see Chap. 15). Similar mechanisms are involved in drug-induced thrombocytopenia and probably agranulocytosis, although aplastic anemia, due to drugs such as chloramphenicol, is unlikely to be immunologic.

2. **Interstitial nephritis.** In some cases of methicillin-induced nephritis, a serum anti–tubular basement membrane antibody as well as immunofluorescence demonstration of IgG, C3, and methicillin antigens in a linear pattern along the renal tubular basement membrane have been demonstrated. Similar findings have been reported in a patient with interstitial nephritis related to phenytoin sodium (Dilantin). These findings suggest type II reactivity.

C. **Type III reactions**

1. **Serum sickness** is the classic example of an **immune complex–mediated** drug reaction. In the past, the widespread use of heterologous serum (e.g., for antitetanus antibody) frequently produced the full serum sickness syn-

Table 12-1. Drug reactions: immunologic classification and clinical implications

Type*	Immune reactants	Examples of clinical reactions	Potential immunologic tests	Major pharmacologic therapy
I: Anaphylactic	Reaginic antibody, primarily IgE	Anaphylaxis Urticaria Angioedema	Immediate skin test (20 min) RAST	Epinephrine Antihistamines
II: Cytotoxic	IgG or IgM antibody against cell-surface antigens; complement	Hematologic Nephritis	Demonstration of antibody in vitro	Corticosteroids
III: Immune complex	Immune complexes; complement	Serum sickness SLE syndrome Vasculitis	Late (Arthus) skin test (6–8 hr) Demonstration of tissue-fixed or circulating immune complexes Demonstration of specific antibody	Corticosteroids
IV: Cell-mediated	Lymphocytes	Contact dermatitis Organ damage	Delayed skin test (24–48 hr) In vitro techniques	Corticosteroids

Key: RAST = radioallergosorbent test; SLE = systemic lupus erythematosus.
* Gell and Coombs' classification.

Table 12-2. A comparison of drug-induced and spontaneous systemic lupus erythematosus

Clinical and laboratory findings	Drug-induced	Spontaneous
Clinical findings		
Age	Older	Younger
Sex	Often seen in males	More common in females
Renal involvement	Less common	More common
Central nervous system involvement	Less common	More common
Rash	Less common	More common
Anemia, thrombocytopenia, leukopenia	Less common	More common
Serositis	More common	Less common
Laboratory findings		
Antibodies to native (double-stranded) DNA	Rare	Often present
Antibody to histones	Primary antinucleoprotein antibody	One of several antinucleoprotein antibodies
Slow acetylators	More susceptible	Probably no increased incidence
Complement levels	Normal	Often reduced

drome 1–3 weeks after antiserum administration. The usual clinical manifestations included skin eruptions (urticarial, maculopapular), fever, and multiple large-joint arthralgia. Lymphadenopathy, peripheral neuropathy, Guillain-Barré syndrome, glomerulonephritis, or multiorgan vasculitis occasionally occurred. The most common cause today for a serum sickness-like syndrome is penicillin, although the exact immunopathogenesis of such reactions is not well defined.

2. **Drug-induced systemic lupus erythematosus (SLE)** resembles naturally occurring SLE, which apparently results from immune complex mechanisms. Several helpful differential points may distinguish these two similar entities (Table 12-2). Hydralazine and procainamide are most commonly associated with drug-induced SLE.

3. **Systemic vasculitis or cutaneous vasculitis** can be secondary to drug-induced immune complex mechanisms. Drug **fever** can be the sole or initial (or both) manifestation of vasculitis. **Cutaneous** vasculitis usually presents with lower extremity palpable purpura, which may be associated with fever and arthralgia. Drug-induced **systemic hypersensitivity angiitis** frequently involves the kidneys and lungs in addition to the skin, can affect additional organs as well, and produces a necrotizing angiitis of small vessels, including veins. Sulfonamides are the drugs most commonly associated with hypersensitivity angiitis.

D. **Type IV reactions**

1. **Contact dermatitis** results from delayed hypersensitivity to topical application of drugs. Not only the drug itself, but also preservatives, such as the parabens, can cause contact sensitivity. In addition, **photosensitivity reactions** appear to involve an interaction between type IV reactivity and a drug made antigenic by solar energy.

2. **Acute pulmonary reactions** to nitrofurantoin may be due primarily to cell-mediated mechanisms. The syndrome consists of fever, dyspnea, and cough, often accompanied by eosinophilia, pulmonary infiltrates, and pleural effusion. The relationship of the immunopathogenesis of acute nitrofurantoin reactivity to nitrofurantoin-induced pulmonary fibrosis is uncertain. Interstitial pneumonitis associated with gold therapy (manifested clinically by

dyspnea, cough, diffuse interstitial infiltrates, restrictive lung disease, and often a rash) may also be related to cell-mediated immune mechanisms. Interstitial pneumonitis and pulmonary fibrosis due to certain antineoplastic drugs, such as bleomycin and busulfan, may be toxic rather than immunologic.

3. **Other reactions.** There is also evidence that some cases of drug-induced interstitial nephritis, encephalomyelitis following live virus vaccination, and possibly hepatocellular damage secondary to certain drugs (e.g., halothane) may be due to cell-mediated immune mechanisms. In addition, certain cases of drug-induced fever or vasculitis may have a type IV component.

II. **Organ system classification.** In the clinical evaluation of patients with possible drug-induced syndromes, classification by organ system is particularly useful. Such a classification, with possible immunologic mechanisms and common examples, is given in Table 12-3.

A. **Immunologic versus toxic organ damage.** It is important to differentiate the immune-mediated drug reactions in Table 12-3 from drug-induced organ-impairment syndromes caused by presumed toxic effects of drugs (not included in the table). The listed drugs cause reactions that occur in a minority of uniquely susceptible persons, are not related to drug dosage, and are often associated with other signs of immunologic reactions (e.g., fever, rash, eosinophilia). In addition, these drugs do not cause injury in experimental animals.

1. Probable examples of toxic effects of drugs not included in this list are chloramphenicol-induced aplastic anemia, antineoplastic drug–induced interstitial pneumonitis and pulmonary fibrosis, anabolic steroid–induced cholestatic jaundice, and acute tubular necrosis caused by many drugs.

2. Although most of the syndromes in Table 12-3 are presumed to be immunologically mediated, idiosyncratic nonimmunologic mechanisms can account for some of these reactions (such as aspirin-induced asthma). Some drugs can produce damage of toxic as well as idiosyncratic or immunologic mechanisms (e.g., drug-induced hepatitis). The **exact** immunologic mechanisms of many of the reactions are as yet unknown.

B. **Associated drugs.** It should be noted that, although certain drugs are commonly associated with certain drug-reaction syndromes, potentially, **any drug** can have such an association. For a convenient reference, consult the *Physicians' Desk Reference* for a listing of the reported syndromes for each drug. A more complete listing of drugs associated with each syndrome is available in reference works on this subject (see Selected Readings).

C. **Cutaneous manifestations** are the most common manifestations of drug allergy (Table 12-4), with maculopapular or morbilliform eruptions most frequently seen. Although clinical or histologic features alone do not usually allow differentiation of a maculopapular rash due to drug allergy from one secondary to other causes, certain features suggest a drug etiology: an acute onset, symmetric distribution, predominant truncal involvement, brilliant coloration, and definite pruritus. A maculopapular drug rash itself can have relatively little morbidity, but it can progress to exfoliative dermatitis, with visceral damage, secondary infection, and even death. In addition, a maculopapular rash can be associated with manifestations of drug allergy in other organ systems.

Diagnosis of Allergic Drug Reactions

I. **Clinical data or history.** The lack of specificity for most of the available laboratory methods for the diagnosis of drug allergy leaves the clinical history as the most important tool in evaluating possible drug-related reactions. Emphasize the following aspects when taking the history:

A. Identify and suspect **all** drugs taken by the patient, even if these drugs are apparently harmless or have been taken previously without incident.

Table 12-3. Classification of drug reactions by organ system

Organ system	Type	Probable mechanism*	Examples
Multisystem involvement	Anaphylaxis	I	Penicillin, allergy extracts, chymopapain
	Serum sickness	III, ?I	Antivenom, antilymphocyte globulin, penicillin
	Fever	?III, ?IV	Penicillin, barbiturates, phenytoin sodium (Dilantin), sulfonamides, quinidine
	Vasculitis	III, ?IV	Sulfonamides, penicillin, allopurinol, iodides
	Systemic lupus erythematosus	?III	Hydralazine, procainamide, isoniazid, phenytoin sodium
Hematologic	Eosinophilia	?	Gold, carbamazepine
	Coombs'-positive hemolytic anemia	II	Penicillin, phenacetin, methyldopa (Aldomet), quinidine
	Thrombocytopenia	II	Quinine, quinidine, sulfonamides, heparin
	Neutropenia	?II	Phenylbutazone, penicillin, antithyroid drugs
	Lymphadenopathy	?	Phenytoin sodium
Pulmonary	Asthma	Nonimmunologic	Aspirin, indomethacin, timolol, propranolol
	Pulmonary infiltrates with eosinophilia	?	Penicillins, sulfonamides, cromolyn sodium, carbamazepine
	Pulmonary edema	?	Opiates, hydrochlorothiazide
	Other	?IV	Nitrofurantoin, gold
Hepatic	Acute hepatitis	?IV	Halothane, isoniazid, methyldopa
	Cholestatic jaundice	?	Phenothiazines
	Chronic active hepatitis	?	Methyldopa, nitrofurantoin
Renal	Acute interstitial nephritis	?II, ?IV	Penicillin, methicillin, nonsteroidal anti-inflammatory drugs
	Chronic interstitial nephritis	?	Analgesics (aspirin, phenacetin)
	Nephrotic syndrome	?	Trimethadione (Tridione), paramethadione (Paradione), gold
Cardiac	Myocarditis	?	Methyldopa, sulfonamides, penicillin
Neurologic	Encephalomyelitis	?IV	Live virus vaccines
	Myasthenic syndrome	II	Penicillamine

*Gell and Coombs' classification (see Table 12-1).

Table 12-4. Cutaneous manifestations of drug reactions

Type	Probable mechanism(s)*	Examples
Urticaria, angioedema	I, ?III	Penicillin, insulin, sulfonamides
Maculopapular, morbilliform	?	Ampicillin, barbiturates, sulfonamides
Contact sensitivity	IV	Antihistamines, neomycin, ethylenediamines, parabens
Fixed drug eruption	?IV	Phenolphthalein, barbiturates, tetracycline
Erythema multiforme (including Stevens-Johnson syndrome)	?	Sulfonamides, penicillin, phenytoin sodium (Dilantin), phenylbutazone
Toxic epidermal necrolysis	?IV	Sulfonamides, phenylbutazone, penicillin
Erythema nodosum	?	Oral contraceptives, iodides
Purpura	?	Sulfonamides, barbiturates, antihistamines
Exfoliative dermatitis	?	Carbamazepine, gold, sulfonamides
Photosensitivity eruptions	IV	Sulfonamides

*Gell and Coombs' classification (see Table 12-1).

    B. Determine the **temporal relationship** between exposure and symptoms. Except for anaphylactic-type reactions, 7–10 days is a common period before symptoms appear.

    C. Determine the **route of administration, duration of treatment,** and **prior drug exposure.** Allergic drug reactions increase in frequency with intermittent, repeated, high-dose parenteral administration of a drug. It is helpful but **not mandatory** to establish that a sensitizing dose was received (as many patients do not recall a prior exposure).

    D. Obtain a detailed history of the **presenting clinical manifestations** and correlate them with the various forms of drug allergy (see Tables 12-3 and 12-4).

    E. A history of symptoms subsiding promptly on discontinuation of the drug suggests allergy to that drug. Symptoms resulting from depot drugs or drugs with long half-lives, however, may persist. Occult sources of continued drug exposure should also be considered.

II. Immunologic tests in drug allergy. To confirm a drug allergy, one must demonstrate a relevant immunologic reaction to the drug or its metabolites. Most drugs, usually simple chemicals (molecular weight approximately 1000 daltons), are not immunogenic but require complexing with a carrier protein to elicit an immunologic response. Often, the organic radicals formed by these complexes do not cross-react antigenically with the parent compound. Thus, the difficulty in immunologic testing for drug allergy lies in the fact that, for most drugs, testing with the drug itself does not utilize the antigen responsible for the symptoms.

    A. Skin testing

        1. Immediate skin tests

            a. Immediate skin tests involve the development of a wheal-and-flare reaction caused by mediator release from mast cells. This mediator release is attributed to an IgE antibody-bridging reaction and requires that the skin test material have at least **two** antigenic determinants per molecule, a property uncharacteristic of most simple univalent drugs. Only a few drugs complex with skin site proteins or form polymers in solution, resulting in the formation of **multideterminant molecules.**

   b. Another problem with immediate-type skin testing is that false-positive reactions may occur if the drug is a **direct histamine releaser** (e.g., codeine) or is **too concentrated.**

   c. The only **simple drug** for which reliable skin test materials are currently available is **penicillin. Large-molecular-weight drugs,** such as toxoids, antisera, insulin, adrenocorticotropic hormone (ACTH), and egg-protein vaccines, are sufficiently antigenic to use as immediate skin test material. Simultaneous normal patient controls are needed to rule out irritant responses if standard protocols are unavailable.

2. **Positive delayed skin tests** reflect previous lymphocyte sensitization. In some individual cases, delayed skin test reactions have been reported to correlate well with delayed-onset reactions to corticosteroids, ampicillin, and local anesthetics. However, delayed skin testing in most clinical situations involving possible drug allergy **has not** been established as a useful diagnostic procedure. In addition, the chances of **sensitizing** or causing a **severe immediate reaction** with intradermal administration of a drug significantly decrease the desirability of such testing.

3. **Patch tests** read at 48–72 hours are of value for diagnosing contact sensitivity to topically applied medicines (see Chap. 8). Their usefulness in evaluating allergic reactions to parenterally or orally administered drugs is questionable. One report states that in a series of 30 patients with drug-related rashes, patch testing with the drug produced negative results in all cases. Other reports, however, have demonstrated positive patch test reactions in patients with maculopapular or eczematoid rashes following oral practolol, diazepam, meprobamate, and penicillin.

B. In vitro tests

1. In vitro tests for **immediate hypersensitivity** include **total serum IgE levels, specific IgE antibody levels,** as measured by the radioallergosorbent test (RAST), and **histamine release** from mast cells or basophils (see Chap. 2).

   a. Total serum IgE has been reported to rise with an acute allergic drug reaction and fall subsequently. The patient's prior serum IgE level must be known to make this test useful.

   b. A RAST for antibodies to antigenic determinants in penicillin allergy correlates well with the results of skin testing and provocative testing.

   c. Rat peritoneal mast cells, after sensitization with serum from penicillin-allergic patients, will degranulate on subsequent exposure to penicillin.

   d. Although these in vitro studies eliminate the risk of skin testing, they require time and special laboratory capability, which limit their usefulness.

   e. In vitro studies are probably less sensitive than skin testing, and a RAST for antibodies to minor determinants of penicillin is not available.

2. In vitro tests for **IgG and IgM** antibodies are indicated in conditions caused by cytotoxic antibodies, such as may occur in hematologic reactions.

3. **Tests for sensitized lymphocytes** can be measured by the **lymphocyte transformation test** or the **production of lymphokines** or both.

   a. The lymphocyte transformation test involves the culture of peripheral blood lymphocytes with an antigen, e.g., a drug. A positive reaction occurs when the lymphocytes undergo transformation or blastogenesis, as evidenced by the incorporation of tritiated thymidine. A positive reaction with appropriate controls indicates a lymphocyte-mediated reaction against the drug. A positive lymphocyte transformation test reaction in well-controlled situations has been reported with the following symptoms:

(1) Fever, rash, edema, lymphadenopathy, impaired liver function, and eosinophilia caused by carbamazepine.

(2) Exofoliative dermatitis caused by phenytoin sodium.

(3) Pulmonary infiltrates caused by nitrofurantoin.

(4) Hepatitis caused by halothane.

(5) Dermatitis caused by nickel salts.

(6) Dermatitis caused by mestranol.

(7) Urticaria and dermatitis caused by certain antituberculosis drugs. Factors limiting the use of the lymphocyte transformation test for diagnosis of drug allergy include the need for specialized equipment, delay in obtaining results, uncertainty about the appropriate hapten-carrier antigen, and the frequent inability to relate positive tests and immunologic mechanisms in suspected drug allergy.

b. **Lymphokine production,** such as macrophage migration inhibition factor, is probably a more specific indicator of lymphocyte sensitization than is the lymphocyte transformation test. Although positive results have been reported, especially with penicillin allergy, the same limiting factors as apply to the lymphocyte transformation test make its clinical usefulness impractical at this time.

c. **Direct challenge** can confirm the relationship of a suspected drug to a given clinical syndrome. **Because of the potential morbidity and mortality involved,** however, **this test is generally unjustified.** When a drug is essential in a patient with a past history of an adverse reaction to it, direct challenge in the form of **incremental challenge testing** (see next section, I.C) can be considered, but only if experienced physicians and resuscitative equipment are available.

Prevention of Allergic Drug Reactions and Approach to Patients with a History of a Prior Reaction

Prevention is the most effective way to minimize morbidity and mortality from drug reactions. Prevention involves two main principles. First, avoid the use of any drugs, especially those that are more likely than others to be associated with drug reactions, unless a definite medical indication exists. Second, obtain a careful history of drugs to which the patient has previously had an adverse reaction and avoid these drugs and those that may cross-react with them. In addition to the well-known relationships between the penicillins and cephalosporins, there is cross-reactivity among the aminoglycosides (streptomycin, kanamycin, neomycin, and gentamycin), and there is potential (although unpredictable) cross-reactivity among the para-aminobenzine derivatives (sulfonamide antibiotics, sulfonylurea hypoglycemics, thiazide diuretics, acetazolamide, procaine, procainamide, and aminosalicylic acid). Prevention is a prime consideration in patients with a history of an adverse drug reaction, since such patients can be at increased risk of a reaction on subsequent exposure to that drug. The magnitude of this risk depends on a number of factors, including the type of previous reaction and the duration since the last exposure to the drug. The physician must determine these factors to weigh the magnitude of the risk of readministration against the risk of not using the drug.

I. **Classification of prior reaction.** Attempt to classify the drug reaction as previously outlined.

A. **A non-drug-related reaction** should occur only if the same psychogenic or coincidental factors are present now.

B. **Dose-related effects** in normal persons can recur if the same dosage is utilized. These reactions should not increase in intensity and may be prevented by dose reduction.

C. **Immunologic reactions** in susceptible persons require special consideration because these reactions can occur on readministration of the drug (unless adequate time has passed to allow loss of immunologic reactivity), can increase in intensity on repeat exposure, and may be fatal.

1. **Immediate-type immunologic reaction.** Because they can potentially become **rapidly fatal,** immediate-type immunologic reactions should be carefully considered.

   a. A history of anaphylaxis, urticaria, or angioedema in the past increases the present risk. On the other hand, a history of a maculopapular rash only (at least for penicillin) may not increase the risk of an immediate-type reaction. However, **histories** of drug "rashes" are often vague and may not allow for accurate differentiation of a maculopapular eruption from an urticarial rash, or a rash associated with serum sickness or vasculitis. A patient with a history of a well-defined, **non-immediate-type** immunologic drug reaction in the past (e.g., serum sickness or vasculitis) may not be at increased risk of a subsequent immediate-type reaction, but this risk cannot be determined **with certainty** by the history.

   b. **Incremental challenge testing.** Because of the limitations of historic data and the current lack of immunologic methods that assess the risk of an immediate-type reaction accurately for most drugs, apply the following approach to patients with histories of possible immune-mediated reactions (refer to approaches to specific, frequently involved drugs under Special Considerations in Drug Allergy):

      (1) The safest approach that proves satisfactory in most clinical situations is to substitute a **non-cross-reactive** drug.

      (2) In clinical circumstances in which a specific drug is essential because there are no adequate non-cross-reacting substitutes, **incremental challenge testing** is recommended. This technique uses small initial doses of the drug, followed by incremental dose increases until a therapeutic dose is reached. Although incremental challenge testing resembles true "desensitization," it is not necessarily desensitization because sensitization has not been proved. Rather, this practical procedure allows the physician to determine, as safely as possible, whether or not a patient who is possibly allergic to an essential drug can tolerate it when no acceptable substitutes exist. When incremental challenge testing is to be done, the following guidelines should be observed:

         (a) Inform the patient carefully and completely regarding the benefits and risks of the incremental challenge testing procedure.

         (b) If possible, obtain consultation from an appropriate specialty service regarding the absolute need for the drug.

         (c) Perform the test in the hospital under the supervision of a physician experienced in the procedure and with personnel and facilities immediately available for treatment of anaphylaxis.

         (d) Generally use the route of administration by which the drug will be administered.

         (e) Administer test doses 15 minutes apart (although a longer interval may be desirable for oral administration). A sample incremental challenge testing protocol is shown in Table 12-5.

   c. **Desensitization.** If during the incremental challenge testing procedure the patient experiences an immediate-type reaction, the decision as to further treatment usually favors **no** treatment with the drug. However, in **rare** life-threatening situations, treatment with the drug may be required. In this situation, true **desensitization** can be attempted.

      (1) If a minimal to a moderate local reaction has occurred, repeat the same dose and then increase cautiously.

      (2) If systemic symptoms or a large local reaction has occurred, decrease the dose and increase in smaller increments.

      (3) Treat anaphylactic manifestations (Chap. 10).

II. In general, **non-immediate-type immunologic reactions** contraindicate readministration because no "desensitization" method has been reported to prevent a type II,

Table 12-5. Sample incremental challenge testing protocol

Dose number	Dilution[a]	Volume (ml)
1	1:100	Puncture test
2	Undiluted	Puncture test
3	1:100,000	0.1[b]
4	1:10,000	0.1[b]
5	1:1000	0.1[b]
6	1:100	0.1[b]
7	1:10	0.1[b]
8	Undiluted	0.1[b]
9	Undiluted	0.5[b]
10	Undiluted	1.0[b]

[a] Serial 10-fold dilutions of the undiluted drug are usually made on a weight/volume basis.
[b] Intradermal.

III, or IV reaction from occurring in a susceptible patient. However, sensitivity may no longer be present, and, if the drug is absolutely essential with no adequate substitute, incremental challenge testing may be attempted.

Treatment of Drug Reactions

I. **Discontinuation of the responsible drug** is the most important treatment in an ongoing drug reaction. Many patients experiencing a drug reaction are taking multiple drugs, and, as discussed earlier, the causative drug may not be readily identifiable. In this situation, discontinue the drugs that are more likely to be causing the reaction (based on the considerations previously discussed) and least essential for the patient's well-being.

II. **Symptomatic therapy.** The pharmacologic or symptomatic treatment of an ongoing drug reaction will depend on the clinical manifestations.

   A. For many reactions, especially cutaneous, **discontinuation** of the responsible drug suffices.

   B. The symptomatic treatment of anaphylaxis, urticaria, asthma, or contact dermatitis due to drug allergy is the same as the treatment when these conditions are the result of other causes.

   C. **Corticosteroids and antihistamines.** Aspirin and antihistamines often suffice in the treatment of serum sickness, but corticosteroids may be necessary. Local treatment of the pruritus associated with maculopapular eruptions is often sufficient, but antihistamines may be useful in addition. Corticosteroids are necessary, however, when exfoliative dermatitis is present. Supportive treatment of hematologic drug reactions may include transfusions, and the addition of corticosteroids may serve to decrease cell destruction. Corticosteroids may also be useful in hastening recovery from vasculitic, hepatic, renal, and pulmonary reactions. Certain patients with vasculitis possibly related to drug reactions may require cytotoxic therapy in addition.

Special Considerations in Drug Allergy

The general rules for the diagnosis and management of possible allergic reactions to drugs have been presented in preceding sections. Several drugs are exceptions because immediate-type reactions to these drugs are not IgE-mediated or because skin test reagents predictive of IgE-mediated reactivity to these drugs are available. These drugs warrant special consideration. Immunizing agents are in this category. However, allergic reactions to these agents are covered in Chap. 19.

I. **Penicillin allergy**

A. **Incidence.** Allergic reactions to penicillin and its derivatives are the most common examples of drug allergy. The frequency of penicillin reactions ranges from 1–10%, with systemic anaphylaxis occurring in about 15 patients per 100,000 treated with penicillin. An estimated 300 lives per year in the United States are lost because of penicillin reactions.

B. **Types of reactions.** Allergic reactions to penicillin have been classified as immediate, accelerated, or late.

1. **Immediate reactions,** which include urticaria and anaphylaxis, usually begin within 30 minutes of receiving the drug and can be life-threatening.

2. **Accelerated reactions** begin 2–72 hours after drug administration and consist of urticaria, pruritis, wheezing, or laryngeal edema.

3. **Late reactions,** occurring after 72 or more hours, are the most common reactions to penicillin and are usually manifested as morbilliform rashes, urticaria, or fever. Penicillin is also the most common cause of serum sickness–type reactions. In addition, it can cause a late reaction consisting of recurrent urticaria and arthralgia without the fever, lymphadenopathy, or splenomegaly that accompany serum sickness. Less common penicillin reactions include hemolytic anemia, nephritis, granulocytopenia, thrombocytopenia, and neuritis.

C. **Antigenic determinants**

1. Penicillin is a simple low-molecular-weight substance that must form multivalent drug-protein complexes to become immunogenic. In vitro, the major degradation product of penicillin consists of benzylpenicilloyl (BPO) haptenic groups. Thus, these groups are known as the **major antigenic determinant.** Benzylpenicillin can react with a synthetic polypeptide (polylysine) to form penicilloyl-polylysine, which is nonimmunogenic (does not sensitize the patient) but produces an immediate positive skin test reaction that is diagnostic in patients with penicilloyl-specific IgE antibody. This major determinant has been associated with accelerated and late urticarial reactions. A penicilloyl-polylysine reagent is marketed commercially for skin testing as Pre-Pen.*

2. Other degradation products of penicillin that can form hapten-protein conjugates are called **minor determinants.** The minor determinant mixture is **not commercially available,** but dilute solutions of fresh and 2-week-"old" penicillin G (10,000 units/ml) are suggested as a substitute for skin testing purposes. The minor determinants are important in immediate and, to a lesser degree, accelerated reactions. Table 12-6 summarizes the role of the various antigenic determinants in penicillin reactions.

D. **Diagnostic approach**

1. Obtain a detailed **history.** Inquire about local anesthetic allergy if procaine penicillin is to be used.

2. Establish a sound, current **indication** for penicillin therapy. If an alternative drug is acceptable, use it in a patient with a positive history since skin testing is not completely without risk or totally reliable. Do **not** do a skin test to satisfy your curiosity or that of the patient. Generally, use skin testing in history-positive patients for whom alternative drugs are not available.

3. Perform testing immediately before institution of penicillin therapy to avoid interim sensitization.

4. Skin tests with Pre-Pen, or a minor determinant mixture, or diluted penicillin G are predictive of immediate and accelerated allergic reactions but

*Kremers-Urban Co., P.O. Box 2038, 5600 W. County Line Road, Milwaukee, WI 53201.

Table 12-6. Immunology of penicillin reactions

Reaction	Primary antigen	Antibody class
Anaphylaxis	MDM	IgE
Accelerated reaction	BPO	IgE
Hemolysis	BPO linked to red cell membrane	IgG, IgM
Interstitial nephritis	BPO linked to tubular membrane	IgG, IgM
Maculopapular rash	?BPO	?IgM Delayed hypersensitivity

Key: MDM = minor determinant mixture (benzylpenicillin, benzylpenicilloate, benzylpenilloate, and alpha-benzylpenicilloyl-amine); BPO = benzylpenicilloyl haptenic group.

have no role in the **predictive** or **post hoc** evaluation of drug fevers, serum sickness, maculopapular eruptions, hematologic reactions, or nephritis. One method of using penicillin skin testing is discussed in **5.**

5. In patients with a **vague history,** perform skin testing first by scratch or prick testing with Pre-Pen and penicillin G (freshly prepared and "old" solutions), diluted 10,000 units/ml in physiologic saline. In patients with a **strong history** of an immediate-type systemic reaction, begin with decreased concentrations of penicillin G (i.e., 10, 100, 1000 units/ml). Use simultaneous saline controls and inquire about prior antihistamine therapy within the preceding 72 hours. If the scratch tests are negative, proceed to intradermal testing using Pre-Pen and dilutions of penicillin G (100, 1000, 10,000 units/ml) sequentially. (Inject a volume of 0.02 ml for intradermal testing.) Read tests 15 minutes after placement. Any positive skin test mandates the discontinuance of further testing and precludes the use of any penicillin drug in that patient unless clinical desensitization is used. Advise all patients whose skin tests are positive that they are **currently** sensitive, they should avoid penicillin derivatives, and they should wear a Medic Alert tag.

6. **Interpretation of the skin tests** and the limits of their predictability have been investigated in a cooperative study by the American Academy of Allergy (*J. Allergy Clin. Immunol.* 60:339, 1977). Of patients with a positive penicillin allergy history, 19% had a positive skin test to Pre-Pen, penicillin G, or both, whereas 7% of patients with a negative history had positive skin tests. Skin tests were positive in 46% of patients with a history of anaphylaxis, 17% of patients with a history of urticaria, and 7% of patients with a history of maculopapular rash. On challenge with penicillin, 6% of patients with a positive history reacted versus 2% of patients with a negative history. In nine challenged patients with a positive skin test, a reaction occurred in six, of whom three were immediate or accelerated reactors. When 346 patients with a negative skin test were challenged, 3% had a reaction, but less than 1% had an early-type reaction thought to be mediated by IgE. Penicillin allergy is a **variable state,** and approximately 75% of all patients thought to be sensitive to penicillin may tolerate the drug at some later date. For this reason, skin testing is more reliable than history alone for predicting **current** allergic status.

E. **Management of patients with positive skin tests**

1. Use alternative antibiotics, if possible, in any patient with a positive skin test reaction to penicillin. Suggestions for alternative antibiotics are found in Table 12-7.

2. The use of **semisynthetic analogs** and **cephalosporins** in penicillin-allergic patients has been incompletely studied. Semisynthetic penicillins contain a six-amino penicillanic nucleus, which accounts for their ability to

Table 12-7. Alternative antibiotics for penicillin-allergic patients

Infection	Antibiotic
Streptococcal prophylaxis	Erythromycin, sulfonamides
Streptococcal infections	Erythromycin
Streptococcus viridans endocarditis	Vancomycin
Pneumococcal pneumonia	Erythromycin
Staphylococcal infection (minor)	Erythromycin
Staphylococcal infection (severe)	Vancomycin
Purulent meningitis (with *Diplococcus pneumoniae, Neisseria meningitidis,* or *Haemophilus influenzae*)	Chloramphenicol
Gonorrhea	Tetracycline or spectinomycin
Syphilis	Erythromycin or tetracycline
Clostridial infections	Clindamycin*
Enterococcal endocarditis	Vancomycin (with gentamycin or streptomycin)

*Some strains of clostridia are resistant to clindamycin.

form antigenic complexes. All patients with presumed or proved penicillin sensitivity should be considered allergic to the semisynthetic analogs of penicillin.

   a. If a specific semisynthetic penicillin is proposed for use, one may test for allergy by doing a prick puncture using the drug. If the results are negative, incremental challenge testing (see p. 251) can be done with the drug, using the proposed route of administration. Because of the unknown relation between penicillin G testing and subsequent administration of semisynthetic penicillins, this may be the safest approach.

   b. Because cephalosporins contain the seven-amino cephalosporanic acid nucleus, they are not chemically defined as penicillins. However, they do share with penicillin the common and highly reactive beta-lactam ring structure, which probably accounts for the partial cross-antigenicity. Patients with a history of penicillin allergy have a fourfold increase in allergic reactions to cephalosporins when compared with patients without a history of penicillin allergy. Moreover, patients with a positive skin test to penicilloyl-polylysine and a positive history have an incidence of reactions to cephalosporins approaching 50%. Although skin tests for cephalosporins have been recommended, the appropriate antigens have not been validated. Therefore, it seems prudent to seek alternatives other than the cephalosporins in penicillin-allergic patients.

  3. Certain clinical situations can mandate penicillin use even in patients with a positive history and positive skin tests. **Enterococcal endocarditis** and other life-threatening infections (when there has been no improvement with alternative antibiotics) may be indications for cautious administration of penicillin **(penicillin desensitization)**.

   a. This procedure has produced fatalities and requires strict physician supervision and intensive care unit monitoring.

   b. In most instances the patients experience allergic symptoms— **controlled anaphylaxis** is the goal. A parenteral desensitization schedule is outlined in Table 12-8. An oral desensitization schedule with less risk of reaction is found in Table 12-9.

   c. Reserve the use of antihistamines, adrenergic drugs, and corticosteroids for the appearance of symptoms. Prophylactic use or simultaneous administration of these agents has not been shown to protect against anaphylaxis and can suppress milder symptoms that precede an anaphylactic reaction.

Table 12-8. Desensitization schedule for cautious parenteral administration of penicillin

A. Preparation of solutions with aqueous crystalline penicillin G:
   1. Dilute 5-million-unit vial to 5 ml = 1 million units/ml (solution 1).
   2. Dilute 1 ml of solution 1 to 10 ml = 100,000 units/ml (solution 2).
   3. Dilute 1 ml of solution 2 to 10 ml = 10,000 units/ml (solution 3).
   4. Dilute 1 ml of solution 3 to 10 ml = 1,000 units/ml (solution 4).
   5. Dilute 1 ml of solution 4 to 10 ml = 100 units/ml (solution 5).
B. Administration
   1. Scratch-test 1 drop of solution 3 on forearm. If negative at 15 min, proceed to 2.*
   2. Administer intradermal test with 0.02 ml of solution 5. If negative,* proceed with penicillin administration as outlined in C. Record blood pressure, pulse, and respiration at 5-min intervals.
C.

Solution number	Concentration (units/ml)	Subcutaneous injections every 15 min	
		Volume	Units
5	100	0.05	5
		0.1	10
		0.2	20
		0.4	40
		0.8	80
4	1,000	0.15	150
		0.3	300
		0.6	600
		1.0	1,000
3	10,000	0.2	2,000
		0.4	4,000
		0.8	8,000
2	100,000	0.15	15,000
		0.3	30,000
		0.6	60,000
		1.0	100,000
1	1,000,000	0.2	200,000
		0.4	400,000
		0.8	800,000

D. Continuous intravenous penicillin G therapy may be started at this point. Serious difficulties with the present course of penicillin therapy are not expected at this point, although delayed or late reactions may occur.

*If positive, decrease to a more dilute solution and begin subcutaneous administration with a dose 10-fold below positive intradermal concentration.

    d. All patients being desensitized should have an indwelling intravenous line for rapid administration of medications and fluids, if necessary, and resuscitation equipment should be available. The treatment of anaphylaxis is discussed in Chapter 10.

II. Aspirin sensitivity. Aspirin is second to penicillin as a cause of adverse drug reactions. Nonallergic adverse reactions that may be due to aspirin include nephrotoxicity related to salicylate abuse, hemolytic anemia in patients deficient in glucose 6-phosphate dehydrogenase, abnormal platelet function, gastrointestinal toxicity, hepatitis, and bone marrow suppression.

Three types of syndromes resembling allergic reactions occur within 2–3 hours of aspirin ingestion: aspirin-sensitive asthma/rhinitis, urticaria/angioedema, and anaphylactoid reactions. The first two reactions are most common.

Table 12-9. Oral desensitization protocol for penicillin

Dose[a]	Penicillin G units	Route
1	100	PO
2	200	PO
3	400	PO
4	800	PO
5	1600	PO
6	3200	PO
7	6400	PO
8	12,500	PO
9	25,000	PO
10	50,000	PO
11	100,000	PO
12	200,000	PO
13	400,000	PO
14	800,000	PO
	Wait 30 min	
15	100,000	IV
16	200,000	IV
17	400,000	IV
18	800,000	IV

[a] Interval between doses, 15 min.
From T. J. Sullivan. Allergic reactions to antimicrobial agents. *J. Allergy Clin. Immunol.* 74:594, 1984. With permission.

A. Aspirin-sensitive asthma

1. **Incidence.** An estimated 2.5% of an allergic population with rhinitis, asthma, or both will experience adverse reactions to aspirin. As many as 28% of children with chronic severe asthma can show a significant reduction in pulmonary function following aspirin ingestion. The prevalence of aspirin sensitivity by oral challenge in the subpopulation of asthma patients afflicted with nasal polyps and sinusitis rises to 30–40%. Females experience more adverse reactions than do males—as high as 2:1 in some studies. The genetics of aspirin sensitivity are not known, but a familial occurrence may exist.

2. **Pathogenesis**

   a. An immunologic mechanism has not been proved in most aspirin-sensitive asthmatic patients. Skin tests with aspiryl-polylysine, agglutinating antibodies to aspiryl-coated erythrocytes, lymphocyte transformation testing with aspirin as the antigen, and complement activation studies indicate no significant difference between aspirin-sensitive patients and control groups.

   b. Aspirin can cause **acetylation** of serum and cellular proteins as it is metabolized to acetic and salicylic acids. Theoretically, this acetylation could change the antigenicity of the protein and evoke autoimmune mechanisms. Also, acetylation could alter neurohumoral or other receptors in the lungs or other tissues. However, the acetylation theory is questionable since nonacetylating drugs such as indomethacin can produce similar symptoms.

   Additional nonimmunologic mechanisms have been suggested, including altered responses of kinin receptors, activation of tissue enzymes by aspirin due to the lack of a hypothetical enzyme inhibitor, and aspirin-induced activation of the alternate complement pathway. There is neither clinical nor experimental support for the first two possibilities, and the results of studies of complement activation during aspirin-induced bronchospasm have been conflicting.

c. **Prostaglandin synthesis inhibition** (through inhibition of the cyclooxygenase pathway for arachidonic acid metabolism) is a function of aspirin, indomethacin, ibuprofen, and mefenamic acid. These seemingly unrelated compounds are all capable of provoking asthma in sensitive patients. The prostaglandin E series produces bronchodilation, while the prostaglandin F series causes bronchoconstriction. An imbalance between the effects of aspirin on the two series could cause asthma in susceptible patients. Alternatively, blockade of the cyclooxygenase pathway might increase the formation of products of the lipoxygenase pathway, particularly leukotrienes C and D, which are also capable of causing bronchospasm.

d. Another potential mechanism involves aspirin-induced nonimmunologic release of mediators from respiratory mast cells. This hypothesis would be consistent with the observations that antihistamines or cromolyn sodium blunt the typical aspirin-induced respiratory response. The final explanation for aspirin idiosyncrasy may relate to the complex interactions between the respiratory mast cell, preformed mediators, prostaglandins, and leukotrienes.

3. **Clinical presentation**
   a. The typical aspirin-sensitive asthmatic patient begins with perennial rhinitis during young to middle age that may be exacerbated by aspirin intake. Subsequently, nasal polyps, hyperplastic and purulent sinusitis, peripheral eosinophilia, and asthma typically develop at variable intervals, leading to the classic "aspirin-triad" of asthma, nasal polyps, and aspirin idiosyncrasy. Aspirin-sensitive asthma can occur in patients without significant rhinitis, polyps, or sinusitis. Although nearly 50% of aspirin-sensitive asthmatics may have positive skin tests, the asthma in such patients is usually triggered primarily by nonallergic or unidentifiable factors.

   b. Acute aspirin-induced asthma may be severe, prolonged, and occasionally fatal; is usually associated with profound nasal congestion, rhinorrhea, and/or ocular injection and is occasionally associated with syncope; and should be treated vigorously, with therapy that includes the use of parenteral corticosteroids.

4. **Diagnosis**
   a. The **history** and **physical findings** in aspirin-sensitive patients can be similar to such findings in other patients with asthma or rhinitis. A history of aspirin intolerance may or may not be elicited from the patient. Nasal polyps, commonly found in patients with the aspirin triad syndrome, are not distinctive for aspirin idiosyncrasy.

   b. **Laboratory** and **radiographic studies** such as nasal and peripheral eosinophilia, sinus x-rays showing hyperplastic sinuses and polypoid changes, a prediabetic glucose tolerance test, and increased sensitivity to inhaled methacholine and histamine have all been observed in aspirin-sensitive patients, but are not specifically revealing. Skin tests with aspiryl-polylysine are not helpful in diagnosing aspirin-induced asthma and **are not recommended** because of the danger of anaphylaxis and sensitization.

   c. **Oral challenge** with aspirin is the only definitive way to diagnose current aspirin sensitivity. Such a challenge can identify reactive patients with no previous history of drug sensitivity.
      (1) A protocol for aspirin challenge is described in Table 12-10. However, aspirin challenge is a potentially hazardous procedure and should generally be considered as an investigative tool to be per-

Table 12-10. Protocol for three-day oral aspirin (ASA) challenge[a]

Time of day	Day 1	Day 2	Day 3
8:00 A.M.	Placebo	ASA, 3 mg or 30 mg[d]	ASA, 150 mg
11:00 A.M.	Placebo[b]	ASA, 60 mg	ASA, 325 mg
2:00 P.M.	Placebo[c]	ASA, 100 mg	ASA, 650 mg

[a] Subject must be symptom free. Challenge should be conducted in a hospital setting by experienced personnel equipped to treat anaphylactic or severe asthmatic reactions.
[b] May substitute tartrazine, 25 mg.
[c] May substitute tartrazine, 50 mg.
[d] Begin with 3 mg in more sensitive patients.
From D.D. Stevenson. Diagnosis, prevention, and treatment of adverse reactions to aspirin and nonsteroidal anti-inflammatory drugs. *J. Allergy Clin. Immunol.* 74:617, 1984. With permission.

Table 12-11. Pharmacotherapy in aspirin-sensitive patients

Drugs to be avoided	Permissible drugs*
Amidopyrine	Acetaminophen
Antipyrine	Choline magnesium trisalicylate
Diflunisal	Choline salicylate
Ditazole	Chloroquine
Fenoprofen	Narcotics (e.g., codeine, meperidine)
Flufenamic acid	Propoxyphene
Ibuprofen	Salicylamide
Indomethacin	Salsalate
Ketoprofen	Sodium salicylate
Meclofenamate	
Mefenamic acid	
Naproxen	
Noramidopyrine	
Oxyphenbutazone	
Phenylbutazone	
Piroxicam	
Sulindac	
Tartrazine-(FD&C yellow dye no. 5) containing drugs	
Tolmetin	
Zomepirac	

*Reactions in some patients have been reported.

formed only at allergy centers by experienced personnel with intensive care units immediately accessible.

  (2) In lieu of performing challenge testing, routinely advise asthmatic patients, especially those who are corticosteroid-dependent or who manifest nasal polyps, to avoid aspirin and other nonsteroidal anti-inflammatory drugs (Table 12-11).

5. Treatment

  a. The patient must avoid all aspirin-containing drugs as well as other anti-inflammatory drugs that work through inhibition of prostaglandin synthesis (Table 12-11). Caution patients to read labels routinely and to note aspirin is also termed acetylsalicylic acid or salicylic acid acetate. Table 12-11 presents guidelines for drug use in the aspirin-sensitive patient.

b. **Tartrazine** (FD&C No. 5), a yellow dye used as a food and drug coloring additive, may cause adverse reactions in some aspirin-sensitive individuals. Such sensitivity can be confirmed using an oral challenge test (see Table 12-10). Tartrazine-sensitive patients should avoid tartrazine-dyed (yellow or orange) foods and drugs (see Appendix XII.D).

c. Aggressive medical treatment of rhinitis, sinusitis, nasal polyps, and asthma, as outlined in Chaps. 4, 5, and 6, is mandatory. Inhalational or systemic corticosteroids or both are often needed to obtain control of symptoms. Either **surgical drainage** of sinuses or **polypectomies** (or both) are necessary if sinusitis or nasal polyps are refractory to medical treatment. There is no evidence that these surgical procedures exacerbate asthma, and there is increasing evidence that control of coexisting rhinosinusitis in patients with asthma benefits the asthma.

d. If aspirin or other nonsteroidal anti-inflammatory drugs are required for management of a concomitant disease in a patient with a history of aspirin sensitivity, aspirin challenge may be advisable. After a positive oral challenge, aspirin desensitization, as described by Stevenson (*J. Allergy Clin. Immunol.* 74:620, 1984), may be considered. The potential therapeutic benefit of such aspirin desensitization for the asthma or rhinitis in aspirin-sensitive patients is under current investigation.

6. **Prognosis.** If aspirin idiosyncrasy is detected early and treated properly with appropriate preventive and therapeutic measures, it should have no worse a prognosis than other late-onset, nonreaginic asthmatic syndromes. Aspirin avoidance has no apparent influence on the general course of aspirin-sensitive asthma other than to prevent aspirin-induced exacerbations.

B. **Urticaria/angioedema**

1. Urticaria/angioedema may be associated with aspirin ingestion through one of several distinct mechanisms.

a. Aspirin and other nonsteroidal anti-inflammatory drugs may aggravate chronic urticaria in a dose-related and apparently pharmacologic manner. Approximately one-third of patients whose urticaria is aggravated by aspirin will also have their urticaria aggravated by tartrazine. Patients with chronic urticaria should be advised to avoid aspirin and other nonsteroidal anti-inflammatory drugs, and patients whose urticaria is aggravated by aspirin should probably be tried on a salicylate- and dye-free diet.

b. Aspirin and other prostaglandin synthetase inhibitors may precipitate urticaria in some patients **without** chronic urticaria. In some of these patients, rhinitis or asthma may occur along with the urticaria.

c. Aspirin may occasionally induce urticaria on an immunologic basis. Aspirin anhydride (a contaminant of commercial acetylsalicylic acid) and the aspiryl hapten have been associated with IgE-mediated responses in some patients with aspirin-induced urticaria.

III. **Local anesthetics**

A. **Classification of reactions.** Adverse reactions following administration of local anesthetics can be classified as shown in Table 12-12. Although adverse reactions commonly occur, true local anesthetic (IgE-mediated) allergy appears to be extremely rare. Coincidental reactions or reactions due to the direct toxic effects of the local anesthetic are probably more frequent. Although the clinical manifestations of the prior reaction can help characterize it and better predict the present risk, many features, such as local swelling, hypotension, tachycardia, and syncope, are seen in nonallergic reactions as well.

B. **Specific drugs.** Local anesthetics can be divided into two groups (Table 12-13): Group I contains the benzoic acid esters, and group II includes drugs with the amide structure. On the basis of **contact dermatitis** studies, it is believed that

Table 12-12. Classification of adverse reactions following local anesthetic administration

Reactions not due to local anesthetic agent
    Psychomotor responses
        Hyperventilation
        Vasovagal syncope
        Endogenous sympathetic stimulation
    Operative trauma
Toxic responses in normal persons
    Central nervous system effects
    Cardiovascular effects
    Local effects
Responses in susceptible persons
    Idiosyncratic
    Allergic

Table 12-13. Local anesthetic grouping

Group I: Benzoic acid esters	Group II: Others
Benzocaine	Bupivacaine (Marcaine)*
Chloroprocaine (Nesacaine)	Dibucaine (Nupercaine)*
Cyclomethycaine (Surfacaine)	Dyclonine (Dyclone)
Hexylcaine (Cyclaine)	Etidocaine (Duranest)*
Procaine (Novocain)	Lidocaine (Xylocaine)*
Proparacaine (Ophthaine)	Mepivacaine (Carbocaine)*
Tetracaine (Pontocaine)	Pramoxine (Tronothane)
	Prilocaine (Citanest)*

*Amides.

group I drugs do not cross-react with group II drugs, and that group II drugs do not cross-react with each other. **Anecdotal** clinical information suggests that reactions occur less frequently with group II drugs than with group I drugs.

C. Approach to the patient
   1. Avoidance of local anesthetic agents may be possible in patients with suspected "caine" allergy. However, avoidance in a patient undergoing a surgical or dental procedure for which a local anesthetic would suffice exposes the patient to increased pain (if no anesthesia is utilized) or increased risk (if general anesthesia is administered). Similarly, no equally effective substitute for lidocaine or procainamide may be available for patients with certain types of cardiac arrhythmia. Avoidance of local anesthetics **may not** be in the patient's best interest, and the risk of not using the drug must be balanced against the risk of a subsequent reaction.
   2. Review carefully the history of the previous reaction. If the history suggests a severe idiosyncratic or allergic reaction, seriously consider anesthetic avoidance.
   3. Because it is often difficult to determine from the history the risk of a subsequent allergic reaction, skin testing and incremental challenge testing have been used to determine whether a patient with a past local anesthetic reaction can tolerate a local anesthetic.
      a. Discuss the benefits and risks of skin testing and incremental challenge with the patient and obtain informed consent.

Table 12-14. Skin testing and incremental challenge
in administration of local anesthetics

A. Skin testing Step*	Route	Volume (ml)	Dilution
1	Puncture		1:100
2	Puncture		Undiluted
3	Intradermal	0.02	1:100

B. Subcutaneous incremental challenge Step*		Volume (ml)	Dilution
4		0.1	1:100
5		0.1	1:10
6		0.1	Undiluted
7		0.5	Undiluted
8		1.0	Undiluted

*Administer at 15- to 30-min intervals.

      b. Although skin tests with local anesthetics are of unproved reliability, review of the literature on the use of local anesthetic skin testing suggests it is reasonable to begin the process of identifying a safe local anesthetic for a patient with a history of a prior reaction with skin testing (Table 12-14). The preparation used for skin testing should not contain a vasoconstrictor (which can mask a positive skin test).

      c. Choose a drug for skin testing and challenge that would not be expected to cross-react with the drug implicated in the prior reaction. If the prior drug is unknown, a group II drug should be chosen.

      d. Since preservatives in local anesthetics (parabens, metabisulfite) can cause adverse reactions, consider skin testing challenge and treatment with preparations free of preservatives, particularly if the history suggests possible paraben or metabisulfite sensitivity. Alternatively, consider that the prior local anesthetic reaction could have been IgE-mediated.

      e. If the intradermal skin testing is negative, proceed to the incremental challenge (Table 12-14). If the history was of a delayed reaction, confirm a negative reaction (1) at 24–48 hours after the skin testing before proceeding to incremental challenge and (2) at 24–48 hours after the incremental challenge before proceeding to clinical use. As always with incremental challenges, it must be performed under careful observation and where facilities are available to treat severe adverse reactions.

      f. If incremental challenge is accomplished without adverse reaction, the risk of an adverse reaction to subsequent administration of that drug is apparently no greater than for the general population.

  IV. Anaphylactoid reactions during general anesthesia

    A. Clinical features. Anaphylactoid reactions during general anesthesia are usually due to either the induction agent or the muscle relaxing agent (Table 12-15). The most common clinical features are cutaneous manifestations (erythema, urticaria, or angioedema), hypotension, bronchospasm, and abdominal symptoms. Reactions are reported to occur more commonly in women, patients with a history of "atopy" or asthma, and patients with a history of a prior reaction during general anesthesia.

    B. Pathogenesis. The agents listed in Table 12-15 are all capable of direct histamine release (with the apparent exception of etomidate). Many reactions occur on first exposure, and increased plasma histamine has been reported during such reactions. Thus, exaggerated direct histamine release or increased target organ responsiveness to the histamine released in susceptible individuals may

Table 12-15. Discriminating dilutions of intravenous anesthetic agents for use in skin testing

Drug	Discriminating dilution*	Volume utilized (ml)
Muscle-relaxing agents		
d-Tubocurarine	3 µg/ml	0.02
Succinylcholine	100 µg/ml	0.02
Pancuronium	200 µg/ml	0.02
Gallamine	200 µg/ml	0.02
d-Allylnortoxiferine	50 µg/ml	0.02
Alcuronium	1:1000	0.02
Fazadinium	1:1000	0.02
Decamethonium	1:1000	0.02
Induction agents		
Thiopentone	1:100	0.02
Althesin	1:100	0.02
Propanidid	1:100	0.02
Etomidate	1:100	0.02

*Patients with prior reactions, but not controls, are reported to be positive (> 10-mm wheal) at these concentrations or less.

explain these reactions; however, other data implicate complement-dependent mechanisms (especially with a mixture of alfaxalone and alfadolone [Althesin]) or IgE-mediated mechanisms (especially with muscle relaxants) instead or in addition.

   C. Diagnosis. Skin testing with induction and muscle-relaxing agents has been recommended as a means of defining the responsible drug in patients experiencing an anaphylactoid reaction during general anesthesia, and potentially as a method of defining safe agents for subsequent use. Dilutions of these agents have been described that allegedly distinguish between normal controls and reactive subjects (Table 12-15).

   D. Approach to patients. Treat anaphylactoid reactions during general anesthesia in the standard manner for treating anaphylaxis (see Chap. 10). Only agents to which the subject has negative skin tests should be considered for use during subsequent general anesthesia. However, repeat general anesthesia in these patients must still be approached with great caution since some patients have been reported to have reactions on separate occasions to separate agents, and negative skin tests have not been systematically validated as ensuring subsequent tolerance of an intravenous anesthetic agent. Therefore, in patients with prior anaphylactoid reactions during general anesthesia who require subsequent surgery, the use of volatile anesthetic agents, regional anesthesia, or pretreatment with antihistamines and corticosteroids using a protocol similar to that for radiographic contrast media (see sec. **V**) should be considered.

V. Radiographic contrast media

   A. Clinical features. Adverse reactions occur in 5–8% of patients following administration of a radiographic contrast medium (RCM). Serious reactions occur in 0.1% of patients, and the rate of fatal reactions is reported to be 1 in 40,000 to 1 in 50,000 procedures (a figure as high as 1 in 10,000 has been reported). The clinical manifestations can be classified by the type of the reaction (anaphylactoid, cardiopulmonary, miscellaneous) or the severity (minor, major) (Table 12-16). These reactions, except for renal failure, usually occur within 3–10 minutes after injection. Certain clinical conditions can increase the risk of certain types of contrast media reactions (Table 12-17). Although contrast media reactions can follow any route of exposure, they are most common with intravascular administration.

Table 12-16. Clinical manifestations of contrast media reactions classified by type and severity of reaction

Type of reaction	Anaphylactoid	Cardiopulmonary	Miscellaneous
Minor	Limited urticaria Pruritus Conjunctivitis Rhinitis	ECG changes	Nausea, vomiting Flushing Arm pain Headache Parotid swelling Mild diaphoresis

Major	Generalized
	    urticaria
	Angioedema
	Bronchospasm
	Shock
		Shock
		Pulmonary edema
		Chest pain
		Cardiac arrhythmia
		Cardiopulmonary
		    arrest
			Convulsions
			Acute renal failure

Most common	Urticaria	ECG changes	Nausea, vomiting

Potentially
    fatal
	Shock
	Bronchospasm
	Laryngeal edema
		Shock
		Pulmonary edema
		Cardiac arrhythmia
		    or arrest
			Convulsions
			Renal failure

Table 12-17. Risk factors for contrast media reaction

Factor	Type of reaction
Age over 50 Preexisting cardiovascular disease	Cardiopulmonary
Preexisting renal failure Increased age Entities associated with potential renovascular impairment (diabetes, myeloma, hypertension, dehydration, hyperuricemia)	Acute renal failure
Personal history of allergy, asthma	Mild or moderate anaphylactoid reaction (small increased risk)
History of prior anaphylactoid reaction	Anaphylactoid reaction (large increased risk)

B. **Etiology.** Although many contrast media reactions mimic IgE-mediated reactions, there is little evidence that these reactions are immunologically mediated. The most likely explanation for anaphylactoid reactions—although it is not proved—is that the RCM causes nonimmunologic mediator release in susceptible patients. Possible causes of the other reactions include direct chemotoxic effects, nonimmunologic complement activation, hemodynamic effects of the hypertonic solution, vagal stimulation, or other mechanisms. The majority of deaths following RCM are not associated with the clinical or pathologic features of anaphylaxis, and autopsies often do not reveal the cause of death. Consequently, the cause of most fatal reactions to RCM is unknown.

C. **Prevention** of RCM reactions is difficult for several reasons. Since the reactions are nonimmunologic, sensitivity tests are not predictive. Furthermore, the cause of these reactions is unknown, and they may occur on the first exposure to RCM. Preventive measures, however, can reduce the risk.

1. In a patient with risk factors (see Table 12-17), consider the feasibility of **alternative techniques** (such as radionuclide scanning or ultrasound) that may provide diagnostic information at less risk.

2. Adequately **hydrate** the patient to lessen the risk of acute renal failure in predisposed patients (although acute renal failure has occurred in adequately hydrated patients following contrast media studies).

3. Carefully monitor **renal function** before and after the study in high-risk renal patients, so that supportive treatment of acute renal failure may be instituted as soon as possible.

4. To reduce the risk of pulmonary edema in patients with cardiac disease, **avoid sodium salts** of contrast media.

5. Use **electrocardiographic monitoring** with cardiac patients during the procedure to allow early diagnosis and treatment of potentially fatal cardiac arrhythmias.

6. In terms of prevention of anaphylactoid reactions, if the RCM study **is essential,** the risk and probably the severity of a subsequent reaction can apparently be reduced by pretreatment with **antihistamines** and **corticosteroids.**

   a. Give **prednisone,** 50 mg orally every 6 hours (1 mg/kg/dose for children), beginning 18 hours prior to the procedure; **diphenhydramine,** 1.5 mg/kg intramuscularly (up to 50 mg) 30 minutes to 1 hour prior to the study; and ephedrine, 25 mg orally (0.5–1.0 mg/kg for children) 1 hour prior to the procedure. Omit ephedrine in patients with unstable angina or hypertension.

   b. Whenever RCM is to be administered to a patient with a history of a prior reaction, obtain the patient's informed consent.

   c. Pretreatment can be given to patients with prior **miscellaneous** reactions, such as nausea, vomiting, or flushing, although these types of reactions may not significantly increase the risk of a subsequent adverse reaction.

   d. **Remember:** Serious anaphylactoid RCM reactions may occur even with pretreatment. Therefore, the repeat test must be **essential** and the study must be performed under **careful observation,** with facilities and personnel immediately available to treat an adverse reaction.

   e. Pretreatment for the prevention of cardiopulmonary reactions, convulsions, or renal failure is not effective and **should not** be relied on to prevent these types of reactions.

D. The **treatment** of RCM reactions depends on the clinical manifestations. Minor miscellaneous-type reactions may require no treatment. Treat reactions mimicking IgE-mediated anaphylactic reactions as anaphylaxis (Chap. 10). Use standard therapy for cardiac complications, convulsions, and renal failure following RCM administration.

V. **Insulin allergy and resistance**

A. **Clinical features**

1. Insulin **allergy** can be divided into local and systemic reactions. Although the exact incidence of insulin allergy is unknown, 5–10% of patients receiving insulin can experience reactions that are usually mild, localized, and transient.

   a. **Local reactions,** including swelling, pruritus, and pain, can occur and subside within an hour after insulin injection or may begin up to 24 hours afterward. Some patients exhibit a clearly biphasic reaction, with an early reaction resolving in 1 hour followed by a later, more persistent reaction beginning after 4–6 hours. Local reactions occasionally progress to painful induration that persists for days. Most commonly, they develop within 2 weeks of the initiation of insulin therapy and usually resolve spontaneously within weeks. Large local reactions, however,

especially ones increasing in intensity, can precede a systemic reaction.

   b. Systemic reactions to insulin are relatively uncommon. The most frequent clinical characteristic is generalized urticaria, although other fe-
   tures of anaphylaxis can be present. Systemic reactions usually occur
   soon after reinstitution of insulin therapy after a period, often year
   without it.

2. Insulin **resistance** can be immunologic or nonimmunologic. Nonimmunologic resistance can be associated with such conditions as obesity, ket
   acidosis, endocrine disorders, or infection. Immunologic resistance is very
   rare. It is most common within the first year of insulin therapy, usually
   develops over several weeks, and is usually temporary, lasting only sever
   days to several months. Immunologic insulin resistance develops in some
   patients with insulin allergy within days of initiating insulin desensitiz-
   tion.

B. Etiology. Insulin allergy and immunologic insulin resistance appear to be
classic antigen-antibody reactions. Certain aspects of the involved antigen an
the pathogenic antibody are clinically relevant.

1. The causative **antigen** can be a **noninsulin** protein contaminant or possib
   a nonprotein component (such as protamine or zinc). However, dermal reactions to human insulin and systemic reactions to highly purified insulin in
   patients with insulin allergy suggest that many reactions are directed toward the **insulin molecule itself** or to closely related higher-molecular-
   weight polymers.

2. Commercially available insulins are usually mixtures of beef and por
   insulin, although preparations of only beef, only pork, or synthetic huma
   insulin are now available. Human insulin appears to be less immunogen
   than animal insulins, and pork insulin is generally less immunogenic than
   beef insulin. The latter finding is ascribed to the fact that beef insul'
   differs from human insulin in three amino acids (including two on the
   chain), whereas pork insulin differs only in one amino acid. The A chains c
   pork and human insulins are identical. Although human insulin seen
   generally less immunogenic than pork insulin, there are patients who, by
   skin test titration, are more sensitive to human insulin than to pork in
   sulin.

3. Insulin purification is defined on the basis of the parts per million (ppm) of
   proinsulin contamination. Conventional insulin (previously called "singl
   peak") usually contains 10–25 ppm, whereas purified insulin contains less
   than 10 ppm.

4. The antibody involved in immunologic insulin reactions depends on
   type of reaction. Specific IgE antibody is responsible for generalized allergic
   reactions and probably for many immediate-type local reactions as well a
   certain late-phase reactions. Late-phase reactions are prominent 2–6 hours
   after injection and are usually preceded by an immediate wheal and flar
   (biphasic reaction). Specific IgG antibody causes immunologic insulin resistance; an IgG-mediated Arthus-type reaction is responsible for some late-
   onset local reactions that are prominent 4–12 hours after injection. Deve
   opment of IgG-"blocking" antibody may be responsible for the transient
   nature of many local allergic reactions and for long-term maintenance of
   tolerance in patients desensitized for insulin allergy. Finally, certain loca
   reactions that are prominent 8–24 hours after injection may be due to
   delayed hypersensitivity to the insulin itself or to zinc.

C. Management of insulin allergy

1. **Local reactions** are usually mild and transient, with no specific therapy
   needed. For more troublesome or persistent local reactions, use the follow
   ing sequential approach:

   a. Administer **antihistamines,** e.g., hydroxyzine, 25–50 mg 3–4 times/da
   (in children, 2–5 mg/kg/day in 4 doses).

Table 12-18. Skin testing protocol for insulin[a]

Dilution[b]	Units/ml	Units administered	Pork	Human
1:100,000,000	0.000001	0.00000002	_____	_____
1:10,000,000	0.00001	0.0000002	_____	_____
1:1,000,000	0.0001	0.000002	_____	_____
1:100,000	0.001	0.00002	_____	_____
1:10,000	0.01	0.0002	_____	_____
1:1000	0.1	0.002	_____	_____
1:100	1.0	0.02	_____	_____
1:10	10.0	0.2	_____	_____
Undiluted	100.0	2.0	_____	_____

Intradermal testing using .02 ml.
[b] Use U-100 regular insulin.

    b. Divide the dose of insulin, using separate sites, until reactions disappear.
    c. Switch to conventional pork insulin, purified pork insulin, or synthetic human insulin without zinc.
    d. An increase in the intensity of local reactions demands **careful surveillance** for the onset of a systemic reaction. In insulin-dependent patients, discontinuation of insulin therapy because of local reactions is not advisable, both from the standpoint of optimal management of the diabetes and because interruption of therapy can increase the chances of a systemic reaction on subsequent readministration of insulin.

  2. Systemic reactions
    a. Treat systemic allergic reactions to insulin in the same manner as anaphylaxis (see Chap. 10). The occurrence of a systemic reaction dictates reassessment of the need for insulin. However, in most diabetic patients in whom insulin therapy is initiated, no substitute exists.
    b. If the patient is evaluated within 24–48 hours of the allergic reaction and if continued insulin therapy is essential,
      (1) Do not discontinue insulin therapy.
      (2) In the hospital, with the patient under careful observation, reduce the dose to one-third or one-fourth of the original dose.
      (3) Gradually increase the dose over several days until a therapeutic dose is achieved.
    c. If there has been an interruption of insulin therapy for more than 48 hours, insulin skin testing and desensitization are indicated.
      (1) By insulin skin testing, determine the least reactive insulin for the patient (purified pork or synthetic human) and the level of sensitivity. Make fresh serial 10-fold dilutions of regular insulins and perform serial intradermal tests until positive reactions occur (Table 12-18).
      (2) To begin **desensitization,** use the least reactive insulin at a concentration one-tenth as strong as the most dilute preparation giving a positive test. A representative and useful desensitization protocol (recommended only with the patient in the hospital) for most circumstances is given in Table 12-19. Use regular insulin initially and add intermediate-acting preparations (of the corresponding animal source) later.
      (3) A more rapid schedule is required in certain patients, such as those in impending or frank ketoacidosis or hyperosmolar coma (Table 12-20). In these situations, give insulin subcutaneously at 15- to 30-

Table 12-19. Representative subcutaneous insulin desensitization schedule

Day	Time	Concentration (units/ml)	Volume (ml)	Dose (units)[a]
1	7:30 A.M.	0.0001	0.1	0.00001[b]
	12 noon	0.001	0.1	0.0001
	4:30 P.M.	0.01	0.1	0.001
2	7:30 A.M.	0.1	0.1	0.01
	12 noon	1.0	0.1	0.1
	4:30 P.M.	10.0	0.1	1.0
3	7:30 A.M.	100.0	0.02	2.0
	12 noon	100.0	0.04	4.0
	4:30 P.M.	100.0	0.08	8.0
4	7:30 A.M.	100.0	0.12	12.0
	12 noon	100.0	0.16	16.0
5	7:30 A.M.	100.0	0.20	20.0

[a] Regular insulin is used initially. Intermediate-acting insulin preparations may be considered on day 3.
[b] The initial dose and source of insulin are based on reactivity to intradermal testing (see text and Table 12-18).

Table 12-20. Rapid insulin desensitization schedule

Dose number[a]	Concentration (units/ml)	Volume (ml)	Dose (units)
1	0.0001	0.10	0.00001[b]
2	0.001	0.10	0.0001
3	0.01	0.10	0.001
4	0.01	0.50	0.005
5	0.1	0.10	0.01
6	0.1	0.50	0.05
7	1.0	0.10	0.10
8	1.0	0.20	0.20
9	1.0	0.50	0.50
10	10.0	0.10	1.0
11	10.0	0.20	2.0
12	10.0	0.40	4.0
13	10.0	0.80	8.0
14	100.0	0.10	10.0[c]

[a] Administered subcutaneously at intervals of 15–30 min.
[b] Initial dose and source of insulin are based on reactivity to intradermal testing (see text and Table 12-18).
[c] Subsequent doses may be doubled until the desired dose is reached.

minute intervals. Determine the starting dose and the source of insulin by preliminary skin testing (see Table 12-18).

(4) Both desensitization protocols must be flexible. If a **local reaction** occurs, before increasing the dose, repeat the same dose until minimal or no reactions are present. If a **systemic reaction** occurs, decrease the dose by one-half and increase at smaller increments. In the slower protocol (see Table 12-19), decreasing the time interval between injections can be useful if reactions occur.

D. Management of immunologic insulin resistance

1. Hospitalize patients with rapidly increasing insulin requirements to rule out nonimmunologic causes and stabilize insulin requirements.

2. For immunologic insulin resistance persisting more than several days, switching to purified pork or synthetic human insulin may be the only therapy necessary. In other patients, switching to more concentrated (U-500 [500 units/ml]) or sulfated insulin preparations may be successful.

3. When unstable diabetes or increasing insulin requirements complicate insulin resistance, corticosteroid therapy (initially to 60 mg of prednisone daily, 1–2 mg/kg/day in children) can be initiated. Watch for hypoglycemia at this time; it may occur as the insulin requirement falls rapidly. When insulin therapy has been stabilized, the prednisone can be converted to an alternate-day regimen, tapered, and possibly discontinued.

VI. Chymopapain chemonucleolysis

A. Clinical features

1. Chymopapain for intradiscal injection treatment of herniated intervertebral disks unresponsive to conservative therapy has been approved by the FDA. Chymopapain is a proteolytic enzyme and is found in meat tenderizer, fruit drinks, soft contact lens cleaning solutions, and the manufacture of beer, thus offering ample exposure to sensitize many people to this protein. Current estimates of anaphylaxis with this procedure are 1%, and patients have developed severe anaphylactic reactions, including death (0.14%), even after following the pretreatment recommendations of the package insert (cimetidine and diphenhydramine). Skin testing and in vitro testing to detect IgE antibody reactive with chymopapain exist, but the reliability of these procedures is unknown at this time. Delayed reactions up to 14 days following chemonucleolysis and sensitization from the procedure itself have occurred.

The recommendations given in B and C below are the procedures used in the authors' clinics and are intended only as advice.

B. Diagnosis

1. Prick testing with chymopapain (Chymodiactin, Discase), 1 mg/ml and 10 mg/ml with a negative control (phosphate buffered saline in 0.4% phenol) and a positive control (histamine, 1 mg/ml), can be done. Intradermal testing with chymopapain is not suitable because it is a proteolytic enzyme. An enzyme-linked immunosorbent assay (ELISA) test for chymopapain-specific IgE exists but is not used routinely because severe reactions to prick skin testing have not been reported. A positive chymopapain prick skin test is a contraindication for chemonucleolysis.

C. Treatment

1. Patients with negative skin tests who undergo chemonucleolysis should be pretreated with cimetidine, 300 mg orally, and diphenhydramine (Benadryl), 50 mg orally, at 13 hours, 7 hours, and 1 hour prior to the procedure (as directed in the package insert) as a precaution. Some treatment centers add prednisone, 50 mg orally for 3 doses, at the times stated above. **Pretreatment requirements for patients with negative skin tests and the recommendations for proper handling of patients with positive skin tests may change as further studies become available.**

2. Patients who experience anaphylactic or generalized allergic reactions during the procedure should be treated according to the procedures discussed in Chap. 10.

Selected Readings

Bernstein, D. I., et al. Prospective evaluation of chymopapain sensitivity in patients undergoing chemonucleolysis. *J. Allergy Clin. Immunol.* 76:458, 1985.

Blagren, S. E. Drug-induced lupus erythematosus. *Semin. Hematol.* 10:345, 1973.

Davidson, J. K. Insulin allergy and immunologic insulin resistance. *Compr. Ther.* 8:46, 1982.

Dawson, A. A. Drug-induced hematological disease. *Br. Med. J.* 1:1195, 1979.

deShazo, R. D., and Nelson, H. S. An approach to the patient with a history of local anesthetic hypersensitivity: Experience with 90 patients. *J. Allergy Clin. Immunol.* 63:387, 1979.

DeSwarte, R. D. Drug Allergy. In R. Patterson (ed.), *Allergic Diseases: Diagnosis and Management.* (3rd ed.). Philadelphia: Lippincott, 1985. P. 505.

Dunagan, W. G., and Millikan, L. E. Drug eruptions. *Med. Clin. North Am.* 64:983, 1980.

Fengolio, J. J., McAllister, H. A., and Myllick, F. G. Drug-related myocarditis. *Hum. Pathol.* 12:900, 1981.

Fisher, M. M., and Munro, I. Life-threatening anaphylactoid reactions to muscle relaxants. *Anesth. Analg.* 62:559, 1983.

Goldstein, R. A., and Patterson, R. (eds.). Drug allergy: Prevention, diagnosis, treatment (Part 2). *J. Allergy Clin. Immunol.* 74:549, 1984.

Grammer, L. C., Chen, P. Y., and Patterson, R. Evaluation and management of insulin allergy. *J. Allergy Clin. Immunol.* 71:250, 1983.

Greenberger, P. A., Patterson, R., and Tapio, C. M. Prophylaxis against repeat radiocontrast media reactions in 857 cases: Adverse experience with cimetidine and safety of beta adrenergic antagonists. *Arch. Intern. Med.* 145:2197, 1985.

Humes, H. D., and Weinberg, J. M. Drug-induced nephrotoxicity. *DM* 28:1, 1982.

Jayasundera, N., and Nicholson, D. P. Pulmonary disease induced by drug therapy. *J. Respir. Dis.* 2:31, 1981.

Kleinknecht, D., et al. Acute interstitial nephritis due to drug hypersensitivity. An up-to-date review with a report of 19 cases. *Adv. Nephrol.* 12:277, 1983.

Lipsky, B. A., and Hirschmann, J. V. Drug fever. *J.A.M.A.* 245:851, 1981.

Meddrey, W. C. Drug-related acute and chronic hepatitis. *Clin. Gastroenterol.* 9:213, 1980.

Rosenow, E. C. Drug-induced pulmonary disease. *Clin. Notes Respir. Dis.* 16:3, 1977.

Schatz, M. Skin testing and incremental challenge in the evaluation of adverse reactions to local anesthetics (Part 2). *J. Allergy Clin. Immunol.* 74:606, 1984.

Schatz, M., and Simon, R. A. Adverse reactions to radiographic contrast media: A practical approach. *Immunol. Allergy Pract.* 1:44, 1979.

Settipane, G. A. Aspirin and allergic diseases: A review. *Am. J. Med.* 74(6A):102, 1983.

Spector, S. L., and Farr, R. S. Aspirin idiosyncrasy: Asthma and Urticaria. In E. Middleton, C. E. Reed, and E. F. Ellis (eds.), *Allergy: Principles and Practice* (2nd ed.). St. Louis: Mosby, 1983. P. 1249.

Stevenson, D. D. Diagnosis, prevention, and treatment of adverse reactions to aspirin and nonsteroidal anti-inflammatory drugs. *J. Allergy Clin. Immunol.* 74:617, 1984.

Sullivan, T. J., et al. Desensitization of patients allergic to penicillin using orally administered β-lactam antibiotics. *J. Allergy Clin. Immunol.* 69:275, 1982.

VanArsdel, P. P. Adverse Drug Reactions. In E. Middleton, C. E. Reed, and E. F. Ellis (eds.), *Allergy: Principles and Practice* (2nd ed.). St. Louis: Mosby, 1983. P. 1389.

Vervolet, D., Nizankowska, E., and Arnauda, A. Adverse reactions to suxamethonium and other muscle relaxants under general anesthesia. *J. Allergy Clin. Immunol.* 71:552, 1983.

13

Food Allergy

Michael K. Farrell

The topic of food allergy and the role of food and food additives as causative factors in hypersensitivity diseases evoke considerable controversy. Numerous reports relate every conceivable symptom to food allergy from anaphylaxis to behavioral problems. There are, of course, certain patients in whom classic allergic symptoms develop after the ingestion of specific foods, e.g., anaphylaxis or urticaria after eating shrimp. However, the scarcity of objective, reproducible, and controlled studies to eliminate personal bias and psychological factors have made food allergy a confusing subject. Part of this confusion results from the failure to distinguish immune-mediated reactions from reactions caused by intestinal enzyme deficiencies, toxins or infections, neurologic or psychologic reactions, and reactions to noxious natural constituents of foods. An understanding of normal digestion and absorption as well as the immunology of the gastrointestinal tract allows a more rational approach to reactions to foods. (Refer to the Selected Readings at the end of this chapter for excellent reviews on these subjects.)

Clinical Features of Food Hypersensitivity

I. **Incidence.** Estimates of the incidence of **IgE-mediated food allergy** range from 0.1–7.0% of the population, with the male-to-female ratio being approximately 2:1. Recent studies suggest that 0.5% of infants may have a hypersensitivity reaction to cow's milk. In a child with proved food hypersensitivity, the probability of food hypersensitivity in subsequent siblings is increased up to 50%.

II. The **clinical manifestations** of food allergy include **classic allergic symptoms** (systemic anaphylaxis, asthma, allergic rhinitis, atopic dermatitis, urticaria, angioedema) or **gastrointestinal symptoms** such as nausea, diarrhea, and abdominal pain. The role of food allergy in conditions such as enuresis, migraine headaches, or the allergic tension-fatigue syndrome is controversial.

III. **Food antigens.** Virtually any food can cause allergic symptoms. In addition, several dyes, flavorings, and preservatives can elicit allergiclike reactions. Tartrazine (FD&C yellow dye No. 5) has been incriminated more often than other FD&C dyes. This dye can be found in orange or green food as well as in drugs that are yellow (see Appendix XII.G). (Its relationship to aspirin sensitivity is discussed in Chap. 12.) Commonly implicated flavorings and preservatives include nitrites and nitrates, monosodium glutamate, sulfiting agents, and sodium benzoate (see Appendix XII.H for a list of foods commonly containing sulfites). Foods can also produce nonimmunologic reactions by a toxic effect (e.g., histamine intoxication with scombroid fish such as tuna and mackerel) or by the presence of endogenous pharmacologic agents (e.g., caffeine, alcohol, or theobromine).

Commonly implicated foods include cow's milk, eggs, wheat, corn, chocolate, citrus fruits, nuts, and shellfish. As a general rule, cooked foods are less allergenic than raw foods. Also, families of foods may share common allergenic properties. Cross-reactivity is more common among some food families than others (e.g., crustaceans).

Table 13-1. Classification of food from plant sources

Grain family
  Wheat
    Graham flour
    Gluten flour
    Bran
    Wheat germ
  Rye
  Barley
    Malt
  Corn
    Corn starch
    Corn oil
    Corn sugar
    Corn syrup
    Cerulose
    Dextrose
    Glucose
  Oats
  Rice
  Wild rice
  Sorghum
  Cane
    Cane sugar
    Molasses

Spurge family
  Tapioca

Arrowroot family
  Arrowroot

Arum family
  Taro
    Poi

Buckwheat family
  Buckwheat
  Rhubarb

Potato family
  Potato
  Tomato
  Eggplant
  Red pepper
    Cayenne
  Green pepper
  Chili

Composite family
  Leaf lettuce
  Head lettuce
  Endive
  Escarole
  Artichoke
  Dandelion
  Oyster plant
  Chicory

Legume family
  Navy bean
  Kidney bean

Lima bean
String bean
Soybean
  Soybean oil
Lentil
Black-eyed pea
Pea
Peanut
  Peanut oil
Licorice
Acacia
Senna

Mustard family
  Mustard
  Cabbage
  Cauliflower
  Broccoli
  Brussels sprouts
  Turnip
  Rutabaga
  Kale
  Collard
  Celery cabbage
  Kohlrabi
  Radish
  Horseradish
  Watercress

Gourd family
  Pumpkin
  Squash
  Cucumber
  Cantaloupe
  Muskmelon
  Honeydew
  Persian melon
  Casaba
  Watermelon

Lily family
  Asparagus
  Onion
  Garlic
  Leek
  Chive
  Aloes

Goosefoot family
  Beet
    Beet sugar
  Spinach
  Swiss chard

Parsley family
  Parsley
  Parsnip
  Carrot
  Celery
  Celeriac

Caraway
Anise
Dill
Coriander
Fennel

Morning glory family
  Sweet potato
  Yam

Sunflower family*
  Jerusalem artichoke
  Sunflower seed oil

Pomegranate family
  Pomegranate

Ebony family
  Persimmon

Rose family
  Raspberry
  Blackberry
  Loganberry
  Youngberry
  Dewberry
  Strawberry

Banana family
  Banana
  Plantain

Apple family
  Apple
    Cider
    Vinegar
    Apple pectin
  Pear
  Quince
    Quince seed

Plum family
  Plum
    Prune
  Cherry
  Peach
  Apricot
  Nectarine
  Almond

Laurel family
  Avocado
  Cinnamon
  Bay leaves

Olive family
  Green olive
  Ripe olive
    Olive oil

Heath family
  Cranberry
  Blueberry

Table 13-1. (*continued*)

Gooseberry family	Marjoram	Mulberry family
Gooseberry	Savory	Mulberry
Currant	Pepper family	Fig
Honeysuckle family	Black pepper	Hop
Elderberry	Nutmeg family	Breadfruit
Citrus family	Nutmeg	Maple family
Orange	Ginger family	Maple syrup
Grapefruit	Ginger	Maple sugar
Lemon	Turmeric	Palm family
Lime	Cardamon	Coconut
Tangerine	Pine family	Date
Kumquat	Juniper	Sago
Pineapple family	Orchid family	Legythis family
Pineapple	Vanilla	Brazil nut
Papaw family	Madder family	Poppy family
Papaya	Coffee	Poppy seed
Grape family	Tea family	Walnut family
Grape	Tea	English walnut
Raisin	Pedalium family	Black walnut
Cream of tartar	Sesame oil	Butternut
Myrtle family	Mallow family	Hickory nut
Allspice	Okra (gumbo)	Pecan
Cloves	Cottonseed	Cashew family
Pimento	Stercula family	Cashew
Guava	Cocoa	Pistachio
Mint family	Chocolate	Mango
Mint	Birch family	Beech family
Peppermint	Filbert	Beechnut
Spearmint	Hazelnut	Chestnut
Thyme	Oil of birch	Fungi
Sage	(wintergreen)	Mushroom
		Yeast
		Miscellaneous
		Honey

*Sometimes placed in composite family.
Source: From J. M. Sheldon, R. G. Lowell, and K. P. Mathews. Food and Gastrointestinal Allergy. In *A Manual of Clinical Allergy*. Philadelphia: Saunders, 1967. With permission.

A classification of foods according to shared allergenic properties from both plant and animal sources is given in Tables 13-1 and 13-2. Dietary sources of cow's milk, egg, wheat, corn, and soybean are listed in Appendix XII.

IV. **Diagnostic approach to food allergy.** A careful diagnostic approach is needed for the patient with suspected food hypersensitivity. This approach includes an accurate history, a detailed physical examination, and application of proved laboratory methods. It is of critical importance to remember that the symptoms of food allergy, especially **gastrointestinal** symptoms, can be mimicked by a variety of other clinical entities.

   A. A **detailed allergy history** is essential in all patients with suspected food hypersensitivity (see Chap. 2).

   1. In particular, note the nature and severity of the symptoms (classic allergic respiratory or cutaneous symptoms versus gastrointestinal symptoms), the age of onset, possible precipitating factors, and the temporal relationship between the ingestion of the suspected food and the syndrome.

Table 13-2. Classification of food from animal sources

Mollusks	Pike	Mammals
Abalone	Pickerel	Beef
Mussel	Muskellunge	Veal
Oyster	Mullet	Cow's milk
Scallop	Barracuda	Butter
Clam	Mackerel	Cheese
Crustaceans	Tuna	Gelatin
Crab	Pompano	Pork
Crayfish	Bluefish	Ham
Lobster	Butterfish	Bacon
Shrimp	Harvestfish	Goat
Squid*	Swordfish	Goat's milk
Amphibians	Sunfish	Cheese
Frog	Bass	Mutton
Fish	Perch	Lamb
Sturgeon	Snapper	Venison
Caviar	Croaker	Horse meat
Anchovy	Weakfish	Rabbit
Sardine	Drum	Squirrel
Herring	Scup	Birds
Smelt	Porgy	Chicken
Trout	Flounder	Chicken eggs
Salmon	Sole	Duck
Whitefish	Halibut	Duck eggs
Chub	Rosefish	Goose
Shad	Codfish	Goose eggs
Eel	Scrod	Turkey
Carp	Haddock	Guinea hen
Sucker	Hake	Squab
Buffalo	Pollack	Pheasant
Catfish	Cusk	Partridge
Bullhead	Reptiles	Grouse
	Turtle	

*Sometimes grouped with mollusks.
Source: From J. M. Sheldon, R. G. Lovell, and K. P. Mathews. Food and Gastrointestinal Allergy. In *A Manual of Clinical Allergy*. Philadelphia: Saunders, 1967. With permission.

2. With gastrointestinal symptoms the possibility of an intercurrent gastrointestinal infection must always be considered. Note the possible role of **food additives** (e.g., tartrazine and sulfites) or **antigenically cross-reacting foods** in the patient's diet (see Tables 13-1 and 13-2). Inquire closely concerning other allergic phenomena and the family history of atopic disease.

3. If gastrointestinal symptoms are present, record the patient's nutritional history. In children and adolescents, serial measurement of weight and height should be obtained if possible and compared with standard growth curves (see Appendix XI). If the patient is not following normal growth curves despite an adequate diet, malabsorption must be excluded; with adequate diet and normal growth, malabsorption is unlikely. In adolescents, calculation of growth velocity (compute growth velocity in centimeters/year and plot against standard growth velocity curves) and assessment of stages of sexual development are useful methods for establishing normal adolescent growth and development.

B. **The physical examination** includes careful inspection, particularly for classic allergic stigmata. In the presence of gastrointestinal symptoms, note the muscle mass and amount of subcutaneous tissue. The patient with malabsorption, especially the young child, has a protuberant abdomen, thin extremities, and wasting of the buttocks. Sparse hair growth and the appearance of lanugo on the back indicate continued caloric deprivation. Peripheral edema suggests hypoproteinemia; hepatomegaly occurs with fatty infiltration of the liver during malnutrition.

C. **Laboratory diagnosis of food hypersensitivity**

1. **Eosinophilia,** either blood or tissue, suggests atopy.

2. An elevated **total serum IgE** can identify the patient as atopic (if parasitic infection is excluded) but does not incriminate specific allergens.

3. **Specific serum IgE** antibodies (e.g., radioallergosorbent test [RAST] measurements) indicate circulating IgE antibody to specific antigens. A positive RAST test must be correlated with a double-blind clinical challenge to document suspected symptomatic hypersensitivity (see **9**).

4. **Epicutaneous (prick or scratch) tests** with commercial reagents can identify the patient as atopic, and, as in RAST testing, a positive result indicates the necessity for double-blind challenge studies for documentation of suspected symptomatic hypersensitivity (see **9**). The reliability of epicutaneous skin tests can vary, depending on the food group. Epicutaneous skin testing for milk, egg, soy, fish, and nuts correlate well with clinical symptomatology.

5. **Intradermal skin tests** with commercial allergens are of limited value because of the large number of false-positive reactions in normal persons. Furthermore, in some patients with certain antigens (e.g., nuts), these tests can be dangerous and have produced anaphylactic death.

6. **Hemagglutinating** and **precipitating antibodies** (e.g., milk precipitins) are commonly found in normal persons. Their presence does not necessarily indicate sensitization, and they may be absent in patients with documented food hypersensitivity.

7. **Peroral intestinal biopsy (before** and **after** food challenge) can exclude other intestinal lesions and help quantitate any mucosal injury due to ingested food. The villous architecture may be altered, ranging from mild inflammation to severe atrophy; intraepithelial lymphocytes may be increased; and IgM, IgA, and IgE plasma cells (by immunofluorescence) may be present.

8. Nonspecific measures of intestinal function, such as D-xylose absorption, fecal fat smears, and serum carotene, identify mucosal injury but not the specific cause of injury. Breath hydrogen excretion following administration of a specific carbohydrate (e.g., lactose) allows documentation of specific carbohydrate intolerance. Proctosigmoidoscopy and biopsy may demonstrate colitis in infants with food-induced rectal bleeding.

9. Use **double-blind food challenges** for the exact diagnosis of food hypersensitivity in order to eliminate physician and patient bias. These challenges allow objective descriptions and interpretations of results by the physician. Although in routine clinical usage diet diaries and food eliminations with subsequent reintroduction into the diet as an open trial can give helpful information, only individual blind food challenges give the most precise information for routine clinical care and are an absolute necessity for clinical research studies. The following method proposed by Boch et al. (*J. Clin. Allergy Immunol.* 62:327, 1978) can be used:

   a. Two weeks prior to the challenge, eliminate suspected foods from the diet using the temporary elimination diet given in Table 13-3.

   b. Obtain dry foods (milk, egg, wheat flour, or peanuts). If necessary, wet foods can be freeze-dried and powdered.

   c. Place the suspected food in opaque, colorless No. 1 pharmacy capsules (the capsules should be filled by someone other than the patient or observer). The initial dose, ranging from 20–2000 mg, depends on the suspected degree of hypersensitivity. Administer the capsules just before a meal consisting of the restricted diet.

   d. In infants and young children unable to swallow capsules, have the

Table 13-3. Elimination diet

Foods allowed at mealtime	
Rice	Honey (2 oz/day)
Puffed Rice	Cane sugar
Rice flakes	Salt
Rice Krispies	Oleomargarine without milk
Pineapple ⎤	Crisco, Spry
Apricots ⎥	A carbonated, dye-free beverage
Cranberries ⎬ Fruit or juice	Snacks
Peaches ⎥	1 box rice cereal midmorning and midafter-
Pears ⎦	noon
Lamb	Foods to avoid
Chicken	Any food and drink suspected of causing reac-
Asparagus	tions or not on this list
Beets	Pepper and spices
Carrots	Coffee
Lettuce	Tea
Sweet potato	Chewing gum
Tapioca	
White vinegar	
Olive oil	

      suspected food hidden in the diet by someone other than the parent or observer.

    e. Symptoms usually occur within 2 hours in immediate food hypersensitivity. If no reactions occur within 24 hours, increase the dose twofold daily until a dose of 8000 mg of dried food is reached. This amount of dried food represents approximately 100 gm (3.5 oz) of food in the wet state.

    f. Assess questionable symptoms by administration of glucose-filled capsules in the same manner, being sure to obscure the order of presentation.

    g. A single unequivocal positive reaction is definitive. Failure to react to 8000 mg of a given food usually implies that this food can be included in the diet without any problems.

V. Therapy for documented food hypersensitivity demands accurate diagnosis by history and double-blind challenge. Without the proper diagnosis, attempts at therapy become empirical and irrational. Other causes of food reactions must be constantly borne in mind.

  A. Elimination of the incriminated food is the primary method of treatment. This treatment also includes elimination of possible cross-reacting food substances (see Tables 13-1 and 13-2).

    1. If several major food groups are implicated, a nutritionally adequate elimination diet must be offered. Consult a professional dietitian in these complex cases.

    2. Patients with food hypersensitivity can lose their symptomatic reaction possibly through development of immunologic tolerance. Especially in infants with milk allergy, the offending food can often be cautiously reintroduced after an appropriate interval (usually after age 2 years). Food reintroduction should be done cautiously and with adequate preparation for treatment of anaphylaxis. **Patients** with proved anaphylaxis, **especially older children and adults, should not be rechallenged.**

    3. Although complete elimination of the offending food is the prime goal, even a reduction of this food in the diet can provide symptomatic relief. Instruct patients to read labels on food products and to be aware of the antigenic similarity between foods.

B. **Pharmacologic therapy** for food allergy can be attempted in patients with multiple food sensitivities not responding to elimination measures, in patients with unavoidable, uncontrolled exposure to offending foods when meals are eaten away from home, or in those in whom significant symptoms continue because the offending food is not recognized.

1. **H₁ receptor antihistamines** can be helpful in adverse reactions to foods that involve histamine release, e.g., urticaria/angioedema, conjunctivitis, or rhinitis. The use of H_1 antihistamines for gastrointestinal symptoms is controversial. Although premedication with these drugs can be attempted to decrease classic allergic symptoms, H_1 antihistamines **cannot** be relied on to prevent life-threatening anaphylactic food reactions.

2. **H₂ receptor antihistamines** such as cimetidine or ranitidine are useful agents in treating peptic ulcer disease. Their exact role in treating food allergies is not clear.

3. **Adrenergic agents.** Epinephrine is indicated for systemic allergic reactions to foods. Patients with a history of severe reactions should be instructed in the use of preloaded syringes of epinephrine (if no medical contraindication exists for their use) and should carry these syringes with them. (See Chap. 10.) The role of other agents (e.g., ephedrine, metaproterenol, or terbutaline) for chronic symptom control has not been defined.

4. **Corticosteroids,** because of their side effects with extended use, have been used only for temporary treatment of severe hypersensitivity response to food and for the treatment of eosinophilic gastroenteritis caused by food sensitivity.

5. **Cromolyn sodium** has been used as an investigational drug for food allergy (not licensed for oral use). Capsules of cromolyn sodium contain 20 mg of lactose, which may affect patients with a lactase deficiency that frequently accompanies gastrointestinal disorders.

   Although several studies suggest benefit from orally administered cromolyn sodium for the treatment of food allergy, especially in children, the findings are still not conclusive, and further studies are required for a definitive answer for the proper indication and the most effective dose.

6. **Prostaglandin synthetase inhibitors** (acetylsalicylic acid, indomethacin, or ibuprofen). Although a preliminary study suggests possible benefit for their use in food allergy, they are currently not FDA-approved for this purpose.

C. The food-allergic patient with malabsorption and poor nutrition should receive prompt nutritional repletion. Elemental formulas or enteral feedings are used in providing adequate nutrition (Table 13-4). Specific nutritional deficiencies (e.g., vitamins, zinc, essential fatty acids) should be replaced. Total parenteral nutrition may be necessary if oral feedings are not tolerated, if severe gastrointestinal symptoms persist, or both.

D. **Immunotherapy** and **oral hyposensitization** are of unproved effectiveness in

Table 13-4. Elemental formulas and enteral feedings

Product	Protein	Fat	Carbohydrate
Nutramigen	Casein hydrolysate	Corn oil	Corn syrup solids, corn starch
Pregestimil	Casein hydrolysate	Medium-chain triglycerides (coconut oil) and long-chain triglycerides (corn oil)	Corn syrup solids, tapioca
Vital*	Hydrolyzed whey, meat, and soy	Safflower oil, medium chain triglycerides	Glucose polymer, sucrose
Vivonex*	Amino acids	Safflower oil	Glucose

*For use in children over 1 year of age and adults.

the treatment of food allergies. An exception is the recommended trial of sub-cutaneous immunotherapy for respiratory sensitivity to inhaled food allergen (e.g., baker's asthma).

E. **Controversial and unproved procedures** are touted for the diagnosis and treatment of food allergies. Leukocytotoxic testing has been proposed for the in vitro diagnosis of food allergies. Likewise, intracutaneous and subcutaneous provocation testing, neutralization testing, and sublingual provocation testing with food extracts have been advocated for diagnosing allergy to foods. These procedures have also been advocated for treatment of food allergies. The American Academy of Allergy and Immunology and the National Center for Health Care Technology have reported that these tests are unproved, unreliable, and without scientific basis.

Conditions that Mimic Food Allergies

I. **Vomiting** is particularly common in infants and children and is often attributed to food allergy. Vomiting is a symptom, not a diagnosis, and its cause may lie outside the gastrointestinal tract. It is important to determine whether or not the vomiting is associated with other gastrointestinal symptoms, such as distention or diarrhea. The differential diagnosis of vomiting is outlined in Table 13-5.

A. **Gastroesophageal reflux** (due to a lax lower esophageal sphincter) is the most common cause of vomiting in an otherwise healthy infant. The onset of vomiting is in the first month of life and may consist of spitting or be projectile. By 1 year of age, 80% of infants recover without therapy. This isolated vomiting, usually

Table 13-5. Causes of vomiting

Gastrointestinal
   Gastroesophageal reflux (chalasia)
   Obstruction
     Pyloric stenosis, antral web
     Malrotation, superior mesenteric artery syndrome
   Peptic ulcer disease
   Hepatitis
   Pancreatitis
   Infections: acute gastroenteritis (usually occurs with diarrhea)
   Motility disturbances
     Idiopathic pseudoobstruction
     Ileus from trauma, Addison's disease
     Hypokalemia, hypothyroidism
     Acute gastric dilatation (trauma, body cast)
Psychogenic
   Psychogenic vomiting
   Anorexia nervosa, rumination
Extraintestinal
   Metabolic
     Reye's syndrome
     Metabolic acidosis, uremia, lead poisoning
     Disorders of fat oxidation
   Toxic
     Ingestion, drug toxicity (e.g., theophylline)
   Infectious
     Meningitis, encephalopathy
   Increased intracranial pressure
     Trauma, tumor, hydrocephalus

Table 13-6. Differential diagnosis of diarrhea

Infections
  Viral (rotavirus), *Salmonella, Shigella, Amoeba, Yersinia, Campylobacter, Giardia, Cryptosporidia*
Chronic inflammation
  Crohn's disease, ulcerative colitis, tuberculosis, histoplasmosis
Abnormality of anatomy or motility
  Surgical short gut, malrotation, intestinal obstruction, Hirschsprung's disease, chronic constipation (overflow diarrhea), idiopathic intestinal pseudoobstruction
Inadequate pancreatic function
  Cystic fibrosis, Schwachman-Diamond syndrome, malnutrition, lipase deficiency
Alteration of the enterohepatic bile salt circulation
  Metabolic immaturity of the liver (prematurity), cholestatic liver disease, ileal resection, Crohn's disease, bacterial overgrowth of the small bowel ("blind loop")
Abnormality of the intestinal mucosa
  Celiac disease, immune deficiencies, postgastroenteritis changes, drug toxicity, cow's milk or soy protein intolerance
  Primary and secondary disaccharidase deficiencies, monosaccharide intolerance
Miscellaneous
  Irritable bowel syndrome, chronic nonspecific diarrhea
Endocrine
  Hypoparathyroidism, hyperthyroidism, neuroblastoma

after meals and without diarrhea, is rarely due to allergy. **Multiple formula changes are not indicated.**

1. If the vomiting is troublesome, if weight gain is inadequate, or if complications such as recurrent pulmonary infections or apnea occur, the child must be evaluated in depth. An upper gastrointestinal series may demonstrate reflux and rule out distal outlet obstruction. Failure to demonstrate gastroesophageal reflux by x-ray does not exclude reflux. If necessary, esophageal manometry, pH studies, and radioisotope studies can be performed.
2. The **treatment** of esophageal reflux consists of frequent small feedings (2–3 oz every 3 hours), maintaining the upright position 24 hours a day, and antacids, 2–5 ml, 1 hour after each feeding. Additional drug therapies include **bethanechol,** which decreases reflux, and **metoclopramide,** which increases lower esophageal sphincter pressure and enhances gastric emptying. Only those infants who do not improve after 6 weeks of **intensive medical therapy** should be considered possible candidates for surgery.

II. **Diarrhea,** a frequently encountered problem, is similarly often ascribed to food hypersensitivity and treated by multiple dietary manipulations without regard to the cause of the diarrhea or the specific dietary component causing symptoms. Unfortunately, these manipulations often result in a diet insufficient to meet caloric requirements. This can perpetuate the diarrhea, causing decreased pancreatic enzyme synthesis and intestinal mucosal function. Weight loss and increasing diarrhea result in increased malnutrition, thus setting up a vicious cycle. In young children, especially infants under 4 months of age, avoid hypocaloric diets for periods longer than 48 hours. If the diarrhea becomes chronic and persistent (> 50 gm of stool/day in children, 100 gm/day in adults), or if it is impossible to achieve adequate caloric intake, a more detailed evaluation should follow, keeping in mind the differential diagnostic possibilities (see Table 13-6).

A. The **history** in a child with diarrhea should include the following:
   1. The **temporal sequence** of abnormal stools, failure to thrive, and caloric intake.
   2. The temporal relationship to the **introduction of cereals** (? celiac disease).
   3. **Changes in feedings,** especially formulas, and correlation of protein and carbohydrate content with symptoms.

4. Previously normal stools followed by persistent abnormal stools after acute gastrointestinal infection.
5. Abdominal pain or distention.
6. Emotional disturbances.
7. Physical and emotional environment (e.g., failure to thrive on a maternal deprivation basis).

B. In the **physical examination,** particular attention should be paid to weight and height, general well-being, irritability, and wasting of the buttocks. Other clues to chronic malabsorption include a protuberant abdomen (best viewed in profile with the patient standing), pallor, reddish tinge to the hair, clubbing of the digits, or edema.

1. Because patients may have biases and misconceptions regarding normal stool characteristics, the physician must examine the stool. The following stool characteristics are helpful:
   a. **Pale color** suggests malabsorption or liver disease.
   b. **Mucous stools** suggest infection, colitis, or irritable bowel syndrome, though this type of stool is often a normal variant.
   c. **Bloody stools** suggest colitis or acute infection (e.g., *Shigella, Salmonella, Campylobacter,* enteropathic *Escherichia coli*).
   d. A **high liquid content** suggests sugar intolerance, bacterial overgrowth of the small intestine, bile salt malabsorption, or neuroblastoma.
   e. **Oiliness** suggests pancreatic insufficiency or celiac disease.
   f. Vegetable matter and meat fibers are of little diagnostic significance.

C. **Laboratory studies**
1. A **stool culture** for common pathogens (e.g., *Salmonella* and *Shigella*), as well as rarer pathogens (e.g., *Yersinia* and *Campylobacter*).
2. Stool analysis for **occult blood.**
3. **Complete blood and reticulocyte count.** Chronic intestinal disorders may lead to occult blood loss and malabsorption of iron, folate, or vitamin B_{12}.
4. The **erythrocyte sedimentation rate** is frequently elevated in inflammatory bowel disease.
5. Examination of the stool for *Giardia lamblia, Cryptosporidia,* and *Entamoeba histolytica.*
6. **Sweat chloride determination.** Cystic fibrosis is a frequent cause of poor weight gain and abnormal stools in young children.
7. **Fecal fat determinations.** If the stool volume is excessive and greasy, fecal fat content should be measured. A 72-hour fecal fat quantitation is more reliable than spot fecal smears. Normal children excrete 5–10 gm of fat/day; adults excrete less than 5 gm/day. These amounts represent less than 5–10% of dietary fat ingested during the study.
8. Examine the watery portion of the stool for **reducing substances. Lactose intolerance** is shown by the presence of reducing substances in the aqueous portion of the stool in a patient on a lactose-containing diet. Place 2 drops of stool and 10 drops of water in a test tube and add a Clinitest tablet. Read the color against the chart provided; a reading greater than 0.5% is significant. Sucrose (found in soy formula, juices) is not a reducing substance. To test for sucrose, hydrolyze the stool with an equal volume of 0.1N HCl. Then perform the Clinitest procedure again.
9. **Intestinal biopsy.** This invasive procedure may be necessary to elucidate the exact cause of diarrhea in complex cases. At the time of the biopsy, duodenal fluid for pancreatic lipase and trypsin determinations, Gram stains and bacterial cultures, and fluid for microscopic examination for *Giardia* and other parasites are obtained.

D. Table 13-6 lists the conditions to be considered in the differential diagnosis of diarrhea. Several points are worth noting. The most common causes of fatty stools are cystic fibrosis, celiac disease, and postinfectious steatorrhea. The most frequent causes of runny, liquid stools are acute infections, carbohydrate intolerance, and chronic nonspecific diarrhea (irritable bowel syndrome).

1. Suspect **cystic fibrosis** in any infant with abnormal stools and poor weight

gain. Respiratory symptoms are not always evident. Confirm the diagnosis with a sweat chloride determination.

2. **Celiac disease** is a permanent intolerance to gluten and is characterized by diarrhea and poor nutrition. Malabsorption and histologic abnormalities of the jejunal mucosa are present. Improvement, determined by clinical observation and biopsy, occurs when gluten is removed from the diet. Reintroduction of gluten results in a relapse that is observable clinically and histologically. The correct diagnosis is crucial, since therapy is lifelong, and a gluten-free diet (see Appendix XII) is difficult to follow; **a gluten-free diet should never be prescribed until the diagnosis of celiac disease has been confirmed by intestinal biopsy.**

3. **Postinfectious steatorrhea** occurs transiently following an acute insult, usually a viral infection, and is usually self-limited; if abnormal stools and weight loss persist, consider a medium-chain triglyceride formula (e.g., Pregestimil).

4. **Carbohydrate intolerance** frequently causes watery stools. The intolerance can be either primary or secondary. Primary lactose intolerance is commonly seen in blacks, Orientals, and whites of Mediterranean ancestry. Secondary lactose or sucrose intolerance occurs following an acute injury to the intestine. Diagnosis is by demonstration of reducing substances in the stool (see **C.8**). Treat by removing the offending sugar from the diet.

5. A frequent cause of loose stools in toddlers is the **irritable bowel syndrome.** Although the exact cause is unknown, it is harmless and self-limited, disappearing by age 3–4 years. The child has an average of four stools/day, ranging from two to seven/day. Growth is normal in these children if the diet is adequate, thus excluding malabsorption. Complex elimination diets are not indicated. Frequently, a history of excessive carbohydrate intake (juices, punches) is obtained. Place the child on a regular diet. A frequent cause of morbidity in these children is multiple dietary manipulations, leading to decreased caloric intake and weight loss.

Cow's-Milk Protein Intolerance

Cow's milk protein can cause a variety of symptoms. Sensitization may occur following a minor intestinal insult and may be perpetuated by a secondary disaccharide intolerance. Diarrhea is a constant feature in cow's milk intolerance, and vomiting may occur. Infants may develop rectal bleeding. Multiple proteins are present in cow's milk, but beta-lactoglobulin is the most antigenic.

Several "hypersensitivity" reactions have been attributed to cow's milk. Milk-induced colitis may occur. Ingestion of large amounts may cause a chronic jejunal inflammation, leading to protein-losing enteropathy and chronic blood loss. The mucosal injury may also result in secondary lactose and fat malabsorption. Heiner's syndrome (iron deficiency anemia, pulmonary hemosiderosis, and cow's-milk protein intolerance) has been attributed to cow's milk. The role of cow's milk in infantile colic remains controversial.

Allergy to cow's-milk and soy protein can cause colitis. Also, colitis has occurred in breast-fed infants whose mothers ingested the proteins. Elimination of the protein from the infant and maternal diet resolves the colitis.

Selected Readings

Anderson, J. A., and Sogn, D. D. (eds.). Adverse Reactions to Foods. American Academy of Allergy and Immunology Committee on Adverse Reactions to Foods and the National Institute of Allergy and Infectious Disease. Washington, D.C.: U.S. Department of Health and Human Services (NIH Publication No. 84-2442), 1984.

Bock, S. A. Natural history of severe reactions to foods in young children. *J. Pediatr.* 107:676, 1985.

Bock, S. A., and May, C. D. Adverse Reactions to Foods Caused by Sensitivity. In E. Middleton, Jr., C. E. Reed, and E. F. Ellis (eds.), *Allergy: Principles and Practice.* St. Louis: Mosby, 1983.

Jenkins, H. R., et al. Food allergy: The major cause of infantile colitis. *Arch. Dis. Child.* 59:326, 1984.

Levine, A. S., Labuza, T. P., and Morley, J. E. Food technology: A primer for physicians. *N. Engl. J. Med.* 312:628, 1985.

McCarty, E. P., and Frick, O. L. Food sensitivity: Keys to diagnosis. *J. Pediatr.* 102:645, 1983.

Metcalfe, D. D. (ed.), Goldblatt, M. J., and Simopoulos, A. P. (assoc. eds.), Symposium Proceedings on Adverse Reactions to Foods and Food Additives (Part 2). *J. Allergy Clin. Immunol.* 78(Suppl.):July 1986.

Silverman, A., and Roy, C. *Pediatric Clinical Gastroenterology* (3rd ed.). St. Louis: Mosby, 1983.

Sinatra, F. R. Food faddism in pediatrics. *J. Am. Coll. Nutr.* 3:169, 1984.

Van Metre, T. E. Critique of controversial and unproven procedures for diagnosis and therapy of allergic disorders. *Pediatr. Clin. North Am.* 30:807, 1983.

Rheumatic Diseases

Robert F. Ashman

Normally, the human immune system is so regulated internally that vigorous immune responses are mounted against foreign antigens, but immune reactions directed to self-antigens are kept under strict control. When these controls are rendered ineffective by disease or aging, the response may be directed against the body's own proteins or tissues. These **autoimmune reactions** result in the tissue-damaging inflammation that characterizes rheumatic disease. The variety of symptoms seen in patients with autoimmune diseases reflects the variety of forms of the immune response, with the site of organ damage dependent on the location of the immune reaction. Frequently, the clinical presentations in patients with rheumatic disease cross traditional diagnostic categories, confusing the clinician.

The term **autoimmune disease** is generally applied to any pathologic condition that is associated with demonstrable autoantibody or cytotoxic cells directed to self-antigens, whether or not this "autoimmune" response is specifically determined to be the cause of the disease. Many useful diagnostic laboratory tests are based on detecting these autoimmune responses. The list of autoimmune diseases grows continually as new autoimmune phenomena are described. In many rheumatic diseases, however, clear evidence of autoimmunity is lacking. Therapy can be directed either at the immune system itself or at the inflammation it produces.

I. **Immunopathologic features of autoimmune disease.** Lymphocytes potentially reactive with self-antigens exist in the body. The lymphocyte precursors of autoantibody-secreting cells and the T lymphocyte precursors of autoimmune cytotoxic T cells are present, but are normally kept in check by regulatory controls, to which T-suppressor lymphocytes make an important contribution (see Chap. 1). When these control mechanisms are rendered ineffective, antibodies to self-antigens may be produced and either may bind to antigens in the circulation to form **circulating immune complexes** or may bind to antigens deposited in certain tissue sites, such as the capillary beds of the kidney and the lung. How the chemical properties of antigen and antibody govern their selective deposition in one organ or another is unknown. Wherever antigen-antibody complexes accumulate, **complement** can be activated, releasing mediators of inflammation that increase vascular permeability and attract neutrophils and other phagocytic cells to the reaction site, resulting in local tissue damage. Alternatively, **cytotoxic T lymphocytes** can directly attack body cells bearing the target antigens, releasing mediators that amplify the inflammatory reaction. Autoantibody and complement fragments coat cells bearing the target antigen, leading to destruction by phagocytes or by antibody-seeking **killer cells (K cells).** Several of these mechanisms may operate in a single disease, and their relative importance may vary with time.

II. **Immunologic tests in autoimmune disease**
   A. **Rheumatoid factor**
      1. **Definition.** Rheumatoid factor (RF) is classically defined as an IgM antibody to human IgG-Fc; it is often present in serum in a complex with IgG.
      2. **Method of detection.** In principle, any particle coated with human IgG should be agglutinated by RF. The antibody-coated human type O erythrocytes or sheep erythrocytes originally used have been replaced by bentonite or latex particles for detecting RF, because the latter tests are more sensitive (Fig. 14-1). Today, many laboratories have improved the detection of

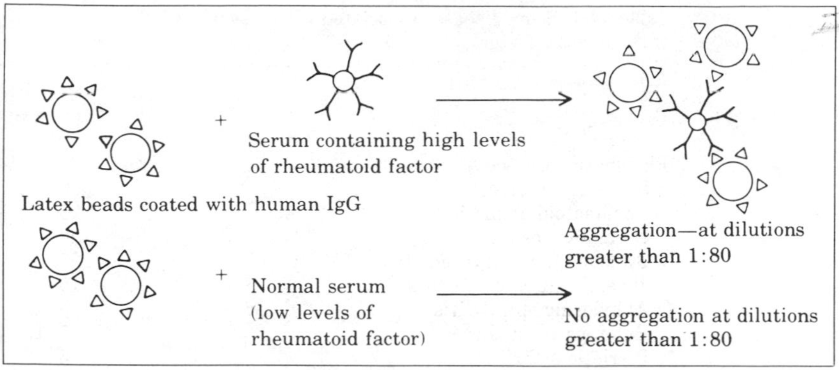

Fig. 14-1. The latex agglutination test for rheumatoid factor, a test commonly performed in the diagnosis of rheumatoid arthritis.

RF by using **nephelometry,** which measures the increasing turbidity of serum containing RF when IgG is added. Serum for RF testing should be stored at $-20°C$ or below unless it is tested promptly.

3. **Interpretation.** The latex agglutination test easily demonstrates small amounts of RF in normal sera, the upper limit of normal usually being a titer of 1:80. The incidence of elevated RF titers in normal individuals increases from 5% below age 60 to 30% in the ninth decade. By latex agglutination, about 75% of rheumatoid arthritis patients have titers of RF exceeding 1:80. The highest titers are generally associated with the most severe and progressive disease. Nodules, systemic vasculitis, Sjögren's syndrome, and other features of extraarticular disease are almost entirely confined to patients with elevated RF levels (i.e., "seropositive" patients). The highest titers often occur with Sjögren's syndrome. Commonly, symptoms are present for 6 months before the rheumatoid arthritis patient becomes RF-positive. Although remission of disease in seropositive patients can be associated with a major decrease in RF titer, reversions to normal RF levels are rare. Rheumatoid factor is not specific for rheumatoid arthritis (Table 14-1).

4. **Other anti-immunoglobulins.** Although the latex agglutination and nephelometry tests preferentially detect IgM, there are also IgG and IgA anti-immunoglobulins in rheumatoid arthritis, especially in patients with systemic vasculitis. In some patients, RF is found in free, IgG-sized IgM subunits, one-fifth the size of the normal IgM molecule. Antibody to the Fab fragment of IgG also is present but is unrelated to the progression of rheumatoid disease. Currently, these other anti-immunoglobulins merit only academic interest.

5. **Pathogenic significance.** In the synovial fluid of the inflamed rheumatoid joint are RF-containing complexes, together with evidence of complement activation, and an abundance of active inflammatory cells. This association suggests that RF may play a role in perpetuating the inflammation, but there is no direct proof that RF causes inflammation in the body.

B. **Antinuclear antibodies**

1. **The antinuclear antibody (ANA) fluorescence test**

    a. **Definition.** The term **antinuclear antibodies** encompasses all the antibodies that can be demonstrated to react with nuclei in tissue sections by the classic indirect immunofluorescence test.

    b. **Method of detection.** A nucleus-rich tissue section (monkey esophagus, rat liver, or fixed cells from a cell line) is overlaid by the patient's serum and incubated, using normal serum as a control. Antibody to nuclear antigens remains fixed to the nuclei when other serum proteins are

Table 14-1. Some diseases associated with elevations of rheumatoid factor

Disease	Percent positive
Rheumatic diseases	
Sjögren's syndrome	90
Rheumatoid arthritis	75
Dermatomyositis	50
Systemic lupus erythematosus	35
Juvenile chronic arthritis	15
Ankylosing spondylitis	5–10
Enteropathic arthritis	5–10
Psoriatic arthritis	5–10
Other inflammatory diseases	
Idiopathic pulmonary fibrosis	60
Subacute bacterial endocarditis	40
Chronic active hepatitis	25
Cirrhosis	25
Leprosy	25
Sarcoidosis	15
Normal individuals	
Normals, age 60 years or less	5
Normals, age 80 years	30

washed away. Then, fluorescein-conjugated antihuman immunoglobulin is incubated with the sections. On washing, this antibody remains bound to nuclei only if the original patient serum contained ANA. The fluorescein is then detected by fluorescence microscopy (Fig. 14-2). Titration of the patient's serum provides quantitation. The criteria for an abnormal test are set by the individual laboratory and may differ with the substrate and fixation method. The use of anti-immunoglobulins directed to other classes has shown that most ANAs are IgG immunoglobulins.

c. **Diagnostic significance.** The main use of ANA is to exclude the diagnosis of systemic lupus erythematosus (SLE), since more than 95% of patients with this disease have positive tests either at the onset of symptoms or within 3 months of onset. The ANA is useful as a screening test for antibody to a wide variety of nuclear antigens but is not specific for SLE. Many chronic inflammatory diseases can produce a positive ANA (Table 14-2). A positive ANA should trigger further diagnostic tests of greater specificity.

(1) The **pattern of staining** of the nuclei differs among diseases and suggests which tests to perform.

(a) **Diffuse** staining indicates that the pattern should be reexamined at a higher dilution. If the pattern **remains diffuse,** deoxyribonucleoprotein is likely to be the antigen, as in SLE.

(b) **Peripheral** staining suggests predominance of anti–deoxyribonucleic acid (anti-DNA) antibody (see **3**).

(c) **Speckled** staining is associated with antibody to extractable nucleoprotein antigens common in scleroderma, mixed connective tissue disease, and drug-induced lupus.

(d) **Nucleolar** staining is associated with antiribonucleoprotein, seen in scleroderma.

These antibodies are described in **3, 4,** and **5** below. The pattern seen is

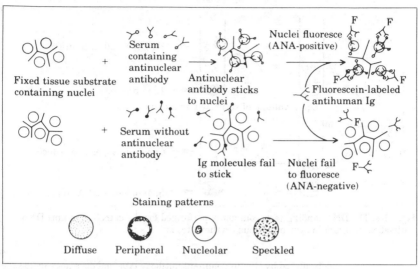

Fig. 14-2. Antinuclear antibody test by indirect immunofluorescence. This screening test is commonly performed in the diagnosis of systemic lupus erythematosus and other rheumatic diseases.

Table 14-2. Diseases associated with a positive ANA test*

Rheumatic diseases
  Systemic lupus erythematosus
  Rheumatoid arthritis
  Juvenile chronic arthritis
  Progressive systemic sclerosis
  Polymyositis
  Sjögren's syndrome
  Chronic active hepatitis

Lymphoproliferative disorders and other neoplasms

Pulmonary diseases
  Fibrosing alveolitis
  Chronic bronchitis
  Tuberculosis
  Histoplasmosis
  Hashimoto's thyroiditis

Miscellaneous conditions
  Pernicious anemia
  Ulcerative colitis
  Chronic membranous glomerulonephritis
  Lepromatous leprosy
  Myasthenia gravis
  Recurrent thrombophlebitis
  Infectious mononucleosis
  Idiopathic autoimmune hemolytic anemia
  Reactions to certain drugs (see sec. **IV.E**)

*Because of differences in technique between laboratories, quoting the incidence of positive antinuclear antibody (ANA) in these conditions is misleading. Normal values should be sought from the laboratory used. The incidence of positive ANA in healthy persons increases after age 70 years to about 20%.

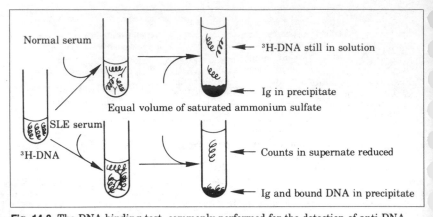

Fig. 14-3. The DNA-binding test, commonly performed for the detection of anti-DNA antibodies in serum in systemic lupus erythematosus.

determined by the predominant antibody type and does not exclude the presence of other antibodies.

(2) The ANA titer correlates poorly with relapses and remissions and is usually not a useful test for following the course of the disease or the response to therapy.

2. LE cell test

a. Definition. A phagocytic cell containing a large homogeneous eosinophilic inclusion is called an **LE cell.** Typical LE cells often form when leukocytes are incubated with serum from SLE patients.

b. Significance. The inclusions are now believed to be partly degraded nuclei, opsonized by antinucleoprotein antibodies and ingested by phagocytes. The LE cell test is laborious and both less sensitive and less specific for SLE than is the ANA. The only advantage of this test is that it requires only ordinary light microscopy, and thus it may still be used to provide suggestive evidence for SLE if facilities for the standard ANA test are not available. Historically, it was the first test developed for SLE.

3. Anti-DNA antibody

a. Method of detection. The subset of ANAs that react with native (double-stranded) DNA can be detected by complement activation, gel diffusion, agglutination of DNA-coated bentonite, and many other techniques. In the standard **DNA-binding test,** patient serum is added to ^{125}I-labeled DNA; then the IgG is precipitated either by anti-Ig or by 50% saturated ammonium sulfate (Fig. 14-3). The conditions are usually set so that sera from healthy persons precipitate less than 20% of the labeled DNA (DNA binding capacity = 20%). Greater precipitation is associated with antibodies to double-stranded DNA.

b. Significance. Antibody to double-stranded DNA is less sensitive than the ANA test in SLE but is much more specific for SLE. Furthermore, it is positively correlated with the risk and severity of nephritis. However, commercial DNA always contains single-stranded as well as double-stranded DNA. Antibody to single-stranded (denatured) DNA is prominent in almost all SLE patients, but also in patients with a variety of other diseases, such as scleroderma, rheumatoid arthritis, dermatomyositis, and chronic active hepatitis. Such antibodies also appear during therapy with a large number of medications, sometimes with SLE-like symptoms. Prominent on this list of medications are procainamide, hydralazine, isoniazid, tridione, alphamethyldopa, and phenothiazines.

Denatured contaminants can be removed by a special type of chromatographic separation, and clinicians in doubt should inquire of their laboratory as to the specificity of their DNA-binding test.

    c. Pathogenic significance. Anti-DNA antibody has been eluted from nephritic SLE kidneys and found in circulating immune complexes. These antibodies are capable of activating complement, the process by which complexes stimulate the destructive activities of phagocytic cells.

4. Antibody to extractable nuclear antigen (ENA)

    a. Definition. Certain antigens of nuclei are readily extractable in aqueous buffers, whereas DNA is not.

    b. Method of detection. The original test devised for anti-ENA demonstrated the decrease in nuclear fluorescence seen after nuclei were extracted to remove ENA, using the standard fluorescence test for ANA described in **1.b.** The extractable antigens will also react with patient sera by forming precipitates in gel. Alternatively, a spot test is available in which serum allowed to bind to a dried spot of antigen on a slide is covered with fluorescein anti-Ig, washed, and compared under an ultraviolet lamp with a spot that has reacted with normal serum. Fluorescence only over the patient's spot indicates that the serum contained antibody to ENA. Antigens identified in ENA include the Sm SS-A(Ro) and SS-B(La) antigens and ribonucleoprotein (RNP). The RNP antigen, but not the Sm antigen, is susceptible to digestion by ribonuclease (RNAase).

    c. Diagnostic significance. Antibody to the Sm antigen is highly specific for SLE. It is reported positive in 25–65% of patients, depending on the study. Antibody to RNP is not specific for SLE and, indeed, is characteristically the dominant ANA in mixed connective tissue disease. About 20% of scleroderma patients and 40% of SLE patients also have anti-RNP antibody. In fact, of the total population who has anti-RNP antibodies, probably a majority are SLE patients, since this disease is much more common than mixed connective tissue disease. SLE patients with a high ratio of anti-RNP to anti-DNA antibodies have a better prognosis, with a lower incidence of nephritis and a greater responsiveness to corticosteroids. Antibody to RNP is thought to be partly responsible for the speckled pattern of nuclear fluorescence and for much of the increased incidence of positive ANA with age.

5. Other nuclear antigens under study

    a. Anti-RNA antibodies promise to have diagnostic significance. Whereas antibody to double-stranded RNA is most common in SLE (51%), antibody to single-stranded RNA appears most frequently in scleroderma, and its presence favors that diagnosis over SLE.

    b. Two nuclear antigens, SS-A and SS-B, first described in Sjögren's syndrome, are detected by gel precipitation. SS-B has high specificity (88% positive) for the sicca syndrome (dry eyes and dry mouth) alone and for sicca syndrome with SLE (73% positive). Most patients with sicca syndrome also have SS-A, as do 65% of SLE patients with sicca syndrome. SS-A is especially common in mothers of infants with congenital heart block and neonatal lupus, and also in subacute cutaneous lupus.

C. Cryoglobulins

    1. Definition. Serum cryoglobulins are proteins that spontaneously and reversibly precipitate at temperatures below normal body temperature.

    2. Method of detection. Serum is drawn at 37°C, allowed to clot, and separated by centrifugation at the **same** temperature. After centrifugation, the serum is placed at 4°C overnight or longer, and the proportion of the volume occupied by resuspended precipitate is determined in a hematocrit centrifuge. For greater accuracy, the washed precipitate from a known volume of serum can be analyzed spectrophotometrically for protein content. The proteins present can be analyzed by gel diffusion techniques using acid buffers.

3. Diagnostic significance. Precipitates containing IgM-RF and IgG are termed **mixed cryoglobulins.**

   a. Mixed cryoglobulins are characteristic of rheumatic disease but are also found in lymphoproliferative disorders, chronic infection, chronic liver disease, and sarcoidosis. Cryoprecipitates with one immunoglobulin class raise the suspicion of myeloma or macroglobulinemia.

   b. Mixed cryoglobulinemia is associated with a variety of manifestations of **vasculitis,** usually with a distal distribution, affecting the colder parts of the body. Unfortunately, the correlation between the quantity of cryoglobulins and the severity of symptoms is poor.

   c. The test is performed at 4°C for maximal sensitivity, but a small amount of protein precipitating at 33–35°C may in fact be considerably more harmful than a large amount precipitating at 4–10°C, since the latter temperature range will not occur in the circulation. Standard methods for measuring small amounts of precipitate at physiologic temperatures are not yet available.

D. Complement

  1. Definition. The complement system is a series of 18 plasma proteins that sequentially activate each other subsequent to the binding of the first component by immune complexes (see Chap. 1), releasing:

   a. Mediators of inflammation.

   b. Fragments that bind complexes to phagocytes.

   c. An aggregate that lyses erythrocytes.

  2. Method of measurement

   a. Total complement activity is a functional test that is usually abnormal if any component is defective. As the complement components are activated, they are consumed. Thus, if a standard antigen and antibody, capable of lysing red cells in the presence of serum with normal complement activity, are added to serum in which complement has already been activated, less lysis than normal occurs at any given serum concentration.

   b. C3 and C4 tests detect the antigenic properties rather than the functional properties of C3 or C4, employing precipitation in gel with specific antibody.

  3. Diagnostic significance. Because of the rapid normal turnover of the complement proteins, within 1 or 2 days of the cessation of complement activation by immune complexes, complement levels return to normal. Thus, low levels suggest that complement has been excessively activated recently, that complement is currently being consumed, or that a single complement component is absent due to a genetic defect. The degree of activation necessary to produce abnormal test results is so great that low "total complements" are seen only in those patients most actively forming immune complexes.

   a. Cases of SLE are reported in which complement levels appeared to predict exacerbations and remissions, but the simple **erythrocyte sedimentation rate** is equally useful for this purpose and is simpler and much less expensive.

   b. Levels of C3 and C4 are useful in distinguishing whether the classic or the alternative pathway of complement activation is dominant (Table 14-3). C4 is destroyed only when the classic pathway is activated; C3 lies at the junction of the two pathways but is much more severely depressed when activation occurs by way of the alternative pathway.

   c. In SLE with nephritis, central nervous system involvement, or hemolytic anemia, serum complement may be reduced. In SLE, although classic pathway activation is most common in acute flares and alternative pathway activation is most common in chronically active disease, any combination may be seen.

   d. Complement may also be depressed in pleural and pericardial effusion fluid in SLE and rheumatoid arthritis.

Table 14-3. Interpretation of complement activation by individual components

Complement determination	Classic pathway	Alternative pathway	Sample improperly stored or too old	Inflammation
CH_{50}	Low	Low, normal	Low	High
C3	Low	Low, very low	Normal	High
C4	Very low	Normal	Low	High

    e. In rheumatoid arthritis, only patients with systemic vasculitis have depressed serum complement, although seropositive (and some seronegative) patients may have depressed complement activity in the synovial fluid of active joints.

    f. In psoriatic arthritis, ankylosing spondylitis, Reiter's syndrome, and enteropathic arthritis, complement is not consumed, and since complement components are among the **acute phase reactants** (serum proteins that increase in a wide variety of infectious or inflammatory states), their level in serum and synovial fluid may actually rise.

E. Erythrocyte sedimentation rate (ESR)

    1. Definition. The **ESR** is the rate of fall of the red cell boundary in a vertical tube of diluted anticoagulated blood under standard conditions.

    2. Diagnostic significance. Rapid sedimentation of erythrocytes in inflammatory conditions is a consequence of red cell microagglutination (rouleaux formation) by elevated levels of fibrinogen, which is one of the **acute phase reactants.** Thus, a high ESR indicates inflammation, but does not favor any particular cause. Once a diagnosis is established by other means, the ESR is the least expensive indicator of disease activity for following exacerbations, remissions, and response to therapy in the majority of patients. The test is useless when red cells have abnormal shapes (as in sickle cell disease and spherocytosis), in hyperviscosity syndromes, and in severe anemia.

        a. By the Westergren method, young adult males should show an ESR of less than 15 mm/hour; for females, the ESR is less than 20 mm/hour.

        b. The meaning of the mildly elevated ESR frequently seen in the elderly (up to 30 mm/hour) is debated, but an ESR of greater than 20 mm/hour in a young person is usually abnormal. At any age, changes are more significant than steady abnormal levels.

        c. An elevated ESR favors an infectious or inflammatory disease (including those in this chapter) over other musculoskeletal conditions, such as osteoarthritis, fibrositis, skeletal fractures, and acute allergic reactions.

        d. The ESR is also elevated in hyper- and hypothyroidism, patients taking birth control pills, and pregnancy, and may remain so for a month postpartum.

        e. When an inflammatory cause for symptoms is suspected, a normal ESR is reassuring, whereas an elevated ESR justifies further workup.

F. C-reactive protein

    1. Definition. C-reactive protein (CRP) is a serum protein and is one of the **acute phase reactants.** C-reactive protein binds the C-polysaccharide of the pneumococcus.

    2. Method of measurement. C-reactive protein is measured by precipitation with specific anti-CRP serum or by agglutination of anti-CRP–coated latex particles.

    3. Diagnostic significance. Although CRP generally parallels the ESR, the former seems to have some peculiarities. Elevation even after mild and sterile tissue injury is rapid and striking. Lack of elevation during some viral diseases, some severe toxic states, and in some forms of chronic inflammatory arthritis renders it less useful in these conditions than the ESR. It is used occasionally to monitor the activity of rheumatic fever. Because of its rapid fluctuations, serial CRP values are more useful than a single determination.

G. Analysis of synovial fluid. Examination of the synovial fluid is mandatory in any patient in whom a joint effusion develops. The only significant complication of aspiration is infection, which may be prevented by proper aseptic technique. Besides its diagnostic significance, removal of excess fluid may have a therapeutic effect, particularly if there is infection or bleeding.

1. **Studies to be done (Table 14-4) include the following:**
   a. A description of the appearance of the fluid with respect to color, turbidity, presence of blood, and viscosity. Marked cloudiness is an immediate clue to an infected fluid. Inflammatory fluids characteristically have low viscosity because of the enzymatic breakdown of hyaluronate by inflammatory cells. Normal fluid is a straw-colored, highly viscous, clear material.
   b. Culture for bacteria, fungi, and acid-fast bacilli.
   c. Complete blood count and differential.
   d. Protein determination to be coupled with a plasma protein measurement.
   e. Sugar determination to be coupled with a simultaneous blood sugar determination.
   f. Examination of the centrifuged sediment for crystals using the polarizing microscope with a red compensator, to permit the diagnosis of gout or pseudogout. If needlelike crystals appear yellow when their long axes are aligned with the compensator (slow ray), they are likely to be urate (gout). Rhomboid crystals appearing blue when their long axes are aligned with the compensator are likely to be calcium pyrophosphate (pseudogout).
   g. Special studies, such as complement and RF determinations, may be done when rheumatoid arthritis, Sjögren's syndrome, or SLE is suspected. In these diseases, joint fluid complement is often low in an acutely inflamed joint ($< 30\%$ of normal serum level), whereas in osteoarthritis, ankylosing spondylitis, Reiter's syndrome, and most other arthritides, it is normal or elevated according to the serum level. An occasional seronegative rheumatoid arthritic patient may also show RF in synovial effusions, but most do not. These tests give inconsistent results in bacterial arthritis and crystal-induced arthritis. Determination of the synovial fluid ANA is not useful. Table 14-4 shows the relationship between synovial fluid findings and the likely diagnoses.

2. **Biopsy of synovium** is indicated when tuberculosis, fungal infection, or tumor is suspected, which occurs when chronic progressive swelling in a single joint remains unexplained after routine examination and fluid culture.

H. HLA antigens. In humans, the cell surface antigens, which determine the acceptance or rejection of tissue grafts, are called **major histocompatibility,** or HLA, antigens (see Chap. 1). In the case of HLA-B27 antigens, their detection may assist in the differential diagnosis of rheumatic disease.

1. **Method of detection.** Different individuals in the species carry different HLA antigens on their cell surfaces, determined genetically like blood group antigens. These antigenic differences can stimulate T cells, which are prominently implicated in graft rejection, but they can also stimulate antibody formation under certain circumstances. Therefore, human antisera that recognize these genetic differences in antigen structure may be obtained from multiply transfused patients or multiparous women. These reagents can be used to detect those same antigens on the surface of white blood cells, a procedure commonly used prior to transplanting kidneys, bone marrow, or other organs. Cells to be typed are mixed with a battery of antisera directed to different HLA antigens and compared with the appear-

Table 14-4. Synovial fluid examination

Class	Degree of inflammation	Appearance	Mucin clot in acetic acid	White blood cell count (per mm³)	Protein (gm/dl)	Glucose	Typical diagnoses
I	None	Clear, slightly yellowish, viscous	Firm, single	≤ 2000 (<25% PMN)	<3	Normal	Trauma, degenerative joint disease
II	Mild	Slightly cloudy	Friable on shaking	2000–5000	>3	Normal	SLE (fluid may have +ANA and/or low complement); pseudogout (calcium pyrophosphate crystals present)
III	Moderate	Definitely turbid	Fragmented	5000–50,000 >50% PMN)	>3	Equivocal	Gout (urate crystals present); rheumatoid arthritis (may have +RF and/or low complement)
IV	Severe	Pus, viscosity poor	None	>50,000 (>90% PMN)	>3	Less than 70% of plasma level*	Septic arthritis (complement usually normal or elevated)

Key: PMN = polymorphonuclear leukocytes; SLE = systemic lupus erythematosus; ANA = antinuclear antibody; RF = rheumatoid factor.
*Glucose less than 20% of plasma level strongly suggests infection. Some rheumatoid arthritis (RA) synovial fluid glucose levels fall in the 20–70% range, overlapping with those of septic arthritis.

ance of typing cells known to carry those antigens in a test tube aggregation reaction.

2. **Relationship to disease.** The estimated relative risks of the development of various diseases may be elevated in individuals bearing certain HLA antigens (Table 14-5). The **relative risk** may be understood as the increased chances that a disease will develop if one has a given antigen, in comparison with the chance of the same disease developing in individuals who lack it.

3. **Importance of HLA-B27.** The only HLA antigen with a disease association strong enough to be useful in differential diagnosis is HLA-B27. Although only 8% of normal whites carry this antigen, 90% of patients with either ankylosing spondylitis (AS) or spondylitis in association with Reiter's syndrome carry it. An elevated percentage of HLA-B27–positive patients is also recorded in juvenile chronic arthritis with spinal involvement, psoriatic arthritis, the arthritis of inflammatory bowel disease, and *Yersinia*-associated arthritis. Major indications for an HLA-B27 test are to rule out AS when back pain develops in relatives of patients with the disease, and to help to distinguish incomplete Reiter's syndrome from gonococcal arthritis, or chronic or atypical Reiter's syndrome from rheumatoid arthritis. A negative test for HLA-B27 does not exclude the diagnosis of AS or Reiter's syndrome.

I. The **Coombs' test** relies on the ability of antisera to IgG or to C3b (a fragment of the third component of complement) to agglutinate erythrocytes that bear these molecules on their surfaces, as occurs in autoimmune and drug-induced hemolytic anemias.

1. In the **direct** Coombs' test, the presence of Ig or C3b on the patient's own erythrocytes is detected by exposing the cells to various dilutions of rabbit or goat antibody to human IgG, IgM, or C3b and scoring agglutination under the microscope. Since C3b remains on the cells long after antibody has escaped, anti-C3b (formerly called anti–non-gamma) may agglutinate cells even when anti-Ig does not, as in about 20% of patients with warm-antibody hemolytic anemia and in most patients with cold agglutinin disease.

2. The **indirect** Coombs' test detects the presence of free antibody to red cell surface antigens in the patient's serum. Standard type O, Rh-negative red cells are exposed to a series of dilutions of patient's serum, washed, and then exposed (as in the direct test) to antibody to IgG, IgM, or C3b. The greatest dilution of patient's serum leading to agglutination is the **indirect Coombs' titer.** If cells are pretreated with proteolytic enzymes, the test's sensitivity is increased.

III. **Rheumatoid arthritis (RA)** is a chronic systemic inflammatory disease of unknown origin that causes inflammation of synovial joints and, less commonly, other structures such as serosal surfaces and small vessels.

A. **Incidence.** Rheumatoid arthritis is the most common autoimmune inflammatory disease, afflicting about 3% of the adult population. In the typical arthritis clinic, 70% of RA patients are female. Onset can occur at any age, but is most frequent between the ages of 30 and 50. No definite racial, geographic, or climatic variation in incidence has been proved.

B. **Clinical diagnosis.** The American Rheumatism Association (ARA) has proposed the criteria shown in Table 14-6 for diagnosing RA and has specified that this diagnosis also requires the specific exclusion of other causes of arthritis by clinical and laboratory criteria.

1. The **onset** of RA may be acute or insidious. Gradual development of symmetric polyarthritis involving the small joints of the hands and feet is typical, but asymmetric, monoarticular, or large-joint presentations are occasionally seen. Fever is an inconsistent feature; weight loss and fatigue are common. Morning stiffness with greater mobility later in the day is a typical complaint.

2. Since RA is a systemic inflammatory disease, it may involve a variety of **extraarticular tissues,** producing vasculitis in the skin (particularly distal)

Table 14-5. Relationship of HLA antigens to disease risk

Antigen and disease	Relative risk[a]
B27	
Ankylosing spondylitis	$100 \times$ [b]
Reiter's syndrome	$40 \times$
Anterior uveitis	$25 \times$
Yersinia or *Salmonella* arthritis	$20 \times$
Psoriatic arthritis with spinal involvement	$11 \times$
Spondylitis associated with inflammatory bowel disease	$9 \times$
Juvenile chronic arthritis with spinal involvement	$5 \times$
B8	
Celiac disease	$9 \times$
Addison's disease	$6 \times$
Myasthenia gravis	$5 \times$
Dermatitis herpetiformis	$4 \times$
Chronic active hepatitis	$4 \times$
Sjögren's syndrome	$3 \times$
Diabetes mellitus (insulin-dependent)	$2 \times$
Thyrotoxicosis	$2 \times$
B5	
Behçet's syndrome	$6 \times$
BW38	
Psoriatic arthritis	$7 \times$
BW15	
Diabetes mellitus (insulin-dependent)	$3 \times$
DR2	
Goodpasture's syndrome	$16 \times$
Multiple sclerosis	$4 \times$
DR3	
Gluten-sensitive enteropathy	$21 \times$
Dermatitis herpetiformis	$14 \times$
Subacute cutaneous lupus erythematosus	$12 \times$
Addison's disease	$11 \times$
Sjögren's syndrome (primary)	$10 \times$
DR4	
Pemphigus (in Jewish individuals)	$32 \times$
Giant-cell arteritis	$8 \times$
Rheumatoid arthritis	$6 \times$
Juvenile diabetes mellitus	$5 \times$
DR5	
Pauciarticular juvenile arthritis	$5 \times$
Scleroderma	$5 \times$
Hashimoto's thyroiditis	$3 \times$

[a]Risk of disease over a lifetime for persons lacking the antigen = 1.
[b]Varies with ethnic group, e.g., 3-fold for Pima Indians and 300-fold for Japanese.

Table 14-6. Criteria for diagnosis and classification of rheumatoid arthritis*

Categories

1. Classic RA: Requires 7 of the 11 criteria, with criteria 1–5 present continuously for 6 wk
2. Definite RA: Requires 5 of the 11 criteria, with criteria 1–5 present continuously for 6 wk
3. Probable RA: Requires 3 of the 11 criteria, with joint symptoms present for 4 wk

Criteria (signs and symptoms) for categories 1, 2, and 3

1. Morning stiffness
2. Pain on motion or tenderness in a joint
3. Swelling of at least one joint observed by a physician
4. Swelling of another joint within 3 months of the first joint
5. Symmetric simultaneous swelling of the same joint or set of joints on the right and left side (excluding the distal interphalangeal joints)
6. Subcutaneous nodules observed by a physician
7. X-ray changes typical of RA
8. Positive RF
9. Poor mucin precipitate from synovial fluid (see Table 14-4)
10. Characteristic histologic changes in synovial membrane (now rarely applied)
11. Characteristic histologic changes in nodules with granulomatous foci in central zones of necrosis, chronic inflammatory cells, and peripheral fibrosis

4. Possible RA: Requires 2 of the 6 criteria and at least 3 wk total duration of symptoms

Criteria (signs and symptoms) for category 4

1. Morning stiffness
2. Pain or tenderness on motion, with recurrence or persistence over a period of 3 wk
3. Joint swelling confirmed by an observer
4. Subcutaneous nodules
5. Elevated ESR
6. Iritis

Key: RA = rheumatoid arthritis; RF = rheumatoid factor; ESR = erythrocyte sedimentation rate.
*As proposed by the American Rheumatism Association.

leg ulcers); Raynaud's phenomenon (painful vasospasm in the hands, frequently induced by cold); lymphadenopathy; episcleritis and conjunctivitis; pleural or pericardial inflammation and effusion; diffuse interstitial pulmonary fibrosis; compression neuropathy (such as carpal tunnel syndrome); other peripheral neuropathies; and a host of other, rarer manifestations. In general, extraarticular manifestations develop late in severe disease.

   C. Laboratory diagnosis
   1. **Radiographic studies.** Early in the disease, x-rays may show only soft-tissue swelling since at least 6 months of continuous inflammation is usually required for bony changes to develop. The earliest changes include periarticular osteoporosis, then narrow joint spaces due to destruction of cartilage, and, finally, **erosions** (loss of bony cortex at articular margins) and, more rarely, subarticular cysts. Periostitis is visible early but gener-

ally disappears with time. Persistent, prominent periostitis suggests a different diagnosis (see secs. **XII** [Reiter's syndrome] and **XIII** [Psoriatic arthritis]) or superimposed infection. As the disease progresses, severe and multiple erosions may produce an irregular articular surface. Subluxation of the joints may occur, and osteoporosis may become generalized. The bone overgrowth and spurs that sometimes appear late in the disease are attributed to superimposed degenerative arthritis rather than to RA.

An adequate **initial radiographic evaluation** of a patient suspected of having RA should include anteroposterior views of the hands, wrists, feet, and knees (standing), as well as lateral extension or fusion views of the neck and any other joints that are clinically involved.

2. **Serologic tests.** The **latex agglutination test** for RF is the main diagnostic aid. Its meaning and limitations are discussed in sec. **II.A.**

3. For following the general degree of inflammatory activity, the **ESR** is useful (see sec. **II.E**), although it usually parallels the physical examination. An elevated ESR favors inflammation over alternative causes of musculoskeletal pain.

4. **Hematology.** Mild leukocytosis is common in acute exacerbations of inflammation. Anemia is typically normochromic, normocytic, with normal marrow iron stores (anemia of chronic disease). Superimposed iron-deficiency anemia due to gastrointestinal blood loss secondary to drug therapy is also common.

5. **Serum chemistry studies.** Serum iron, iron-binding capacity, and degree of saturation are often low. Serum cholesterol is usually low, as in chronic infections. Serum protein electrophoresis shows an increase in gamma globulin or other globulin fractions. Serum alkaline phosphatase is commonly slightly elevated (subclinical liver dysfunction has been postulated). Uric acid, calcium, and phosphorus are generally normal.

6. **Synovial fluid.** See Table 14-4.

D. **Treatment.** In the early stages, management of RA encompasses anti-inflammatory medication, maintenance of range of motion, muscle function through exercise, the application of physical therapy, and patient education. Later in the course of disease, the emphasis often shifts to rehabilitation and corrective surgery. Throughout the course of the disease, successful management is critically dependent on the active participation of the patient and the centralization of ongoing care in the hands of one primary physician.

Therapeutic decisions depend on careful clinical assessment of disease activity. Examination of the number of joints showing the four major signs of inflammation (swelling, tenderness, redness, and warmth) is fundamental for documenting clinical progression or response. Duration of morning stiffness is also a useful indicator of disease activity. Changes in range of motion, grip strength, 50-foot walking time, and effusion size may be used to assess progression of the disease.

1. **Salicylate therapy.** Every patient with RA initially deserves an adequate therapeutic trial of salicylates. Salicylates are anti-inflammatory, analgesic, and antipyretic and relieve stiffness as well as pain.

   a. Both therapeutic and toxic effects depend on the serum **free salicylate level.** As the dose of salicylate increases, there is little change in plasma salicylate level until certain liver enzymes are exhausted, at which point a small increment in salicylate intake may cause a major increase in free salicylate level. The dose needed to saturate liver enzymes varies greatly among individuals. **Low plasma albumin and low urine pH** also predispose to more rapid and greater increases in free serum salicylate.

   b. **Dosage.** Adult patients on aspirin should begin with eight 325-mg tablets (two taken on arising, at lunch, at dinner, and at bedtime). The total daily dose is increased by two tablets every 5–7 days. This schedule allows for the full increment in serum salicylate level to be achieved before the decision is made to raise the dose. The small increments prevent major increases in plasma salicylate, which could cause toxicity (see sec. **VI.D** for aspirin dosage in children). In many patients (except the elderly), tinnitus is an effective warning that therapeutic levels have been reached. However, where possible, it should be established that the plasma salicylate level is stable in the therapeutic range of 20–30 mg/dl. Many patients can regulate their own salicylate levels by noting mild tinnitus about an hour after each dose that then disappears.

c. Patients should be told that the use of aspirin in RA is very different from its use for headache; it should be taken on a regular schedule, not just when pain is intense. Acute pain should be treated by other modalities or analgesics.

d. In the event that a patient does not respond to aspirin, the serum salicylate level will document that an adequate therapeutic trial was achieved.

e. Aspirin **side effects** include dyspepsia (extremely common) and gastroduodenal hemorrhage (direct erosion of the mucosa). Occult blood in the stool is present in about 70% of patients, and the risk of bleeding is increased by alcohol. Tinnitus and hearing impairment are almost always reversible but indicate that the dose should be reduced. Hypoprothrombinemia and potentiation of bleeding are seen in patients who are also on anticoagulant therapy. Such therapy should not be combined with the use of aspirin. Rarer side effects include hypersensitivity reactions (urticaria, bronchospasm) and liver enzyme elevations, even hepatitis.

f. For patients with gastrointestinal toxicity whose inflammation responds to aspirin, a variety of **modified aspirin** derivatives are available, including enteric-coated aspirin and nonacetylated salicylates such as salsalate (Disalcid), choline magnesium salicylate (Trilisate) and diflunisal (Dolobid).

2. None of the more recent **nonsteroidal anti-inflammatory drugs** (Table 14-7) predictably exceeds aspirin in effectiveness. Yet many of these agents have a lower incidence of side effects than aspirin, especially gastrointestinal bleeding, and are useful in patients who cannot tolerate aspirin.

Because patient's react to these medications in a highly individual way with respect to therapeutic response and toxicity, there is no basis for recommending any particular order of trial. The dose is gradually increased at 1- to 2-week intervals toward the maximum until improvement is seen. A therapeutic trial should consist of 2 weeks of administration of the maximal dose of the drug. There is no proved benefit from combining any of the agents in Table 14-7 with aspirin or with each other.

The agents listed in Table 14-7 provide many chances to achieve satisfactory control when aspirin has failed, before progressing to more dangerous agents or while waiting for an antirheumatic drug to take effect. They are all much more expensive than aspirin. In elderly patients, both efficacy and toxicity may appear at lower doses than those given in Table 14-7.

3. The **antirheumatic agents,** mainly **gold** and **penicillamine,** may actually halt the progressive joint destruction in some patients with RA. Both require a commitment from patient and physician to regular clinic visits for drug administration over many months, with repeated blood and urine tests to detect dangerous side effects. Thus, they are appropriate for patients in whom the disease appears to be severe and unremitting, with an unsatisfactory response to other nonsteroidal anti-inflammatory drugs.

a. **Gold.** In the form of gold sodium thiomalate (Myochrysine) or thioglucose (Solganal), gold salts are given by deep intramuscular injection at weekly intervals.

(1) **Dosage.** To test for idiosyncratic reactions, the dose is increased from 10 to 25 to 50 mg over the first 4 weeks (see sec. **VI.D.2** for dose in children). The dose of 50 mg a week is maintained until response or toxicity occurs. Responses with less than 3 months of treatment are unusual. Between 3 months and 1 year, 75% of patients will

Table 14-7. Nonsteroidal anti-inflammatory drugs

Agent	Adult dose	Toxicity	Effect
Indomethacin (Indocin)	50 mg bid, then tid with meals; of no extra benefit in patients on aspirin; available in sustained release (SR) and suppository form	Headaches, (crushing), mental confusion, gastrointestinal pain, ulcers, salt retention	Greater in spine and large joints than in small joints, greater if taken between meals
Phenylbutazone (Butazolidin)	100 mg tid–qid (for periods < 2 wk to avoid toxicity)	Agranulocytosis (sometimes fatal), potentiates anticoagulants, ulcers	Best for large joints, acute gout or other brief flares
Ibuprofen (Motrin, Rufen, Advil, Nuprin)	200–600 mg qid	Less gastrointestinal toxicity than with aspirin, headache, rash	Similar to aspirin in RA
Fenoprofen (Nalfon)	200 800 mg qid	Similar to ibuprofen	Similar to aspirin in RA
Naproxen (Naprosyn)	250–500 mg bid–tid	Similar to ibuprofen	Similar to aspirin in RA, better analgesic than sulindac
Tolmetin (Tolectin)	400–600 mg tid (for children 2 yr and older, 15–30 mg/kg/day)	Less gastrointestinal toxicity than aspirin, rash	Similar to aspirin in RA and indomethacin in AS, least potentiation of anticoagulants
Sulindac (Clinoril)	150 or 200 mg bid	Less gastrointestinal toxicity than aspirin, tinnitis, headache, rash, hepatic toxicity (rare)	Similar to aspirin in RA and indomethacin in AS
Meclofenamate (Meclomen)	50–100 mg qid	Less gastric toxicity than aspirin, but more diarrhea	Similar to aspirin in RA
Piroxicam (Feldene)	20 mg/day (single tablet)	Less gastrointestinal toxicity than aspirin, rash	Similar to aspirin in RA
Ketaprofen (Orudis)	150–300 mg/day in 3–4 divided doses	Gastrointestinal toxicity, renal toxicity, and CNS side effects	Similar to aspirin in RA

Key: RA = rheumatoid arthritis; AS = ankylosing spondylitis.

improve, and 25% will experience a nearly complete remission. If there is no benefit from a 2-gm cumulative dose, gold should be stopped. Once response is achieved, it can often be maintained even though the interval between 50-mg doses is increased to 2 or even 3 weeks to reduce the risk of toxicity.

    (2) Side effects include rash or stomatitis; marrow toxicity, manifested as thrombocytopenia followed by neutropenia and anemia; and renal toxicity, beginning as proteinuria. If gold is not discontinued, the hematologic and renal manifestations can be fatal. Thus, weekly visits include skin inspection, a complete blood count, and urinalysis prior to injection. After a rash clears, gold may often be restarted at a reduced dose without further difficulty, but marrow and renal toxicity mandate **permanent discontinuance.** Eosinophilia is common but does not necessarily predict toxicity. Rarely, thrombocytopenia may occur months after gold is discontinued.

    (3) Auranofin (Ridaura) is a gold preparation taken orally (3 mg twice a day). Efficacy appears equal to intramuscularly administered gold in some studies, a little less in others. Serious side effects appear less frequently, but diarrhea is more common.

  b. Penicillamine. As with gold, the onset of benefit may be delayed several months, the risk of toxicity is substantial, and one-third of patients may receive no benefit. However, neither gold toxicity nor penicillamine toxicity alters the risk of toxicity from the other agents.

    (1) Dosage. The recommended adult regimen consists of one 250-mg tablet/day for 12 weeks, two times/day for 12 more weeks, then 3 times/day until remission of symptoms. For maintenance, the dosage is reduced to the level associated with the first clinical improvement and may be continued indefinitely if effective.

    (2) Sites of serious **toxicity** include the bone marrow, kidneys, and gastrointestinal tract. Reduction or alteration of taste sensation is common but reversible when the drug is stopped. A complete blood count and urinalysis are done weekly to check for thrombocytopenia, neutropenia, proteinuria, and hematuria. If any of these conditions occurs, the drug must be stopped.

4. Antimalarials may be used in conjunction with other anti-inflammatory or antirheumatic drugs to obtain additional relief. For adults, chloroquine phosphate (250 mg/day) or hydroxychloroquine sulfate (Plaquenil Sulfate) (200 mg twice a day; in children 6 mg/kg/day based on ideal body weight) is prescribed, and improvement is generally evident by 3 months. Important side effects are described in sec. **V.C.**

5. Corticosteroids

  a. Systemic corticosteroids (see also Chap. 4). Formerly, systemic corticosteroids were so widely used in the treatment of RA that their severe side effects constituted the most significant cause of mortality associated with this disease. Although these agents immediately reduce the pain of inflammation, the dose necessary to control symptoms often progressively increases into the toxic range, and rapid withdrawal often produces a violent relapse.

    (1) Early dose-related **side effects** of systemic corticosteroid therapy include euphoria, glucose intolerance, and hyperlipidemia. Additional complications become significant when doses greater than 10 mg/day of prednisone (or equivalent) are used longer than 4 weeks. These complications include edema, striae, "buffalo hump," truncal and facial obesity, plethoric face, hirsutism, acne, posterior subcapsular cataracts, glaucoma, ecchymoses, gastrointestinal ulceration, aseptic necrosis (especially of the femoral head), increased incidence of infection (especially tuberculosis), hypertension, "hot flashes" and menstrual disorders, myopathy (presenting as proximal muscle weakness), osteoporosis, pancreatitis (especially in children), and a variety of psychiatric manifestations ranging from insomnia to psychosis.

(2) **Indications and contraindications.** Chronicity of inflammation is a general contraindication to systemic corticosteroid use, applying especially in RA. There are instances in which systemic corticosteroids in high doses (40–60 mg of prednisone/day) for several weeks can be of benefit, especially in severe cases of Felty's syndrome (RA with neutropenia), iritis or episcleritis, serositis, or vasculitis. In patients with chronic joint inflammation only, the balance of benefit to risk with 5–10 mg/day of prednisone is still debated. Side effects are less common at this dose (osteoporosis, hyperglycemia, and gastritis may still occur), and adrenal suppression is minimal. After improvement is noted, dose reductions of 1 mg/day every week should be used to find the minimum dose that maintains improvement. In no instance should doses greater than 10 mg of prednisone a day (or equivalent) be used chronically (longer than about 4 weeks) to control joint inflammation.

(3) **Tapering of corticosteroid dose** (also see Chap. 4). A common management problem is to withdraw patients from inappropriately high doses of corticosteroids. This effort requires carefully timed small decreases in dose (tapering), since abrupt discontinuance may precipitate Addisonian crisis, manifested as fatigue, weakness, sore joints, headaches, gastrointestinal cramps, or even life-threatening vascular collapse. Such symptoms are potentiated by tranquilizers. In patients who have taken 20 mg/day of prednisone for a long period (over 6 months), begin tapering by reducing the dose on alternate days, keeping the total dose over each 2-day period constant. If the patient can tolerate less than 20 mg of prednisone on the low-dose day, adrenal suppression and toxicity will be much less. Dose changes every 2–6 weeks are safest. If the patient begins to feel improvement on the low-dose day or if the low dose reaches zero, reduction of the "high"-day dose should ensue. If the initial dose is 60 mg of prednisone/day, decrease the dose to 40 mg/day, then to 30, 25, and 20 mg/day, then by 2-mg steps to 12 mg/day and by 1-mg steps thereafter, with plateaus longer than 6 weeks when control is marginal. Relapses occur in some patients, dictating that their maintenance dosage must remain for a while at the level that last relieved symptoms. If high-dose steroids were used for less than 6 months, a more rapid tapering schedule may be used.

(4) **Supplementation after withdrawal.** After corticosteroid withdrawal, adrenal gland suppression varies in severity and duration among patients, depending on the duration of treatment. For example, a patient successfully withdrawn from 10 years of high-dose corticosteroids may not have an adequate adrenal response to the stress of severe illness or surgery for 2–5 years after the last dose. Corticosteroid supplementation is needed during surgery in such patients: 100 mg of hydrocortisone before anesthesia the morning of surgery, 15 mg of methylprednisolone given intravenously every 8 hours the next day, and 10 mg every 8 hours the third day. By the fourth day, oral prednisone can often be substituted; no significant corticosteroid side effects or need for prolonged tapering should arise if corticosteroids are discontinued by 1 week.

b. **Local injection of corticosteroids.** The injection of slow-release corticosteroid preparations into the synovial cavity of an inflamed joint can be beneficial. The major indication is one joint that produces a major share of the pain and disability, provided there is no infection.

(1) Strict **aseptic** technique is advised, since the consequences of introducing pathogens into a joint are severe. A 21- or 22-gauge needle long enough to reach the joint cavity is adequate for injection, al-

though aspiration of large effusions may require an 18- to 20-gauge needle.

(2) After fluid is removed, use 0.3 ml of Hydeltra-TBA (40 mg/cc) (Depo-Medrol and Aristospan are alternatives) for small joints (finger, wrist, elbow), 1 ml for medium-to-large joints (ankle, shoulder), and 2 ml for the knee. The benefit may last from 2 days to several months. Generally, one medium or large joint at a time is the limit. The same joint should not be injected more often than once in 2 months or 4 times in 1 year. Restrict the total number of injections to about one/month, or 10 ml/year. Cautioning the patient against the overuse of successfully treated joints may prevent joint damage.

6. Physical therapy

a. **Hot applications** with wet towels or paraffin are often effective in reducing morning stiffness.

b. Although exacerbation of intense inflammation requires a period of **rest** and immobility, prolonged immobility is the route to total disability. Thus, partial control of inflammation justifies instituting **passive range-of-motion exercises** to prevent contracture. When inflammation subsides further, begin the **active range-of-motion** and **isometric exercises;** their regular use contributes significantly to the long-term maintenance of joint function. Pain lasting more than 1 hour after exercise is an indication to decrease the vigor of the exercise but not the frequency. **Quadriceps strengthening exercises** are especially useful when the knee joints are involved.

7. Occupational therapy

a. Analysis of **activities of daily living** should be conducted to identify and prioritize problems caused by joint inflammation occurring at home or on the job.

b. Significant benefit may be derived from **joint protection training.** This training may enable patients to improve their daily living skills considerably while reducing joint stress and pain.

c. **Splinting** of wrists and other painful joints for pain relief at night or during use may be coupled with active range-of-motion exercises.

d. A variety of ingenious **assistive devices** are available to extend the range of activities patients can perform independently, thereby decreasing their dependence on others.

E. **Patient education.** The patient should understand the disease well enough to take an active role in management; this understanding is essential for success. Expectations should be brought into line with reality. Every patient reporting the recent onset of symptoms suggesting RA should be told the following:

1. About half the patients who have symptoms resembling those of RA for less than 6 months recover and do not progress to chronic inflammatory disease.

2. Severe deformities and extreme disability occur in only 5–10% of RA patients. However, after 3 years of continuous symptoms, a complete remission is not to be expected.

IV. **Systemic lupus erythematosus (SLE)** is a systemic inflammatory disease involving immune complex deposition affecting many organs. In many ways, it is the prototype of autoimmune disease. Of patients with the disease, 90% are women. The onset in most patients is between the ages of 20 and 45 years. Although it can be familial and although there is an association between SLE and deficiencies in several of the early classic pathway complement components (especially C2), the genetic mechanisms determining predisposition to the disease have not yet been determined.

A. **Clinical diagnosis.** The symptoms and pathologic features of SLE are determined by the site and extent of immune complex deposition. Thus, patients may differ dramatically in the relative severity and pattern of organ involvement; in fact, two patients with this diagnosis may have no symptoms in common. A variety of clinical features are seen in SLE:

1. **Arthralgias** are often a presenting feature and develop in about 90% of patients.
2. An **arthritis** superficially resembling RA may develop, but objective signs are usually much milder than in RA, pain is more often migratory, and bone erosions or deformities (other than ulnar deviation and subluxation of fingers at the metacarpophalangeal joints) are rare.
3. **Avascular necrosis** of the femoral head can occur even without corticosteroid therapy.
4. In a few patients, **muscle weakness** from inflammatory myositis may develop.
5. Continuous or intermittent **fever** is common; rarely, the fevers cause shaking chills.
6. A characteristic, erythematous, malar butterfly **rash** is common and is often exacerbated by exposure to sunlight. A maculopapular eruption may involve the face, neck, and arms. In its most severe form, the rash presents with induration, epidermal plugs, and scaliness, resulting finally in loss of dermal appendages, scarring, atrophy, and pigmentary changes, as in discoid lupus erythematosus (see sec. **V**).
7. All the lesions typical of systemic **vasculitis** can occur, including distal leg ulcers, involution and scarring of the fingertips and nail beds, and gangrene of the fingertips. **Alopecia** and short hairs at the hairline are also seen.
8. **Cardiac** manifestations (usually subclinical) occur in 50% of patients, most commonly pericarditis or pericardial effusion. Myocarditis usually presents as an arrhythmia.
9. Fifty percent of patients develop some degree of **renal involvement,** manifested as glomerular inflammation, which results from immune complex deposition and complement activation. Eventually, through the destructive activities of inflammatory cells, the glomerular capillary basement membrane may be destroyed, leading to proteinuria and nephrotic syndrome, hematuria, or all three. Later, progressive uremia ensues, but hypertension is only occasional. Persistent proteinuria may be seen in remission because of permanent basement membrane damage.
10. The **lung** is involved in 50% of patients (often subclinically). Platelike atelectasis at the lung bases, pleurisy, and small effusions are common. With time, serosal inflammation may lead to fibrosis. In some patients pleural adhesions result in partial obliteration of the pleural space, elevation of the diaphragm, and reduction in vital capacity.
11. The **nervous system** is involved in about 20% of patients. Peripheral neuropathy can be symmetric or of the "mononeuritis multiplex" variety. Cranial nerve palsies, seizures, or transverse myelitis may occur. Rarely, central nervous system involvement progresses to coma and death. Subtle behavior changes often occur in SLE, and, in an occasional patient, frank **psychosis** develops, often with manic-depressive features. White exudates in the superficial layer of the retina (cytoid bodies) rarely cause symptoms.
12. Antibodies to platelets may cause **thrombocytopenia,** and autoimmune **hemolytic anemia** and **lymphopenia** are often seen.
13. Half of the patients with SLE have **lymphadenopathy,** occasionally of marked degree.
14. The polyserositis of SLE may cause **abdominal pain. Gastrointestinal ulceration** and ulcers in the mouth and oropharynx occur.
15. The American Rheumatism Association has proposed that patients meeting four of the fourteen criteria presented in Table 14-8 be considered to have SLE.

B. **Laboratory diagnosis**
   1. **Tests for autoantibodies, ANA** (see sec. **II.B.1**), and **DNA binding** (see sec. **II.B.3**) are the major diagnostic tests in SLE. Tests for syphilis are often false-positive, but the *Treponema* immobilization test is almost always negative. Antibodies to thyroglobulin or to human IgG (RF) occur, each in

Table 14-8. Systemic lupus erythematosus (SLE): American Rheumatism Association preliminary criteria*

1. Arthritis without deformity
2. LE cells
3. Facial erythema
4. Alopecia
5. Pleurisy or pericarditis
6. Hemolytic anemia, leukopenia, or thrombocytopenia
7. Photosensitivity
8. Cellular casts in urine
9. Raynaud's phenomenon
10. Discoid LE
11. Oral or nasopharyngeal ulcers
12. Proteinuria (3.5 gm/24 hr)
13. Psychosis or seizures
14. False-positive test for syphilis for 6 mo

*Criteria are listed in approximate order of incidence. If four or more criteria are present, SLE is the presumptive clinical diagnosis, but the antinuclear antibody (ANA) should also be positive.

about 20% of the patients. Antibodies to red cell antigens can cause autoimmune hemolytic anemia and can be demonstrated by a positive direct or indirect Coombs' test (see sec. **II.I**). Antiplatelet antibodies can cause thrombocytopenia, and antibodies to lymphocytes may cause depletion of one or more lymphocyte subclasses. Circulating anticoagulants prolong the partial thromboplastin time and prothrombin time, are associated with thromboses and spontaneous abortions, but rarely cause clinical bleeding. A variety of other autoantibodies may also be present. The total immunoglobulin in the serum is elevated in active disease, yet primary immune responses to vaccines may be poor.

2. **Other findings**
   a. The **ESR** is usually raised in active SLE.
   b. Fibrinogen, gamma globulin, and other immunoglobulin fractions are generally elevated. Cryoglobulins (see sec. **II.C**) and cold agglutinins may be present.
   c. Total **complement activity** (see sec. **II.D**) is frequently depressed in active disease, but may be normal when the disease is relatively quiescent. Either the classic or the alternative pathway (or both) may be activated; therefore, both C3 and C4 may be low. SLE patients show an increased incidence of genetic defects affecting the levels of certain complement components, namely, C1, C2, C4, and C5. In the case of C2, the most common deficiency, the histocompatibility alleles HLA-A10 and B18 are associated. Except for C3 and C4, tests for these components are not readily available.
   d. Renal involvement leads to elevated serum **creatinine** and diminished **creatinine clearance.** Urinalysis frequently reveals **proteinuria** and **hematuria.**
   e. For synovial fluid findings, see Table 14-4.
C. **Pathologic features.** Besides the typical LE cell, other characteristic pathologic features are seen in SLE. These features include the following:
   1. The verrucous endocarditis of Libman and Sacks.
   2. Irregular thickening of the basement membrane of the glomeruli, associated with lumpy deposits (visible by electron microscopy) containing immunoglobulin and complement components (revealed by immunofluorescence). These changes in the basement membrane appear as "wire-loop" lesions by light microscopy. Glomerular changes may range from a thick-

ened basement membrane to mesangial hypercellularity, to focal glomerulitis, to diffuse glomerulonephritis with extensive electron-dense deposits and crescent formation. None of these changes is diagnostic of SLE.

3. **Vacuolar myopathy** associated with muscle weakness is seen in some patients.

4. Concentric **fibrosis** ("onion-skin lesion") is seen in the arteries of the spleen.

D. **Therapeutic management**

1. Arthralgia and serositis are best treated with **salicylates** (see sec. **III.D.1**), or, in patients who cannot tolerate aspirin, with other nonsteroidal anti-inflammatory drugs (see Table 14-7).

2. Chloroquine or hydroxychloroquine or other **antimalarials** (see sec. **V.C**) are especially effective in SLE skin involvement but are ordinarily inadequate to control the renal disease. Treatment continues as long as symptoms persist, unless prohibited by side effects.

3. Damage to major organ systems (e.g., the kidneys, central nervous system, or heart) or hemolytic anemia or thrombocytopenia mandates treatment with systemic **corticosteroids**, beginning with at least 60 mg/day of prednisone or its equivalent.

   a. Control of disease sufficient to begin gradual reduction of the corticosteroid dose is achieved when the ESR returns to 20 mm/hour, hematuria ceases, proteinuria decreases, complement returns to normal, creatinine clearance rises, anemia improves, or central nervous system symptoms remit. Early in the disease, proteinuria and renal function should return to normal, but after several relapses, cumulative damage may result in the persistence of proteinuria and creatinine elevation, even when active inflammation is minimal.

   b. Once the disease is controlled, corticosteroids should be tapered slowly to the greatest extent consistent with maintaining clinical improvement (see the discussion of corticosteroid tapering in sec. **III.D.5**).

   c. Clinical relapse, increased hemolysis, or renal function deterioration indicates the need to return to the most recent dose that controlled disease activity, with subsequent tapering more gradual than before.

4. Patients whose disease is incompletely controlled on corticosteroids or who require more than 2 months of doses over 40 mg of prednisone a day (despite attempts to taper) should be considered for immunosuppressive therapy with **azathioprine** or **cyclophosphamide.** These drugs greatly increase the incidence of infection, and their effect on the long-term prognosis of the disease is still being evaluated. In general, their use should be directed by experienced specialists.

5. **Rest** during periods of active inflammation is important.

6. It is not necessary to advise all SLE patients to avoid sunlight, but those who have shown solar sensitivity in the form of a skin rash should be so advised. Sunscreens (commercially labeled sun protection factor [SPF] of 10–15) to protect the skin from ultraviolet radiation should be used by sun-sensitive patients.

E. **Drug-induced SLE syndrome.** Although medications such as isoniazid, procainamide, and hydralazine can induce positive ANA, they have not been shown to affect the course of SLE. They may, however, induce an SLE-like syndrome, presenting as fever and aching, with serositis, arthralgias, or arthritis, and occasionally anemia. The ESR and alpha globulins are elevated. The incidence of positive ANA, however, is much greater than the incidence of symptoms. For example, about 75% of individuals treated with procainamide have positive ANA, but symptoms develop in only 30%. Symptoms are related to the dose and duration of the medication and are generally reversible. Renal involvement is extremely rare. The ANA is not directed to double-stranded DNA as in SLE, but mainly to ribonucleoproteins and histones. The sex incidence of drug-induced ANA is equal. **Treatment** is usually confined to withdrawal of the offending medication. Salicylates can be added until symptoms abate.

V. Discoid lupus erythematosus

A. Clinical features. Discoid lupus erythematosus is a syndrome in which skin lesions similar to those of SLE in appearance, distribution, and pathologic features are seen without the disseminated visceral manifestations. The malar area and scalp are often involved first, followed by the rest of the face, the shoulders, and the backs of the hands. Since the natural history of discoid lupus rarely involves progression to the systemic form of the disease, it is best considered as a separate entity.

B. Pathologic and laboratory diagnosis. Under the microscope, hyperkeratotic plugging of hair follicles, edema in the dermis, dilation and tortuosity of capillaries, and cellular lymphocytic infiltrates around the deeper blood vessels are all characteristic. The deposition of Ig and C3 along the basement membrane of the skin is reported in about 60% of biopsy specimens taken from involved areas, but uninvolved sites do not show this change. This result contrasts with SLE, in which 90% of involved skin and 60% of uninvolved skin show Ig and C3 deposits.

C. Therapy. The treatment of choice is hydroxychloroquine, 400–600 mg/day (not to exceed 6 mg/kg/day), or chloroquine, 250 mg/day, until a satisfactory response is induced. Thereafter, the dose should be reduced as tolerated for maintenance. The drug should be withdrawn if symptoms completely disappear.

Periodic **retinal examinations** (twice yearly by an ophthalmologist) should lead to drug withdrawal if a pathologic condition is seen. Early macular pigment changes can spread, producing a retinitis pigmentosa–like picture, with retinal and optic atrophy. Skin rash, gastrointestinal toxicity, hearing impairment, and anemia may also necessitate stopping the drug.

VI. Juvenile rheumatoid arthritis

A. Clinical features. Juvenile rheumatoid arthritis (JRA), also termed **juvenile chronic arthritis,** is a chronic polyarthritis with onset before age 16 years. Many of its clinical features differ from those of RA in that it usually remains asymmetric, involves large joints early, remains mainly in one or a few joints, produces systemic symptoms out of proportion to the degree of joint pain, and, finally, shows a much lower incidence of RF elevation. Table 14-9 summarizes the difference between the three major forms of JRA: systemic, pauciarticular and polyarticular. A syndrome resembling the systemic form of JRA (Still's disease) can present in adulthood. These patients respond to salicylate therapy.

B. Laboratory features. Elevated acute phase reactants (e.g., ESR) are the only characteristic laboratory abnormalities in active disease. The prognosis is worse in the 15% of patients in whom RF eventually develops. ANAs are characteristic mainly of the patients in whom chronic iritis develops, although a positive ANA can develop in some of the seronegative polyarticular patients. These patients lack IgM rheumatoid factor, but may have IgG rheumatoid factor.

C. Prognosis. Usually, JRA follows a remitting but progressive course during childhood, with progression halting in adolescence, except in the small RF positive group (Table 14-9).

D. Treatment

1. Aspirin is the initial drug of choice for the treatment of JRA, beginning with 80 mg/kg/day in divided doses. If high fevers or joint symptoms persist, the dose can be increased to 120 mg/kg/day. Serum salicylate levels can guide therapy (20–30 mg/dl is therapeutic) but are not as reliable a guide for avoiding toxicity as they are in adults. Because liver toxicity is more common than in RA, serum AST (glutamic oxaloacetic transaminase [SGOT]), serum ALT (glutamic pyruvic transaminase [SGPT]) and bilirubin should be monitored every 6 months or if symptoms of liver toxicity (e.g., vomiting) occur. Tinnitus is not as reliable an indicator of toxicity as in adults.

2. Because high-dose corticosteroids alter growth, they are rarely justified in JRA, except for short courses in patients with iritis or high fevers refractory to salicylates. Gold therapy is sometimes effective (1 mg/kg/month), but rash, proteinuria, and hematologic complications are more common (see sec. **III.D.3.a**).

Table 14-9. Features of juvenile rheumatoid arthritis (juvenile chronic arthritis)

Form	Approximate percentage of cases	Most prominent symptoms	Laboratory findings	Prognosis
Systemic	20	Fever and chills, rash, myalgias, abdominal pain, lymphadenopathy, serositis, often arthritis later	Anemia, liver function abnormalities, leukocytosis; ANA and RF are negative	Chronic, progressive; one-third are disabled
Pauciarticular (four or fewer joints)	35	Knees, ankles, elbows, fingers; chronic anterior uveitis in 30%	ANA positive in 90% of iritis patients but only 30% of patients without iritis	Bone destruction and mild disability
Axial type	15	Sacroiliitis; spine, hip, knee involvement; acute iritis; aortitis	HLA-B27–positive	
Peripheral type	20	Hips and shoulders involved late or not at all	HLA-B27–negative	
Polyarticular	45	Small and large joints involved, tendonitis, periostitis; premature epiphyseal closure, leading to growth disturbance		
Seronegative	30		RF-negative, 25% are ANA-positive	Only one-sixth are disabled
Seropositive	15 (older at onset)	Frequent RA features, such as nodules, vasculitis, tendon rupture; but minimal fever and rash	RF-positive, ANA-negative	Rapidly progresses to disability; persists into adulthood

Key: ANA = antinuclear antibody; RF = rheumatoid factor; RA = rheumatoid arthritis.

3. Other agents effective in JRA include tolmetin, naproxen, and ibuprofen, but most of the agents in Table 14-7 have not been given an adequate trial in this disease. The use of idomethacin is discouraged because of the possibility of liver toxicity. Phenylbutazone is effective but is not recommended because it produces more bone marrow and liver toxicity in children than in adults.

VII. Mixed connective tissue disease

A. **Clinical features.** Mixed connective tissue disease combines the clinical features of scleroderma, RA, polymyositis, and SLE. In most patients the greatest clinical resemblance is to scleroderma. The symptoms, in decreasing order of incidence, include arthritis or arthralgias (96%), swollen hands (88%), Raynaud's phenomenon (84%), abnormal esophageal motility (77%), myositis (72%), and lymphadenopathy (68%). The incidence of fever, enlarged spleen or liver, and serositis ranges between 20 and 33%. Renal disease is extremely rare in this condition.

B. **Laboratory features.** Mixed connective tissue disease is characterized by high titers of antibodies to ribonucleoprotein (RNP), which is one of the extractable nuclear antigens (see sec. **II.B.4**). Thus, these patients are ANA-positive and show a speckled pattern of immunofluorescence. Antibodies to the other extractable nuclear antigens and to DNA are characteristically missing.

C. **Treatment** varies with the symptoms present, combining the measures described under the component diseases.

VIII. Myositis

A. **Incidence.** Myositis, the major inflammatory disease of muscle, can begin at any age, with a peak incidence in the 50- to 70-year age group, much later than RA or SLE. Two-thirds of the patients are women.

B. **Clinical features**. The following five categories of inflammatory myositis have been distinguished:

1. Typical **polymyositis** has an acute, sudden onset of proximal muscle weakness and fever, with or without pain, leading rapidly to contractures; or there may be a chronic, insidious development of weakness and wasting, with very few systemic symptoms. Weakness is nearly always evident first in the legs, particularly when the patient gets up from a chair. Pectoral girdle weakness commonly follows. Dysphagia occurs in only 2% of patients, and progression to respiratory difficulty is rare except in the childhood form. Prominent arthralgias are seen in 15%, and 7% manifest fevers, chills, and Raynaud's phenomenon, which often misleads the clinician into an incorrect initial diagnosis. The response to corticosteroids is moderate.

2. **Dermatomyositis** shows the same modes of onset as polymyositis. However, it also involves a typical erythematous or purple-colored skin rash that is prominent around the orbits and malar area and over the knuckles. When the rash becomes more extensive, it may involve the knees, elbows, and malleoli and show a "shawl" distribution around the neck and shoulders. After prolonged involvement, the skin may become atrophic and scaly, and rarely it becomes necrotic. The skin presentation may precede or accompany the muscle involvement. There are rare patients with the typical skin rash and no myositis.

3. **Myositis with malignancy.** The incidence of malignancy associated with dermatomyositis is sufficiently high in patients over the age of 40 years (especially men) to warrant an extensive search for a neoplasm. The tumors are mainly carcinoma, especially of the lung, prostate, stomach, bowel, and, in women, the genitalia and breasts. A few cases of lymphoma have been reported. Characteristically, these patients respond poorly to corticosteroids.

4. **Childhood dermatomyositis** differs from the adult form in that almost all patients have the rash, and muscle pain is more prominent. Progression is often relentless, and the functional prognosis is worse than in the other forms of myositis. Muscular atrophy and contractures are more common; calcinosis or even muscle ossification is seen. A unique feature of the child-

hood form is the extensive vasculitis and thrombosis, not only in muscle but also in the gut, with a high incidence of abdominal pain, ulceration, bleeding, and perforation, which may be a cause of death.

    5. Polymyositis associated with other inflammatory diseases, particularly Sjögren's syndrome, mixed connective tissue disease, and RA, may occur.

C. Diagnosis. Myositis is the original diagnosis in only 20% of these patients. The correct diagnosis is based on the clinical presentation, the presence in serum of elevated levels of muscle enzymes such as creatine phosphokinase (CPK) and aldolase, an abnormal electromyogram, and a typical muscle biopsy. However, any of these features can be normal in a given patient.

    1. Electromyographic features include a mixture of neuropathic and myopathic changes: spontaneous fibrillation, sharp waves, and insertional irritability resembling denervation, but also complex polyphasic, low-amplitude potentials.

    2. Muscle biopsy shows variation in fiber diameter from degeneration, vacuolization and necrosis of fibers, and a tendency for affected fibers to be peripheral in the muscle bundles. Basophilia and centrally placed nuclei indicate regenerating muscle fibers. Often chronic inflammatory cells are present among the muscle fibers or in vessel walls, but their absence does not rule out the diagnosis.

    3. Serologic tests are rarely useful in diagnosing myositis. Rheumatoid factor elevation is found in a minority of patients, and ANA is positive in about 20%. A nuclear antigen called PM1 appears to be responsible for the ANA-positive cases. Antibody to muscle antigens occurs. Unfortunately, because muscular dystrophy and neurogenic muscular atrophy can also show positive ANAs and antibodies to muscle antigens, these findings have no diagnostic value.

    4. A promising clue to the mechanism of autoimmunity in myositis is the demonstration that myositis patients have T cells cytotoxic for muscle cells. However, this test is not suitable for routine diagnosis.

D. Treatment

    1. Doses of **corticosteroids** equivalent to 60 mg of prednisone/day are initially used to suppress the inflammation. Gradual reduction of dose (tapering) ensues when the patient's course permits. Ordinarily, a fall in CPK, aldolase, or ESR is evident weeks before muscle strength is noticeably improved. Although most patients may require 10–20 mg of prednisone/day to maintain remission, some can be maintained on an alternate-day regimen, thus avoiding many corticosteroid side effects.

    2. Patients who do not respond to corticosteroids within 6 weeks, or in whom severe progression continues after 3 weeks of treatment, may be brought into remission with **methotrexate,** beginning with 5 mg administered intravenously each week and increasing the dose by 10–15 mg each week to 50 mg/week (1 mg/kg/week in children), with monitoring by weekly liver function tests and white blood cell counts. **Azathioprine,** 2–3 mg/kg/day, is the second choice, requiring monthly blood cell counts and liver function tests every 3 months.

    Cyclophosphamide, in a daily dose of 4 mg/kg for 3 days, is an alternative. Leukopenia will usually result, and when the white blood cell count begins to rise again, maintenance cyclophosphamide, 1–2 mg/kg/day, may be given. To minimize the risk of hemorrhagic cystitis, fluid intake should be increased to at least 3 liters/day. Alopecia, inappropriate antidiuretic hormone secretion, and infertility can also occur secondary to treatment. Cases of malignancy have been reported.

    These immunosuppressive drugs should be administered by a specialist familiar with their side effects.

IX. Scleroderma (progressive systemic sclerosis) is a generalized disorder characterized by an increase in collagen thickness in the dermis of the skin and by narrowing the small blood vessels.

A. Clinical features

1. Often, the earliest symptom in scleroderma is **Raynaud's phenomenon**. Patients in whom this symptom develops should be examined periodically to detect the development of other characteristics of scleroderma.

2. One-third of scleroderma patients present with **arthritis** (or **arthralgia**) and finger stiffness, which may initially lead to the tentative diagnosis of RA. Others may present with **muscle weakness** as the chief complaint.

3. **Involvement of the skin** is the most typical and diagnostic manifestation. The affected skin passes through an edematous stage to nonpitting induration and atrophy, sometimes with subcutaneous calcinosis. The fingers are involved early and, in many patients, exclusively, but the disease can progress up the arms and also involve the face and upper trunk. Rarely, the legs or the entire body may be involved. Chemically, the increased collagen deposited in the skin is of type III, the fetal type.

4. **Esophageal involvement** is the most common visceral manifestation of scleroderma and often the only one. Altered esophageal motility, diagnosed by barium swallow, is evident in 90% of the patients. Peptic esophagitis, stricture, and dysphagia can result. The lower third of the esophagus is most affected (80% of patients with esophageal involvement).

5. Dyspnea on exertion is the first symptom of **lung involvement,** followed by chronic cough and pleurisy. Fine interstitial fibrotic changes in the lower third of the lung are seen on x-ray. Decreased diffusion capacity is the earliest alteration in pulmonary function. Later, decreased compliance and obstructive disease become prominent, with an increased residual volume and a decreased vital capacity.

6. In patients with **cardiovascular involvement, pulmonary hypertension** is common. **Arrhythmias** are due to conduction defects within the heart muscle itself, rather than to direct pathologic involvement of the conduction system. Pericarditis and pericardial effusion occur.

7. **Gastrointestinal involvement** consists of sequelae of mucosal wall thickening and hypomotility, which can occur throughout the stomach and intestine, leading to bacterial overgrowth, anemia due to folate or vitamin B_1 deficiency, malabsorption, ileus, or volvulus. Wide-mouthed colonic diverticula are characteristic but rare x-ray features. Patients may experience bloating, cramps, diarrhea, or constipation.

8. **Kidney involvement** is the most common cause of death in scleroderma. The renal lesion involves intimal proliferation in small renal arteries, leading to excess renin production and malignant hypertension. The glomeruli also show inflammation and fibrinoid necrosis. Renal failure can be sudden and refractory to therapy. The response to corticosteroids is characteristically poor. Once renal involvement has begun to produce renal insufficiency, life expectancy is only a few months unless the associated hypertension is successfully treated.

9. **Anemia** may be due to poor food intake, malabsorption, gastrointestinal bleeding, vitamin B_{12} deficiency, autoimmune hemolysis similar to that of SLE, or microangiopathy similar to that of other vasculitides; or it may be the anemia of chronic disease.

10. The subgroup of patients who fail to progress beyond sclerodactyly, calcinosis, telangiectasia, Raynaud's phenomenon, and mild or no esophageal involvement has an excellent prognosis.

B. Laboratory features are generally nondiagnostic. The ESR is usually normal or slightly raised, hypergammaglobulinemia is often present, and the muscle enzymes are usually normal. Rheumatoid factor is positive in 40% of the patients, and about 20% have elevated ANA. The most common nuclear antigen in scleroderma is single-stranded RNA, and the reaction of scleroderma antibody with this antigen is inhibited by uracil. The immunofluorescence pattern of the ANA is generally speckled. Immune complex levels may be elevated. Renin and angiotensin levels are high in hypertensive crises.

C. Therapy. There is no satisfactory therapy for altering the progression of scleroderma. Lubrication of the skin and protection from abrasions and extremes of temperature are important to the patient's comfort. The use of penicillamine and the calcium-chelating agents for calcinosis is still experimental. Also experimental, but promising, is the use of angiotensin-converting enzyme inhibitors (e.g., Captopril) in hypertensive crises. Amputation of gangrenous fingers can be lifesaving. Treatment of congestive heart failure and pulmonary insufficiency is by conventional measures. Systemic corticosteroids are not effective except in rare patients with a marked inflammatory component (usually arthritis).

D. Localized forms

1. **Linear scleroderma** begins in childhood either as a linear streak of thickened skin extending the length of an upper or lower extremity or as a "coup de sabre" streak on the forehead or scalp. Biopsies show fibrosis and lymphocytic infiltration of the thickened dermis. Laboratory abnormalities associated with diffuse scleroderma can occur. Contractures around joints may require surgical correction.

2. **Morphea** is a localized form of scleroderma presenting with isolated plaques or patches of erythematous skin that later become sclerotic. In general, the lymphocyte infiltration and inflammatory nature of these lesions are more marked than in other forms of scleroderma. Penicillamine treatment is used in active disease (see sec. **III.D.3.b**).

3. **Eosinophilic fasciitis** is characterized by the subacute onset of pain, swelling, and tenderness in the hands, forearms, feet, and legs that is not confined to periarticular tissues. Induration and scarring of subcutaneous tissues can produce flexion contractures or carpal tunnel syndrome and can extend to the trunk and face. In contrast to the usual case of scleroderma, Raynaud's phenomenon is absent.

   On histologic examination, inflammation and fibrosis are found throughout all layers of the skin, fascia, and muscle. The inflammatory cells may include many eosinophils. Most patients show peripheral eosinophilia and diffuse hypergammaglobulinemia. Spontaneous remission usually occurs after a few years of continuous involvement. Corticosteroids in modest doses (10–20 mg/day of prednisone or its equivalent) provide relief of symptoms.

X. Sjögren's syndrome

A. Clinical features. Sjögren's syndrome is a combination of keratoconjunctivitis sicca (KCS) and features of other rheumatic diseases, usually RA. The cardinal feature of KCS is dry eyes and dry mouth caused by a lymphocytic infiltrate in lacrimal, salivary, and many other exocrine glands present throughout the gastrointestinal and respiratory tracts. In half of the patients with KCS, the morning stiffness, arthralgias, or arthritis typical of RA develops. A few patients may show symptoms of SLE or polymyositis instead. The remainder of KCS patients never acquire the rheumatic manifestations of Sjögren's syndrome.

B. Diagnosis

1. The diagnosis of the KCS component of Sjögren's syndrome is made by demonstration of decreased tear and salivary secretion. **Schirmer's test** of tear secretions employs a special filter-paper wick. When hung on the lower eyelid, it must be wet to a distance of 15 mm in 5 minutes to demonstrate normal tearing; 10 mm is normal in patients over age 60 years. In Sjögren's syndrome patients, the wick is usually wet no more than 5 mm. Absence of the normal salivary pool under the tongue and the patient's report of difficulty in chewing or swallowing dry foods (e.g., soda crackers) are common features.

2. **Laboratory test findings** are highlighted by the demonstration of an antibody to salivary duct epithelium by immunofluorescence of salivary gland tissue in 50% of patients. However, this antibody test is performed in only a few laboratories. In one-half of the patients, IgG levels are elevated. Cryoglobulins are common, and RF is positive in 90% of the patients who develop arthritis, sometimes in advance of the arthritis. Positive ANA in a speckled or diffuse pattern is found in 70% of patients. The ANA is usually directed

to single-stranded DNA or other nuclear antigens rather than to double-stranded DNA. Titers of ANA and RF in some patients are extremely high—much higher than ordinarily seen in RA and SLE. Antibody to thyroglobulin is demonstrated in 35%, and 50% show a decrease in lymphocyte phytohemagglutinin stimulation or delayed hypersensitivity skin test responses.

3. **Biopsy** of lower lip minor salivary glands shows a lymphocytic infiltrate. If the hyperglobulinemia disappears or if the RF titer falls, a search for extranodal lymphoproliferation should be undertaken since lymphoma has eventually developed in some of these patients, especially lymphoma of the undifferentiated or histiocytic type. Waldenström's macroglobulinemia can also occur.

C. **Treatment.** In most patients, treatment appropriate for RA, plus ad lib use of 0.5% methylcellulose eye drops (5 times/day is usual) and frequent sips of water while eating, constitutes the total therapeutic regimen. When the oropharynx is so dry that it is in danger of ulceration, 1% glycerine in water from a plastic squeeze bottle can be gargled ad lib; room humidification will increase comfort. Conjunctival and corneal ulcers are best treated with boric acid ointment and an eye patch. Topical corticosteroids are helpful for acute episodes, but repeated use increases the risk of fungal or bacterial infections. Dental caries are accelerated, so attentive dental care is necessary. Oral corticosteroids and cyclophosphamide are indicated only for extranodal lymphoid proliferation, which is best managed by a specialist. Other cytotoxic agents or irradiation is added to the regimen if a malignancy is found.

XI. **Ankylosing spondylitis (AS).** Ankylosing spondylitis is more an inflammation of fibrous tissue than of synovium. It tends to follow an axial distribution, with peripheral joints involved less frequently than the spine.

A. **Incidence.** There are about 6 cases/1000 adult males. The incidence of AS is approximately 10% of the incidence of RA in the general population, although the incidence of AS and RA is equal in young adult males. About 16% of patients are female.

B. **Clinical features.** After 3 months of low back pain and stiffness unrelieved by rest, the disease is usually diagnosed by demonstration of the appropriate features by physical examination and x-ray studies.

1. **Sacroiliitis** is the earliest feature seen on x-ray before clinical involvement extends to the lumbar spine. The onset is insidious in 80% of the patients, but the other 20% may present with sharp, jolting pains in the buttocks or hips, often exacerbated by coughing. Paravertebral muscle spasm, aching, and stiffness are common, but some patients may have slow progressive limitation of motion with no pain at all. The disease typically involves ligamentous insertions, fibrocartilage, and the invertebral disks.

2. **Peripheral joint involvement** occurs in 25% of patients, usually (but not always) after involvement of the spine. Typical extraspinal sites include the manubriosternal joint, the symphysis pubis, and the shoulder and hip joints. Even in patients with severe peripheral joint disease, the fingers and metatarsophalangeal joints are only mildly affected compared with the larger, more central joints.

3. **Cardiovascular involvement** follows a different pattern than in RA. **Aortitis** can involve the proximal ascending aorta, with elastic fiber destruction in the medial layer. The fibrosis may extend into the mitral valve, the septum, or the atrioventricular node, leading to arrhythmias due to conduction defects. Pericarditis can occur. Long P–R intervals and first-degree heart block are seen. Aortic insufficiency and left ventricular hypertrophy may ensue late in the disease. The heart is involved in less than 5% of total cases, but patients who have active disease for more than 30 years have a higher incidence.

4. **Anterior uveitis** with synechiae and cataracts are more common extraarticular manifestations and occur in 25% of patients.

5. **Lung involvement** is generally confined to mild upper lobe fibrosis. Typically, the diffusion capacity is normal at a time when compliance is clearly impaired by the limited motion of the costovertebral joints.

C. **Laboratory features**

1. The ESR is less useful as an index of activity than in RA. Patients may have a mild secondary anemia. There are no typical autoantibodies in this disease.

2. Testing for the histocompatibility antigen **HLA-B27** is valuable in differentiating the occasional AS patient with mainly peripheral joint involvement from gonococcal arthritis or RA; 88% of AS patients are HLA-B27–positive, compared with 8% of the normal population. In AS, A2-B27, A10-B27, and A28-B27 are the most common haplotypes, whereas in Reiter's syndrome the most common haplotype is A3-B27.

3. **X-ray features** of the disease are helpful in diagnosis. Sclerosis, erosions, and blurring of the margins of the sacroiliac joints are the most common initial abnormalities. The anterosuperior margin of the vertebral bodies may be eroded by granulation tissue invading the insertion of the longitudinal ligaments, and the anterior vertebral margins may be squared. Later, bone spurs called **syndesmophytes** form, following the margin of the annulus fibrosis. These bone spurs may form a bridge between vertebrae, finally fusing them to form a "bamboo" spine. Some patients may have inflammation of the disks, with destruction of adjacent vertebral bodies that radiographically resembles tuberculosis.

D. **Treatment and prognosis**

1. **Drug therapy.** In patients with mild disease, **aspirin** is the drug of choice (see sec. **III.D.1**). In severe cases, indomethacin is more effective. For patients who have side effects to indomethacin, sulindac, tolmetin, or another nonsteroidal anti-inflammatory drug (see Table 14-7) is a useful alternative. Phenylbutazone is also effective, but the hematologic side effects preclude its use in a chronic disease such as AS for more than 2 weeks unless it is the only medication that is successful. Gold and antimalarial agents are useless, and the use of corticosteroids is unwarranted.

2. **Exercise.** The difference between ultimate success and failure in preserving function lies with the postural exercise program and the quality of the patient's participation. Daily exercises should be directed toward maintaining a straight spine and erect posture, preserving as much mobility as possible. Breathing exercises and Hubbard tank therapy are useful.

3. **Irradiation** therapy is not used currently in AS because of the danger of leukemia.

XII. **Reiter's syndrome.** The triad of arthritis, conjunctivitis, and nonspecific urethritis defines Reiter's syndrome, although some patients develop only two of the three symptoms.

A. **Incidence.** Reiter's syndrome occurs mainly in young adult males. When it occurs in a female, HLA-B27 positivity is almost 100%. The initial cases were described following dysentery (*Yersinia, Salmonella, Shigella*). Other cases of Reiter's syndrome have been associated with venereal infection with *Chlamydia*. In most cases, however, there is no association with infection.

B. **Clinical features**

1. **Urethritis,** when present, is generally the first symptom, preceding other symptoms by one or more weeks. The discharge is mucopurulent, prostatitis is common, and, in rare cases, hemorrhagic cystitis may be present. Generally, cultures are negative.

2. The **conjunctivitis** and **iritis** are usually bilateral, as opposed to the anterior uveitis of AS, which is often unilateral. The incidence of iritis is 10% in the first attack, but this symptom eventually develops in 20–25% of patients with the typical arthritis. Rare cases of optic neuritis occur.

3. The **arthritis** typically begins in the weight-bearing joints, is not symmetric, and generally runs a course of weeks to months. It may vary in severity

from absence to extreme joint destruction. Involvement of the feet and spine is most common and is associated with HLA-B27 positivity. More than 50% of patients with Reiter's syndrome have at least two attacks. Patients who have chronic joint involvement usually have several attacks before the chronic phase begins; thus, a long follow-up is needed to demonstrate the chronic nature of the disease.

4. One-third of patients with Reiter's syndrome have sacroiliac x-ray change. that may be asymmetric and are similar to those in AS. Small-joint involvement, especially in the feet, is more common in Reiter's syndrome than ir AS and is often asymmetric. Heel pain is a particularly ominous predictor o eventual disability.

5. **Skin involvement** includes balanitis circinata and keratoderma blennor rhagica (inflammatory hyperkeratotic lesions of the toes, nails, and soles of the feet) resembling psoriasis.

The various manifestations of the syndrome (presented in **1–5**) are usually not present simultaneously.

C. Laboratory features include sterile pyuria, elevated ESR and white cell count and synovial fluid that may be clear to grossly purulent. Typical **radiographic features** include erosions (apparent after at least 2 months, often resembling RA), and periosteal proliferation (a common feature seen in the calcaneus, knees, and metatarsal bones). Antibodies to gonococci or *Chlamydia* are no more frequent than in the general population. HLA-B27 is present in most patient: with axial disease, distinguishing them from patients with recurrent gonococcal arthritis.

D. Treatment of this condition is primarily with **salicylates** (see sec. III.D.1). In some patients, indomethacin or phenylbutazone is more effective than salicylates, especially if there is spinal involvement (see Table 14-7). Risk of bon marrow toxicity limits phenylbutazone use to 2 weeks.

XIII. Psoriatic arthritis

A. Clinical features. Psoriatic arthritis is the form of arthritis associated with the skin disease psoriasis and is difficult to diagnose in the absence of skin involvement. The arthritis occurs in 5–7% of psoriasis patients.

1. About 50% of psoriatic arthritis patients have a distal distribution of arthritis, which is distinguished from RA by the early and more severe involvement of the distal interphalangeal joints (before involvement of the metacarpophalangeal joints) and the typical nail changes (pitting). Erosions can be extensive and are accompanied by more bone proliferative changes than those seen in RA. Other patients show a distribution more typical of RA. A third group may have an axial distribution.

2. Psoriatic arthritis often remains asymmetric throughout its course and may retain its original monoarticular or oligoarticular distribution. New bone formation is prominent. Ossification of the anterior spine ligament may be visible as it passes a disk, only later connecting to the corner of a vertebral body. In contrast to Reiter's syndrome, psoriatic arthritis characteristically involves the upper extremities earlier and more severely than the lower extremities. Aortic insufficiency may occur.

B. Laboratory features. There are no characteristic autoantibodies or immune abnormalities.

C. Treatment is the same as that described for AS and Reiter's syndrome. Gold is of unproved benefit even when the clinical features resemble those of RA. An increased incidence of toxic skin reactions to gold in these patients has been reported. Antimalarial agents are contraindicated because of their tendency to exacerbate the skin lesions. **Methotrexate** should be tried in the most refractory cases.

XIV. Systemic vasculitis. The term **vasculitis** encompasses a variety of disorders characterized by chronic inflammatory reactions that destroy the walls of blood vessels. For each disease discussed in this section, the diagnosis of vasculitis must be based on **biopsy.**

A. Polyarteritis nodosa

1. **Incidence.** Onset is at any age but is most frequent between 20 and 50 years of age. polyarteritis nodosa is approximately 25% as common as SLE and 50% as common as dermatomyositis or scleroderma. Males constitute 70% of the patients.

2. **Pathologic features.** The disease is typically concentrated in the muscular layer of medium- and small-sized arteries. Polymorphonuclear leukocytes predominate, but lymphocytes and eosinophils are also present. Fibrinoid necrosis begins in the media but progresses to involve the full wall thickness in a focal manner, such that the wall opposite the lesion may be normal. Aneurysms or strictures commonly result. A single biopsy may show several stages in the evolution of the lesions. The arteries of the kidney and heart are most commonly involved, followed by the peripheral nerves. The gastrointestinal tract, skin, central nervous system, liver, spleen, testes, and adrenal glands are less commonly involved, and the lungs are usually spared.

3. **Clinical features.** In most patients the disease begins with vague symptoms of fever, fatigue, and weight loss. Beyond these general symptoms, it is impossible to describe a typical case because of the variety of types of organ involvement. Kidney involvement presents as proteinuria, leading to hematuria and renal failure or sometimes to hypertension. Abdominal pain, melena, and bowel infarction occur. Angina and myocardial infarction may occur. Myalgias and muscle wasting, central nervous system symptoms, mononeuritis multiplex (involvement of first one nerve and then another in a seemingly disorganized pattern), and arthritis are also common features.

4. **Laboratory features.** The diagnosis is based on biopsy findings. The ESR is elevated. Anemia is common. Hepatitis B antigen is demonstrated in 20–40% of the patients, but a cause-effect relationship is unproved. Hepatitis B antigen, immunoglobulin, and C3 are present in vessel-wall deposits in some patients. Characteristic aneurysms of medium-sized vessels are evident on angiography in some patients.

5. **Treatment** is often unsatisfactory, but 60 mg/day or more of oral prednisone commonly ameliorates symptoms early in the course of the disease. Adding cytotoxic agents such as cyclophosphamide improves survival. The 5-year survival rate has improved to about 50%, with most deaths occurring in the first year. Patients whose kidneys survive the first year appear to have a better prognosis.

B. Allergic vasculitis (Churg-Strauss vasculitis)

1. **Incidence.** There are no age or sex restrictions. Atopic individuals are most commonly involved.

2. **Pathologic features.** Venules as well as arterioles are involved early. Generally, involved vessels are smaller than those involved in polyarteritis nodosa, but there is some overlap. Typically, the lesions seen on biopsy are all at the same stage of evolution. The inflammation begins in the intima, rather than in the media, and eosinophils are extremely prominent, even in early lesions. Veins may be involved before arteries or without arterial involvement. Involvement of any of the organs seen in polyarteritis nodosa can occur. But typically, lung involvement is the most prominent feature and may be the only feature, especially early in the course of the disease.

3. **Clinical presentation.** Cough, asthma, and pulmonary infiltrates with eosinophilia characterize this disease, but other symptoms resembling those of polyarteritis nodosa may occur. Palpable purpura and urticaria are also seen.

4. **Laboratory features.** Allergic vasculitis is characterized by a high ESR and peripheral eosinophilia. Serum IgE is often elevated. Biopsy shows necrotizing small-vessel vasculitis, eosinophilic infiltrates, and granulomata.

5. **Treatment.** In general, the response to corticosteroids in these patients is

better than in patients with polyarteritis nodosa. Any drugs suspected of provoking the reaction should be withdrawn, but often no inciting cause is apparent.

C. Takayasu's arteritis

1. **Incidence.** Onset of this rare condition has been recorded in individuals between 9 and 45 years of age. Females constitute 85% of cases, with a predominance of Orientals.

2. **Pathologic features.** The aorta and the large elastic arteries branching from it are the main sites of involvement in Takayasu's arteritis. The elastic lamina disintegrates first, followed by medial necrosis with thrombosis and scarring, leading to constrictions. Compromise of the vasa vasorum and infarction of the artery wall may help to cause this condition. The aortic arch, carotids, and brachial arteries are involved in 58% of the patients. In 12%, the abdominal aorta and renal and mesenteric arteries are mainly involved, but 30% have involvement in both thoracic and abdominal areas.

3. **Clinical features**

   a. A "prepulseless" phase occurs, consisting of shortness of breath, tachycardia, and a cough resembling that of influenza or chronic respiratory infection. In some patients this phase is followed by an acute phase of arterial inflammation, with arteries that are tender on direct pressure. Most patients have a more chronic course, without pain.

   b. In a few patients, onset is subacute, with fever, sweats, and nausea, but no overt arterial tenderness. Striking progression of the disease can occur in asymptomatic patients.

   c. Arm and jaw claudication, muscle wasting, hair loss, ulceration of the nose and tongue, and syncope can occur in the late stages in patients with severe arterial narrowing ("pulseless disease"). After 5 years of activity, the disease usually fails to progress, and the patient is left with the results of the arterial scarring, including multiple arterial bruits.

4. **Laboratory features.** Apart from an elevated ESR in the acute stages, no laboratory abnormalities are characteristic. The diagnosis is made by physical examination and arteriography, because the involved arteries are too large to biopsy.

5. **Treatment.** In general, the response to corticosteroids is poor, although patients with acute inflammatory symptoms may respond. (As in other diseases, the corticosteroid response appears to be proportional to the intensity of the inflammation.) Some patients respond to immunosuppressive agents. Most patients survive, but 10% of patients die of central nervous system ischemia.

D. Giant-cell arteritis

1. **Incidence.** Most patients are beyond 50 years of age, with the greatest incidence in the eighth decade. The disease occurs equally in both sexes.

2. **Pathologic features.** Large elastic and medium-sized muscular arteries are most severely involved. Variants of this condition are named for the arteries primarily involved, e.g., **temporal** or **cranial** arteritis. Inflammation typically begins in the adventitia and progresses to involve the whole wall. Generally, occlusion occurs by focal narrowing, due to swelling of the wall without thrombosis or aneurysm formation. Giant cells are commonly found, but are not required for the diagnosis. After a period of active inflammation, the lumen is permanently narrowed by scarring. Adjacent areas may be uninvolved. The carotid branches, including the ophthalmic arteries, are more commonly involved than are the mesenteric or renal arteries.

3. **Clinical features** of giant-cell arteritis include tenderness and inflammation along the course of the temporal artery, bruits in the cranial or neck area, and reduced temporal artery blood flow measurements. In addition, typical symptoms include jaw claudication, atrophy of temporal and tongue muscles, transient visual blurring, diplopia, eye pain, and persistent unilateral headache. Forty percent of patients with giant-cell arteritis eventually

develop visual symptoms. Episodes of blurred vision are reversible, but the major danger is irreversible **sudden blindness** which occurs in 30% of untreated patients.

Alternatively, the disease may begin with the symptoms of **polymyalgia rheumatica** with fever, malaise, and pain in the shoulder girdle muscles, without any demonstrable abnormalities by physical examination such as muscle wasting or weakness. Both symptom complexes can occur in the same individual, or each can occur separately.

4. **Laboratory features.** Significant elevation of the ESR is characteristic, and normochromic, normocytic anemia is common. Immunoglobulins are normal, and immune complexes are not found. In giant-cell arteritis, lymphocytes proliferate in response to elastin, other arterial wall antigens, or muscle. Biopsy of the temporal artery shows focal granulomatous arteritis, often with giant cells and "skip areas" of normal arterial wall. Biopsy of a clinically inflamed nodule should confirm the diagnosis, but if there are no clinically obvious lesions, a 4-cm segment should be examined. In a patient with suggestive symptoms and a negative biopsy, diagnosis may be confirmed by a biopsy of a similar segment on the opposite side.

5. **Treatment**
    a. The danger of blindness constitutes the major justification for high-dose corticosteroid therapy in giant-cell arteritis. Patients with typical temporal arteritis symptoms and a high ESR should undergo temporal artery biopsy. Patients with positive biopsies should receive 60 mg of prednisone/day until the disease is suppressed, at which time cautious tapering can begin (see sec. **III.D.5**). As long as clinical symptoms and the ESR improve, slow tapering toward a 10-mg/day dose can continue. Relapses call for an increase of at least 10 mg/day. Because of the high rate of clinical relapse, daily prednisone therapy should be continued for at least 2 years. Administration of high-dose prednisone less than 1 week before biopsy will not alter the interpretation. Patients who have lost vision in one eye must be immediately treated to save the other eye. Blind patients should not be treated with prednisone unless there are signs of active disease elsewhere.
    b. Patients manifesting only polymyalgia rheumatica symptoms should be treated with 10 mg (in rare cases, 20 mg) of prednisone/day, since this symptom complex characteristically responds to that dose. Such patients should be followed closely to identify the few patients who later develop symptoms of inflammation in cranial arteries, necessitating temporal artery biopsy. Less than 5% of patients with only polymyalgia rheumatica symptoms develop severe eye problems.

E. **Wegener's granulomatosis**
    1. **Incidence.** Onset can occur at any age, and 60% of these patients are female.
    2. **Pathologic features.** Inflammation characteristically begins in small arteries, arterioles, and veins, with necrotizing and granulomatous vasculitis. The diagnosis depends on finding both necrotizing and granulomatous changes on biopsy specimens. Several stages of evolution are seen in the same biopsy specimen. The sinuses, lungs, and kidneys are the most prominent sites of involvement.
    3. **Clinical features.** In most patients the disease begins with sinusitis and fever, simulating an upper respiratory infection, and progresses to involvement of the lung and kidneys. After repeated episodes, the granulomatous inflammation may involve the peripheral nerves, central nervous system, joints, heart, eyes, middle ear, and skin, with much variation among patients. The incidence of involvement of each of these other systems ranges from about 25–50% of these patients. Some patients have only respiratory system involvement (limited Wegener's).
    4. **Laboratory features.** The ESR and the white blood cell count are elevated. Often serum IgA is elevated, and serum IgM is depressed. Anemia is com-

mon. Rheumatoid factor is present in 50% of these individuals. A few patients have glomerular deposits of immunoglobulin and C3 on biopsy. Antinuclear antibody is not observed.

  5. **Treatment.** Death occurs in 90% of patients within 2 years unless they are treated. The corticosteroid response is generally poor, but the response to **cyclophosphamide** combined with corticosteroids is excellent (see sec. VIII.D.2).

F. **Rheumatoid vasculitis**

  1. **Incidence.** Rheumatoid vasculitis occurs in about 5% of RA patients, typically in patients with severe seropositive disease for 10 years or more.

  2. **Pathologic features.** Capillaries and arterioles are the principal sites of involvement. The inflammation first involves the adventitia, then may progress to fibrinoid necrosis of the vessel wall. The infiltrate consists mainly of lymphocytes and primarily involves the skin, peripheral nerves, and serosal surfaces.

  3. **Clinical features.** Purpura and slow-healing skin ulcers on the lower extremities are common. The asymmetric peripheral sensory and motor neuropathy is characteristically refractory to most analgesics. Pericarditis that sometimes leads to hemopericardium can occur.

  4. The **laboratory features** are identical to those in other patients with severe seropositive RA. Cryoglobulins may be found.

  5. **Treatment.** Rheumatoid vasculitis is one of the few indications for high-dose corticosteroid therapy in RA. **Prednisone,** 60 mg/day, is given and is followed by tapering when control is achieved (see sec. III.D.5). Cytotoxic agents may be helpful in some patients.

G. **Henoch-Schönlein purpura**

  1. **Incidence.** The peak age of onset is 3 years. Onset after 50 years of age is exceedingly rare.

  2. **Pathologic features.** Most inflammation begins in the capillaries and consists of a neutrophil infiltrate, with local hemorrhage behind thrombi. The skin, kidneys, joints, and gastrointestinal tract are the major sites of involvement.

  3. **Clinical features.** Purpura and urticaria, with arthralgia or arthritis, may occur. Involvement of the lower extremities is more common and more severe than that of the hands. Abdominal pain is probably due to similar lesions in the gastrointestinal tract. Hematuria and proteinuria may occur, and 10% of patients become hypertensive. A single episode is usual, although some cases involve two or three episodes, with complete recovery between episodes and no residual damage. Usually, these recurrences happen within 2 years of the initial episode, and purpura is the most common symptom. Permanent renal damage is rare.

  4. **Laboratory features.** Despite the inflammation, complement is usually normal. Deposits of IgA in the glomeruli and skin are a characteristic feature. An elevated serum IgA level may be observed.

  5. **Treatment** is primarily supportive. Corticosteroids may be beneficial in children who are systemically ill, especially with abdominal pain.

H. **Mixed cryoglobulinemia**

  1. **Pathologic features.** Biopsy specimens from skin lesions demonstrate a leukocytoclastic vasculitis. Immunofluorescence studies may show immunoglobulin and complement in vasculitic lesions of the kidney and skin.

  2. **Clinical findings** include palpable purpura, arthralgia, fatigue, and weakness; and symptoms are often similar to Henoch-Schönlein purpura and systemic lupus erythematosus. Diffuse glomerulonephritis occurs frequently and may lead to renal failure.

  3. **Laboratory findings.** The presence of mixed cryoglobulins containing IgG and IgM immunoglobulins characterize this disease. The IgM component often has anti-IgG (rheumatoid factor) activity. Serum complement levels may be decreased. Hepatitis B antigen and coccidioidin antigen have been

demonstrated in the cryoprecipitates of some patients with mixed cryoglobulinemia. These laboratory findings, especially the presence of cryoglobulins, distinguish this disease from Henoch-Schönlein purpura. The absence of antibody to double-stranded DNA and the absence of immunoglobulin deposition at the dermoepidermal junction on skin biopsy separate mixed cryoglobulinemia from SLE.

4. **Treatment.** Patients usually respond well to corticosteroids. Prognosis is worsened in patients who have significant renal lesions, and cytotoxic agents may be required in those with progressive renal failure.

I. **Hypocomplementemic vasculitis**

1. **Pathologic features.** Biopsy of cutaneous lesions usually demonstrates a leukocytoclastic vasculitis. In patients with renal involvement, kidney biopsies may reveal mild glomerulonephritis with immunoglobulin and complement deposition on the glomerular basement membranes.

2. **Clinical manifestations** of hypocomplementemic vasculitis include recurrent episodes of urticuria, arthritis, abdominal pain, and, in some patients, symptoms of kidney involvement. Severe renal impairment does not occur.

3. **Laboratory findings.** The characteristic features of this disease are a reduction of serum complement levels and an absence of ANAs.

4. **Treatment.** Patients usually respond well with corticosteroids.

J. **Polyarteritis in childhood**

1. **General clinical features.** Polyarteritis in childhood differs from the adult form of the disease in sparing the central nervous system and involving the skin, muscle, and kidneys less frequently. Instead, the characteristic site of involvement is the coronary arteries, often resulting in either arterial rupture during the acute active stage or subsequent myocardial infarction due to thrombosis.

2. **Kawasaki disease** (the mucocutaneous lymph node syndrome) is a variant of childhood polyarteritis. The cause is unknown, although viral or toxic agents are suspected. The rickettsial-like structures found in many of the lymph node biopsy specimens in Kawasaki disease suggest a possible pathogenesis. It occurs in a male-female ratio of 1.5:1.0, with the highest incidence at about 1 year of age.

   a. Kawasaki disease presents as an acute febrile illness with the following major clinical features:

   (1) **Fever** lasting 5 days or more.

   (2) Bilateral **conjunctival** injection.

   (3) **Changes of the lips and oral cavity:** dryness; cracked lips; glowing red lips; hypertrophy of the tongue papillae with a "strawberry" tongue appearance; diffuse reddening of the oropharyngeal mucosa.

   (4) **Changes of the peripheral extremities:** reddening of the palms or soles or both; edema of the hands or feet or both; generalized desquamation; desquamation from the fingertips.

   (5) **Polymorphous exanthem.**

   (6) Acute nonpurulent **cervical lymph node swelling.**

   The Centers for Disease Control state that the presence of fever and four of the other five major features are necessary to make a diagnosis of Kawasaki disease, providing other explanations for the illness have been excluded. The presence of one of the findings listed under features **3** or **4** above is sufficient to establish that particular feature.

   b. In 70% of patients there are electrocardiographic or physical signs of cardiac abnormalities.

   c. Inflammation of vessels in the joints, kidney, gastrointestinal tract, and central nervous system may occur.

   d. Although aneurysms of most major arteries can occur, the coronary arteries are the most common site of angiographic abnormalities.

   e. The **mortality** is 1–2%, with death usually resulting from coronary thrombosis. Death can occur long after an uneventful recovery (weeks to years); 50% of deaths occur within 1 month of onset, 95% within 6 months. Males under 1 year of age are at greatest risk.

   f. Because of the significant risk of mortality, **cardiac complications** must be diagnosed early and appropriately monitored and treated. All patients with suspected Kawasaki disease require careful assessment by physical examination as well as electrocardiographic and echocardiographic studies to rule out cardiac involvement. Patients with signs of cardiac involvement, especially those patients with echocardiographic evidence of coronary artery involvement, may require coronary angiography.

3. Pathologic and laboratory features. Microscopically, the arteritis of Kawasaki disease is identical to that of polyarteritis. Because the changes are often confined to the coronary arteries, which cannot be biopsied, diagnosis of polyarteritis in childhood depends on the clinical presentation, electrocardiogram, echocardiogram, and angiography.

4. Treatment. High-dose aspirin therapy (100 mg/kg/day) can be started in the acute stage of polyarteritis and Kawasaki disease. The response is variable. Treatment should be continued for 2 months. Many patients with polyarteritis respond to corticosteroids (prednisone, 1–2 mg/kg/day). Corticosteroids in Kawasaki disease produce a variable response and may aggravate coronary lesions in some patients. Heparinization similarly yields variable results. High-dose intravenous gamma globulin therapy (400 mg/kg/day on 4 consecutive days) in conjunction with aspirin therapy has been reported to reduce the prevalence of coronary-artery abnormalities when administered early in the course of disease (Newburger, J. W., et al. *N. Engl. J. Med.,* 315:341, 1986). Patients with Kawasaki disease must be observed closely during the first 6 months after recovery for possible coronary thrombosis. Acute electrocardiographic changes usually return to normal despite residual coronary arteritis.

XV. Behçet's syndrome
   A. Clinical features
      1. The **three symptoms** of classic Behçet's syndrome are as follows:
         a. Recurrent, sharply defined, painful ulcerations of the **oral mucosa.**
         b. Similar ulcerations of the **genitalia.**
         c. Iritis.
      2. Inflammation of various other tissues is frequently seen in association with two or all three of the classic symptoms.
         a. Skin lesions, including pyoderma, erythema nodosum, or the appearance of pustular lesions at the site of skin trauma.
         b. Other ocular symptoms, including conjunctivitis, keratitis, retinal thrombophlebitis, and optic atrophy.
         c. A large-joint inflammatory arthritis in which effusion and soft-tissue swelling are out of proportion to the resulting bone damage or deformity; the knees are often involved with sparing of the small joints of the hands and feet.
         d. Intestinal and rectal **ulcerations.**
         e. Vasculitis, including thrombophlebitis of superficial or large veins and occlusions or aneurysms of major arteries.
         f. Neuropsychiatric symptoms, including meningitis, myelitis, and organic brain syndromes.
         g. Diffuse pulmonary infiltrates.
      These diverse symptoms can occur simultaneously or years apart, and generally follow a course of exacerbation and remission.
   B. Pathologic and laboratory features. All the organ systems involved may manifest vasculitis that is not distinctively different from other types. Abnormalities commonly include elevated ESR and C-reactive protein, anemia, polyclonal IgG elevation, and circulating immune complexes. Antibodies against oral mucosal antigens are found. Cryoglobulins occur in 25% of patients. Calcium-dependent

rosetting of platelets around neutrophils may be visible on blood smears during acute exacerbations. Rheumatoid factor and ANA are absent. There is no definitive diagnostic test for Behçet's syndrome, and diagnosis is usually based on long-term clinical observation of the patient.

  C. **Treatment. Corticosteroids** or **immunosuppressive agents** in therapeutic doses as previously described are used to treat active disease. Despite such treatment, many cases are progressive. Therapeutic benefits from blood transfusions are not confirmed. Unnecessary needle punctures of the skin **should be avoided.**

XVI. **Familial Mediterranean fever** is inherited as an autosomal recessive trait and occurs mainly in Sephardic and Iraqi Jews, and in Turks, Armenians, and Levantine Arabs.

  A. **Clinical features.** Beginning with the first attack in childhood or adolescence, the course of the disease consists of recurrent, unpredictable attacks lasting 4 days to several months, with symptom-free intervals. Attacks consist of fever and arthritis, with or without bursitis, and abdominal crises. Erysipelaslike skin lesions about the ankle, pleuritis, and pericarditis can occur. Characteristics of the arthritis include acute onset, asymmetric distribution, and pain and tenderness of the joints that are more prominent than warmth or swelling. The abdominal crises resemble acute peritonitis.

  B. **Laboratory diagnosis.** There are no consistent abnormalities in peripheral blood count or serologic findings, but the ESR and fibrinogen levels are elevated during an attack.

  C. **Treatment.** Prophylactic treatment with 0.6 mg of colchicine 2 or 3 times/day reduces the number and severity of attacks, but neither colchicine nor corticosteroids are effective during an acute attack. Physical therapy is important in preventing disuse atrophy in patients with recurrent joint pain. The use of narcotics and surgical exploration of the abdomen should be avoided during a crisis. The long-term **prognosis** is favorable, except that permanent damage to the hip joint can occur, and renal amyloidosis causes premature death in some patients.

XVII. **Relapsing polychondritis**

  A. **Incidence.** Onset in middle life and equal incidence in males and females characterize this rare rheumatic disease.

  B. **Pathologic features.** Invasion of cartilaginous structures by chronic inflammatory cells results in the destruction of cartilage and its replacement by fibrous tissue.

  C. **Clinical features.** Although any cartilaginous structure in the body can be the site of inflammation, the disease characteristically follows a focal, asymmetric, and episodic course. The destruction of cartilage may be slow and painless, or it may be acute and accompanied by clinical signs of inflammation. In the order of decreasing frequency, the disease may involve ear cartilage; nasal cartilage; articular cartilage; cartilage of the trachea, larynx, and auditory canal; and costochondral cartilage. Fifty to sixty percent of patients develops ocular involvement with conjunctivitis or episcleritis, and an equal number develop defective hearing. Twenty-five percent or less develop labyrinthine vertigo or aortic insufficiency. The interval from diagnosis to death ranges from 10 months to over 20 years. Respiratory failure from either tracheal collapse or infectious complications causes death more frequently than aortic insufficiency.

  D. **Laboratory findings** are nonspecific, consisting of increased ESR, mild to moderate anemia, increased immunoglobulins, and a low incidence of positive RF.

  E. **Treatment.** Oral prednisone at 60 mg/day is the standard treatment for an acute attack. Cautious tapering to a maintenance level of 10 mg/day begins only after the inflammation has subsided. Many patients require maintenance prednisone for years to suppress the inflammation. Prosthetic valve replacement is the only effective treatment for aortic valve involvement.

XVIII. **Enteropathic arthritis**

  A. **Incidence.** A peripheral arthritis develops in 20% of patients with regional enteritis, 12% of patients with ulcerative colitis, and about 30% of patients who have undergone intestinal bypass surgery for morbid obesity. Sexes are equally affected, and the usual onset is in the third to fifth decade.

A disease resembling ankylosing spondylitis may occur in association with ulcerative colitis or regional enteritis, with a male-to-female ratio of 2:1 in contrast to the 9:1 ratio seen in ordinary ankylosing spondylitis.

B. Clinical features. In most patients, the onset is abrupt and limited to one to three joints, often with an asymmetric and migratory pattern. Knees and ankles are most commonly affected (except in the HLA-B27–positive patients who tend to develop a disease resembling ankylosing spondylitis). Attacks usually last less than 2 months but may last longer than a year, often appearing to parallel the intensity of enterocolitis. Arthritic episodes prior to the onset of bowel symptoms are unusual (10% of patients). Swelling, redness, and effusion may be present or there may be no objective findings. Patients with inflammatory bowel disease who have uveitis, recurrent oral ulcerations, pseudopolyps, or perianal involvement are 3–4 times more likely to have arthritis than patients lacking these symptoms.

About 25% of patients with the spondylitic form have symptoms before the onset of their bowel disease, and the symptoms frequently do not parallel the intensity of the enterocolitis. The arthritis associated with intestinal bypass surgery is symmetric, polyarticular, and often involves inflammation of muscle and tendon sheaths.

C. Laboratory features. Elevated ESR, anemia, and leukocytosis are common, but RF and ANA are characteristically absent. Both marginal erosions and periostitis may be evident on x-rays, but serious bone damage and deformity are unusual. Circulating antibodies to colon epithelium are found in both ulcerative colitis and regional enteritis patients, and lymphocytes have been shown to be cytotoxic for colon epithelial cells in vitro. Whether these autoantibodies occur in response to damaged colon tissue or whether the diseases are autoimmune is unknown. Intestinal bypass patients frequently show immune complexes with cryoglobulin characteristics that may contain antigens derived from intestinal bacteria. Seventy-five percent of these patients with spondylitis are positive for HLA-B27, whereas patients with peripheral arthritis maintain the normal HLA distribution (8% HLA-B27–positive).

D. Treatment. The peripheral joint disease improves when the bowel disease is treated with surgery or systemic corticosteroids. However, the status of the bowel disease, not the arthritis, should govern such therapeutic decisions. Otherwise the use of salicylates or other nonsteroidal anti-inflammatory drugs and physical therapy as described for rheumatoid arthritis (see sec. **III**) are helpful. The patients with spondylitis should be treated as described for ankylosing spondylitis (see sec. **XI**).

XIX. Rheumatic fever is a poststreptococcal disease characterized by nonsuppurative inflammation of various organs, principally the heart, joints, central nervous system, skin, and subcutaneous tissues.

A. Incidence. Acute rheumatic fever occurs primarily in school-age children and young adults. Its incidence peaks at approximately 8 years of age, affecting both sexes equally.

B. Clinical and laboratory features. The clinical features vary considerably. Acute attacks, whether initial or recurrent, are always preceded by a mild to severe (or subclinical) group A streptococcal infection, usually pharyngitis. Fever and arthritis are the most frequent symptoms.

The diagnosis of rheumatic fever is by clinical criteria; there is no single laboratory test or diagnostic sign. (Because of the long-term therapeutic implications, the diagnosis should be made with caution.) The modified Jones criteria (American Heart Association Report, 1955) serve as a diagnostic guide. Major criteria include carditis, polyarthritis, chorea, subcutaneous nodules, and erythema marginatum. Minor criteria include fever, arthralgia, prolonged PR interval on electrocardiogram, increased ESR or C-reactive protein, and previous rheumatic fever. Two major criteria or one major and two minor criteria are considered suggestive of rheumatic fever, but no combination is absolutely diagnostic. Supporting evidence of a previous streptococcal infection must also be present, e.g., a history of recent scarlet fever, a positive throat culture for group A streptococci, or an increase in antistreptococcal antibody titers (see Chap. 18).

C. Treatment

1. **Eradication** of streptococci is accomplished with penicillin, which is given at the time of initial diagnosis (benzathine penicillin G, 600,000–1.2 million units intramuscularly; erythromycin, 250 mg orally 4 times/day for 10 days in patients with penicillin sensitivity).

2. **Bed rest** is indicated during active carditis.

3. **Salicylates** are used for symptomatic relief, especially for fever and arthritis. In adults, 5–8 gm of aspirin/day in 4–6 divided doses is administered (in children, 60–120 mg/kg/day in 4–6 divided doses) for the duration of the attack, usually 6–12 weeks. The dose must be adjusted by clinical response and by serum salicylate level determination (maintain the level between 20 and 30 mg/dl).

4. **Corticosteroids** are indicated for patients with severe carditis to reduce morbidity and mortality. Prednisone is administered (40–60 mg/day in adults, 2 mg/kg/day in children) for 4–6 weeks and tapered over 2 months.

5. **Tranquilizers** (e.g., haloperidol) can be used to treat neurologic symptoms. Treatment of congestive heart failure with **digitalis** and **diuretics** may be necessary.

6. **Prophylaxis** for recurrent streptococcal infections is mandatory in patients with documented rheumatic fever. Benzathine penicillin G (1.2 million units intramuscularly once a month), penicillin G (200,000 units), or phenoxymethyl penicillin (250 mg) orally 2 times/day (erythromycin, 250 mg 2 times/day in patients with penicillin sensitivity) is continued for life, especially in high-risk patients (military or health care personnel, or persons frequently exposed to children).

D. Prognosis. Severe, fulminant carditis is an uncommon cause of mortality. The morbidity in acute rheumatic fever relates to residual cardiac damage; two-thirds of patients with carditis develop residual damage. Disability is often related to recurrent, acute attacks with additive cardiac damage, indicating the need for antistreptococcal prophylaxis.

Selected Readings

Bryant, N. J. *Laboratory Immunology and Serology.* Philadelphia: Saunders, 1986.

Cohen, A. S. (ed.). *Laboratory Diagnostic Procedures in the Rheumatic Diseases* (2nd ed.). Boston: Little, Brown, 1975.

Cohen, A. S. (ed.). *The Science and Practice of Clinical Medicine* (Vol. 4). *Rheumatology and Immunology.* New York: Grune & Stratton, 1979.

Gupta, S., and Talal, N. *Immunology of Rheumatic Diseases.* New York: Plenum, 1985.

Kelley, W. N. (ed.). *Textbook of Rheumatology.* Philadelphia: Saunders, 1981.

McCarty, D. J. (ed.). *Arthritis and Allied Conditions* (10th ed.). Philadelphia: Lea & Febiger, 1985.

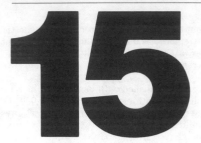

Immunohematology and Transfusion Therapy

Kwan Y. Wong and
Manley McGill

An enormous number of antigens are present in blood components. Red cell blood groups contain close to 400 antigens; neutrophils and platelets share HLA antigens in addition to their own specific antigens; and plasma proteins are antigenically different, even within their own classes. Immune reactivity to these antigens can result in a wide variety of clinical disorders.

Immunologic Disorders of the Erythrocyte

I. **Basic considerations**
   A. **Agglutination** of red blood cells (RBCs) by antibody, a basic technique in immunohematology, has allowed definition of RBC antigens. The agglutination process is preceded by the coating of RBCs with antibody (sensitization), which is dependent on the concentrations of antigen and antibody as well as on the pH, temperature, and ionic strength of the reacting medium. Agglutination occurs when the **antibody** attached to the RBC overcomes the repelling force between two RBCs (caused by an ionic cloud of negative charges on the cell surface—the zeta potential). A **complete antibody** (e.g., IgM, a large molecule with 10 binding sites) produces agglutination in a saline suspension. An **incomplete antibody** (e.g., IgG, a small molecule with only two binding sites) cannot bridge the gap between two RBCs unless the zeta potential is reduced by suspending RBCs in a colloidal medium (bovine albumin) or by removing sialic acid residues from the RBC membrane with proteolytic enzymes (ficin, papain, bromelin, or trypsin). Agglutination also depends on **antigen availability**—its number and location on the RBC membrane. The common A and B antigens, glycoproteins on the RBC membrane, are easily bound by anti-A or anti-B antibodies. However, many blood group antigens are proteins located within the RBC membrane. Enzyme treatment of the RBC can increase the accessibility of these antigens, notably the Rh antigens.
   B. **Antiglobulin test.** A practical application of the agglutination reaction is the antiglobulin test (Coombs' test).
      1. The **direct Coombs' test** detects **antibody** or **complement** on the **RBC surface** in the following steps:
         a. Antiglobulin serum (Coombs' serum) is prepared by injecting human serum or purified human globulin into an animal (usually a rabbit). The antibody produced is harvested and can be further absorbed to possess specificity against only one type of protein, e.g., anti-IgG or anticomplement.
         b. Red cells are adequately washed with saline to remove any trace amount of serum that could neutralize the antiglobulin and produce a false-negative result.
         c. If antibody or complement is present on the RBC surface, the addition of antiglobulin serum will produce agglutination.
      2. The **indirect Coombs' test** detects antibody **in the serum.** The serum is first

incubated with a mixture of type O red blood cells, and then the direct Coombs' technique is used as in **1.**

C. Red cell antigens. Antigens found on RBCs can be divided into two classes: polysaccharide and protein antigens. Polysaccharide antigens include the ABO, MN, Ii, and P systems; protein antigens include the Rh, Kell, Kidd, and Duffy systems.

    1. Polysaccharide antigens have the following characteristics:

        a. They usually elicit an IgM antibody response.

        b. They may stimulate warm-reacting (37°C) or cold-reacting (4°C) antibodies.

        c. They are responsible for isoantibodies (isoagglutinins); type A blood has anti-B isoantibodies, type B blood has anti-A isoantibodies, type O blood has anti-A and anti-B isoantibodies, and type AB has neither.

        d. They may elicit antibodies causing **immediate** transfusion reactions.

    2. Protein antigens elicit primarily IgG and warm antibodies and, rarely, cold antibodies or isoantibodies. Transfusion reactions due to these antibodies are often of the delayed type.

II. Hemolytic anemias mediated by immune mechanisms. Hemolytic anemias result from an increased rate of RBC destruction due to intracorpuscular defects or extracorpuscular agents. Immune mechanisms play a significant role in hemolytic disorders caused by extracorpuscular factors. These disorders include autoimmune hemolytic anemia, cold hemagglutinin disease, and paroxysmal cold hemoglobinuria. Erythroblastosis fetalis and ABO incompatibility, seen in newborn infants, are due to placental transfer of maternal blood group antibodies (IgG). **Other causes of hemolysis may be present and must be recognized for effective management.** These include congenital abnormalities of the RBC membrane, RBC enzymes, or hemoglobin and mechanical fragmentation of the RBC.

    A. Autoimmune hemolytic anemia. Antibody directed against a person's own RBC antigen(s) produces autoimmune hemolytic anemia. This condition may be the sole manifestation of autoimmune disease (20%) or secondary to an underlying systemic disorder (80%), such as lymphoid malignancy or collagen vascular disease. Most cases of autoimmune hemolytic anemia are due to warm-reacting antibodies (at 37°C), usually of the IgG class. IgM and IgA antibodies occur less frequently and usually in association with an IgG antibody. The clinical severity varies and can be **life-threatening.** Mortality is less than 40% for patients with idiopathic autoimmune anemia; mortality in the secondary type reflects the prognosis of the underlying disease.

        1. Clinical picture. The onset of anemia is often insidious, with no associated symptoms unless there is an underlying disease. Severe hemolysis causes fever, chills, nausea, vomiting, and pain in the abdomen, back, and chest. Jaundice may develop 24 hours later. The severe anemia can produce weakness, lethargy, and cardiac decompensation. The spleen may be palpable.

        2. Diagnosis

            a. The complete blood count shows normochromic, normocytic anemia with increased polychromasia, nucleated red cells, spherocytes, and, occasionally, fragmented red cells.

            b. The urine may be positive for urobilinogen or blood (due to hemoglobinuria).

            c. The **diagnostic test** is the direct Coombs' test. Using specific antisera against immunoglobulin or complement, three patterns of red cell coating are identified: immunoglobulin alone (20–40%), immunoglobulin(s) and complement (30–50%), and complement alone (30–50%). In 2–4% of patients with the clinical manifestations of autoimmune hemolytic anemia, the Coombs' test may be negative. By determining the reactivity pattern, it may help to exclude some diagnostic possibilities. For example, systemic lupus erythematosus is unlikely if RBCs are coated with IgG alone. There is **no correlation** between the severity of the hemolysis and the degree of positivity of the Coombs' test. **IgG subclass**

determination has clinical correlation in that in vivo hemolysis usually occurs with IgG_3-coated red cells, while in vivo hemolysis with IgG_4-coated red cells is rare.

d. Antibody can be eluted from the surface of the RBC and tested for blood group specificity. If only IgG is involved, it usually reacts against antigen(s) of the Rh system. If the eluate contains a mixture of antibodies, specificity probably exists against multiple red cell antigens, making cross-matching for transfusion extremely difficult.

3. Therapy of autoimmune hemolytic anemia must be directed at correction of the underlying disease process, if present. In children, hemolysis is usually transient and secondary to viral infection. In all other cases, the natural course of the disease consists of periods of exacerbation resulting in severe anemia, which can be a medical emergency.

a. Corticosteroids. Corticosteroids are the **drugs of choice.** Once the diagnosis of autoimmune hemolytic anemia is made, start prednisone, 40–60 mg/sq m daily in divided doses. Higher doses of prednisone (4–6 mg/kg/day) for 3–5 days may be necessary for control of severe acute hemolysis. With improvement, reduce dosage slowly over a 6- to 8-week period to a dose that maintains remission. (Some patients require a small dose of 10–20 mg **every other day,** while others may require larger doses for prolonged periods.) Adrenocorticotropic hormone (ACTH) has no advantage over corticosteroids.

b. Splenectomy should be considered if the patient is not responding to corticosteroids, or if high-dose corticosteroids (> 20–40 mg prednisone **daily**) are required to maintain a remission. There is no correlation between the antiglobulin reaction pattern and the response to splenectomy.

c. Immunosuppressive agents should be considered when splenectomy fails to control hemolysis. **Cyclophosphamide,** 2–3 mg/kg/day orally, or **azathioprine,** 2.0–2.5 mg/kg/day orally, can be used alone or with corticosteroids. Monitor the **white blood cell count** periodically.

d. Blood transfusion with packed red cells should be given **only if hemolysis is rapid, resulting in severe anemia.** Start corticosteroids at the same time as the transfusion. The benefit from blood transfusion is only transitory because of the subsequent destruction of transfused cells, and it is often hard to find compatible blood. With multiple transfusions, alloantibodies are formed in addition to autoantibodies. This added sensitization may further complicate the cross-matching process.

B. Cold hemagglutinin disease. Cold antibodies, usually IgM or, rarely, a mixture of immunoglobulins, react optimally at low temperature (4°C). They produce hemolysis by fixing complement to RBCs when the blood circulates to portions of the body exposed to cold ambient temperatures (the peripheral cutaneous microcirculation can normally reach 30°C).

1. Classification

a. Over one-half of the cases of cold agglutinin disease are classified as **chronic idiopathic** or **chronic cold agglutinin disease.** In this disorder, the cold antibody is monoclonal in origin, most often with kappa light chains, has specificity against the I antigen of adult RBCs with titers over 1:1000, and reacts over a wide temperature range, with substantial activity at 30–32°C (skin temperature).

b. Cold antibodies **secondary to systemic disease** are usually polyclonal, with low titers and a narrow thermal amplitude. IgM anti-I antibodies are associated with mycoplasma infection and some viral infections; anti-i antibodies are found in patients with infectious mononucleosis or lymphoreticular disease.

c. Cold agglutinins can also be found in **healthy persons.** These antibodies are usually polyclonal, in low titers (less than 1:64), and have anti-I specificity.

2. Clinical symptoms include a Raynaud-like phemomenon of the hands and feet (acrocyanosis, skin mottling, and numbness). These symptoms are often worse in the winter, or during the summer if the patient is exposed to excessively cool air conditioning. The spleen may be enlarged.

3. **Laboratory diagnosis**
   a. A **complete blood count** may show reduced hemoglobin and hematocrit, with polychromasia and spherocytes on blood smear. Erythrophagocytosis may occasionally be seen. Cold agglutinin disease **should be suspected** if a RBC count cannot be performed because of agglutination at room temperature.
   b. The **diagnostic test** is to demonstrate the cold antibody in the serum. The direct Coombs' test is usually negative, but it may be positive with anticomplement if there is evidence of hemolysis. Collect blood in the following manner:
      (1) Draw blood into prewarmed syringes and into prewarmed tubes, and allow it to clot at 37°C.
      (2) Use an anticoagulant such as EDTA to inhibit fixation of complement onto RBCs.
      (3) Titer the cold antibody at 4, 22, and 37°C to estimate the thermal amplitude of the reaction.

4. **Therapy**
   a. Patients should avoid exposure to low temperatures. In patients with cold antibodies secondary to infection, avoid the use of **cooling blankets** to control fever. A warming coil should be used for transfusion of RBCs in patients whose antibodies show significant activity at low body temperatures.
   b. Corticosteroids and splenectomy are not helpful.
   c. Immunosuppressive agents, in particular, chlorambucil (2–4 mg/day) may be helpful. Monitor white blood cell counts.
   d. If blood transfusions are indicated because of severe anemia, the crossmatching should be done only after absorption of the cold antibody with the patient's own RBCs. This absorption allows detection of other alloantibodies. Blood warmers (37°C) should be used with these transfusions. The following precautions should be observed:
      (1) Do not allow an excessive length of tubing between the warmer and the intravenous needle. This will cool the blood again.
      (2) The warmer should be well monitored. Overheated RBCs are rapidly destroyed in vivo and can be lethal.

C. **Paroxysmal cold hemoglobinuria** is a rare form of immunohemolytic anemia resulting from a biphasic reaction involving an IgG cold antibody, the **Donath-Landsteiner antibody**. In the first phase, IgG fixes complement onto the red cell at a low temperature; this is followed by complement-mediated lysis on rewarming of the cells to 37°C. The antibody has specificity against the P blood group antigen.

   1. **Clinical presentation.** This anemia, which is often associated with syphilis (particularly congenital syphilis), can be a complication of viral infections such as measles, mumps, chickenpox, infectious mononucleosis, and "flu" syndromes. Exposure to cold produces pallor, hemoglobinuria, and other symptoms of hemolysis. The prognosis is good, since resolution is usually spontaneous. This disease rarely becomes chronic with intermittent episodes of hemolysis.
   2. **Laboratory diagnosis** is made by demonstrating the Donath-Landsteiner antibody. Mix test serum with normal type O red blood cells. Incubate the mixture at 4°C for 30 minutes (complement fixing), then at 37°C for an additional 30 minutes (complement lysis). For a negative control, reverse the incubation conditions or use heat-inactivated serum (devoid of complement).
   3. **Therapy.** Patients should avoid cold exposure. Corticosteroids and splenectomy are not helpful. If blood transfusions are needed, use blood warmers.

D. **Paroxysmal nocturnal hemoglobinuria** (PNH) is a rare myeloproliferative dis-

Table 15-1. Drugs commonly associated with hemolytic anemia

Immune complex (innocent bystander)
  Aminosalicylic acid
  Chlorpromazine
  Isoniazid
  Phenacetin
  Quinidine
  Quinine
  Rifampin
  Stibophen
  Sulfonamides
  Thiazides

Hapten type
  Penicillin
  Cephalosporins
  Tetracycline

Aggregation of serum protein on red blood cell (RBC)
  Cephalosporins

Autoimmune type
  Levodopa
  Mefenamic acid
  Methyldopa

---

order that can terminate in acute leukemia. Red blood cells are abnormally sensitive to the lytic action of complement. Using low concentrations of cold antibodies with high concentrations of complement, PNH cells, but not normal cells, are lysed. The results of direct and indirect Coombs' tests are usually negative (C3 may occasionally be found on RBCs). There is no specific treatment, and therapy is directed at prevention and management of the three major complications: thrombosis, infection, and aplastic or hemolytic crises.

E. **Drug-related immunohemolytic anemia.** Antibodies to drugs can interact with RBCs to produce hemolysis on an immune basis, accounting for approximately 20% of all cases of acquired immune hemolytic anemia.

1. Four possible mechanisms have been proposed (Table 15-1).

   a. **Immune complex (innocent bystander).** Drug-antibody complexes attach to the RBC membrane **nonspecifically** and fix complement to produce hemolysis. The direct Coombs' test is often positive for complement only; occasionally, IgG may be present. Antibodies in the serum may be demonstrated by incubating normal RBCs with the patient's serum in the **presence of complement and the suspected drug.** This immune complex mechanism is responsible for the majority of drug-induced hemolytic anemias (see Table 15-1). Small doses of drug readministered after a latent period can produce acute intravascular hemolysis with hemoglobinemia, hemoglobinuria, and even renal failure.

   b. **Hapten-type reactions** result from a drug binding to the RBC membrane, becoming immunogenic, and stimulating antibody production (usually IgG). The direct Coombs' test is strongly positive for IgG. To demonstrate the antibody in the patient's serum, normal cells must be preincubated with the suspected drug before adding the test serum. A classic example of a hapten-type reaction is associated with high-dose penicillin therapy (> 10 million units/day). Although the direct Coombs' test becomes positive in approximately 3% of these patients, hemolysis develops in only a few patients. The hemolysis produced is not intravascular but extravascular (through erythrophagocytosis). The high titers of antipenicillin IgG present in these patients **do not correlate** with the presence or absence of IgE-mediated penicillin allergy.

   c. **Red blood cell membrane alteration with nonspecific adsorption** of aggregates of normal serum protein (IgG and complement) can produce a positive direct antiglobulin test. No reaction occurs if the patient's serum is mixed with normal RBCs. The cephalosporins produce this reaction; reports of hemolytic anemia are rare.

   d. An **autoimmune** type of reaction results when a drug stimulates production of antibodies (with Rh specificity), which then react with RBCs. The direct Coombs' test is positive for IgG. Incubation of the patient's serum with normal RBCs **without a drug** leads to IgG coating the RBCs. Drugs definitely implicated in this reaction are methyldopa, levodopa, and mefenamic acid. The direct Coombs' test becomes positive in approximately 15% of patients receiving methyldopa, but less than 1% of the patients will have a hemolytic anemia. The incidence of a positive direct Coombs' test appears to be dose related. Anemia usually develops gradually after several months of treatment; intravascular hemolysis has not been reported.

  2. **Therapy. Stop the offending drug.** In reactions of the immune complex type, prompt recovery occurs unless renal failure has developed. In autoimmune-type reactions, clinical recovery may take several weeks, and the antiglobulin test may remain positive for 1–2 years.

F. Erythroblastosis fetalis. Blood group incompatibility between mother and infant can produce hemolytic disease in the fetus and newborn infant. Severe anemia may lead to congestive heart failure in the fetus, resulting in hydrops fetalis. In all instances except ABO incompatibility, the mother must have been previously sensitized by the blood group antigen she lacks in order to produce specific antibody. During normal pregnancy, the amounts of fetal RBCs that enter the maternal circulation are insufficient to stimulate antibody production. However, during the third stage of labor, as much as 1 ml of fetal blood can enter the maternal circulation with resulting maternal immunization. Hemolytic disease of the newborn due to blood group incompatibility is unusual with the first pregnancy unless the mother has been previously transfused or sensitized as a result of abortion or amniocentesis. (In ABO incompatibility, in which anti-A and anti-B antibodies are naturally present, the first child can be affected by the placental transfer of these naturally occurring isoantibodies.) The most common cause of erythroblastosis is the D antigen of the Rh system (CDE/cde). Approximately 15% of white persons and 7% of black persons lack the D antigen and are termed Rh negative. Other antigens that may be implicated included c (hr′ or Rh4), E (rh″ or Rh3), Kell (K1), Duffy, and M, S, and U of the MN system.

  1. **Clinical presentation in the fetus.** Hemolysis and anemia occur in the fetus and, in severe cases, lead to heart failure and hydropic stillbirth. Hyperbilirubinemia does not occur in utero because bilirubin is freely transported across the placenta into the maternal circulation. **In the newborn infant,** the major problem is hyperbilirubinemia, which can lead to kernicterus and brain damage. Hepatosplenomegaly can be present. The differential diagnosis includes neonatal hepatitis, infection, metabolic disorders, and hemorrhage.

  2. **Diagnosis**

   a. Early in the pregnancy, a prenatal maternal ABO and Rh blood type should be determined and the serum screened for unusual blood group antibodies. If the mother is Rh-negative, the probable Rh genotype of the father is determined. The anti-D titer in maternal serum should be monitored periodically to detect sensitization.

   b. In sensitized mothers, amniocentesis and spectrophotometric analysis of amniotic fluid (see **3**) are more reliable means to assess the severity of the disease than the maternal anti-D titers.

   c. At birth, immediately determine the hemoglobin and serum bilirubin of the cord blood in a known case of blood group incompatibility.

   d. Perform the direct Coombs' test with the infant's RBCs. If the Coombs' test is positive, the specificity of the eluate from the infant's cells should be determined. If this specificity does not correspond to that of the maternal antibody, further evaluation of the cause of the positive direct Coombs' test is necessary.

3. **Prenatal therapy.** Early, aggressive **prenatal** therapy can lead to decreased morbidity and mortality in the newborn infant. The following guidelines should be used:

   a. When the titer of anti-D antibody exceeds 1:8 in the mother, amniocentesis should be performed to measure the bilirubin level or the bilirubin-protein ratio in the amniotic fluid. These determinations reflect the severity of the hemolysis.

   b. If the fetus is severely affected, as indicated by the bilirubin measurement (*Pediatrics* 35:815, 1965) or a bilirubin-protein ratio of 0.55 or more (*Obstet. Gynecol.* 26:826, 1965), transfuse with type O Rh-negative RBCs if the gestational age is over 24 weeks. (Inject RBCs into the peritoneal cavity of the fetus, and they are absorbed into the circulation.) Usually, a transfusion is required at 2- to 3-week intervals as determined by repeat amniocentesis studies. The production of RBCs by the fetus may be partially or completely suppressed after repeated intrauterine transfusions.

   c. The fetus can be delivered by cesarean section when the gestation weight is estimated to be adequate (around 33–36 weeks).

   d. Determine the infant's blood type and the direct antiglobulin test immediately after delivery. (A successful intrauterine transfusion may result in an Rh-negative typing in the infant.)

   e. Infants with a positive direct Coombs' test at birth will probably require subsequent exchange transfusions.

4. **Postnatal therapy.** Postnatally, hyperbilirubinemia must be treated with exchange transfusions or, in the appropriate setting, phototherapy.

   a. Exchange transfusions

   (1) Indications for exchange transfusion after delivery are as follows:

   (a) A hemoglobin level less than 14 gm/dl, or a serum bilirubin level greater than 4 mg/dl in the cord blood.

   (b) A rapid increase in the serum bilirubin level (about 4 mg/dl every 8 hours) within the first 24 hours.

   (c) A bilirubin level greater than 20 mg/dl for normal infants and 12–16 mg/dl for premature infants or sick term babies.

   (2) Remove small volumes (10–20 ml) of the infant's blood and replace it with donor blood. An exchange transfusion with twice the blood volume of the infant should reduce the bilirubin and anti-D antibody to about 55% of the original value. (Complete reduction is not possible because the extravascular pool slowly equilibrates with the plasma pool.) Approximately 90% of the infant's RBCs are replaced by donor RBCs.

   (3) The **blood** to be used for exchange transfusions should be compatible in cross-match with the mother's serum and as fresh from collection as possible to minimize the metabolic changes associated with the storage of blood.

   (4) An exchange transfusion can be associated with a number of **complications** (Table 15-2) and should be performed by experienced personnel using the following guidelines:

   (a) Perform the exchange transfusion in a clean room with resuscitation facilities and heating devices to keep the baby warm.

   (b) Catheterize the umbilical vein or saphenous vein using sterile surgical techniques.

   (c) Measure the venous pressure. If the volume of blood in the umbilical catheter is over 8 cm above the umbilicus, remove an extra 10–20 ml of blood before the exchange procedure.

   (d) Withdraw 10–20 ml of blood from the venous catheter, discard

Table 15-2. Complications of exchange transfusions

Bleeding
  Overheparinization of donor blood
  Thrombocytopenia
  Perforation of umbilical vein
Cardiac
  Heart failure due to hypervolemia and transfusion overload
  Cardiac arrest due to hyperkalemia, hypocalcemia, and/or
    citrate toxicity
Embolism and thrombosis
  Air emboli
  Portal vein thrombosis
Infection
  Bacterial sepsis
  Hepatitis from donor blood
  Necrotizing enterocolitis

---

and then replace with an equal volume of donor blood. (This can
be done with a three-way or four-way stopcock system.)

- **(e)** Monitor the heart rate and respirations during the entire procedure. **Keep the baby warm.**
- **(f)** Inject 1 ml of 10% calcium gluconate slowly with every 100 ml of
  exchange blood.
- **(g)** After completion of the exchange transfusion, remove the catheter and close the wound with a purse-string suture.

b. Phototherapy (blue light that decomposes bilirubin to water-soluble
products) can be used with caution as an **adjunct** to exchange transfusion (either before or after transfusion) **but should not be substituted
for a complete diagnostic evaluation** of the cause of jaundice. During
phototherapy, serum bilirubin monitoring is essential since the infant
may not appear as jaundiced but may still have severe hemolysis. Protect the eyes of the infant with bandages to prevent retinal damage.

c. Packed red blood cell transfusions may be necessary after intrauterine transfusions or exchange transfusions to correct anemia (hemoglobin
< 7–10 gm/dl). Sometimes, anti-D–coated cells are slowly removed
from the circulation, and, 3–6 weeks after birth, a late anemia rather
than hyperbilirubinemia may occur.

d. Passive immunization of the mother. The incidence of Rh sensitization
is markedly reduced if anti-D immunoglobulin (RhoGAM) is given to an
Rh-negative mother within 72 hours after delivery of an Rh-positive
baby. Also, give RhoGAM following abortion or amniocentesis in which
fetal cells can enter the maternal circulation. One ampule of anti-D (300
μg) is capable of "neutralizing" about 15 ml of D-positive cells. Higher
doses are necessary if greater fetal-maternal bleeding is suspected and
confirmed by staining for fetal RBCs in the mother's blood (Betke
method).

G. ABO incompatibility. Hemolytic disease due to ABO incompatibility is usually
seen in type A or B infants with type O mothers who have naturally occurring
isoagglutinins (anti-A and anti-B antibodies) in their serum. Prenatal diagnosis
is not possible. A high maternal titer of anti-A or anti-B is not predictive of ABO
hemolytic disease in the newborn.

1. **Clinical picture.** The first pregnancy can be affected. In the full-term infant,
   severe anemia and hydrops fetalis are rare. In some infants, jaundice can
   develop on the first day of life, but hemolysis is not as severe as in Rh
   incompatibility. As is the case with Rh incompatibility, **other causes of
   hyperbilirubinemia must be excluded.**

2. Diagnosis

a. The blood smear shows spherocytes and, occasionally, fragmented cells (ABO hemolytic disease may be difficult to differentiate from hereditary spherocytosis).

b. A direct Coombs' test on the infant's RBCs is usually negative or weakly positive because of the small number of A or B antigenic sites on fetal RBCs and the relative insensitivity of the current manual method of performing the direct Coombs' test. Eluates from the infant's RBCs react normally against adult A or B cells.

3. Therapy for ABO incompatibility is directed toward reduction of hyperbilirubinemia. The use of phototherapy, with close monitoring of bilirubin levels, has reduced the need for exchange transfusions, and the latter procedure is necessary in fewer than 1 in 3000 infants with ABO incompatibility. Low-titer (of anti-A and anti-B) type O blood is used.

Immunologic Disorders of Platelets

Immune destruction of platelets can occur in a fashion similar to that in immunohemolytic anemia, although less is known about the immunology of specific antiplatelet antibodies. Demonstration of antiplatelet antibodies is difficult, and the technique is not routinely available in clinical blood banks or serology laboratories. Methods of demonstrating platelet antibodies include agglutination, complement fixation, consumption of antiglobulin, platelet lysis, inhibition of clot retraction, platelet factor 3 release, serotonin release, and immunofluorescence. The complement fixation and antiglobulin consumption techniques usually give more consistent results than the other methods.

One method is to use radiolabeled *Staphylococcus* protein A. IgG-coated platelets first react with anti-IgG; *Staphylococcus* protein A then binds with the Fc portion of anti-IgG. The result can be quantified by determining the radioactivity.

Immune-mediated mechanisms are responsible for acute idiopathic thrombocytopenic purpura, chronic idiopathic thrombocytopenic purpura, isoimmune neonatal thrombocytopenia, and some forms of drug-induced thrombocytopenia.

I. Acute idiopathic thrombocytopenic purpura (ITP) is predominantly a disease in children between the ages of 2 and 6 years. The majority of children have a history of antecedent febrile illness, with or without a viral exanthem, days or weeks before the onset of purpura. Immunization with live virus vaccines can also be associated with acute ITP. The bleeding manifestations are usually cutaneous, with sudden onset of widespread petechiae and bruising. Epistaxis, hematuria, oozing from the gums, and gastrointestinal bleeding can occur, usually within the first week of illness. Intracranial bleeding is rare and is commonly associated with bleeding from mucosal surfaces. Mild splenomegaly (palpable spleen tip) is present in 5–10% of the children with acute ITP.

A. Diagnosis. Acute ITP is diagnosed by exclusion of other disorders.

1. The **complete blood count** is usually normal except for thrombocytopenia. Occasionally, mild eosinophilia or atypical lymphocytes are present.

2. Bone marrow examination shows no specific diagnostic features. The number of megakaryocytes may be normal or increased. Eosinophilic myeloid precursors may or may not be increased, and, if there is an associated anemia, hyperplasia of the RBC precursors is present. With the typical history of onset of the illness and absence of abnormal white blood cells on the blood smear, the diagnosis of ITP can often be made on clinical grounds without a bone marrow examination. However, bone marrow examination is definitely necessary to exclude other causes of thrombocytopenia if treatment with corticosteroids or splenectomy is considered or the diagnosis is not certain.

B. Therapy
1. **General treatment measures** for acute ITP include avoidance of trauma, especially to the head, and avoidance of intramuscular injections, which can cause painful hematomas or even blood loss. Withhold drugs that inhibit platelet aggregation (e.g., salicylates). Enemas, hard toothbrushes, and abrasive foods should be avoided.
2. Bleeding is most severe during the first week. During this time it may be necessary to observe the child **in the hospital.**
3. Corticosteroid therapy for acute ITP is controversial. There is no consensus of opinion as to what dose or how long corticosteroids should be used. Corticosteroid treatment does not accelerate the rate of recovery or influence the prognosis. However, an increase in platelet count may be seen as a result of blocking the ability of the reticuloendothelial system to remove antibody-coated platelets. Generally, prednisone, 1–2 mg/kg/day, is used in patients with bleeding from the mucosal surfaces because of the potential risk of intracranial hemorrhage. Another consideration to use prednisone is the activity of the child. It is not practical, if not impossible, to keep a close eye on an active youngster constantly. It may be advisable to use low doses of corticosteroids, such as an every-other-day regimen, to minimize the side effects from prolonged corticosteroid treatment.
4. If there is persistent or increased mucosal bleeding, **emergency splenectomy** is recommended. The result is often satisfactory, with a return of normal platelet count in 1–3 days in the majority of patients.
5. The use of high dose intravenous gamma globulin (400 mg/kg/day for 3–5 days or 1 gm/kg/day for 2 days) can be used in patients with acute ITP in whom corticosteroid therapy is contraindicated or in patients with chronic ITP who are unresponsive to corticosteroid therapy. The response to intravenous gamma globulin is variable.
6. Platelet transfusion is rarely indicated—the survival of transfused platelets is very short (see p. 341, sec. **E.4.**, for indications).
7. The child may return to normal activity when clinical signs of bleeding subside, even if the platelet count has not returned to normal. Body-contact sports, riding bicycles, or climbing heights should be avoided until the platelet count becomes normal.
C. Prognosis. The disease is self-limiting in the majority of patients. About 50% of children with ITP will recover within 4 weeks; 85% will recover within 4 months. The remaining patients recover spontaneously within a year; in a few instances, after several years. Recovery is usually permanent, although the disease may recur in a small number of children following a viral infection or live virus vaccine. Arbitrarily, patients with persistent thrombocytopenia for over a year are considered to have the chronic form of ITP.
II. **Chronic idiopathic thrombocytopenic purpura** is predominantly seen in adults and older children, with a slightly greater incidence in young women. The onset is insidious, and a history of antecedent infection is rarely obtained.
A. Diagnosis of chronic ITP is by exclusion of other causes of chronic thrombocytopenia, such as thrombocytopenia associated with bone marrow disease, systemic lupus erythematosus, drug-induced thrombocytopenia, transfusion-associated purpura, or thrombocytopenia secondary to other miscellaneous causes. **Bone marrow examination is mandatory.**
B. Therapy
1. **Corticosteroids** are often given initially (prednisone, 1–2 mg/kg/day) with a response expected after 1–2 weeks (see sec. **I.B.5.** above for indications for intravenous gamma globulin). If there is no improvement after 3–4 weeks, splenectomy is the treatment of choice. Splenectomy results in improvement in 70–90% of patients and produces permanent normal platelet counts in two-thirds. No reliable method of predicting the response to splenectomy is available.
2. **For splenectomy failures,** control of bleeding may be possible with corticosteroids or other immunosuppressive treatment. Vincristine can be given

Table 15-3. Drugs commonly associated with platelet destruction

Acetaminophen	Ethylchlorvinyl	Phenylbutazone
Acetazolamide	Furosemide	Quinine
Acetylsalicylic acid	Gold salts	Quinidine
Aminosalicylic acid	Heparin	Rifampin
Carbamazepine	Hydantoins	Stibophen
Cephalothin	Indomethacin	Sulfonamides
Chlorthalidone	Isoniazid	Sulfonylureas
Cimetidine	Levodopa	Thiazide diuretics
Digitoxin	Methyldopa	Valproate sodium

intravenously every 7–10 days at 1.5 mg/sq m, with a maximal single dose of 2 mg. Alternatively, vinblastine (0.1–0.3 mg/kg) can be given as an intravenous bolus injection or infusion over 4–6 hours every 7–10 days. Azathioprine, 2.0–2.5 mg/kg/day orally can also be tried. These immunosuppressive measures should be tried if there is a contraindication for splenectomy in those patients who have failed corticosteroid therapy. The use of danazol is still investigative.

III. **Isoimmune neonatal thrombocytopenia.** Destruction of fetal platelets by maternal antibodies can occur in a manner similar to that in Rh incompatibility. The Pl^{A1} (Zw^a) platelet antigen accounts for the majority of the cases of isoimmune neonatal thrombocytopenia. In contrast to Rh incompatibility, firstborn infants are affected in approximately 50% of the cases. Bleeding manifestations, which start shortly after delivery, range from petechiae and bruises to gastrointestinal or intracranial hemorrhage.

A. **Diagnosis.** Serologic incompatibility between maternal serum and fetal or paternal platelets can be demonstrated with the techniques of platelet antibody detection (paternal platelets are more readily obtainable for study than those of the infant). Other causes of neonatal thrombocytopenia must be excluded: infection, hemangioma, congenital absence of megakaryocytes, maternal ITP, and maternal drug therapy, e.g., thiazide.

B. **Therapy.** The disease is self-limiting, with recovery of normal platelets within a few days or up to 2 months, when maternal antibodies disappear. If there is active bleeding, the following treatment should be considered:

1. Random donor platelet transfusion may not be effective since the Pl^{A1} antigen occurs in 98% of the population. **Administration of washed maternal platelets** is the treatment of choice to stop bleeding.

2. **Exchange transfusion** may be performed to remove antibodies. This is followed by platelet transfusion.

3. **Prednisone,** 1 mg/kg/day, may be tried to decrease the rate of platelet destruction.

IV. **Drug-induced thrombocytopenia.** The immune complex mechanism is the most frequent cause of immune destruction of platelets (innocent bystander). The antibody in the patient's serum reacts with platelets only in the presence of the drug. Occasionally, the drug binds directly to platelets to form a primary antigen (hapten), which then reacts with the antibody. Some of the common drugs causing thrombocytopenia on an immune basis are listed in Table 15-3.

A. **Clinical presentation.** Bleeding manifestations (petechiae, purpura, and bleeding from the gastrointestinal and urinary tracts) appear within hours after administration of the offending drug. The duration of symptoms depends on the rate of excretion of the drug. After stopping the drug, the platelet counts usually return to normal in approximately 7 days.

B. **The diagnosis** is often difficult to confirm by in vitro demonstration of specific antibodies against suspected drugs. A skin patch test of the suspected offending drug may cause local purpura in sensitized patients. However, the diagnosis is usually made by temporal correlation of drug administration and resulting thrombocytopenia.

C. Therapy
   1. Observe the general measures of the management of thrombocytopenia (see sec. **I.B.1**).
   2. **Stop all drugs** unless the drug is essential to the patient's welfare. Avoid related compounds.
   3. Platelet transfusion is usually not helpful because transfused platelets are similarly affected.
   4. Corticosteroids may help by reticuloendothelial blockade (see sec. **I.B.3**).
   5. It is essential to avoid reexposure to the drug.
V. Familial thrombocytopenia may be related to congenital abnormalities of platelet morphology or platelet function. In these patients, autologous platelets have a shortened survival, whereas platelets from normal donors survive normally. It is of immunologic interest that Wiskott-Aldrich syndrome, an X-linked immunodeficiency disease, has an associated thrombocytopenia. The variation in the severity of Wiskott-Aldrich syndrome leads to the speculation that isolated X-linked thrombocytopenia may be a variant of this syndrome.

Immune-Mediated
Coagulation Disorders

Congenital disorders of coagulation result from the absence of a coagulation factor or the presence of a dysproteinemia (coagulation protein is present but functionally abnormal). **Acquired disorders** are related to decreased synthesis of coagulation factors secondary to systemic disease (e.g., liver disease or amyloidosis) or the acquisition of anticoagulants. Most acquired anticoagulants inhibit the activity of factor VIII (antihemophilic factor) and are characteristically IgG antibodies, although some are IgM or IgA antibodies. The cause of anticoagulant production is unclear. It may be due to a genetic predisposition or related to polymorphism of the factor VIII molecules.

I. The following clinical conditions are associated with circulating factor VIII inhibitors:
   A. An inhibitor to injected factor VIII develops in about 10% of patients with severe hemophilia. There is no correlation between the incidence of inhibitor and the degree of exposure to factor VIII. Factor VIII inhibitors are less commonly seen in patients with mild hemophilia than in patients with severe hemophilia.
   B. Patients with systemic lupus erythematosus, rheumatoid arthritis, ulcerative colitis, or regional enteritis may have anticoagulants.
   C. Previously healthy postpartum women may demonstrate anticoagulants for days to several months after childbirth.
   D. Healthy persons may have documented anticoagulants.
II. Diagnosis. The presence of factor VIII inhibitor can be demonstrated by mixing the patient's plasma with normal plasma in varying concentrations and measuring the partial thromboplastin time (PTT) and factor VIII functional activity. Strong inhibitors affect normal plasma immediately on mixing, although it is often necessary to incubate the mixture of test plasma and normal plasma for 1–2 hours to demonstrate the inhibitor activity. (Include a control incubation of normal plasma with saline to determine spontaneous loss of factor VIII activity with time.) For standardization of the measurement of factor VIII inhibitors, incubate the patient's plasma with an equal amount of pooled normal human plasma at 37°C for 2 hours, and then determine the residual factor VIII activity. When the patient's plasma produces a residual factor VIII activity of 50%, it is considered to contain 1 Bethesda unit of inhibitor/ml (*Throm. Diathes. Haemorrh.* 34:869, 1975).
III. Therapy
   A. Treatment should be directed to managing the underlying disease process if possible.

B. In the event of bleeding, large quantities of **factor VIII concentrate** (200–300% correction) can be given to overcome the antibody activity. An anamnestic response can be expected 2–4 days after reexposure to factor VIII, reaching a maximum within 2 weeks.

C. In patients with high titers of inhibitors, **exchange plasmapheresis** or **exchange transfusion** (for children) may be necessary to lower the titer of inhibitor, followed by large doses of factor VIII concentrate.

D. Another approach to patients with factor VIII inhibitor is to administer **activated vitamin K-dependent factors** (prothrombin complex, 75 factor IX units/kg, repeat in 12–24 hours if indicated), bypassing the factor VIII-dependent steps in intrinsic coagulation. Thrombosis may be a complication of this type of treatment, especially in the presence of liver disease. An anamnestic rise in inhibitor can also occur secondary to contamination with factor VIII in this preparation.

E. The use of corticosteroids has been unsuccessful in **hemophiliac patients** with factor VIII inhibitor. Long-term treatment with corticosteroids or other immunosuppressive agents may be helpful in **nonhemophiliac patients.**

F. Factor VIII inhibitors are often species specific. Bovine or porcine factor VIII preparations (investigational in the United States) can be effective in securing hemostasis in the event of life-threatening bleeding. Anaphylaxis is expected with repeated use of these preparations.

Immunologic Disorders of the Neutrophil

Immune destruction of the neutrophil has not been well studied until recently, mainly because of the complexity and lack of reliability of methods for testing neutrophil antibodies. Leukocyte-agglutinating antibodies were originally observed in multiparous women and patients who had had multiple transfusions. From these observations evolved the identification of the HLA system and tissue-typing techniques. Neutrophils have specific antigens as well as shared antigens. The neutrophil-specific antigens are regulated at two independent genetic loci: NA and NB. The shared antigens include HLA antigens (platelets, lymphocytes, and other tissues) and the 5b antigen (red cells, lymphocytes, monocytes, eosinophils, platelets, spleen, and lymphoid tissues that are independent of HLA).

Detection of specific neutrophil antibodies is mainly by an agglutination technique, which is more tedious than RBC agglutination, requiring special attention to the method of cell separation, the type of medium used, the temperature of reaction, and the physiologic state of the cell. Another method of detecting neutrophil antibodies is by testing the opsonic activity of the serum by macrophage ingestion of sensitized neutrophils.

I. Isoimmune neonatal neutropenia results from maternal antibody directed against the infant's neutrophils and becomes apparent when an infection develops. Affected infants with mild neutropenia remain asymptomatic and undiagnosed. Firstborn infants can be affected.

A. Diagnosis

1. The total **white blood cell count** may be normal, increased, or slightly decreased. The neutrophil count is very low or nonexistent. There is moderate monocytosis and occasionally an increase in eosinophils.

2. The **bone marrow** is hypercellular, with maturation of the myeloid cells "arrested" at the metamyelocyte or band stage.

3. Demonstration of the **specific antibody** (anti-NA1, anti-NA2, or anti-NB1) can be done in some medical centers. The diagnosis is often made by exclusion of other causes of neutropenia.

B. Treatment. The neutropenia usually lasts 2–17 weeks, with a mean duration of 7 weeks. Treatment is supportive, with prompt institution of antimicrobials when infection occurs. Corticosteroids are not helpful.

II. Autoimmune neutropenia is usually part of an autoimmune disease and is often associated with hemolytic anemia, or thrombocytopenia, or both. Autoantibodies reactive with neutrophil-specific antigens NA_2 and ND_1 can be demonstrated and the detection of these antibodies can elucidate some cases of "idiopathic" neutropenia as actually cases of isolated autoimmune neutropenia. Treatment is with **corticosteroids,** as in autoimmune hemolytic anemia.

Paraproteinemias

Paraproteinemias include a number of disorders of the B lymphocytes and plasma cells that result in overproduction of an immunoglobulin or subunit of an immunoglobulin. The protein produced is usually homogeneous (i.e., monoclonal and designated as the M component).

I. **Clinical and immunochemical findings common to these disorders** include the following:
   A. Large lymph nodes infiltrated by immature lymphocytes and plasma cells (hepatosplenomegaly may also be present).
   B. A **hyperviscosity syndrome,** associated with the increase in serum protein concentration, producing visual disturbances, ischemic neurologic symptoms, and a bleeding tendency. (The Sia water dilution test is a simple screening test. Add a drop of the patient's serum to a cylinder of distilled water. A filmy white precipitate indicates a positive result.)
   C. A **single spike,** revealed by serum protein electrophoresis and indicating the monoclonal nature of the protein. (The exception is in heavy-chain disease, in which a broad band occurs in gamma and alpha types. In mu heavy-chain disease, the serum protein electrophoretic findings are usually normal or show some degree of hypogammaglobulinemia.)
   D. Bence Jones protein in the urine, as well as in the serum.

II. **Benign monoclonal gammopathy** is a common immunoglobulin disorder, found in 1% of healthy adults over 25 years of age and 3% of persons over 70. There are no associated clinical symptoms, nor does the disease progress. The major importance of benign monoclonal gammopathy is the need to distinguish it from multiple myeloma. With early myeloma without lytic bone lesions or increased numbers of plasmacytoid cells in the marrow, the distinction is often difficult and occasionally impossible. No treatment is necessary for this condition.

III. **Plasma cell myeloma (multiple myeloma)** is the most common form of plasma cell neoplasm. The neoplastic cells produce excessive amounts of monoclonal immunoglobulins. The myeloma protein is IgG in 50% of the patients, IgA in 20%, IgM in 10%, light chain in 10%, and, rarely, IgE or IgD. Non-immunoglobulin-producing myelomas are rare.
   A. The **clinical symptoms** depend on the extent of involvement of the disease. Back pain, rib pain, or pathologic fractures occur commonly with skeletal involvement. Hypercalcemia is common if there are extensive osteolytic lesions. Impaired renal function results in azotemia (especially with light-chain disease). Bone marrow involvement results in a leukoerythroblastic blood picture or varying degrees of cytopenia. Hyperviscosity is common (especially with IgG myeloma).
   B. The **diagnosis** is made by demonstrating the monoclonal protein in the serum and urine, together with demonstration of the typical bone lesions by x-ray. The M component in the serum is often greater than 3.0 gm/dl.
   C. **Therapy** is designed to prolong survival and partially ameliorate symptoms.
      1. The use of **immunosuppressive agents** may produce transient improvement. Commonly used drugs include prednisone, melphalan, cyclophosphamide, chlorambucil, and nitrosoureas.
      2. **Radiotherapy** to pathologic fractures and extramedullary plasmacytomas may alleviate pain.
      3. **Maintain adequate urine output** in patients with hypercalcemia and hyperuricemia. Hypercalcemia can be treated with either calcitonin, 100–200 units subcutaneously every 12 hours, or prednisone, 40–80 mg daily.

4. The **hyperviscosity syndrome** can be treated with **plasmapheresis.**

D. The **prognosis** in plasma cell myeloma is best for IgM myeloma and worsens progressively for patients producing kappa chains only, IgG, IgA, lambda chains only, and IgD.

IV. Waldenström's macroglobulinemia is a disorder with proliferation of a clone of B lymphocytes, forming immature plasma cells that secrete monoclonal IgM. This disease, common in the sixth or seventh decade of life and with a slight male predominance, can present with fatigue and weakness. Raynaud's phenomenon, cold urticaria, and cold hypersensitivity are major symptoms in those with serum cryoglobulins. In some patients a bleeding tendency may be related to abnormal platelet function or decreased levels of clotting factor. The hyperviscosity syndrome may be present. The lymph nodes are enlarged, as are the liver and spleen.

A. Diagnosis

1. Anemia, usually due to hemodilution, is a common finding.

2. The direct Coombs' test is always negative.

3. The M component is readily demonstrated by electrophoresis.

4. There may be an associated decrease in the levels of normal immunoglobulins. The activity of the macroglobulins in certain patients resembles that of cold agglutination antibody or anti-IgG antibody (forming cryoprecipitable IgM-IgG complexes).

B. Therapy. The course of Waldenström's macroglobulinemia is variable, but usually progresses slowly over several years. Plasmapheresis is indicated for those with hyperviscosity syndrome. The use of chlorambucil, cyclophosphamide, or melphalan may be helpful.

V. Heavy-chain disease is a group of disorders in which a defective immunoglobulin heavy chain is synthesized (the Fd portion of the heavy chain is deleted, but the Fc portion is intact). The abnormal protein is monoclonal in origin. Four types of abnormal heavy chains have been identified: gamma, alpha, mu, and delta. The abnormal protein reacts with antisera to the corresponding immunoglobulin, but not with antisera to kappa or lambda light chains. The clinical picture resembles that of malignant lymphoma, with lymphadenopathy and hepatosplenomegaly. The bone marrow is diffusely infiltrated by activated lymphocytes, plasma cells, eosinophils, and histiocytes. Surface immunoglobulin is not observed on the lymphocytes. The causes of these disorders are unknown.

A. Gamma heavy-chain disease is usually found in patients over 40 years of age, although it has been identified in a few patients between 12 and 40 years of age. Fever, lymphadenopathy, and anemia are common presenting features. The serum concentrations of normal immunoglobulins are usually decreased; the levels of the abnormal proteins exceed 2 gm/dl. There is no satisfactory treatment for this disorder. The course of the disease is variable—patients may survive for a few months to years. In the terminal phase, there is a marked increase in the number of plasma cells in the bone marrow—a picture like that of plasma cell leukemia.

B. Alpha heavy-chain disease, the most common form of heavy-chain disease, is seen in persons under 50 years of age, with the peak incidence in the second and third decades. The abdominal lymphoid tissue is commonly involved, with markedly enlarged mesenteric lymph nodes and infiltration of the intestinal mucosa by lymphocytes and plasma cells. Villous atrophy is present. Chronic diarrhea and malabsorption are common symptoms. Some patients respond to treatment regimens for malignant lymphoma, whereas others achieve complete remission with antimicrobials alone.

C. Mu heavy-chain disease is rare since nearly all affected patients have chronic lymphocytic leukemia. Lymph node enlargement is uncommon. Vacuolated plasma cells are present in the bone marrow. Most patients excrete large amounts of kappa light chains in the urine. The diagnosis is made by demonstrating the abnormal monoclonal protein by careful immunochemical studies. The treatment is directed to the underlying disease, chronic lymphocytic leukemia.

D. Delta heavy-chain disease has been reported in only one patient. This patient presented with renal insufficiency, osteolytic lesions, and a bone marrow picture of myeloma. Electrophoresis demonstrated a peak between the gamma and beta regions, reactive with anti-delta but not with anti-kappa or anti-lambda sera.

Blood Transfusion Therapy

Blood transfusion therapy can be used for erythrocyte, leukocyte, platelet, or plasma protein disorders. The use of satellite plastic bags in a closed system has allowed fractionation of a unit of blood into three or four components: (1) Plasma can be separated from the RBCs by centrifugation within 2 hours of collection. (2) Packed RBCs with a hematocrit of 70–75% can be stored like whole blood without affecting the survival of transfused RBCs. (3) The buffy coat (containing platelets and white blood cells) can be further centrifuged to separate the platelet concentrate from the rest of the plasma. (4) Factor VIII can be extracted from the remaining plasma by cryoprecipitation. Cryoprecipitate-extracted plasma can serve either as volume expander or as replacement therapy for factor IX deficiency (hemophilia B). Component therapy is economical and medically advantageous in that sensitization of the recipient to unwanted components can be decreased.

Before deciding on any transfusion therapy, several considerations help to determine the necessity of the transfusion and the type of blood products to be used:

Anemia is a frequent indication for transfusion therapy. However, if anemia is due to a treatable cause (e.g., severe iron deficiency anemia), try medical treatment first. The absolute indications for transfusion with red cells include (1) symptoms referable to anemia, (2) acute onset and progression anticipated, and (3) associated complications such as severe pneumonia, cerebrovascular accident, or congestive heart failure.

Hepatitis is one of the complications from transfusion therapy. Screening blood donors for hepatitis B antigen has virtually eliminated the incidence of hepatitis B due to blood transfusion. However, it is estimated that over 10% of all blood recipients develop hepatitis described as non-A, non-B. The incubation period for this form of hepatitis has been reported as 2–15 weeks. The medical consequences of non-A, non-B hepatitis are uncertain at the present time. Screening blood donors for serum alanine aminotransferase (ALT or SGPT) does not reduce the incidence of non-A, non-B posttransfusion hepatitis. An etiologic agent has not been identified, and no screening test is yet available.

Primary cytomegalovirus (CMV) infection may follow transfusion of blood products from CMV-seropositive donors and has a high mortality among immunocompromised patients who are CMV-seronegative (CMV-SN). This complication may be prevented by using blood products from CMV-SN donors. Some blood centers have donor testing programs to provide CMV-SN red cell concentrates, fresh-frozen plasma, random donor platelet concentrates, and apheresis products. All products should be tested before transfusion since about 6% of donors will convert to CMV-seropositive within a year. In some parts of the United States, CMV-SN blood components may be difficult to obtain since greater than 90% of blood donors are CMV-seropositive. Clinical situations for which CMV-SN blood products are indicated include (1) newborn infants born of CMV-SN mothers and weighing 1250 gm or less, (2) CMV-SN pregnant women, (3) patients with severe combined immunodeficiency, (4) patients receiving intensive chemotherapy or immunosuppressive treatment who are CMV-SN, and (5) bone marrow transplant patients who are CMV-SN.

The etiologic agent of **acquired immunodeficiency syndrome (AIDS)** has been identified as a human T-cell leukemia virus (HTLV-III) termed the human immunodeficiency virus (HIV). Transfusion-associated AIDS has been reported in a small number of patients, mainly hemophiliacs. Although the current antibody tests for HIV (see Chaps. 17 and 18) are sensitive and specific, a negative antibody test does not guarantee that a person is free of virus, especially if the exposure was recent. Individuals at high risk for AIDS should not donate blood. Despite the screening of all blood products for HIV antibody, physicians should strictly adhere to medical indications for transfusions. All individuals identified as HIV antibody–positive should be counseled by blood bank or public health service staff specifically trained to deal with the psychological stress associated with positive test results. **Graft-versus-host disease** may follow transfusion of blood products containing viable donor lymphocytes in patients with impaired immune function. This disease has also been reported with intrauterine transfusion and exchange transfusion for hemolytic disease of the newborn. Irradiation of blood products prior to transfusion can prevent this complication. Blood products are treated with 3000 rads, which has no effect on RBC, granulocyte, or platelet function. Irradiated blood products should be used in patients with cell-mediated immunodeficiency states and patients undergoing intensive chemotherapy or bone marrow transplantation. In some medical centers, irradiated blood products are used for all neonates.

I. Indications for component therapy

A. Whole blood is indicated for the following:

1. The treatment of acute blood loss associated with **hypovolemic shock.** If the volume of replacement is equal to, or in excess of, the blood volume of the patient, use components (e.g., red cells, fresh-frozen plasma, platelet concentrates) because labile clotting factors and platelets can be depleted by multiunit transfusions. For lesser degrees of blood loss unassociated with hypovolemia, treat with packed RBCs.

2. **Septic shock.**

3. **Exchange transfusions** for neonatal hyperbilirubinemia or removal of toxic substances from the blood as in poisoning in children. It is also indicated for reducing alloantibody concentration prior to transfusion of a specific blood component (e.g., in patients with platelet antibodies who require platelet transfusion for the control of life-threatening hemorrhage).

4. **Priming renal dialysis units** or **heart-lung circuits.**

B. Packed red blood cells are indicated in the following conditions:

1. Anemia due to **poor marrow function** or marrow failure; e.g., marrow replaced by malignant cells, aplastic anemia, patients on chemotherapy, patients with a chronic disease such as uremia. Maintain the hemoglobin level above 10 gm/dl in this group of patients.

2. **Acute hemolytic anemia,** which can be a medical emergency. A rapid drop (a decrease of 2–3 gm/dl of hemoglobin within 6 hours) is an indication for transfusion.

3. **Thalassemia major.** Attempt to maintain hemoglobin levels above 10 gm/dl. Transfuse patients with other types of **chronic hemolytic anemia** if there is significant decrease from the usual hemoglobin level due to infection or aplastic or hemolytic crises. Use packed RBCs in patients with **sickle cell anemia** to reduce the hemoglobin S level to less than 40% prior to undergoing general anesthesia in order to avoid cerebrovascular complications.

4. Severe iron deficiency is **not** an indication for transfusion **unless** there is an associated condition such as pneumonia or congestive heart failure. **Start iron therapy** immediately.

Use 10–15 ml/kg of packed cells for children and 500–1000 ml for adults. Perform exchange transfusion, using packed RBCs, if the patient is in severe heart failure.

C. Leukocyte-poor red blood cells should be used for the same conditions as for packed RBCs in a patient who has experienced febrile nonhemolytic transfusion reactions. Leukocyte-poor RBCs can be obtained by washing RBCs with normal saline to remove the white blood cells and platelets. Alternatively, the unit of RBCs can be centrifuged at high speed to agglutinate the leukocytes, and the unit is then administered through a microaggregate filter.

D. In **frozen-thawed red blood cells,** leukocytes and platelets are destroyed by a freezing-thawing process and removed by washing procedures. They may be used:

1. For the same conditions as for packed RBC transfusions, but in patients who have experienced nonhemolytic reactions despite the use of leukocyte-poor packed RBCs.

2. For persons with rare blood types who have units of their own blood preserved in the frozen state for "autotransfusions" when necessary.

E. Platelet concentrates. Three types of platelet products are available for transfusion: (1) pools of random donor platelets processed from units of whole blood, (2) platelet concentrates collected from single donors by apheresis, and (3) platelets frozen in liquid nitrogen for long-term storage, usually autologous platelets. Platelets can be stored at 22°C for up to 7 days, but the posttransfusion increment is about half that seen with platelets after 1 day of storage. An 8-unit pool of random donor platelets contains about 4.4–6.5 $\times$ 10^{11} platelets. In an average sized adult, transfusion of an 8-unit pool (about 4–5 units/sq m) should produce an increase in platelet count by 40,000–80,000/mm^3 1 hour after transfusion. However, response to platelet transfusions are dependent on variables, including storage time before transfusion, storage temperature, associated clinical conditions, and the presence or absence of lymphocytotoxic or HLA antibodies. Fever, sepsis, and splenomegaly can decrease the yield from platelet transfusion. Lymphocytotoxic or HLA antibodies develop in about 40–50% of patients requiring regular platelet transfusions. A one-hour posttransfusion platelet count is a reliable way to assess the efficacy of platelet transfusion. **Indications** for platelet tranfusion are as follows:

1. Patients with bleeding due to nonproduction of platelets, e.g., leukemia and aplastic anemia.
2. Patients who require massive blood replacement (equal to or greater than the patient's blood volume).
3. Patients with bleeding problems due to congenital or acquired platelet dysfunction.
4. Platelet transfusion is generally **not** useful in thrombocytopenia due to destruction of platelets (immune thrombocytopenia or ITP, disseminated intravascular coagulation). However, platelets may be given to secure hemostasis for a brief period, as in the immediate postoperative period after splenectomy for ITP before the platelet count improves.

For patients requiring frequent platelet transfusions, ABO type-specific platelet concentrates should be used to avoid hemolytic anemia secondary to coating of the A or B cells by anti-A or anti-B antibodies. (ABO incompatibility does not affect posttransfusion platelet survival.) Rh-negative patients, particularly women with good long-term prognosis, should receive platelet concentrates from Rh-negative donors. Patients refractory to random donor platelet concentrates may respond to **fresh** random donor platelets. If this is not successful, single-donor platelet concentrates from HLA-matched donors should be tried. Experience with large populations of alloimmunized patients indicates that, for 100 patients, a donor pool of 2500 HLA-typed donors supplies an average of only nine donors with no mismatched antigens. Twenty-five percent of the patients may not have HLA-matched donors. Added to difficulties in locating suitable donors is the fact that, for reasons that are unclear, 25% of all HLA-matched platelet concentrates do not produce acceptable posttransfusion increments. In some blood centers, alloimmunized patients can have their own platelets harvested when they are in remission and frozen in dimethyl sulfoxide (DMSO) for subsequent autologous transfusion.

F. Fresh-frozen plasma can be used for the following:

1. As a volume expander in the treatment of **shock** and **dehydration,** although plasma protein fractions can serve the same purpose.
2. Single-donor plasma can supply **clotting factors** in patients in whom a single factor deficiency is not identified (e.g., in liver disease) or in patients requiring massive blood transfusions.
3. Factor IX deficiency (hemophilia B) can be treated with plasma unless the volume of infusion is large and commercial concentrates can be used.
4. Frozen plasma can be used for the treatment of **antibody-deficiency states** as a source of immunoglobulins and opsonins (20 ml/kg every 4 weeks). Patients with associated IgA deficiency may produce anti-IgA antibodies, which can lead to anaphylaxis when reacting with IgA. In patients with T

cell deficiency, the plasma should be irradiated before administration to avoid possible graft-versus-host disease (see p. 340 and Chap. 17).

G. **Cryoprecipitate.** When frozen plasma is thawed at 4°C, the protein that remains in a precipitated form is rich in factor VIII. One unit of factor VIII is defined as the amount of factor VIII in 1 ml of normal plasma. The average amount of factor VIII in the cryoprecipitate from 1 unit of blood is about 100 units. For treatment of bleeding in a hemophiliac patient, attempt to increase the factor VIII level to 50%; 1 unit/kg of factor VIII will increase the level by 2%. Cryoprecipitate also contains a significant amount of fibrinogen and can be used for replacement in afibrinogenemia or dysfibrinogenemia.

H. **Albumin.** A 5% albumin preparation is used as a plasma expander. The 25% concentration of albumin should not be used in the presence of dehydration but can be used in hypoalbuminemic states.

I. **Gamma globulin.** Commercial gamma globulin preparations contain mainly IgG at a concentration of about 165 mg/ml and are given intramuscularly. Intravenous preparations of gamma globulin are available. (See Chaps. 17 and 19.)

II. **Hazards of blood transfusion therapy.** The use of blood or blood products is not without potential risk to the recipient. The incidence of adverse reactions with transfusion therapy is about 5% in adults. Some of the delayed complications may not have been recorded, and the incidence may be higher. However, the use of specific components certainly can lower the incidence of reactions.

A. **Nonimmunologic complications**
 1. **Acute problems** related to transfusion therapy include the following:
  a. Bacterial contamination, which leads to high fever, chills, and shock.
  b. Air embolism.
  c. Heart failure due to fluid overload.
  d. Acidosis due to massive use of acidified plasma.
  e. Cerebral anoxia due to the massive use of stored blood low in, 2,3-DPG.
 2. **Delayed complications** include the following:
  a. Transmission of diseases such as malaria, hepatitis, cytomegalovirus infections, or AIDS.
  b. Hemosiderosis from multiple blood transfusions.

B. **Immunologic complications**
 1. **Acute transfusion reactions** can be due to the following:
  a. Hemolysis as a result of incompatible blood transfusion. The antibody-RBC reaction triggers the production of anaphylotoxin from activation of the complement system. There is intravascular hemolysis, resulting in free hemoglobin in the plasma, formation of methemalbumin (a brown pigment), and hemoglobinuria. Clinically, there is an acute onset of fever, chills, back pain, chest pain, shock, and renal failure. These symptoms may occur after a small amount of blood is infused. The majority of acute hemolytic reactions are due to ABO incompatibility as a result of clinical error. Thus, it is of utmost importance to label the cross-matched specimen properly and check patient identification before blood is administered.
  b. Anaphylaxis due to IgA—anti-IgA reaction.
  c. Reactions, such as urticaria, diffuse rash, fever, chills, and wheezing of undetermined etiology, possibly allergic.
 2. **Delayed transfusion reactions** include the following:
  a. Delayed hemolysis due to alloantibody. The hemolysis may take place several days after transfusion.
  b. Isoimmunization and formation of antibodies against cellular as well as serum protein antigens.

C. **Investigation of a transfusion reaction**
 1. When signs and symptoms of a transfusion reaction develop, **stop the transfusion immediately.**
 2. Obtain a blood sample from the container for **smear** and **culture** for bacteria. Similarly, culture a sample of blood from the patient for bacteria.

3. The unit of blood should not be discarded. Return the unit to the blood center with a sample of blood from the patient for a direct antiglobulin test, repeat ABO and Rh typing, repeat cross-matching, and screen for antibodies in the serum.
4. Appropriate **blood chemistries** should be done to monitor renal function.
D. **Treatment of transfusion reactions**
1. Treat **shock** with a plasma expander. Another unit of blood should be carefully cross-matched and transfused, with careful observation of the patient.
2. With **acute intravascular hemolysis,** maintain an adequate urine output and consider **alkalinization** of the urine. (Hemoglobin is more soluble in alkaline than in acid urine.) Infusion of **mannitol** is recommended to maintain renal blood flow and glomerular filtration.
3. If **bacterial contamination** is highly suspected, **antimicrobials** should be initiated immediately.
4. Urticaria can be treated with **parenteral diphenhydramine.** Parenteral epinephrine and corticosteroids should be used if wheezing, laryngospasm, or hypotension is present (see Chap. 10).

Selected Readings

Adler, S. P., et al. Prevention of transfusion-associated cytomegalovirus infection in very-low-birthweight infants using frozen blood and donors seronegative for cytomegalovirus. *Transfusion* 24:333, 1984.

Bove, J. R. Transfusion-associated AIDS—A cause for concern. *N. Engl. J. Med.* 310:115, 1984.

Boxer, L. A. Immune neutropenias: Clinical and biological implications. *Am. J. Pediatr. Hematol. Oncol.* 3:89, 1981.

Chaplin, H., Jr. Clinical usefulness of specific antiglobulin reagents in autoimmune hemolytic anemia. *Prog. Hematol.* 8:25, 1974.

Conrad, M. E. (guest ed.) Transfusion therapy. *Semin. Hematol.* 18(2):79, 1981.

Honig, C. L., and Bove, J. R. Transfusion-associated fatalities: Review of Bureau of Biologics Reports 1976–1978. *Transfusion* 20:653, 1980.

Issitt, P. D., and Issitt, C. H. *Applied Blood Group Serology* (2nd ed.). Oxnard, CA: Spectra Biologicals, 1975.

Miescher, P. A., and Graf, J. Drug-induced thrombocytopenia. *Clin. Haematol.* 9:505, 1980.

Moss, R. A. Drug-induced immune thrombocytopenia. *Am. J. Hematol.* 9:439, 1980.

Petz, L. D. Drug-induced immune haemolytic anaemia. *Clin. Haematol.* 9:455, 1980.

Queenan, J. T. (ed.) *Modern Management of the Rh Problem* (2nd ed.). New York: Harper & Row, 1977.

Schiffer, C. A, et al. Potential HLA-matched platelet donor availability for alloimmunized patients. *Transfusion* 23:286, 1983.

Shapiro, S. S., and Hultin, M. Acquired inhibitors to the blood coagulation factors. *Semin. Thromb. Hemost.* 1:336, 1975.

Swisher, S. N. (guest ed). Autoimmune hemolytic anemia. *Semin. Hematol.* 13(4):247, 1976.

Yeager, A. S., et al. Sequelae of maternally derived cytomegalovirus infections in premature infants. *J. Pediatr.* 102:918, 1983.

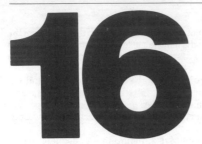

The Immune System and Neoplasia

Paul M. Zeltzer

The interaction of macrophages, lymphocytes, and their products plays an important role in tumor rejection. Successful immunization with tumor-specific antigens (TSAs) against tumor recurrence has been documented in mice and guinea pigs, but many aspects of the rodent tumor-antigen interaction have not been applicable to human tumors. This chapter will focus on the practical aspects of the interaction between human cancers and the immune system and the ways in which immunologic methods can be utilized to diagnose, monitor, and treat patients with cancer.

I. **Etiologic factors in human cancer.** The factors that cause the majority of cancers are unknown, but the interplay between environment (carcinogens encountered in the workplace, life-style, personal habits) and the susceptible host (heredity, sex, age) probably accounts for the majority of neoplasms. The separation of these factors is for purposes of discussion only (Table 16-1).

   A. **Environmental factors.** The majority of human cancers occur in tissues exposed to the agents we ingest and the environment in which we live and breathe.

      1. The overwhelming proportion of lung, oral cavity, and laryngeal cancers (90%) are correlated with **cigarette use.** Esophageal, bladder, and pancreatic cancer risk is also increased by smoking. Skin cancer, the most common squamous epithelial malignancy, is associated with contact with coal tar and ultraviolet radiation exposure.

      2. **Aerosolized pollutant** exposure, in addition to nicotine and tar, is associated with lung cancer. These pollutants include lead, copper, zinc, arsenic, and cyclic aromatic hydrocarbons; these suggested agents may be responsible for the high incidence of lung cancer seen in some southern coastal cities of the United States. Exposure to asbestos (silica), an insulating material commonly used in shipbuilding, is strongly associated with pleural mesotheliomas and lung cancer; even a 1-month exposure increases this cancer risk, which is further aggravated by cigarette smoking.

      3. **Industrial chemicals** that increase the risk of cancer are vinyl chloride in plastics manufacturing (liver angiosarcomas) and benzene in printing (leukemia). Bladder cancer is associated with aniline and coal-tar derivatives.

      4. The continuous use of certain **drugs** is associated with cancer.

         a. **Immunosuppressive drugs,** such as cyclophosphamide, azathioprine, and methotrexate, used to treat cancer, renal transplant rejection, and severe inflammatory diseases (e.g., rheumatoid arthritis and psoriasis) increase the risk of the development of a lymphoma 100-fold.

         b. Long-term administration of **hydantoin anticonvulsants** is also related to the development of lymphomas, some of which regress after the drug is stopped.

         c. Therapeutic use of **oral contraceptives** and **androgens** is related to the development of carcinoma and adenoma of the liver, and **rauwolfia drugs** are associated with breast cancer. The decreased administration of **estrogens to postmenopausal women** correlates with a reduced incidence of endometrial cancer. Clear cell carcinoma of the vagina in a young woman should prompt an inquiry into in utero exposure to stil-

Table 16-1. Known etiologic factors in cancer

Factor	Type of cancer
Environmental exposure	
Aerosol and/or industrial pollutants	
Asbestos (silica)	Mesothelioma
Lead, copper, zinc, arsenic, cyclic aro-matics, tobacco	Lung cancer
Vinyl chloride	Liver angiosarcoma
Benzene	Leukemia
Aniline dyes, coal	Skin, bladder carcinoma
Drugs	
Androgenic steroids	Hepatocellular carcinoma
Stilbestrol (prenatal)	Vaginal adenocarcinoma
Estrogen (postmenopausal)	Endometrial carcinoma
Rauwolfia	Breast carcinoma
Hydantoins	Lymphoma
Chloramphenicol, alkylating drugs	Leukemias, lymphomas
Radiation	
Ultraviolet	Skin cancer
Ionizing (fallout, industrial exposure)	Leukemias, thyroid tumors
Isotopes, radium	Osteogenic sarcoma
Therapeutic	Osteogenic sarcoma, fibrosarcoma, skin, breast, thyroid carcinomas
Infections	
Herpesvirus (Epstein-Barr virus)	Burkitt's lymphoma, nasopharyngeal carcinoma
Herpesvirus type 2	Cervical cancer
Human immunodeficiency virus (HIV)	Kaposi's sarcoma
	Non-Hodgkin's lymphoma
	Primary lymphoma of the brain
Parasites	Bladder cancer
Geographic	
China	Nasopharyngeal carcinoma
Iran	Esophageal carcinoma
Russia, Japan, Iceland, Finland	Gastric carcinoma
United States, Western Europe	Colon, breast carcinoma
Africa	Hepatocellular carcinoma, Burkitt's lymphoma
Host	
Chromosomal abnormalities	Leukemias
Primary and secondary immunodeficiency	Lymphomas, leukemias

bestrol derivatives; the latency period is long, and cancer may develop 7–21 years after exposure.

5. **Radiation** increases the risk of human cancer.
   a. Persons exposed to **ionizing radiation** from atomic bombs have a 6–40 times greater incidence of acute lymphoblastic, acute myelogenous, and chronic myelogenous leukemia and benign and malignant thyroid nodules.
   b. Watch-face painters using radium previously suffered from osteosarcomas; because of awareness and worker protection, this is no longer a problem.
   c. **Therapeutic irradiation** also increases the risk of **second** tumors (e.g., osteosarcoma, fibrosarcoma, skin cancer). For example, in 10% of chil-

dren treated for rhabdomyosarcoma or retinoblastoma, a second recurrence of the primary cancer develops near the portal of irradiation years following treatment.

d. Irradiation to the fetus increases the leukemia risk 50%. Similarly, children who receive neck irradiation to treat cough due to enlarged tonsils or to treat croup associated with a large thymus now have an increased risk of benign and malignant thyroid nodules developing after a latency period of 10–30 years. Spinal irradiation for spondylitis increases the risk of acute myelogenous leukemia 10-fold.

6. **Two herpesviruses** are strongly associated with cancer: Epstein-Barr virus (Burkitt's lymphoma and nasopharyngeal carcinoma) and venereally transmitted herpesvirus type 2 (cervical cancer). The human immunodeficiency virus (HIV), the cause of acquired immunodeficiency syndrome (AIDS), is associated with an increased incidence of Kaposi's sarcoma, non-Hodgkin's lymphoma, and primary lymphoma of the brain.

7. Infection of the bladder with *Schistosoma* is also linked with later development of cancer in that organ.

8. **Geographic differences** in cancer incidence may be due to host factors, environmental factors, or both, although immigrants usually assume the cancer risk of their adopted country. Gastric cancer predominates in people eating smoked foods and fish, while colon and breast carcinoma are more common in western societies, in which more protein and fat are ingested. In Africa, liver cancer is related to spoiled food (aflatoxins), while Burkitt's lymphoma occurs in limited areas having cofactors of both endemic malaria and Epstein-Barr virus infection.

B. Host factors

1. A dramatic increase in leukemia is seen in abnormalities of **chromosome number** or **arrangement** (e.g., Fanconi's anemia, Bloom's syndrome, Down's syndrome) and in disorders of **improper repair of DNA** damaged by electromagnetic irradiation (xeroderma pigmentosum).

2. Cancer incidence in the **immunodeficiency syndromes** is 10,000-fold greater than expected, and 80% of the cancers are lymphomas. The preponderance of lymphomas in congenital, acquired, and drug-induced **immunosuppression** is consistent with the failure of immune surveillance or antigenic overstimulation, with loss of normal feedback control. The link between genetic abnormality and leukemia is consistent with a germinal or somatic mutation in a stem cell line.

C. Immune surveillance. The theory of immune surveillance proposes that the host's cellular (T lymphocyte) immune response evolves as a defense against incipient neoplastic change and eliminates clones of cancer cells as they appear. A corollary requires that neoplastic cells have new or altered cell-surface antigens (TSAs) against which this immune response develops.

This theory makes the following predictions:

1. **At periods of relative immunodeficiency** (infancy, old age), **malignancy occurs with greater frequency than during middle life.** Leukemia and brain tumors predominate in childhood; skin, breast, colon, and uterine cancers are major cancers in the elderly. However, these cancers are not the lymphomatous cancers that occur in immunodeficient persons (see Table 16-1).

2. **Drug-induced or genetic depression of the immune system leads to a greater incidence of all malignancies.** In immunosuppressed persons, 80% of cancers are lymphomatous and not the frequently occurring types. If immune surveillance were a significant control mechanism, this theory would predict polyclonal neoplasms. However, most cancer is monoclonal, as determined by isoenzyme analysis. Families with multicentric, polyclonal tumors are seen (multiple endocrine adenomatosis, basal cell carcinoma with brain tumors, thyroid medullary carcinoma with pheochromocytoma), but these tumors are rare.

3. **Spontaneous regression occurs in persons with intact immunity, and tumors with a lymphocytic infiltration have a better outcome.** Spontaneous regression (neuroblastoma) as well as responses to minimal chemotherapy (Burkitt's lymphoma) are documented. However, direct proof that TSAs cause this rare occurrence of spontaneous regression is lacking. Lymphocytic infiltration of tumors and draining regional lymph nodes are correlated with a good outcome; although suggestive, these characteristics alone are not proof of immunity to TSAs, since infectious agents cause similar responses.

4. In summary, since a specific defect of immune surveillance or TSA(s) (or both) related to cancer **has not been documented,** immune surveillance is now conceptualized as a possible defense operative through a variety of mechanisms: the T cell; the "natural killer" cell (a null cell activated by interferon); the macrophage; or an antibody. Tumor-specific antigens, if present, are weak immunogens and may have a positive or negative influence on an established tumor.

D. **Immune depression and neoplasia.** There is a general tendency for patients in the advanced stage of any cancer to have diminished immune responses. In Hodgkin's disease and head and neck cancer, immune response may be diminished in seemingly minimal disease, and this defect may persist in Hodgkin's disease for years after a "cure." In acute lymphoblastic leukemia, there is a mild immune defect in B cell– and T cell–dependent function. Apart from these observations, T-cell and B-cell quantitation and T-cell functional assays (e.g., in vitro phytohemagglutination responsiveness and delayed hypersensitivity skin tests) are not clinically helpful in predicting or determining a clinical response or serving as criteria to change therapy in the individual patient with nonlymphoid malignancy.

II. A **tumor marker** is the characteristic of a neoplastic cell by which it can be detected or operationally differentiated from a normal cell (Table 16-2). An example is alpha fetoprotein (AFP), which is secreted by certain tumors and circulates in levels that reflect tumor mass. Other examples include carcinoembryonic antigen (CEA) and beta subunit human chorionic gonadotropin (B-hCG). Markers also allow classification of tumor subsets, e.g., leukemias and breast cancer.

Although not tumor-specific, markers can be used for **diagnosis, monitoring,** and **prognosis.** If the histopathology is nondiagnostic or unavailable, a known tumor marker may limit the diagnostic possibilities and suggest a further search for a primary site. Serial changes in serum levels of these markers allow assessment of positive or negative responses to therapy. In childhood leukemia, surface markers of leukemia cells allow grouping of the leukemias into high-risk and low-risk types, with markedly different treatment approaches and success.

A. **Solid-tumor markers**
1. **Hormones** (e.g., adrenocorticotropic hormone [ACTH], calcitonin, catecholamines) may be secreted by differentiated tumors of endocrine organs and squamous cell lung tumors. Oat cell carcinomas may produce B-hCG, antidiuretic hormone (ADH), serotonin, calcitonin, parathyroid hormone, and ACTH, which may be used to follow the response to therapy. Some breast cancers have progesterone or estradiol receptors or both, which are strongly correlated with positive responses to hormone therapy. Similarly, neuroblastomas and pheochromocytomas secrete catecholamine metabolites (vanillylmandelic acid [VMA], homovanillylmandelic acid [HVA], metanephrine) that can be detected in urine. Neuroblastomas also release neuron-specific enolase and ferritin, which can be used for diagnosis and prognosis.
2. **Alpha fetoprotein,** an age-related product of the fetal liver that is synthesized up to birth, is secreted into serum in nanogram to milligram quantities by the following tumors: hepatocarcinoma, endodermal sinus tumors, and teratocarcinomas of the testis, ovary, mediastinum, and sacrococcyx (Table 16-3). In 10–15% of patients with gastric and pancreatic cancers with liver metastasis, the concentration of AFP also may be elevated. Non-

Table 16-2. Summary of useful markers for diagnosis, prognosis, and monitoring of tumors

Type of cancer	Serum markers					Cell surface markers	Clinical use*
	AFP	CEA	B-hCG	Neuronal enolase	Other hormones		
Adrenocortical	–	–	–	–	+	–	D, M
Breast	–	+	–	–	–	–	(D), M
Carcinoid	–	–	–	+	+	–	D, M
Choriocarcinoma	–	–	+	–	–	–	D, M
Colorectal	Rare	+	–	–	–	–	(D), M
Endodermal sinus	+	–	+	–	–	–	D, M
Esophageal	–	+	–	–	–	–	M
Gastric	Rare	+	–	–	–	–	(D), M
Hepatoma	+	–	–	–	–	–	(D), M
Leukemias	–	–	–	–	–	+	D, P
Lymphoma (non-Hodgkin's)	–	–	–	–	–	+	D, P
Neuroblastoma	–	–	–	+	+	–	D, M, P
Ovarian	Rare	Rare	–	–	+	–	M
Pancreatic	Rare	+	–	–	Rare	–	(D), M
Parathyroid	–	–	–	–	+	–	D, M
Pheochromocytoma	–	–	–	–	+	–	D, M
Pituitary adenoma	–	–	–	–	+	–	D, M
Pulmonary (oat cell)	–	–	+	+	+	–	M
Pulmonary (squamous)	–	+	+	+	–	–	M
Seminoma	–	–	–	–	–	–	none
Sézary syndrome	–	–	–	–	–	+	D, (P)
Teratocarcinoma	+	–	+	–	–	–	D, M
Thyroid (colloid)	–	–	–	–	+	–	D, M
Thyroid (medullary)	–	–	–	+	+	–	D, M

Key: + = useful; – = not useful; AFP = alpha fetoprotein; CEA = carcinoembryonic antigen; B-hCG = beta subunit human chorionic gonadotropin.
*Diagnosis (D), prognosis (P), and monitoring of response to therapy (M) are the suggested uses for the serum and cell surface markers of these tumors. Parentheses indicate a lack of specificity for the indicated marker.

Table 16-3. Serum alpha fetoprotein (ng/ml) by age and disease[a,b]

Disease	Range (ng/ml)	Percentage of patients > 20 ng/ml
Cancerous conditions		
Endodermal sinus	390–210,000	100
Teratocarcinoma	20–130,000	75
Seminoma	20	0
Hepatocellular carcinoma	20–5,000,000	70
Pancreatic, gastric carcinoma with liver metastases	20–500	15
Noncancerous conditions		
Hepatitis		
Neonatal (0–3 mo)	40,000–290,000	100
Viral	21–4400	31
Chronic active	23–4210	33
Persistent	21–267	10
Chronic hepatitis B antigenemia	33–36	18
Primary biliary cirrhosis	20	0
Ataxia telangiectasia	44–2800	95
Cystic fibrosis	56–8800	?
Tyrosinemia	20,000–300,000	100

[a]The following laboratories make alpha fetoprotein determination by radioimmunoassay: Smith Kline Bio-Science Laboratories, 7600 Tyrone Avenue, Van Nuys, CA 91405; Roche Clinical Laboratories, 5 Johnson Drive, Raritan, NJ 08869. Send 1–2 ml of serum by airmail.
[b]Normal values at birth (in ng/ml) are 60,000–120,000; at 0–2 months, 25–1000; at 2–6 months, 25–100; and at 6 months, 20. In a normal pregnancy they are 18–113 in the first trimester, 160–550 in the second, and 100–400 in the third.

cancerous conditions, with modest serum elevations of AFP (20–2000 ng/ml), are hepatitis, cystic fibrosis, and ataxia-telangiectasia; high elevations occur with prematurity and tyrosinemia.

Alpha fetoprotein is a very reliable marker for following the response to chemotherapy and radiation therapy. The level should be obtained every 2–4 weeks (metabolic half-life in vivo is 4 days). Both AFP and B-hCG should be quantitated initially in all patients with teratocarcinoma, since one or **both** markers may be secreted in 85% of patients and recurrent tumors may secrete AFP or B-hCG.

3. **Carcinoembryonic antigen,** unlike AFP, is a cell surface protein found predominantly on fetal endocrine tissues in the second trimester (Table 16-4). Of endodermally derived gastrointestinal neoplasms, 75% shed CEA in excess of 2.5 ng/ml of plasma. Though stable or elevated levels usually indicate progression, and decreasing CEA suggests a response in patients with metastatic colorectal disease, CEA does not correlate with clinical status in 35% of these patients. Of patients with head, neck, and breast carcinomas, 50% also have CEA in excess of 2.5 ng/ml; and 20% of smokers and 7% of former smokers have CEA in excess of 2.5 ng/ml, as do many patients with active inflammatory bowel disease. Thus, CEA is not a cancer screening test and **must** be used with caution. Two plasma specimens should be obtained 2–4 weeks apart to detect a trend.

Estimation of CEA helps to differentiate benign from malignant pleural and ascites effusions. In conjunction with cytology, levels greater than 12 ng/ml are strongly correlated with malignancy and suggest malignancy even when the cytologic findings are negative.

4. **Beta subunit human chorionic gonadotropin** (metabolic half-life in vivo is 16 hours), detected specifically by radioimmunoassay, is a sensitive tumor

Table 16-4. Carcinoembryonic antigen (ng/ml) and distribution in total population[a,b]

Disease state	0–2.5 ng/ml (%)	2.6–5.0 ng/ml (%)	5.1 or more ng/ml (%)
Healthy subjects			
Nonsmoker	97	3	0
Former smoker	93	5	2
Smoker	81	15	4
Carcinoma			
Colorectal	28	23	49
Pulmonary	24	25	51
Pancreatic	9	31	60
Gastric	39	32	29
Breast	53	20	27
Other	51	28	21
Noncarcinomatous malignancy	60	30	10
Nonmalignant disease			
Benign breast tumor	85	11	4
Rectal polyps	81	15	4
Cholecystitis	77	17	6
Cirrhosis	29	44	27
Acute ulcerative colitis	69	18	13
Emphysema	43	37	20

[a]Plasma CEA and B-hCG are determined by the following laboratories: Smith Kline Bio-Science Laboratories, 7600 Tyrone Avenue, Van Nuys, CA 91405; Roche Clinical Laboratories, 5 Johnson Drive, Raritan, NJ 08869.
[b]Heparin interferes with CEA analysis. Use EDTA as an anticoagulant.
Source: Adapted from test information sheet on 2000 subjects, Roche Clinical Laboratories, Nutley, NJ.

marker, while antisera to **whole** human chorionic gonadotropin cross-react with luteinizing hormone, follicle-stimulating hormone, and thyroid-stimulating hormone. Any serum level of B-hCG greater than 1 ng/ml strongly suggests pregnancy or a malignant tumor such as endodermal sinus cancer, teratocarcinoma (with endodermal sinus elements), choriocarcinoma, molar pregnancy, testicular embryonal carcinoma, or oat cell carcinoma of the lung. B-hCG analyses can be obtained from the laboratories listed in Tables 16-3 and 16-4.

5. **Neuron-specific enolase** is an isoenzyme that is specific for all tumor cells derived from the neural crest. It has been detected in neuroblastoma, pheochromocytoma, oat cell carcinomas, medullary thyroid and C-cell parathyroid carcinomas, and other neural crest–derived cancers. Serum levels are frequently raised in disseminated disease.

6. **Tumor-specific antigens** have been claimed to be present in melanoma, osteogenic sarcoma, lung, brain, breast, and ovarian cancers. The documentation and distribution of TSA, as well as evidence that the immune response to these antigens is related to tumor control, must await further investigation.

B. **Leukemias.** Knowledge of lymphocyte surface markers has had a dramatic impact in defining the prognosis and treatment of acute lymphoblastic leukemia (ALL) (Table 16-5).

1. **T-cell (thymus-derived) leukemia** is defined by the ability of sheep erythrocytes to form rosettes and attach to sheep-erythrocyte receptors on large lymphoblasts. It typically occurs in males over 7 years old and may be

Table 16-5. Lymphocyte surface markers in malignancy

Type of malignancy	Markers[a,b]		
	T cell (%)	B cell (%)	Non-T, non-B ("Null cell") (%)
Leukemias			
Acute lymphoblastic	25	1	74
Chronic lymphocytic	2	96	2
Hairy cell	0	+	+
Myeloid	0	0	100
Sézary syndrome	+		
Mycosis fungoides	+		
Non-Hodgkin's lymphoma	5	75	20
Immunoblastic lymphadenopathy		+ (polyclonal)	

[a]Available in reference laboratories and most university medical centers and large hospitals.
[b]A plus (+) indicates association, but only a few patients were studied.

associated with a mediastinal mass and eventual central nervous system involvement. Remissions have been difficult to maintain, prompting the development of newer, aggressive chemotherapies. Sézary syndrome in adults is a T-cell leukemia whose lymphoblasts function as a T "helper" subset. A few leukemias in childhood have been found to have T "suppressor" activity, with resulting low immunoglobulin levels.

2. **B-cell leukemia.** Acute lymphoblastic leukemia (ALL) of the B-cell type, unlike T-cell leukemia, expresses surface-membrane immunoglobulin and occurs in elderly persons or at any age as the leukemic phase of a lymphoma; it has a poor prognosis. In adults, chronic lymphocytic leukemia (CLL) and hairy cell leukemia resemble mature lymphocytes and are membrane immunoglobulin positive. In contrast to CLL and the immature B cell in ALL, the cells in multiple myeloma and the macroglobulinemias are more mature cells, which secrete their monoclonal cytoplasmic immunoglobulin products and usually do not have membrane immunoglobulin. Interestingly, the few patients with immunoblastic lymphadenopathy whose cases have been reported were membrane immunoglobulin positive, and this immunoglobulin was polyclonal, in contrast to the monoclonal immunoglobulin in other B-cell disorders.

3. **"Null cell" leukemia** lymphoblasts neither form rosettes with sheep erythrocytes, nor do they possess membrane immunoglobulin, but most have a surface antigen reactive with a "null cell" antiserum, also called **common acute lymphoblastic leukemia antigen (CALLA).** This is the most common type of leukemia in childhood. Children between the ages of 2 and 7 years and with leukocyte counts less than 10,000/mm³ have the best prognosis (75% cure rate).

4. **Myeloid leukemias** are derived from myelomonocytic precursors and have surface markers in common with their normal counterparts, i.e., receptors for complement (C3) and the Fc portion of IgG, but no membrane immunoglobulin. Cytochemical enzyme markers, such as nonspecific esterase (monocytic) and peroxidase (myeloid and monocytic), can help differentiate myeloid leukemias from PAS-positive, esterase-, and peroxidase-negative lymphoblastic leukemias.

5. Advances in **treatment** have been dramatic, and protocols are currently being developed to attain maximal survival without the attendant morbidity of chemotherapy. For all the leukemias, surface markers usually remain

Table 16-6. Effect of chemotherapy on immune responses

Drug	Antibody		Delayed hypersensitivity	
	Primary response	Secondary response	Primary response (initial exp.)	Secondary response (recall)
Corticosteroid	0	0	+ +	+
Methotrexate	+ +	+	+	0
6-Mercaptopurine, azathioprine, 6-thioguanine	0 0 0	+ + +	+ + +	0 0 0
Cytosine arabinoside	+	+ +	0	0
Cyclophosphamide	+ +	0	+	0
L-Asparaginase	+	0	0	0
Daunomycin	+	0	+	0

Key: 0 = no effect; + = slight effect; + + = significant effect.

constant, and relapse occurs in the same cell type seen at diagnosis. To give optimal treatment, surface markers performed prior to therapy should be determined in all leukemic patients. Repeat analysis of these markers usually is not helpful or appropriate in the evaluation of therapy.

6. An increase above normal in the **percentage** and **absolute number** of cells with markers must be demonstrated. Leukemia with a normal leukocyte count or only a few blast forms, or both, cannot be accurately typed.

C. **Non-Hodgkin's lymphomas.** Luke's and Collins' classification relates cell morphology to the observed and theoretic cell types seen in lymphocyte development and activation. Surface-marker characterization of the non-Hodgkin's lymphomas provides insight into their causes and is prognostically useful. The majority of lymphomas are of the B-cell type, and, if a leukemic phase develops, it too has B-cell characteristics. However, T cell– and B cell–derived lymphomas respond to quite different therapies.

D. **Hodgkin's lymphoma** might be considered as a war between T cells and Reed-Sternberg cells on the lymph node battleground. The Reed-Sternberg cell has been described as either a transformed macrophage or an altered T cell that is attacked by normal, activated T cells. Depressed T-cell function, which is common, may be secondary to the loss of T cells by phagocytosis or neoplastic transformation of the T cells. Even Hodgkin's lymphoma patients with minimal disease, and those thought to be cured, have impaired T-cell function as measured by phytohemagglutinin responsiveness, suggesting a primary or secondary immune defect. Tumors that are predominately lymphocytic on histologic examination have the best prognosis. This observation suggests an immunologic response though the mechanism is unclear.

III. **Drug-induced immunosuppression.** Infection secondary to immune suppression is a major cause of death in cancer patients in clinical remission as well as those beginning therapy. Drugs used to treat leukemia and solid tumors have a profound suppressive effect on the inflammatory response, delayed hypersensitivity (T cell), and/or specific antibody production (B cell). Drug effects vary markedly in different species. **Only data on humans** are presented in Table 16-6.

A. **Corticosteroids.** The T lymphocyte is the major immune target cell for corticosteroid action, although a combined and absolute lymphomonocytopenia occurs 4 hours after administration of cortisone. Cortisone causes a depletion of T lymphocytes by blocking egress from the bone marrow into the circulation. Cutaneous delayed hypersensitivity (e.g., to tuberculin protein) may be diminished, but recovers within a week of stopping the drug. Even on alternate-day corticosteroid administration, delayed hypersensitivity (e.g., to tetanus toxoid) is diminished.

B. **Other chemotherapeutic agents**

1. Folate antagonists and purine analogs have a more profound effect on antibody response than on delayed hypersensitivity. These effects vary with the immunizing agent, timing of administration, and length of time over which the chemotherapeutic agent is administered. With **combination** chemotherapies for leukemia, delayed hypersensitivity to recall antigens in vitro rebounds with an "overshoot" phenomenon 10–20 days after each course. However, after 2 years of chemotherapy, recovery of recall (secondary) delayed hypersensitivity and antibody response is delayed 12–36 weeks.

2. **Antibody responses** are poor during initial induction of leukemia. Responses to killed poliovirus and influenza vaccines during the maintenance phase of chemotherapy are suppressed but still measurable. Thus, patients receiving chemotherapy are at risk of infections, especially those cleared by antibody (e.g., encapsulated bacteria). A recent trial of attenuated varicella-zoster vaccine demonstrated that most children with leukemia respond with antiviral antibody when immunized after 1 year of treatment with chemotherapeutic agents. For these reasons, live attenuated virus vaccines should **not** be administered to patients receiving chemotherapy except under carefully monitored controlled situations. Vaccines using killed organisms (e.g., diphtheria-pertussis-tetanus, pneumococcal vaccines) can be safely given because they do not propagate in vivo.

IV. **Immunotherapy.** The concept of immune control over neoplasia began over 100 years ago, when dramatic regressions of cancer were noted following streptococcal infections. More recently, lung cancer patients with empyema were noted to live longer than those without this infection.

Although immunotherapy for cancer has made significant strides in recent years, it remains primarily at the research level. Immunotherapy has the theoretical advantage of killing the "last" neoplastic cell, while chemotherapy can only kill a percentage of the cancer cells present. Only small numbers of cells (about 10^5) are affected by specific immunotherapy, and thus it will be most useful when used in combination with chemotherapy.

A. Immunotherapy may have the following **beneficial effects** (even though the identity of tumor-specific rejection antigens is still speculative).

1. Many cancer patients have a general depression of immune function. If this immune function could be augmented, resistance to infection might be increased, which would allow more potent chemotherapy and radiation therapy.

2. Surgery, anesthesia, radiation, and chemotherapies have direct toxic effects on immunocompetent cells. These effects may be modified or prevented by immunotherapy.

3. Immunotherapy also may act through nonspecific mechanisms, such as increased reticuloendothelial clearance of immune complexes, antigens, and toxins, or through macrophage activation against tumor cells.

4. Immunotherapy may modify a weak antigen and make it more immunogenic, subjecting the cell to lymphocyte-mediated or antibody-mediated killing, or both.

B. **Agents and methods in immunotherapy**

1. **Immunomodulators** or **stimulators** are microbial products that heighten the immune response (Table 16-7). For example, the immunostimulator levamisole can restore a lowered level of thymus-dependent immunity (increase T rosettes) in some patients. These agents may be used alone (nonspecific therapy) or combined with tumor cells (specific therapy) to induce immunity by modifying weak antigens or by providing optimal exposure for immunization. Local injection of chemical haptens, viruses, or bacteria can induce an inflammatory response that preferentially kills tumor cells at the site. These locally injected materials are most successful in primary and secondary skin cancers.

Table 16-7. Immunotherapy in malignant disease*

Approach	Agent	Proposed mechanism	Localized	Widespread
Active				
Specific	Modified or unmodified tumor cells, cell extract	Cellular and/or humoral response	+ (lung, melanoma)	0/+ (leukemia)
Nonspecific				
Systemic	Calmette-Guérin bacillus (BCG)	General immunocompetence	+ (leukemia)	0
	Methanol-extracted residue (MER) of mycobacteria skeletal wall	Increased reticuloendothelial activity	+ (melanoma)	0
	Corynebacterium parvum	Same as MER	0	0
	Pseudomonas vaccine	Same as MER	0	0
	Levamisole	Restores immunocompetence	0	0
	Interferon	Restores immunocompetence	+ (brain)	+
Local	BCG	Macrophage activation	++ (skin cancer)	++ (skin cancer)
	Virus	Killing of tumor with bystander effect	+	++ (metastases in skin)
	Bacterial vaccine	Unknown	+	+
	Hapten (DNCB)	Killing of tumor with bystander effect	0	0
Passive	Allogeneic or xenogeneic antibody	Removes soluble antigen or directly kills target cell	0	0
	Targeted monoclonal antibody	Conjugated with antitumor drug or radioisotope	+ (melanoma)	+ (brain)
Adoptive	Lymphocyte	Transfer of specific immunity	+ (bladder)	0/+ (melanoma)
	Lymphocyte extract Immune RNA Transfer factor	Transfer of specific immunity		0
	Lymphokine-activated killer cells	Cytolysis of tumor cells	+ (lung)	+

*Effect on cancer regression: 0 = no effect; + = some effect; ++ = significant effect.

Source: Adapted from J. Gutterman. Immunotherapy of human solid tumors: Principles of development. In J. E. Castro (ed.), *Immunologic Aspects of Cancer.* Lancaster, England: MTP Press, 1978.

2. **Adoptive immunotherapy** attempts to transfer immunity (against infectious agents or tumors) by giving lymphocyte products from an immune to a nonimmune person. Current research is directed toward the use of lymphokine- or mitogen-(phytohemagglutinin) activated killer cells (LAK or PAK). This involves the in vitro incubation of autologous killer cells obtained from spleen or hematopoietic tissue with interleukin-2 (T-cell growth factor) or with mitogen to enhance proliferation of cytolytic cells that attack tumor cells. The use of interleukin-2 in conjunction with in vivo antigen stimulation of killer cell activity is also being investigated.

3. **Passive immunotherapy (serotherapy)** uses immune serum to remove tumor antigen or directly attack the neoplastic cell. Though theoretically promising and simple in design, this method has shown no positive effect. The manufacture, dose, timing, interval, and route of administration of the agents are critical to obtain any beneficial effect. Current research is directed toward the development of monoclonal antibodies conjugated with antitumor drugs or high-dose radioisotopes and directed to specific tumor cells.

C. **Immunotherapy results**

1. **Malignant melanoma.** In localized disease, regression of nodules injected directly with the Calmette-Guérin bacillus (BCG) occurs in 60–90% of patients. Although the disease-free interval is prolonged and a few patients are long-term survivors, relapse occurs in most patients. In widespread disease, chemotherapy and immunotherapy may prolong survival, but they do not affect mortality. Response to BCG most strongly correlates with general immunocompetence. Reports of BCG, *Corynebacterium parvum*, and levamisole used in widespread disease describe no significant effect on tumor regression or mortality. Conjugated monoclonal antibody targeted to melanoma cells has shown positive results.

2. **Other tumors.** The Calmette-Guérin bacillus has shown small but encouraging effects in the treatment of localized lung cancer, lymphoma, and colon carcinoma when used in combination with chemotherapy. In acute myelogenous leukemia treated with BCG and allogeneic leukemia cells, there is a prolongation of remission, but more important, survival after the second reinduction from relapse appears to be enhanced.

Selected Readings

Aisenberg, A. C. Cell lineage in lymphoproliferative disease. *Am. J. Med.* 74:679, 1983.

Bergsma, D. (ed.). *Immunologic Deficiency Diseases in Man* (vol. 11). White Plains, NY: National Foundation March of Dimes, 1975.

Calabresi, P., Schein, P. S., and Rosenberg, S. A. (eds.): *Medical Oncology.* New York: Macmillan, 1985.

DeVita, V. T., Hellman, S., and Rosenberg, S. A. (eds.): *Important Advances in Oncology 1986*. Philadelphia: Lippincott, 1986.

Evans, A., D'Angio, G., and Seeger, R. Advances in neuroblastoma. *Prog. Clin. Biol. Res.* 175:XXIII, 1985.

Hancock, B. W., and Ward, A. M. (eds.). *Immunologic Aspects of Cancer.* Baltimore: University Park Press, 1985.

Knudson, A. G. Genetics and the etiology of childhood cancer. *Pediatr. Res.* 10:513, 1976.

Pierce, G. B., Shikes, R., and Fink, L. *Cancer: A Problem of Developmental Biology.* Englewood Cliffs, NJ: Prentice-Hall, 1978.

Ritz, J., and Schlossman, S. F. Utilization of monoclonal antibodies in the treatment of leukemia and lymphoma. *Blood* 59:1, 1982.

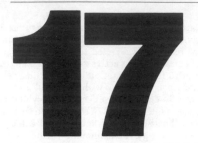

Immunodeficiency Diseases

Alan P. Knutsen and
Thomas J. Fischer

The immune system includes a number of defense mechanisms that provide protection from infection: (1) physical barriers such as skin and mucous membranes, (2) nonspecific humoral factors such as tissue lysozymes and interferon, (3) specific humoral factors (antibodies), (4) specific cell-mediated immunity (T lymphocytes, lymphokines, and macrophages), (5) phagocytic neutrophils and macrophages, and (6) complement proteins. Defects in one or more of these systems can produce a spectrum of clinical manifestations, depending on the system(s) affected and the extent of involvement. These defects can be congenital or acquired, occur in children or adults, and be primary defects or secondary to an underlying disorder (lymphoproliferative and other malignancies; viral induced acquired immunodeficiency syndrome [AIDS]; malnutrition; aging; immunosuppressive therapy; and conditions causing loss of immunoglobulin or leukocytes from the body, e.g., nephrotic syndrome or intestinal lymphangiectasia).

Recurrent infection without obvious underlying disease is a common clinical problem, especially in children. Opportunistic infections and certain forms of malignancy are especially prevalent in adults and children with AIDS (see p. 375). Despite the importance of identifying immunodeficiency, many patients with recurrent infections are not immunodeficient, and exclusion of immunodeficiency does not complete the evaluation. Other disorders in which there is increased susceptibility to infection are listed in Table 17-1. A logical, orderly evaluation is needed to provide an accurate diagnosis and determine the correct therapy.

Classification of Primary Immunodeficiency

To evaluate a patient for immunodeficiency adequately, a basic understanding of the immune system is required (see Chap. 1). Although exact categorization is often difficult in this complex, interwoven system, primary immunodeficiencies can be classified into five major areas. Under these major headings, recognized clinical syndromes can be grouped according to the predominant effector mechanism that is defective. It must be realized that other interacting mechanisms can also be defective.

I. **Antibody deficiency or dysfunction** (B cell deficiency) comprises 50–60% of all primary immunodeficiencies. Immunoglobulins of one or all classes can be completely absent, or their concentration below normal values. An occasional patient can have normal levels of immunoglobulins with inadequate antibody function to one or more specific antigens.

II. **Combined antibody and cellular deficiency** (T-cell and B-cell deficiency) represent 10–20% of primary immunodeficiencies. The wide range of clinical symptoms and other immunologic findings demonstrates the heterogeneity of this type of immunodeficiency.

III. **Primary cell-mediated deficiency** (T-cell deficiency) accounts for 5–10% of primary immunodeficiencies. Although it is operationally useful to classify isolated (pure) T-

Table 17-1. Disorders in which susceptibility to infection is increased

Type of disorder	Conditions
Primary immunodeficiency	B cell, T cell, combined, phagocytic, complement
Secondary immunodeficiency	Malnutrition, prematurity, infiltrative and hematologic diseases (e.g., lymphoma and leukemia), splenectomy, uremia, immunosuppressive therapy, protein-losing enteropathy, infections, such as acquired immunodeficiency syndrome (AIDS), aging, surgery, and trauma
Circulatory	Sickle cell disease, diabetes mellitus, varicose veins, congenital cardiac defects
Obstructive	Ureteral or urethral stenosis, bronchial asthma, allergic rhinitis, blocked eustachian tubes, cystic fibrosis
Integument defects	Eczema, burns, skull fractures, midline sinus tracts, immotile cilia
Unusual microbiologic factors	Overgrowth secondary to antibiotics, chronic infection with resistant organisms, continuous reinfection (water supply, infectious contact, contaminated inhalation therapy equipment)
Foreign bodies	Ventricular shunts, central venous catheters, artificial heart valves, urinary catheters, aspirated foreign body

Source: Adapted from E. R. Stiehm. Immunodeficiency Disorders: General Considerations. In
E. R. Stiehm and V. A. Fulginiti (eds.), *Immunologic Disorders in Infants and Children* (2nd ed.).
Philadelphia: Saunders, 1980.

cell disorders, there are very few of them. The majority of T-cell immunodeficiency
disorders are associated with some difficulty in the ability to form antibody.

IV. **Disorders of phagocytic cells** (granulocytes, monocytes, or both) constitute approximately 10–15% of all primary immunodeficiencies. However, these disorders are
often associated with severe infections because the protective effects of both antibody and complement are mediated largely by the phagocytosis of pathogens.

V. **Deficiency or dysfunction of complement proteins** results in inadequate opsonization of microorganisms, leading to infection. Although complement disorders account for a small percentage of primary immunodeficiencies (< 2% of the total), they
frequently coexist with systemic lupus erythematosus (SLE) and other diseases
associated with an immunopathologic process.

Clinical Findings in Primary Immunodeficiency

The history and physical examination are of prime importance in evaluating the
type and severity of immunodeficiency, the extent of laboratory investigation
needed, and the response to specific treatment to be expected. It is still not completely possible to exclude a diagnosis of immunodeficiency by laboratory tests
alone.

I. **History**

A. **Recurrent infection,** especially of the respiratory tract, is a common symptom of
immunodeficiency. Immunodeficient patients are extraordinarily prone to otitis
media, rhinitis, tonsillitis, sinusitis, bronchitis, and pneumonia. Although six to
eight upper respiratory infections a year are not uncommon in normal young

children (especially if there is exposure to older siblings or to other children, e.g., at day-care centers), the common characteristics of infections in immunodeficient children differ from those of infections in normal children in the following ways:

1. Bacterial infections are **severe** (e.g., pneumonia, meningitis, sepsis).
2. **Repeated** respiratory infections occur, especially in infants under 3 months of age.
3. **Repeated** respiratory infections occur in infants under 9 months of age with no increased exposure to infection, e.g., older siblings. (Acquired immunodeficiency can occur at **any age,** and the absence of a history of repeated or severe infections in an adult or older child does not rule out immunodeficiency of **recent onset.**)
4. Infections are **chronic** and lead to **complications** such as mastoiditis or bronchiectasis.
5. **Unusual opportunistic infections** (e.g., *Pneumocystis carinii, Aspergillus fumigatus, Candida albicans,* or *Serratia marcescens)* are common.
6. Episodes of infection **do not completely clear** or **respond inadequately to treatment.**
7. A seasonal allergy pattern is absent, and a family history of allergy is often absent (atopic symptoms can mimic immunodeficiency).

B. **Failure to thrive** is common. Recurrent or chronic infections produce underweight, short children in whom the developmental milestones are delayed. An active, robust patient is not likely to have a **significant** immunologic deficiency.

C. **Chronic or prolonged diarrhea,** malabsorption, or vomiting is frequently present in all types of immunodeficiency disorders.

D. Review of the **past history** also reveals problems associated with immunodeficiency disorders. Direct specific inquiries to the following:

1. **Maternal illness during pregnancy.** Congenital rubella and dysgammaglobulinemia are associated.
2. **Length of gestation and birth weight.** Infants small for their gestational age are more susceptible to infection than normal-sized infants.
3. **Neonatal course.** Hypocalcemic seizures and cardiovascular abnormalities occur in the Di George syndrome.
4. **Immunizations.** Live virus vaccines may have had adverse effects, especially in cell-mediated immunodeficiency.
5. **Surgery.** Tonsillectomy, adenoidectomy, ventilatory tubes, or abscess drainage may have been necessary for recurrent infection. A retrospective pathology review of tonsils or adenoids can help determine the presence of plasma cells or germinal centers or both.
6. **Prior treatments for infection.** The need for repeated courses of antibiotics or gamma globulin, and the **apparent effect,** are significant.
7. Sexual habits, intravenous drug abuse, and a history of blood transfusion suggests possible exposure to the human immunodeficiency virus (HIV).

E. A detailed **family history** may reveal important clues such as the following:

1. Early infant deaths, recurrent or chronic infections, lymphoreticular malignancy, or autoimmune disorders in near or distant relatives. Because X-linked recessive trait transmission is found in various disorders (Wiskott-Aldrich syndrome, chronic granulomatous disease, some forms of hypogammaglobulinemia and severe combined immunodeficiency syndrome), the family history on the maternal side demands careful scrutiny. A history of consanguinity should be sought, and if possible, a genetic tree constructed.
2. **Racial background.** The finding of hemoglobinopathies such as sickle cell disease in family members may suggest a cause for the repeated infections.
3. Atopic disease or cystic fibrosis in family members can suggest other causes of recurrent infection. General differences in the features of allergic and immunodeficiency diseases are listed in Table 17-2.

II. **Physical examination** of a patient with significant immunologic deficiency usually

Table 17-2. General differences between allergic and immunodeficiency diseases

Feature	Allergic disease	Primary immunodeficiency disease
Family history	Atopy	Early death, frequent infections
Febrile episodes	No	Yes
Response to antibiotics	No	Yes
Response to bronchodilators	Yes	No
Purulent secretions	No	Yes
Same-site involvement	Yes	No
Lymphadenopathy	Yes	No
Wheezing	Yes	No
Seasonal pattern	Yes	No

reveals a pale, irritable, thin patient who appears chronically ill. As noted, an active, well-nourished, well-developed child is unlikely to have a **significant** immunologic deficiency. Other specific aspects of the physical examination include the following:

A. **Serial plotting of heights and weights** for age can help in the estimation of the extent and time of onset of growth failure and can serve as a guide to the effectiveness of therapy (see Appendix XI for growth charts).

B. It is common to find **small** or **absent tonsils** or small amounts or absence of other lymphoid tissues, especially in antibody deficiency syndromes. However, as a result of chronic infectious stimulation, massive lymphadenopathy and hepatosplenomegaly can occur in certain syndromes with infiltration by other cells such as histiocytes.

C. **Ears draining purulent material,** perforations of the tympanic membrane, and purulent rhinitis are frequent.

D. **Oral or cutaneous candidiasis** persisting after 6 months of age, resistant to standard topical antifungal therapy, and without appropriate inducing events (breast-feeding, broad-spectrum antibiotics) often is the initial manifestation of a T-cell disorder or a combined T-cell and B-cell immunodeficiency disorder.

E. **Clubbing** of the nails, increased anteroposterior chest diameter, and persistent rales suggest chronic pulmonary infections and complications such as bronchiectasis. These clinical features are also seen in pediatric AIDS patients with lymphoid interstitial pneumonitis.

F. **Recurrent cutaneous abscesses** are common in patients with host-defense defects. Other cutaneous findings include the following:

   1. **Seborrheic dermatitis-like conditions:** severe combined immunodeficiency, Leiner's disease (dysfunction of C5 protein).

   2. **Cutaneous candidiasis:** severe combined immunodeficiency, chronic mucocutaneous candidiasis, congenital thymic aplasia (Di George syndrome), and myeloperoxidase deficiency.

   3. **Lupus erythematosus-like** rashes: selective IgA deficiency and complement protein deficiencies (C1r, C2, C5, and C7). Genetic carrier mothers of boys with chronic granulomatous disease have lesions characteristic of chronic cutaneous discoid lupus erythematosus.

   4. Rashes of the **atopic dermatitis** type: hyperimmunoglobulin E syndrome and Wiskott-Aldrich syndrome.

G. **Chronic encephalitis** can lead to severe dementia and death in patients with severe combined immunodeficiency.

H. **Chronic conjunctivitis** or **arthritis/arthralgia** is present occasionally.

Table 17-3. Special clinical features associated with immunodeficiency disorders

Clinical features	Disorders
Biochemical	
Adenosine deaminase deficiency	T-cell, B-cell immunodeficiency
Nucleoside phosphorylase deficiency	T-cell immunodeficiency
Dermatologic	
Eczema	Wiskott-Aldrich, T-cell, B-cell immunodeficiency
Sparse, hypopigmented hair	Short-limbed dwarfism with immunodeficiency
Telangiectasia	Ataxia-telangiectasia
Petechiae	Wiskott-Aldrich syndrome
Oculocutaneous albinism	Chédiak-Higashi syndrome
Endocrinologic	
Hypoparathyroidism (congenital)	Di George syndrome (congenital thymic aplasia)
Hypoparathyroidism (acquired)	Chronic candidiasis
Hypothyroidism, Addison's disease and diabetes	Chronic candidiasis
Gonadal dysgenesis	Chronic candidiasis and ataxia-telangiectasia
Hematologic	
Thrombocytopenia	Wiskott-Aldrich syndrome
Anemia (pernicious)	Chronic candidiasis
Anemia (Coombs' positive)	Wiskott-Aldrich syndrome
Skeletal	
Short-limbed dwarfism	Short-limbed dwarfism with immunodeficiency
Abnormalities of bone	Immunodeficiency with adenosine deaminase deficiency

  III. Special clinical features are often found in certain patients that strongly suggest a specific immunodeficiency disorder. These features are listed in Table 17-3.

Screening Laboratory Tests for Primary Immunodeficiency

General screening laboratory tests can detect more severe and common disorders of immune function. These tests, readily available in a physician's office or clinical laboratory, can provide an adequate laboratory evaluation if their results are supported by the history and the physical findings.

However, when questions of immune competence persist, other, more complex tests are required to detect more subtle abnormalities.

  I. A **complete blood count** may detect anemia, leukopenia, or thrombocytopenia. The total absolute polymorphonuclear leukocyte count should be greater than 1200 cells/mm^3; the total absolute lymphocyte count should exceed 1200 cells/mm^3 (for patients less than 2 years of age the lymphocyte count should be greater than 2500 cells/mm^3). Because T cells constitute approximately 75% of peripheral blood lymphocytes, lymphopenia can be equated with decreased T cells. Both neutropenia and lymphopenia can be secondary to infection, drug usage (especially immunosuppressive agents), and autoimmune disease. When neutropenia or lymphopenia is present, repeat serial determinations are indicated.

II. **Quantitative immunoglobulins** (IgG, IgM, IgA) can be obtained by simple radial immunodiffusion techniques or automated immunoprecipitation techniques. Neither protein electrophoresis nor immunoelectrophoresis is sensitive enough to provide exact information about the levels of individual immunoglobulins. Interpret quantitative immunoglobulin results according to age-related standards (see Appendix VII). Immunoglobulin levels within 2 S.D. of the mean for age are normal. As a general rule, marked deficiencies of IgG are diagnosed if values are below 200 mg/dl; deficiencies of IgM and IgA are indicated by values below 10 mg/dl. Panhypogammaglobulinemia should be diagnosed only when total IgG, IgM, and IgA are less than 400 mg/dl.

III. **Total serum IgE levels** by radioimmunoassay or enzyme-linked immune assays can help distinguish atopic disease from immunodeficiency. However, markedly elevated IgE levels can be found in immunodeficient states, especially in cell-mediated immunodeficiency. Similarly marked elevations can be found in parasitic disorders and allergic bronchopulmonary aspergillosis. IgE levels must be interpreted according to the method used and compared with age-matched normal subjects (see Appendix VI).

IV. **Saline isohemagglutinin** (anti-A, anti-B, or both) determinations are a measure of IgM antibody function and can be readily performed in most clinical laboratories. With the exception of persons with blood group AB, who lack isohemagglutinins, most immunologically competent persons over 6 months of age have titers of at least 1:8 against A-erythrocyte antigens and 1:4 against B-erythrocyte antigens. Over 1 year of age, anti-A titers usually exceed 1:16, and anti-B titers usually exceed 1:8. The result is difficult to interpret within 30 days of gamma globulin administration or in infants up to 6 months of age who still have maternal IgG isohemagglutinins.

V. **Sweat chloride** determinations should be done as a screening test, especially in a patient with a history of repeated respiratory infections, malabsorption (characterized by bulky, greasy stools), and failure to thrive. Values greater than 60 mEq/liter are abnormal. When elevated levels are obtained, repeat sweat determinations by alternative methods should be done for absolute documentation. In questionable cases, trypsin activity of intestinal fluid should be measured (stool trypsin activity is not as reliable).

VI. An evaluation of chronic infection should include an **erythrocyte sedimentation rate, appropriate cultures,** and **x-rays** that are indicated by the history and physical findings. Lateral nasopharyngeal x-rays may demonstrate decreased lymphoid tissue in the nasopharynx (common in hypogammaglobulinemia); a chest x-ray in the newborn period can demonstrate the presence of a thymus, making a significant T-cell deficiency less likely. (However, stress can shrink the thymus, and its absence **may not** indicate immunodeficiency.)

VII. **Skin tests for delayed hypersensitivity** using specific antigens placed by intradermal injection help define the presence of competent cell-mediated immunity. In approximately 85% of adults, the reaction will be positive (> 5 mm of induration) to one or more of these antigens. In the pediatric population this percentage is lower, although there is a progressive increase in the frequency of cutaneous response with age. Only one-third of infants (< 1 year of age) will react to *Candida* or streptokinase-streptodornase antigens; four-fifths of 1- to 5-year-old children will have positive induration reactions to at least one of these antigens. As a general rule, the child under 1 year of age who has had severe *Candida* dermatitis and thrush resistant to therapy should have a positive skin reaction.

The delayed hypersensitivity skin test sheet in Table 17-4 can be a helpful adjunct to routine delayed hypersensitivity skin testing. For proper use of these tests; observe the following guidelines:

A. Ascertain the **activity** of the skin test antigen by testing a normal person sensitive to the particular antigen.

B. **Corticosteroids** and **other immunosuppressive agents** can interfere with these tests and produce false-negative results.

C. Check for a **history** of a **severe local** reaction to skin tests in the past to avoid exaggerated reactions in sensitive patients. If exaggerated responses have been obtained in the past, the skin test **should be avoided** or, if necessary, given at a

Table 17-4. Delayed hypersensitivity skin test sheet

Name: _____   Date: _____

Antigen	Erythema and induration (mm) (intermediate test strength)			Erythema and induration (mm) (second test strength)		
	Strength	24 Hr	48 Hr	Strength	24 Hr	48 hr
Candida[a]	1:100			1:10		
Mumps[b]						
PPD	5 TU			250 TU		
Trichophyton[c]	1:30					
Tetanus toxoid[d]	1:10					
Multi-test CMI[e]						

[a]*Candida* (Dermatophyton O, Hollister-Stier Laboratories, N. 3525 Regal, Spokane, WA 99207)
[b]Mumps, Eli Lilly and Company, 307 E. McCarty, P.O. Box 618, Indianapolis, IN 46206. (FDA states efficacy is undetermined and further evaluation is required.)
[c]*Trichophyton*, Hollister-Stier Laboratories, N. 3525 Regal, Spokane, WA 99207.
[d]Tetanus toxoid, fluid, Wyeth Laboratories, P.O. Box 8299, Philadelphia, PA 19101.
[e]Multi-test CMI, Merieux Institute, Miami, FL, is a kit that contains eight individual tines applying seven antigens (*Candida albicans,* tetanus toxoid, diphtheria toxoid, streptokinase, old tuberculin, trichophyton, and proteus) simultaneously, with a glycerol control.

        more dilute concentration. Try also to document any previous exposure to the antigen.
  D. Perform the test as follows:
    1. Use a sterile 1-ml tuberculin syringe with a 0.5-in. 27-gauge needle for each injection.
    2. Draw a little over 0.1 ml of the antigen solution into the syringe, expressing air bubbles (these will give inaccurate results), and make sure the needle is filled (it will hold almost 0.05 ml).
    3. Use the forearms as the injection site. If the arms are not usable, the back may be used.
    4. A bleb 5–10 mm in diameter should be raised immediately. The absence of bleb formations indicates that the injection was subcutaneous rather than intracutaneous. Repeat the injection at another site.
    5. Mark and circle each site.
    6. Record the skin test results at **24 and 48 hours.** If they are negative at 24 hours, it is safe to apply the second-strength antigens.
  E. A kit for quantitatively determining delayed hypersensitivity skin tests is available (Multi-test CMI, Merieux Institute, Miami, FL). The user of this kit, which contains eight individual tines, applies intradermally seven antigens (*Candida albicans,* tetanus toxoid, diphtheria toxoid, streptokinase, old tuberculin, *Trichophyton* and *Proteus*) and a glycerol control simultaneously. The number of positive reactions (edema > 2 mm) and the sum of induration are recorded. Normal values for children and adults are established for comparison.
VIII. Tests for **complement proteins,** although not routinely included in the screening tests, are indicated if there is a history of familial deficiency of complement proteins or autoimmune disease.

A. **A total hemolytic complement (CH_{50})** measures the functional complement activity of C1 through C9 of the complement cascade and is a useful screening procedure. However, individual complement abnormalities or abnormalities in the alternative pathway can exist despite a normal CH_{50} value.

B. Assays for **serum C3 and C4** are routinely available by radioimmunodiffusion, using precipitating antibody to measure the amount of specific protein in the serum. These assays do not measure **functional activity**.

C. By testing for total hemolytic complement (CH_{50}), C3, and C4, many complement-related disorders predisposing to infection can be better delineated. The four general types of findings and their interpretation are as follows:

1. Reduced C3 and C4 implies that the classic activation unit has been initiated and the functional unit activated (e.g., active viral hepatitis and immune complex formation—seen in various disorders).

2. Normal C3 with low C4 suggests a deficiency of C4 (e.g., hereditary angioneurotic edema, malaria, and certain patients with systemic lupus erythematosus).

3. Normal C4 and low C3 suggests a congenital deficiency of C3, deficiency of C3b inactivator, or activation of the functional unit by the alternative pathway (e.g., gram-negative endotoxemia). Low C3 is also seen in neonates, thermal injuries, and malnutrition.

4. Normal C3 and C4 but low CH_{50} indicates an isolated deficiency of another complement component. Further testing is indicated.

Advanced Laboratory Evaluation

Advanced laboratory evaluation is indicated if abnormalities are noted in the screening test results. If clinical observations and the usual screening test findings do not agree, a more sophisticated immune analysis is indicated to detect subtle defects. Also, because defects in one part of the host-defense mechanism can be associated with other deficiencies, a complete evaluation of the whole immune system is generally required if a defect in one branch of the system is noted. It is imperative that specific therapy not be instituted until an accurate diagnosis is made. Advanced tests of immune function, usually available in specialized laboratories, can be grouped into five categories.

I. Advanced laboratory evaluation for **antibody (B-cell) deficiency**

A. **Quantitation of B cells.** Lymphocytes in the peripheral blood can be identified specifically as B cells by the presence of immunoglobulin receptors on their surface (SmIg). In normal control subjects, 10–20% of peripheral blood lymphocytes have detectable surface immunoglobulins by this technique. Interpretation, however, must be carefully based on the normal values for each laboratory because small variations in technique can alter the final results.

B lymphocytes also have surface complement receptors and receptors for aggregated immunoglobulins (EAC rosettes). However, macrophages, natural killer cells (NK cells), and certain subsets of T cells can also express these receptors, and EAC rosettes are therefore less accurate than SmIg for specific determination of B-cell numbers. Monoclonal antibodies that detect cell surface antigens are also used to identify B cells, macrophages, and NK cells as well as T cells (Table 17-5).

B. **Preexisting antibodies.** Determination of functional antibody production can be made by measuring antibody to a previous immunization or natural infection. Antibody can be measured in vitro to tetanus, diphtheria, *Streptococcus*, poliovirus, measles, rubella, and other antigens, depending on the availability of the facilities in the area. State health laboratories will often perform these tests or know where they can be done.

C. **Antibody response to injected antigens.** In addition to measuring preexisting antibody, it is helpful to demonstrate specific antibody formation to an injected antigen at the time of the immune evaluation. **(Do not give live or attenuated**

Table 17-5. Tests distinguishing different populations of mononuclear cells

Test	Predominant cells identified
Monoclonal antibody[a]	
CD3 (OKT3, Leu 4)	Pan T cell
CD4 (OKT4, Leu 3)	T helper/inducer cells
CD8 (OKT8, Leu 2)	T suppressor/cytotoxic cells
CD2 (OKT11, Leu 5)	E rosette receptor, T cell and some natural killer cells
CD 16 (Leu 11c)	Natural killer cells
OKT9	Transferrin receptor
CD1 (OKT6, Leu 6)	Thymocyte, activated T cell
OKT10, Leu 17	Thymocyte, activated T cell
CD11 (OKM1, Leu 15)	Monocyte
CD20 (B1, Leu 16)	B cell
E rosette	T cell
SmIg	B cell
EBV binding	B cell
EAC rosette	B cell, monocyte, some activated T cells
IgG(Fc) binding	B cell, monocyte, some activated T cells
Peroxidase	Monocyte
Esterase	Monocyte

[a]Monoclonal antibodies available commercially from Ortho Diagnostic Systems, Raritan, NJ 08869 (OK series) and from Becton-Dickson, 2375 Garcia Mountain View, CA 94043 (Leu series)
Key: CD = antigen cluster designation; E = sheep erythrocytes; EAC = E sensitized with antibody and complement; SmIg = cell surface membrane immunoglobulin; EBV = Epstein-Barr virus.

virus vaccines to document antibody formation. Limit immunization to highly purified, nonreplicating antigens.) Optimally, antibody formation to polysaccharide antigens (e.g., pneumococcus or *Haemophilus influenzae* type B polysaccharide vaccines) and protein antigens (e.g., tetanus or diphtheria or both) should be documented. A normal response is a fourfold rise from the level in preinjection serum samples in serum antibody titer obtained 3–4 weeks after injection of antigen (see p. 370 for precautions with typhoid vaccine).

D. **Lymph node biopsy** can be helpful in the diagnosis of equivocal cases of immunodeficiency or to exclude reticuloendothelial malignancy in known immunodeficient patients with marked lymphadenopathy. (Routine biopsy is not indicated because of the possibility of infection and the anesthetic risk.) It is best to perform the biopsy after local antigenic stimulation; e.g., give a tetanus or typhoid immunization in the anterior thigh and obtain a biopsy specimen from an inguinal node on the same side 5–7 days later. Specimens from patients with antibody deficiency show a few plasma cells, an increased number of primary lymphoid follicles, cellular disorganization, a thin cortex, and absence of germinal centers. An increased number of histiocytes and other reticuloendothelial elements may be present.

E. **Secretory antibody studies.** Selective secretory deficiencies **without** serum deficiency are rare. In patients with suspected secretory deficiency and a suspicious clinical history, but with normal serum antibody as determined quantitatively and qualitatively, measurement of antibodies in the secretions is indicated (tears are the easiest secretions to obtain and measure).

F. **IgG subclass level measurements** are indicated in patients with repeated infections who have normal or mildly subnormal IgG levels or selective IgA deficiency, or both. IgG2 deficiency, which comprises approximately 20% of the total IgG serum, alone or in association with selective IgA deficiency or IgG4 deficiency, is well recognized. Antibody formation to polysaccharide antigens, such as *Pneumococcus* or *H. influenzae* type B vaccines or both, should be performed if IgG2 deficiency is found.

G. **Metabolic studies,** using radiolabeled tracer immunoglobulins, are useful in patients with suspected loss of immunoglobulins through the gut.

H. Sophisticated in vitro studies of antibody synthesis or release (or both) and of T cell–B cell interaction (suppressor and helper T-cell function) can be used for better elucidation of the pathophysiology of immunodeficiency. These tests are available only in research laboratories with an investigative interest in immunodeficiency.

II. Advanced cell-mediated (T cell) evaluation

A. **T-cell markers.** Thymus-derived lymphocytes have the property of binding sheep red blood cells to their surface membranes, forming so-called E-rosettes. Other T-cell surface antigens have been identified using monoclonal antibodies. T cells can be phenotypically classified using monoclonal antibodies that correlate with their function (Table 17-5).

Monoclonal antibodies (MoAb) identifying cell surface antigens are useful in the identification of T cells, B cells, and monocytes. As the technology has progressed, determination of cell surface antigens by MoAb has become useful in analyzing the differentiation and maturation of T and B cells.

Monoclonal antibodies are produced by a single clone of hybrid cells called hybridomas. Splenic B cells, obtained from mice immunized with a particular antigen, are fused with a murine neoplastic plasma cell. The hybrid cells are cloned to establish individual cell lines that produce specific antibodies to the immunized antigen. The advantages of MoAb versus polyclonally generated antibodies are the production of large quantities of antibody with identical specificity to a particular antigen and the elimination of cross-reacting, contaminating antibodies.

B. **In vitro proliferative lymphocyte response**

1. In animal models and humans there are multiple subpopulations of thymus-derived lymphocytes with specific cell functions. Among these functions are the following:

   a. **T-cell suppressor function,** which allows the body to differentiate cells from noncells and acts to regulate other immune functions.

   b. **T-cell helper function,** which influences B cells to respond to antigen stimulation with specific antibody formation.

   c. **T-cytotoxic cells,** which react to foreign antigen stimulation by blast transformation to damage other cells directly.

   d. **Lymphokine-producing cells,** which react to foreign antigen by releasing one or more of a variety of substances, termed **lymphokines** (e.g., macrophage activation factor [MAF], leukocyte inhibiting factor [LIF], and γ-interferon [IFN-γ]) which amplify immunologic reactivity to foreign antigen.

   e. In addition, interleukins (IL), substances that cause activation, proliferation, or differentiation of lymphoid cells, have been identified: **IL-1,** previously named LAF (lymphocyte activating factor), causes activation of T cells; **IL-2,** previously named TCGF (T-cell growth factor), causes proliferation of T cells; **BCGF** and **BCDF,** B-cell growth factor and differentiation factor, respectively, stimulate B cells.

2. **Advanced laboratory tests** that are generally available to measure T-cell function include the in vitro response to **mitogens** (e.g., phytohemagglutinin, concanavalin A, or pokeweed mitogen), **antigens** (e.g., *Candida albicans*), or **allogeneic cells** (mixed-leukocyte culture).

   a. For screening, delayed hypersensitivity skin tests (e.g., with *Candida*) should always be used first. A **positive skin test in a patient with a normal total lymphocyte count usually excludes the possibility of severe cellular immune deficiency.** However, in patients with a suspicious clinical history whose skin tests are positive, an in vitro evaluation is indicated for better definition of subtle defects.

b. When unstimulated lymphocytes are exposed to mitogen, antigens, or allogeneic cells, they are transformed into large, blastlike cells, with synthesis of DNA and eventual cell division (blastogenesis). In the laboratory, lymphocyte activation is usually measured by the uptake of a radiolabeled nucleic acid into DNA, precipitation of the radiolabeled DNA, and subsequent counting of this label. Accurate interpretation of these results requires knowledge of certain technical points.

(1) Normal peripheral blood lymphocytes respond to different doses of either mitogen or antigen with varying degrees of response. **Normal values for a dose-response curve must be established.**

(2) Normal human peripheral blood lymphocytes respond to mitogens, antigens, or allogeneic cells in a time-response curve, a variable that must be included for accurate interpretation.

(3) Results can be presented as **counts/minute,** reflecting the amount of radioactively labeled material taken up by the DNA and thus the extent of stimulation; i.e., the more counts/minute, the greater the stimulation. Results can also be expressed as the ratio of counts/minute of stimulated cells to counts/minute of resting cells (the **stimulation index**). This index is simply a ratio that is affected by elevated resting counts and therefore may not reflect the true status of the patient's T-lymphocyte function. Elevated resting counts have been seen in patients who have received multiple blood transfusions, some normal newborns, and in allergic persons. For accurate interpretation, the results should be reported not only in terms of the stimulation index, but also as counts/minute for resting and stimulated cells.

(4) Mitogens such as phytohemagglutinin stimulate the production of large numbers of T lymphocytes, resulting in high counts for normal persons. Specific antigens, on the other hand, stimulate fewer cells because of reduced exposure and thus produce lower counts. In vitro results must be compared with normal values for each antigen or mitogen from each laboratory.

(5) In vitro stimulation of lymphocytes by specific antigens is more sensitive than delayed hypersensitivity skin tests in determining previous exposure and reactivity to a particular antigen. Thus, a person with suspected normal cellular immunity to a particular antigen can demonstrate a positive in vitro response but have a negative delayed hypersensitivity skin reaction to that antigen.

(6) Mixed leukocyte cultures can be used to evaluate the ability of T lymphocytes to recognize foreign cells (allogeneic cells). The mixture consists of peripheral blood lymphocytes from a patient and from an immunologically nonidentical donor. The donor cells, treated with mitomycin C or irradiation (to block blastogenesis of the donor cells), can act as a stimulus to blastogenesis, which is measured by radiolabeled DNA incorporation. As with specific antigen stimulation, only a subpopulation of T cells is stimulated by foreign cells, and counts/minute are usually lower than with mitogen stimulation. The results must be compared with normal values from the laboratory.

C. Active sensitization with 2,4-dinitrochlorobenzene (DNCB) can be used to assess cellular immunity. However, since burns can occur during sensitization, and the chemical is potentially carcinogenic, this procedure is rarely used.

D. Biopsy. Deficiencies of lymphocytes in the thymus-dependent deep cortical areas of lymph nodes are noted in cellular immune deficiencies. Because of the anesthetic and infection risk, lymph node biopsy should not be done when there is unequivocal laboratory evidence of cellular immunodeficiency.

In certain cases of severe combined immunodeficiency, a biopsy of the thymus gland is necessary to confirm the diagnosis (islands and nests of endodermal

cells that have not become lymphoid; absent Hassall's corpuscles). This procedure is not difficult in the hands of a skilled thoracic surgeon.

E. In severe T cell-deficient patients who have received white blood cell transfusions from donors of the opposite sex, **chromosome determinations** may demonstrate sex chromosome chimerism because of the ability of the donor's lymphocytes to establish a viable graft in the recipient host. If the engrafting-cells'
donor and the recipient are of the same sex, HLA typing can be used to detect
chimerism.

F. In certain forms of combined immunodeficiency, enzymes of the purine pathway
(adenosine deaminase [ADA] or nucleoside phosphorylase [PNP]) are deficient
and can be assayed in specialized laboratories. Likewise, levels of various thymic hormones (e.g., thymosin; factor thymic sérique) have been low in certain
cellular immunodeficiencies and have been measured in research laboratories.

III. Advanced laboratory evaluation for **phagocytic deficiencies** is indicated primarily
for patients with chronic, recurrent bacterial infections, especially if normal antibody or cellular function (or both) has been documented. The following six serial
steps are involved in phagocytosis and killing: random cell movement; chemotaxis;
opsonization and bacterial fixation; ingestion of organisms; metabolic activation of
the phagocytes to kill the organisms; and destruction or digestion of the organisms.
Defects can occur at each step, leading to increased susceptibility to infection.

A. The **nitroblue tetrazolium test** is a dye reduction assay for chronic granulomatous disease and is based on the increased metabolic activity of normal granulocytes during phagocytosis. If the results of a screening nitroblue tetrazolium test
(slide test or tube test) are abnormal, a quantitative test should be done.

B. **Bacterial phagocytosis and killing tests** are the definitive assays for assessing
the functional activity of granulocytes (and monocytes in selected patients), as
well as for testing serum opsonic activity.

  1. Procedure

   a. Peripheral leukocytes are isolated, washed, counted, and suspended in a
   medium containing normal serum (as an opsonic source) and an equal
   number of freshly grown bacteria (usually *Staphylococcus aureus* or
   Escherichia coli).

   b. Following incubation and agitation at 37°C for 2 hours, aliquots are
   removed from the leukocyte-bacteria suspension at 0, 30, 60, and 120
   minutes. Then the number of viable bacteria is assayed by pour-plate
   techniques.

   c. After 120 minutes the mixture is centrifuged so that the leukocytes (and
   any phagocytized bacteria) are in the cell button, and free bacteria are
   in the supernatant. Both the cell button and the supernatant are then
   assayed for viable bacteria.

  2. Results. Normal leukocytes phagocytose and kill 95% of the bacteria within
  120 minutes. Leukocytes from patients with chronic granulomatous disease
  kill less than 10% of the bacteria, and viable bacteria are also found within
  the leukocyte, indicating that phagocytosis has occurred but intracellular
  killing is still deficient. In an opsonic defect, viable bacteria are found in the
  supernatant fluid.

C. **Leukocyte chemotaxis.** The directed migration (chemotaxis) of effector cells,
usually granulocytes or monocytes, to sites of antigen challenge allows for the
rapid degradation of foreign material. Increased susceptibility of the host to
infection results if there is an intrinsic cellular defect of chemotaxis, if cell-
directed inhibitors of chemotaxis exist, or if there is an abnormality (absence,
inhibition, or dysfunction) of the serum or tissue factors that provide a chemotactic gradient for the cell.

  1. In vivo localization: Rebuck skin windows. The skin is abraded with a
  scalpel blade over an area of 4 sq mm to produce fine capillary bleeding.
  Coverslips are placed over the site and then are changed at various intervals (every ½–2 hours) over a 24-hour period. The coverslips, with the
  adhering leukocytes, are then stained and analyzed. There should be an

initial influx of polymorphonuclear granulocytes within 2 hours. Within 12 hours these granulocytes are replaced by mononuclear cells. Various modifications of this technique are currently employed.

2. **In vitro chemotaxis tests.** Granulocytes or monocytes can be separated from peripheral blood and exposed to a variety of different chemotactic factors. The number of cells moving toward the factor (or moving randomly without chemotactic factor) can be quantitated by using an assay with a millipore filter (Boyden-chamber method) or assays employing agarose in a plastic Petri dish.

D. The **spleen** plays a major role in host defense (phagocytic and humoral), as is evident in asplenic patients, who can suffer overwhelming sepsis. Absence of the spleen should be suspected in the patient with episodes of sepsis, bizarre red blood cell forms, or in whom a peripheral blood smear demonstrates Howell-Jolly bodies. A spleen scan will fail to demonstrate radioisotope localization in the left upper quadrant of the abdomen in affected patients.

E. **Other tests** of leukocyte function are indicated for patients with suspected subtle defects of leukocyte function or when a complete evaluation of patients with known immune defects is required for investigative purposes. Such tests include enzyme studies for myeloperoxidase, glutathione peroxidase, lysozyme, glucose 6-phosphate dehydrogenase, and pyruvate kinase; quantitative iodination; measurement of chemiluminescence; and electron-micrographic studies. In neutropenic states further studies include serial white blood cell counts (for a cyclic pattern); white blood cell response to corticosteroids, adrenalin, or endotoxin; measurement of leukocyte antibodies; and bone marrow examination.

F. A **bone marrow examination** is indicated for persistent leukopenia or leukocytosis, unusual vacuolization of the cells, or when myelocytes are present in the peripheral blood.

G. A deficiency of a cell-surface glycoprotein, complement receptor type 3 (CR3), present on phagocytic cells, resulting in delayed cord separation, pyogenic infections, and periodontitis, has been identified. The monoclonal antibodies OKM1, Leu 15, or mac-1 can be used to detect this glycoprotein.

IV. Advanced laboratory evaluation for **complement and opsonic deficiencies.** If the complement screening test results are abnormal, or the clinical history suggests a complement deficiency (Table 17-6), other, more detailed studies can be done in selected research laboratories: measurement of individual complement components (immunochemical and functional assessment); assays of the nonclassic, alternative complement pathway; and assays of the patient's serum to determine its ability to generate chemotactic factors as well as to provide opsonic activity. An opsonic deficiency is demonstrated by the inability of the test serum to enhance phagocytosis of yeast particles or bacteria by normal leukocytes.

General Measures in the Treatment of Immunodeficiency Disorders

Patients with immunodeficiency require extraordinary amounts of medical care to maintain general health and nutrition, to prevent emotional problems related to their chronic disability, and to treat their numerous infectious episodes.

I. **Diet.** No special dietary limitations are necessary except in patients with malabsorption and diarrhea. In these patients, professional dietary consultation is helpful to ensure that the diet is adequate for normal growth and development. Chronic malnutrition can further depress a variety of immune functions.

II. **Avoidance of pathogens.** Patients with immunodeficiencies, especially the severe combined B cell–T cell variety, should be protected from unnecessary exposure to infection.

A. "Germ-free" care of infants with severe combined immunodeficiency, although effective in reducing or eliminating contact with microorganisms, is technically

Table 17-6. Complement deficiency in humans

Complement deficiency	Associated diseases
C1q	SLE-like syndrome; decreased secondary to agammaglobulinemia
C1r	SLE-like syndrome, dermatomyositis, vasculitis, recurrent infections and chronic glomerulonephritis, necrotizing skin lesions, and arthritis
C1s	SLE, SLE-like syndrome
C1 INH	Hereditary angioedema, lupus nephritis
C2	Recurrent pyogenic infections, SLE, SLE-like syndrome, discoid lupus, membranoproliferative glomerulonephritis, dermatomyositis, synovitis, purpura, Henoch-Schönlein purpura, hypertension, Hodgkin's disease, chronic lymphocytic leukemia, dermatitis herpetiformis, polymyositis
C3	Recurrent pyogenic infections, SLE-like syndrome, arthralgias, skin rash
C3b inactivator	Recurrent pyogenic infections, urticaria
C4	SLE-like syndrome, SLE, dermatomyositis-like syndrome, vasculitis
C5	Neisserial infections, SLE
C5 dysfunction	Leiner's disease, gram-negative skin and bowel infection
C6	Neisserial infections, SLE, Raynaud's phenomenon, scleroderma-like syndrome, vasculitis
C7	Neisserial infections, SLE, Raynaud's phenomenon, scleroderma-like syndrome, vasculitis
C8	Neisserial infections, xeroderma pigmentosa, SLE-like syndrome

Source: Adapted from J. T. Cassidy, and R. E. Petty. Immunodeficiency and Arthritis. In J. T. Cassidy (ed.), *Textbook of Pediatric Rheumatology.* New York: Wiley, 1982, pp. 131–168; R. J. Wedgewood, F. S. Rosen, and N. W. Paul. Primary immunodeficiency diseases. *Birth Defects* 9:345, 1983; and R. Pahwa, et al., Treatment of the immunodeficiency diseases. *Springer Semin. Immunopathol.* 1:355, 1978.

demanding and extremely expensive. Less vigorous isolation is usually not very helpful because ubiquitous organisms of low pathogenicity from healthy persons can often cause disease in these patients. However, patients with milder immunodeficiency or patients with severe immunodeficiency who cannot be provided a germ-free environment may be benefited if exposure to potentially serious pathogens is partially reduced. For example, at home, patients should sleep in their own beds, preferably have rooms of their own, and be kept away from persons with respiratory or other infections.

B. Since many patients with **antibody deficiency** can have a normal life span with gamma globulin therapy, patients should not be overprotected and turned into emotional cripples. The affected child should be encouraged to go outdoors, to play with other children in small groups, and to attend nursery school and regular school. Much as with the diabetic child, the ultimate goal is to teach the child to live as normal a life as possible.

III. **Genetic counseling** is limited by the inability to identify the heterozygote in most hereditary immunodeficiencies. However, parents of an affected child with an autosomal recessive disorder (e.g., ataxia-telangiectasia syndrome, Chédiak-Higashi syndrome) or an X-linked disorder (e.g., chronic granulomatous disease, Wiskott-Aldrich syndrome, congenital X-linked agammaglobulinemia) can be counseled as to the likelihood that other children in the family will have similar problems. Also, adenosine deaminase and nucleoside phosphorylase deficiencies (which are associated with severe combined immunodeficiency) can be detected prenatally. This service can be offered to parents with a family history of severe combined immuno-deficiency. Obtain immunoglobulin levels on the members of the immediate family of a patient with antibody deficiency to assess any possible familial patterns. Similarly, complement abnormalities should prompt study of other family members. If any are found to have suggestive histories, a detailed history, a physical examination, and appropriate screening laboratory tests are indicated. Follow newborn siblings of affected patients carefully for manifestations of a similar disorder.

IV. Infectious complications
  A. Chronic otitis media must be managed aggressively by surgical intervention (ventilatory tubes) in addition to antibiotic therapy. Special attention should be directed to hearing loss, and a routine audiologic evaluation should be incorporated into the treatment plan.
  B. Patients with **chronic pulmonary disease** should be followed with yearly pulmonary function testing (or more often if there is evidence of deterioration of pulmonary function). The importance of a home treatment program of postural drainage and inhalation therapy (see Chap. 6, **V.A.6**) should be emphasized in patients with respiratory involvement.
  C. Sinusitis requires aggressive antibiotic therapy and topical decongestant therapy during acute episodes. If symptoms continue, surgical lavage is warranted for treatment as well as to recover the infecting organism. Radical sinus operations should be avoided unless absolutely needed, especially in the young child.

V. Psychosocial support. Because of the severe psychological and financial demands placed on severely affected patients and their families, attention must be paid to these areas. The school should be made aware of the problems and provide tutors to help make up for school absences. Financial counselors can give the patient or the family information about agencies that can provide partial or complete financial support for the patient's medical needs. Agencies for crippled children in many states can provide help for immunodeficient patients. The Immune Deficiency Foundation (P.O. Box 586, Columbia, MD 21045) provides educational information to patients and helps sponsor patient support groups through its regional affiliates.

VI. General precautions
  A. Avoid whole blood transfusions in patients who have, or are **suspected** of having, cellular immunodeficiency, since infused donor lymphocytes may cause a graft-versus-host reaction. If transfusion is necessary, the blood should be first irradiated (3000 rad) before administration.
  B. Avoid the administration of live virus vaccines (e.g., poliovirus, measles, mumps, and rubella) and Calmette-Guérin bacillus (BCG) in all immunodeficient patients, but especially in those with a cellular immunodeficiency. These vaccines carry the risk of vaccine-induced infection. In the past, parents, siblings, and other household members were not given smallpox vaccine (when widely used) because of the high risk of spreading to the patient. Similarly, oral live attenuated poliovirus vaccine should be withheld from household members to prevent spread; Salk vaccine, a killed virus preparation, can be substituted for it (see Table 19-3).
  Vaccines using killed organisms have, in general, been harmless, and their use for stimulating a measurable antibody response is of some diagnostic value. However, less-purified killed vaccines such as typhoid and paratyphoid have produced shock in patients with Wiskott-Aldrich syndrome, probably on the basis of endotoxic activation of complement by the alternative pathway in patients whose titers of "natural" antibodies are too low to prevent this reaction. In light of this problem, **such vaccines should be used with caution in immunodeficient patients.**
  C. Tonsillectomy and adenoidectomy should be performed rarely and then only with strict indications. Similarly, **splenectomy is contraindicated** except in the most severe and unusual circumstances. The addition of the phagocytic defect (absence of the spleen) to an already existing immunologic defect can significantly increase the risk of sudden, overwhelming sepsis.
  D. Corticosteroids and other immunosuppressive agents usually should be avoided in immunodeficient patients.

E. Antibiotics

1. **Use in acute illness.** Before antibiotics became available most patients with significant immunodeficiencies often succumbed to their initial infection. Antibiotics, because of their lifesaving potential, should be started **immediately** for fevers and other manifestations of infection after blood and other appropriate cultures have been obtained. **(These cultures are absolutely mandatory to direct further therapy if the infection does not respond to the initial antibiotic chosen.)** The choice and dose of antibiotic for a specific infection are identical to those used in immunocompetent patients. If the infection does not respond to antibiotics, consider the possibility of fungal, mycobacterial, viral, or protozoan infection (e.g., *P. carinii*).

2. **Prophylactic antibodies** can be of benefit in immunodeficiency syndromes, especially in disorders characterized by rapid overwhelming infections, e.g., Wiskott-Aldrich syndrome.

   A variety of regimens are employed for chronic antibiotic therapy. One useful regimen employs several antibiotics in alternating cycles at 1- to 2-month intervals. This regimen allows suppression of infection while preventing emergence of resistant organisms. A satisfactory combination of antibiotics in children can include amoxicillin, erythromycin, trimethoprim and sulfamethoxazole, or a cephalosporin; in adults, amoxicillin, trimethoprim and sulfamethoxazole, tetracyclines, or a cephalosporin can be useful.

Specific Treatment of Immunodeficiency Disorders

I. Specific treatment for antibody deficiency

A. Gamma globulin, commercially prepared, is the primary means of replacing IgG antibody passively (it contains less than 1% of IgM and IgA). Many patients with antibody deficiencies are treated successfully with repeated administration of human gamma globulin; other patients, often with other immunologic or hematologic defects, remain chronically ill or have progressive degeneration. Gamma globulin is of limited value in combined antibody and cellular immunodeficiency and of no value in the treatment of isolated cellular immunodeficiencies.

1. **Dosage**

   a. The use of intravenous gamma globulin (IVIG), available commercially as Sandoglobulin (Sandoz, East Hanover, NJ 07936), Gammagard (Travenol Laboratories, Glendale, CA 91202), and Gamimune-N (Cutter Biological, Berkeley, CA 94710), has widely replaced the use of intramuscular immune serum globulin (ISG). The three preparations of IVIG have been processed from ISG, are predominantly monomeric IgG, and are biologically intact. The usual dosage of IVIG is 100–400 mg/kg/month. Individualization of the dose and dosing frequency is based on the clinical response and the determinations of serum IgG levels. The advantages of IVIG versus ISG are (1) it is less painful, (2) larger doses are more easily administered, and (3) higher serum levels are achieved. For proper administration of these preparations, the product insert instructions must be closely followed.

   b. The usual intramuscular dosage is 100 mg/kg/month, equivalent to 0.7 ml/kg/month of the commercially available 16.5% gamma globulin (165 mg/ml). Give in divided doses every 3–4 weeks, following an initial loading dose 2–3 times the maintenance dose. Maintenance doses in an adult should not exceed 20 ml at a time, or 40 ml/month. Because of the large intramuscular dose, once-a-month administration is often painful. If intramuscular gamma globulin is given, many patients prefer divided doses every 1–2 weeks given at multiple sites—5 ml/site in a large child or an adult. (No more than 20 ml should be given at one time, even in an adult.) The buttocks are preferred, but the anterior thighs can also be used. More frequent dosing may also improve the control of infection and maintain serum levels of IgG above 200 mg/dl. (The 200 mg/dl figure is the general approximation. The increase in the IgG level after a standard gamma globulin dose varies from patient to patient and from dose to dose because of different rates of absorption, local proteolysis at the injection site, and distribution within the tissues.) Serial immunoglobulin assays are generally not necessary to gauge the effectiveness of treatment. During acute infections, gamma globulin metabolism increases, and extra injections may be required.

2. **Adverse effects**
   a. **Local reactions,** especially with intramuscular gamma globulin, include tenderness, sterile abscesses, fibrosis, and rare sciatic nerve injury. **Avoid** the use of intramuscular gamma globulin in patients with bleeding disorders because of the risk of hematoma formation.
   b. **Systemic reactions.** Fever, chills, nausea, vomiting, and back pain can occur with IVIG and are often related to the rate of infusion or concomitant host infection. Similar reactions are seen with intramuscularly administered gamma globulin. More severe reactions, such as anaphylactic reactions (hypotension, flushing, or bronchospasm) are unusual but can be fatal. They usually are due to aggregated IgG (if ISG is used) or to anti-IgA antibodies (IgE isotype). All severe systemic reactions require immediate treatment (see Chap. 10). For subsequent gamma globulin administration in these patients with severe reactions, the following measures should be taken:
      (1) Critically reassess the need for gamma globulin. Is the patient truly IgG deficient and will he or she benefit from gamma globulin administration?
      (2) If gamma globulin is needed, test with small intradermal doses (0.02 ml) of gamma globulin from different manufacturers, looking for local and systemic reactions. Assays for determination of anti-IgA antibodies (IgE or IgG) are available in certain research laboratories. If the reaction is due to anti-IgA antibodies, IVIG depleted of IgA (Gammagard) can be used with caution. If there is no reaction, give the dose cautiously in a setting in which anaphylaxis can be immediately treated. Slow intramuscular (2–3 ml/hour) administration of the dose of ISG by an infusion pump through a 23-gauge "butterfly" needle has been used to reduce the number and severity of the reactions. Pretreatment with corticosteroids and diphenhydramine (Benadryl) several hours before administration has been recommended. Be aware, however, that pretreatment can mask early systemic manifestations.
      (3) If reactions occur, plasma transfusions from a single related donor (usually the father) can often be tolerated.

B. **Hyperimmune gamma globulin preparations,** prepared from normal donors who have titers of specific antibody, are useful in preventing or decreasing the severity of attacks in immunodeficient patients exposed to varicella (zoster immune globulin) or to vaccinia (vaccinia immune globulin) (see Chap. 19).

C. **Frozen plasma** may be helpful for selected antibody-deficient patients in whom satisfactory infection control with intramuscular gamma globulin injections every 1–2 weeks has not been achieved; for patients who have experienced serious local or systemic reactions to intramuscular or intravenous therapy; and for patients who cannot be given intramuscular injections because of bleeding disorders or extensive skin lesions. Patients with severe, life-threatening infections and refractory diarrhea can also be excellent candidates for fresh-frozen plasma.

1. The **advantages** of intravenous plasma therapy are as follows:
   a. Compared with intramuscular gamma globulin, intravenous plasma therapy achieves higher levels of serum immunoglobulin with more rapid equilibration between body fluid compartments.

    b. All classes of immunoglobulins are administered.

    c. Catabolic losses due to local proteolysis by muscle enzymes are avoided.

    d. Plasma donors can be immunized to provide high titers of specific antibodies.

  2. The **disadvantages** of intravenous plasma therapy include the risk of serum-transmitted infection and transfusion reactions. To minimize the risk of transmitted infections, restrict plasma donors to one or two donors, preferably family members of the same blood group whose blood has been carefully screened for exposure to agents such as hepatitis B virus and HIV.

  3. Dosage. The usual dose for plasma is between 15 and 20 ml/kg every 3–4 weeks, depending on the patient's clinical status. An initial loading dose of 2–3 times the maintenance dose should be given. Do not cause fluid overload. The initial loading dose should be given over several days. Monthly maintenance volumes can be given over several hours, observing for fluid overload. In patients with an antibody deficiency associated with deficiency of cell-mediated immunity, plasma should be irradiated (3000 rad) prior to administration to avoid possible induction of graft-versus-host disease.

II. Specific treatment for cellular deficiency. Specific treatment for T-cell deficiency is complicated because these disorders often involve heterogeneous defects, especially disorders of severe combined immunodeficiency. This heterogenicity has often made it difficult to determine the exact requirements for complete immunologic reconstitution. As a result, a number of treatment approaches are currently employed. Because of the complexity of diagnosis and treatment, such patients are usually cared for by referral centers with an investigative capacity and interest in immunodeficiency diseases.

  A. Bone marrow transplantation. Bone marrow contains the pluripotent cell that differentiates into the hematopoietic, lymphoid, phagocytic, and megakaryocytic cell series. Bone marrow, theoretically providing precursors for a variety of cell systems, has been used successfully to treat severe combined immunodeficiency and Wiskott-Aldrich syndrome, as well as aplastic anemia, leukemia (acute myelogenous, acute lymphoblastic), chronic granulomatous disease (X-linked form), and congenital neutropenia.

  The bone marrow transplantation procedure entails the following: Multiple small aspirates are made from the iliac crest of the donor under general anesthesia. A large volume (300–500 ml) of marrow is collected in a heparinized container and filtered through fine wire mesh to remove bone spicules. This preparation (approximately $3–5 \times 10^8$ mononuclear cells/kg) is then given to the patient intravenously.

  Although this procedure is relatively simple, successful bone marrow transplantation requires detailed tissue typing and matching to avoid fatal graft-versus-host disease. Transplanted haploidentical bone marrow (usually from a parent) that has been treated with soy-lectin agglutination or by monoclonal antibody to remove postthymic T cells can successfully reconstitute severe T-cell deficiencies. This procedure has permitted treatment for virtually all severe T-cell immunodeficiencies.

  Extensive medical support is required to care for the severely immunosuppressed host before and after transplantation. Bone marrow transplantation should be done in medical centers willing and able to provide adequate clinical and research services.

  B. Fetal thymus transplantation, experimentally available, has been used in a variety of disease states in which thymus-dependent immunity is depressed. The best results have been seen in the Di George syndrome, as manifested by relatively rapid, complete, and permanent reconstitution of T-cell immunity. The fetal thymus tissue (obtained from a fetus of < 14 weeks' gestation in order to minimize the possibility of graft-versus-host disease) has been given subcutaneously as an organ implant into a muscle in the anterior abdominal wall; as a cell suspension, either by the intravenous or intraperitoneal route; or as thymic fragments by the intraperitoneal route.

C. **Fetal liver transplantation,** experimentally available, has been used in the treatment of severe combined immunodeficiency with varying degrees of success. Severe graft-versus-host disease is a problem, especially when liver cells from fetuses of more than 12 weeks' gestation are used. Based on experimental evidence in mammals and limited clinical experience in humans, successful reconstitution is usually associated with high doses of liver cells (from fetuses of 10–12 weeks' gestation) given intraperitoneally to the patient as early in life as possible.

D. **Cultured thymic epithelium** is an experimental procedure that involves culturing thymic tissue in vitro for 3 weeks and implanting the epithelial monolayers devoid of lymphocytes (which have the potential for provoking graft-versus-host disease) either subcutaneously or intraperitoneally into the patient. Pieces of postnatal thymus are obtained incidentally (with informed consent) from immunocompetent children undergoing thoracotomy for the correction of cardiac lesions. It appears that cultured thymic epithelial grafts can be effective in immunodeficient patients when the primary defect resides in the thymus and not in the stem cells.

E. **Replacement therapy** for cellular immunodeficiency is an attempt to replace substances critical for immunologic competence without transplantation of viable, replicating donor cells (analogous to gamma globulin or plasma therapy for antibody deficiency).

   1. **Transfer factor** is a dialyzable substance of low molecular weight ($< 10,000$ daltons), which is derived from leukocyte lysates of normal donors whose skin tests are positive for common antigens, e.g., PPD or *Candida*. In addition to enhancement of T-cell response to specific antigens, it produces nonspecific immune enhancement by mechanisms of action not yet known. Evidence that it has successfully treated immunodeficiency comes primarily from anecdotal reports, not from controlled studies. At best, the results have been highly variable, with the most dramatic reports of improvement noted for patients with chronic mucocutaneous candidiasis. Improvement has not occurred in patients with severe combined immunodeficiency. It is of concern that lymphoproliferative disorders have appeared in some patients after transfer factor therapy was begun. Whether or not these effects are causally related to transfer factor administration is unknown; however, the possible benefits and risks must be carefully assessed before any transfer factor therapy is begun.

   2. **Thymic hormones.** A variety of peptide hormones, some probably of thymic origin, others thymus-dependent, have been purified. **Thymosin,** one of these hormones, exerts in vitro and in vivo effects that appear to require the presence of a precursor cell responsive to thymosin. In most cases of severe combined immunodeficiency, no response to thymosin has been observed, while in other isolated and less severe T-cell deficiencies, the early results with thymosin therapy have been encouraging. The **side effects** are tolerable, although skin reactions at the site of injection eventually develop in approximately one-third of these patients.

   3. **Enzyme replacement.** The autosomal recessive form of severe combined immunodeficiency can occur in conjunction with an adenosine deaminase deficiency. Transfusion of frozen irradiated normal red blood cells as a source of adenosine deaminase in this form of severe combined immunodeficiency has resulted in clinical improvement and increases in peripheral blood counts and serum immunoglobulins, as well as development of normal responses to mitogens and allogeneic cells.

   4. **Trace elements.** An inborn error of metabolism that prevents the normal absorption of zinc from the gastrointestinal tract results in a form of severe combined immunodeficiency associated with acrodermatitis enteropathica. The clinical manifestations of this disease include severe skin lesions, gastrointestinal malfunction with malabsorption and diarrhea, and bizarre, irritable behavior. Treatment with zinc in sufficient amounts by parenteral

or oral routes corrects all manifestations of the disease, which is often fatal if untreated.

III. **Specific treatment of phagocytic disorders.** Specific cellular or enzyme replacement for phagocytic disorders, such as chronic granulomatous disease, mycloperoxidase deficiency, and Chédiak-Higashi syndrome, is less well defined than for T-cell disorders. Bone marrow transplantation has been used in chronic granulomatous disease and congenital neutropenia; the awareness of enzymatically different forms of chronic granulomatous disease may allow specific enzyme replacement in the future. For the present, "specific" treatment includes antibiotics, granulocyte transfusions, and vitamin C.

A. **Antibiotic therapy**
   1. Antibiotic therapy for **acute illness** should be given early and by the intravenous route during an active infection after taking appropriate cultures. Patients with phagocytic disorders are at a significant risk of fulminant, overwhelming sepsis and should be treated aggressively during acute illnesses.
   2. **Long-term** administration of sulfonamides or antistaphylococcal drugs appears to decrease the number of infections in most patients.

B. **Granulocyte transfusions,** together with antibiotics, may be beneficial during the course of severe infection.

C. The use of **vitamin C** (ascorbic acid) in those patients with Chédiak-Higashi syndrome (partial oculocutaneous albinism, neutropenia, recurrent pyogenic infection, and giant lysosomes in all lysosome-containing cells) appears to correct neutrophil defects and decrease susceptibility to infection.

IV. **Specific treatment for complement deficiency**

A. **Fresh-frozen plasma** from normal donors can replace specific complement components in patients with isolated complement component defects and increased susceptibility to a wide range of microorganisms. Patients with deficiency or dysfunction of C5 protein and patients with C3 or C3b inactivator deficiency show clinical and laboratory improvement following **plasma infusions.** Plasma infusions may benefit patients with C1-esterase inhibitor deficiency (hereditary angioedema—see Chap. 9) during acute attacks.

B. **Anabolic steroids** such as danazol can induce production of normal C1-esterase inhibitor and prevent dangerous attacks of angioedema (see Chap. 9). This treatment is a form of therapy for immunodeficiency, using molecular engineering.

Acquired Immunodeficiency Syndrome

An illness occurring in young previously healthy men, now recognized as **acquired immunodeficiency syndrome (AIDS),** was first reported in 1981 by the Centers for Disease Control. The disease was initially observed to occur in homosexuals and intravenous drug abusers but has subsequently been reported in other populations and from other countries. The incidence of AIDS has steadily increased since first reported; over 24,000 cases had been diagnosed in the United States by January 1987. The predominant risk groups still comprise homosexual or bisexual males (65%) and intravenous drug abusers (17%), but also include transfusion recipients, patients with hemophilia, those having heterosexual contact with a person with AIDS, and infants infected transplacentally or during the perinatal period.

Human immunodeficiency virus-1 (HIV), previously named human T lymphotropic virus-type III (HTLV-III) and lymphadenopathy-associated virus (LAV), has been shown to be the causative agent of AIDS and AIDS-related diseases. It is estimated that approximately one million individuals in the United States have been exposed to HIV. Furthermore, with an estimated incubation period of 2–6 years or longer, HIV-related illnesses are likely to increase (see Chap. 18 for serologic determination of HIV).

Table 17-7. Clinical findings in AIDS

Chronic interstitial pneumonitis*
Infections: opportunistic and bacterial* organisms
Hepatosplenomegaly
Diffuse lymphadenopathy
Failure to thrive* or weight loss
Chronic diarrhea
Small for gestational age*
Peculiar facies*
Parotitis*
Rash (eczema-like)
Thrombocytopenia
Malignancies: Kaposi's sarcoma, lymphoma
Neurologic manifestations, acute and/or chronic

*Predominantly seen in children with AIDS.

The diagnosis of AIDS is based on (1) clinical criteria of infection(s) with opportunistic organisms and/or malignancies such as Kaposi's sarcoma or central nervous system lymphoma, (2) a cellular immune deficiency, and (3) HIV infection. *Pneumocystis carinii* pneumonia is the most frequent opportunistic infection. However, mucocutaneous candidiasis, toxoplasmosis (disseminated or central nervous system infection), disseminated cytomegalovirus infection, mucocutaneous herpes simplex, *Mycobacterium avium intracellulare* infections, cryptococcal meningitis, and cryptosporidosis have all been reported (reviewed by J. B. Green and M. J. Slepian. A Clinical Approach to Opportunistic Infections Complicating the Acquired Immune Deficiency Syndrome. In A. E. Friedman-Kien and L. J. Laubenstein (eds.), *AIDS. The Epidemic of Kaposi's Sarcoma and Opportunistic Infections.* Chicago: Year Book Medical Publishers, 1984. Pp 89–95). (See Table 17-7.)

Both an acute and a chronic encephalitis are seen in patients with AIDS due to HIV infection. Also, central nervous system infections due to papovavirus (causative agent of progressive multifocal leukencephalopathy), cytomegalovirus, *Cryptococcus neoformans,* and *Toxoplasma gondii* can occur.

Patients with AIDS have an increased incidence of secondary cancers. Most commonly observed are Kaposi's sarcoma, non-Hodgkin's lymphoma, and primary lymphoma of the brain.

HIV infection is also associated with other symptoms, such as persistent generalized lymphadenopathy, fever of unknown origin, idiopathic thrombocytopenic purpura, night sweats, weight loss, herpes zoster infection, or thrush, sometimes called **AIDS-related complex (ARC).** More extensive classification systems of HIV related diseases have been proposed by Haverkos et al. (see Table 17-8) and the Centers for Disease Control (Table 17-9).

Pediatric acquired immune deficiency syndrome (PAIDS) was first reported by Oleske et al. (*J.A.M.A.* 249:2345, 1983), Rubenstein et al. (*J.A.M.A.* 249:2350, 1983), and Scott et al. (*N. Engl. J. Med.* 310:76, 1984). Subsequently, PAIDS has been frequently diagnosed in children in the United States, approximately 1% of the total AIDS cases. This, however, reflects only a fraction of children infected with HIV. Thus, the full impact of HIV-related diseases in children is still to be determined.

The risk factors for development of PAIDS are (1) parent with or at risk for AIDS (75.8%), (2) blood transfusion recipient (14.3%), and (3) hemophilia (4.8%). In the first group, clinical disease may be manifested at birth with abnormal facies (microcephaly, boxlike forehead, hypertelorism, flat nasal bridge, blue sclerae, triangu-

Table 17-8. Proposed stratification of human immunodeficiency virus-1 (HIV)–related illnesses

Category	Clinical features
1	Asymptomatic
2	Idiopathic thrombocytopenic purpura
3	Unexplained* palpable lymphadenopathy at two or more noncontiguous, noninguinal sites, of greater than 4 months duration
3A	Systemic symptoms absent
3B	Fevers low grade (< 38.5°C), intermittent, or continuous for greater than 1 month or night sweats (four or more nights in the last month)
4	Minor opportunistic infection (OI), unexplained thrush or herpes zoster in individuals < 60 years of age
4A	No adenopathy
4B	Adenopathy as above
5	Systemic prodrome defined as intermittent or continuous fevers > 38.5°C for one or more months or watery diarrhea for two or more weeks or sustained weight loss more than or 10% of body weight; no etiology established
6	AIDS with Kaposi's sarcoma, no OI
7	AIDS with OI with or without Kaposi's sarcoma

*Common causes of lymphadenopathy, including syphilis, tuberculosis, cytomegalovirus, infectious hepatitis, and lymphoma should be considered and appropriate diagnostic studies performed.
Source: Adapted from Haverkos, H. W., et al., *J. Infect. Dis.* 152:1095, 1985.

lar-shaped philtrum, and patulous lips) and subsequently with infections by 6–8 months. PAIDS associated with transfusions in the newborn period usually present by 7–8 months of age, but children infected at an older age seem to have an incubation period similar to adults, approximately 2–6 years or longer.

The clinical manifestations of PAIDs are similar to those in adults with AIDS (see Table 17-7). Opportunistic infections are similar to those reported in AIDS, namely *P. carinii* pneumonia, mucocutaneous candidiasis, and cytomegalovirus infections. Chronic interstitial pneumonitis, parotitis, and bacterial infections, principally due to *Streptococcus pneumoniae*, *S. aureus*, and gram-negative bacteria, are particular problems in PAIDS. Both an acute and a chronic encephalitis can occur. Milder symptoms, such as zoster infection, idiopathic thrombocytopenic purpura, fever of unknown origin, and generalized adenopathy (ARC), are also seen in PAIDS.

The laboratory abnormalities seen in AIDS and PAIDS are outlined in Table 17-10. HIV infection results in a partial combined immunodeficiency disorder. The hallmark of AIDS is decreased percentage and absolute number of T-helper cells due to HIV destruction, which differentiates this disease from most other primary pediatric T-cell immunodeficiency disorders in which T-helper/suppressor populations are present in normal ratios. T-cell immune function is similarly decreased as assessed by delayed hypersensitivity skin testing; decreased in vitro lymphoproliferative responses to mitogen, antigen, and alloantigen stimulations; and decreased in vitro synthesis of gamma-interferon and IL-2. Specific T-cell and natural killer cell cytotoxicities are also deficient. Although hypergammaglobulinemia, principally IgG and IgA, is seen, abnormal de novo antibody synthesis to specific antigens is also reported. Increased circulating immune complexes are frequently observed. Antibody to HIV and/or identification of the virus also differentiates PAIDS from other immune deficiencies.

Table 17-9. Classification system for human immunodeficiency virus-1 (HIV)–related diseases

Group 1	Acute infection defined as a mononucleosis-like syndrome with or without meningitis
Group 2	Asymptomatic infection defined as the absence of signs or symptoms of HIV infection
Group 3	Persistent generalized lymphadenopathy defined as adenopathy of 1 cm or greater at two or more extrainguinal sites
Group 4A	Constitutional disease defined as one or more of the following: persistent fever > 1 mo, weight loss > 10%, diarrhea > 1 mo
4B	Neurologic disease defined as dementia, myelopathy, or peripheral neuropathy
4C-1	Opportunistic infections due to one of twelve specified infectious diseases listed in the surveillance of AIDS: *Pneumocystis carinii* pneumonia, cryptosporidiosis, toxoplasmosis, candidiasis, histoplasmosis, mycobacterial infection with *M. avium* or *kansasii*, cytomegalovirus and herpes simplex infections, cryptococcosis, strongyloidiasis, isosporiasis, progressive multifocal leukoencephalopathy
4C-2	Symptomatic disease due to one of six secondary infectious diseases: oral hairy leukoplakia, herpes zoster, Salmonella bacteremia, nocardiosis, tuberculosis, oral candidiasis
4D	Secondary cancers defined as Kaposi's sarcoma, non-Hodgkin's lymphoma, or primary lymphoma of the brain
4E	Other conditions attributable to HIV infection such as chronic lymphoid interstitial pneumonitis

Source: Adapted from Centers for Disease Control. *M.M.W.R.* 35:334, 1986.

Table 17-10. Abnormalities of immunity in patients with AIDS

1. Lymphopenia
2. Decreased T helper/inducer lymphocyte number and percentage
3. Anergy or hypoergy of delayed hypersensitivity skin tests
4. Decreased to absent lymphoproliferative responses to mitogens, antigens, and alloantigens
5. Decreased T cell and natural killer cell cytoxicities
6. Hypergammaglobulinemia (especially IgG and IgA)
7. Elevated circulating immune complexes
8. Decreased to absent antibody responses to antigen immunizations, especially to neoantigens
9. Increased serum beta-2 microglobulin
10. Abnormal thymic structure

Although no definite treatment for AIDS is currently available, the most likely therapy is a combination of antiviral drugs and immune enhancers or modulators. To be effective, antiviral agents must cross the blood-brain barrier. Most antiviral agents in current trials are inhibitors of reverse transcriptase (HIV is a retrovirus). These drugs (suramin, azidothymidine [AZT], HPA-23, ribavirin, and foscarnet) inhibit viral replication and, if effective, will likely have to be taken life-long. Though antiviral drugs may be effective alone in ARC and milder disease, immune enhancers or reconstitution is likely to be necessary in AIDS patients. Clinical trials with thymic hormones, lymphocyte transfer, bone marrow transplantation, and isoprinosine are being evaluated. Immune modulators, such as gamma- and alpha-interferons and IL-2, have had only limited success. Currently, IVIG is given to PAIDS patients to replace the antibody defect and may improve T-cell immune function. Research is being directed toward the development of a vaccine against HIV.

The risk to other children and adults of HIV transmission from a child with AIDS is extremely low. Current guidelines from the Centers for Disease Control recommend school attendance if the child has control of stool and urine; body excretions such as vomit are readily disinfected with 10% household bleach (e.g., Clorox); contact with blood from cuts can be avoided by wearing gloves and other protective coverings. Whether to give children with PAIDS live viral immunizations is currently under study.

Selected Readings

Buckley, R. H. Gammaglobulin replacement. *Clin. Immunol. Allergy* 5:141, 1985.

Buckley, R. H. Immunodeficiency. *J. Allergy Clin. Immunol.* 72:627, 1983.

Buckley, R. H., et al. Development of immunity in human severe primary T cell deficiency following haploidentical bone marrow stem cell transplantation. *J. Immunol.* 136:2398, 1986.

Gupta, S., and Gottlieb, M. S. Treatment of the acquired immune deficiency syndrome. *J. Clin. Immunol.* 6:183, 1986.

Rosen, F. S., Cooper, M. D., and Wedgwood, R. J. The primary immunodeficiencies (Parts I and II). *N. Engl. J. Med.* 311:235, 300, 1984.

Scientific Group on Immunodeficiency, WHO. Primary immunodeficiency diseases. *Birth Defects* 19:345, 1983.

Selwyn, P. A. AIDS: What is now known. I. History and immunovirology. *Hosp. Pract.* 21:67, 1986.

Shannon, K. M., and Ammann, A. J. Acquired immune deficiency syndrome in childhood. *J. Pediatr.* 106:332, 1985.

Stiehm, E. R. Immunodeficiency Disorders: General Considerations. In E. R. Stiehm and V. A. Fulginiti (eds.), *Immunologic Disorders in Infants and Children* (2nd ed.). Philadelphia: Saunders, 1980. Chap. 11.

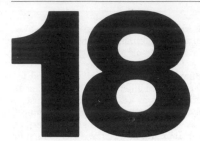

Immunologic Methods Useful in the Diagnosis of Infectious Disease

Mary J. Spencer

I. The immune response in infectious diseases. The immune response is described as the total of responses initiated by a foreign antigen that results in an inflammatory response. The rate at which a patient can mount an immune response to an invading organism will affect the course and outcome of the infection.

   A. Physical barriers that protect the host include cutaneous epithelium, mucosal cells, ciliated respiratory and gastrointestinal epithelium, and vascular endothelium.

   B. Macrophages, which are fixed in either the spleen or the liver, or free macrophages, which are migratory and are present in alveolar and peritoneal tissue, are barriers to dissemination of infectious agents. Organisms are either killed or ingested by macrophages.

   C. Antibody production (humoral immunity) is a primary mechanism preventing the spread of infectious diseases to other organs.

   1. **IgM antibody** is the earliest antibody produced by the host after antigenic challenge and is found primarily in the intravascular compartment. The function of IgM is to assist the reticuloendothelial system by clearing the blood of organisms by opsonization and agglutination.

   2. **IgA antibody** is found in the serum and, more important, is also the primary antibody present on mucosal surfaces and in tears, saliva, and nasal and gastrointestinal secretions.

   3. **IgG antibody** constitutes about 80% of serum immune globulin. It is the major antibacterial, antifungal, and antiviral antibody.

   D. Cell-mediated immunity can achieve destruction of a pathogen in two ways: by direct destruction of organisms by sensitized lymphocytes or by contact between the antigen and antigen-reactive lymphocytes, which leads to release of lymphokines that attract macrophages. Patients with defective cell-mediated immunity but intact humoral immunity are subject to severe infections such as tuberculosis, measles, varicella, and *Candida.*

   E. Lymphocytes. There are two major types of lymphocytes.

   1. **B lymphocytes** are derived directly from the bone marrow and produce immunoglobulins.

   2. **T lymphocytes** arise in the bone marrow and mature under the influence of the thymus. These lymphocytes have the ability to recognize antigens and differentiate in at least three ways:

      a. They can become helper or cooperating T cells, which have the capacity to assist B lymphocytes in promoting antibody synthesis.

      b. They can become suppressor T cells that impede or suppress B-cell synthesis of immunoglobulins.

      c. They can become effector T cells that may be involved with cell-mediated immunity and produce the typical delayed hypersensitivity skin reaction.

   F. Complement is a group of circulating plasma proteins with complex stimulatory or inhibitory functions. Complement promotes phagocytosis of microorganisms by the formation of antigen-antibody-complement complexes.

   G. Interferon is a protein substance that enhances host resistance to viruses by release into the bloodstream or by its presence in uninfected cells.

II. Immunologic techniques in the diagnosis of infectious diseases

A. Historical aspect of infectious diseases.
It is important in the interpretation of serologic tests to consider the following:

1. History of the illness.
2. History of previous infection.
3. Vaccination history (i.e., date and type of immunization).
4. Travel history.
5. The geographic area where the patient resides and contact with the environment.
6. History of contact with others.
7. Season of the year.
8. History of animal contact.

B. Collection of specimens.
Specimens may be obtained from any body fluid or tissue: whole blood, serum, urine, pleural fluid, peritoneal fluid, joint fluid, cerebrospinal fluid (CSF), bone marrow, mucosal secretions, or extracts of tissues. A sufficient quantity of the specimen must be obtained, the amount varying with the type of serologic test. Both an acute and a convalescent specimen must be obtained; the time interval between the two varies with the specific disease (usually 10 days to 2 weeks).

III. The serologic methods of measuring antigen-antibody reactions
are listed in Table 18-1.

A. Radioimmunoassay
is an extremely sensitive method that involves competition between labeled and unlabeled antigen for combining sites on antibody. The test is specific for the detection and the quantification of microquantities of compounds.

Table 18-1. Serologic methods of measuring antigen-antibody reactions

Specific serologic tests
  Radioimmunoassay
  Immunofluorescence techniques
  Immunodiffusion
    Radial immunodiffusion
    Double immunodiffusion
  Electrophoresis
    Counterimmunoelectrophoresis
    Immunoelectrophoresis
  Agglutination test
    Direct agglutination tests
    Indirect passive agglutination tests
    Indirect hemagglutination
  Complement-fixation tests
  Enzyme-linked immunosorbent assays
  Precipitating antibody tests
    Capillary precipitation
    Double gel diffusion
    Crossed immunoelectrophoresis
    Circumlarval precipitation

Miscellaneous tests
  C-reactive protein
  Cold agglutination
  Febrile agglutinins
  Weil-Felix
  Sabin-Feldman dye test
  Quellung phenomenon
  Limulus lysate assay
  Bentonite flocculation test

B. Immunofluorescence techniques are used to demonstrate specific antigen or the presence of specific antibody. The test employs immunologic agents that have been labeled with fluorescent dyes without affecting the protein's biologic or immunologic properties. The fluorescent antibody reaction consists of antigen-antibody union made visible by a fluorescent dye, usually fluorescein isothiocyanate, incorporated into the system. The technique can identify a microorganism or antibody in serum. There are three types in use.

1. **The direct fluorescent antibody** procedure identifies unknown antigens by employing fluorescein-labeled specific antibody that is layered on the slide to be examined. The reaction of an unknown antigen with labeled antibody is observed with a fluorescence microscope.

2. The **inhibition fluorescent antibody** technique enables the detection of reaction between an unknown antibody and a specific antigen.

3. The **indirect fluorescent antibody** technique is used to detect antibody in unknown serum. It involves exposing unlabeled antibody to unlabeled antigen followed by anti–gamma globulin labeled with fluorescent dye, which will react with the unlabeled antibody fixed by antigen. The antibody content of an unknown serum can be detected.

C. Immunodiffusion (precipitin assay) techniques are used to detect the reaction of antigen and antibody by the precipitation reaction. The test involves the direct interaction of a soluble antigen with its corresponding antibody (precipitin), which yields a visible precipitate. The use of pure antigens provides a precise quantitative measurement of antigen-antibody interaction.

1. **Precipitate in solution.** If increased amounts of a soluble antigen are added to a constant amount of antiserum, a precipitate curve is formed. Antigen-antibody precipitate first appears in the zone of antibody excess, reaches a maximum in the equivalence zone, then diminishes in the zone of antigen excess.

2. **Precipitate in gel** is the most common method of demonstrating a precipitin reaction between a soluble antigen and its corresponding antibody.

    a. **Radial immunodiffusion** is based on the principle that there is a quantitative relationship between the amount of antigen placed in a well surrounded by antibody uniformly dispersed in a thin layer of agar and the resulting precipitate. The area of the precipitation ring is proportionate to the antigen concentration. The test is primarily used to measure immunoglobulins.

    b. **Double immunodiffusion** is a simple semiquantitative test based on the principle that antigen and antibody diffuse through gel (agar) and form immune complexes that can be visualized. Antigen and antiserum are placed in separate wells and allowed to diffuse through the gel. A visible band of precipitate appears where the antigen and antibody meet at the zone of equivalence.

3. **Electrophoresis**

    a. **Immunoelectrophoresis** involves a combination of the methods of immune precipitation and electrophoresis. It is used primarily for identification of serum proteins. The serum is placed in a cell on a slide coated with agar, and an electric current is applied across the long axis of the slide to cause separation of the individual components. A trough cut into the agar parallel to the axis of the electric current is filled with antisera to the specific protein components (antigen) to be tested. Separated antigen diffuses radially, while the antisera diffuse as a band. A precipitant arc forms between each specific antigen-antibody component.

    b. **Counterimmunoelectrophoresis** is a variation of the immunodiffusion test. Serum and antigen are placed in apposed wells (as in the immunodiffusion test), and an electric current is passed through the gel substrate (purified agar or agarose), which brings antigen and antibody reactants together rapidly. A precipitation line forms where antigen and antiserum meet in the zone of equivalence. This test is useful for detecting antigens for rapid diagnoses.

D. The **agglutination test** is a semiquantitative test that achieves a high degree of sensitivity through the use of antigen-coated or antibody-coated particles. An aggregation of suspended particulate antigen (or particles coated with antigen) is observed when mixed with antibody (agglutinin). The quantity of insoluble antigen is constant, and the serum to be tested is serially diluted, allowing determination of antibody titer.

    1. The **direct agglutination test** is used for the detection of antigens located on the surfaces of formed blood elements or on microorganisms. The test is performed by mixing dilutions of antiserum with a suspension of particulate material containing surface antigens. The relation between antigen and antibody is manifested by agglutination or aggregation of particles in a test tube, or wells, or on a slide. It is more sensitive than precipitation tests because the bulk of the combining mass is provided by the cells or the microorganism that contains the surface antigens. These tests are independent of temperature except in the case of cold agglutinins, which contain antibodies that agglutinate bacteria or erythrocytes more efficiently at temperatures below 37°C.

    2. In the **indirect (passive) agglutination test** soluble antigens are bound to the surfaces of red blood cells or other inert carrier particles such as latex or bentonite. Antibody is measured by making serial dilutions of serum with a saline solution and mixing each dilution with equal amounts of the coated red blood cells or other inert particles. This technique is highly sensitive for the detection of antibody present in low concentration.

E. Complement-fixation tests. The hemolytic complement-fixation test is based on the principle that a standard amount of complement, when added to a mixture of antigen and antibody, is fixed by the antigen-antibody complex that is formed. The consumption of complement in vitro can be used as a test to detect and measure antigens, antibodies, or both.

F. The **enzyme-linked immunosorbent assay (ELISA) test** is a safe, economical, and highly sensitive test. It is based on the premise that when antigen or antibody is chemically (covalently) linked to an enzyme, the resulting conjugate retains its immunologic and enzymatic activity, which can be measured.

G. Miscellaneous tests

    1. C-reactive protein is a specific beta globulin that appears rapidly after the onset of inflammation or tissue injury. Any positive reaction is considered abnormal. Levels of C-reactive protein in this nonspecific test may be elevated in acute bacterial infection (including tuberculosis) and viral infection, as well as in acute myocardial infarction and malignant and rheumatic diseases.

    2. Cold agglutination is a nonspecific reaction seen in certain diseases in which antibodies agglutinate erythrocytes at 4°C. These reactions occur in *Mycoplasma pneumoniae* and, less commonly, in influenza, adenovirus, other acute viral respiratory infections, and African trypanosomiasis. A titer of 1:32 in a single specimen of a more than fourfold antibody titer rise within 7–14 days is significant.

    3. Febrile agglutinins are used in the diagnosis of several febrile diseases (salmonellosis, paratyphoid, brucellosis, tularemia, rickettsial diseases). The test is a titration of the patient's serum antibody by agglutination of suspensions of known killed bacterial cells (antigen). The titer is the highest dilution of a patient's serum that will cause agglutination of a known bacterial antigen. Paired acute and convalescent phase sera are collected 10–21 days apart; a fourfold titer rise is significant.

    4. The **Weil-Felix test** is an agglutination test used to make a presumptive diagnosis of rickettsial diseases. It depends on the agglutination of OX-19, OX-2, and OX-K strains of *Proteus vulgaris* by serum antibody produced by typhus and the spotted fever rickettsial diseases.

5. The **Sabin-Feldman dye test** is used in the diagnosis of toxoplasmosis. This test depends on the ability of specific antibodies to block the uptake of alkaline methylene blue into the cytoplasm of *Toxoplasma gondii*.

6. The **Quellung phenomenon** occurs as a result of type-specific antisera causing the polysaccharide capsules of *Haemophilus influenzae, Streptococcus pneumoniae,* and *Neisseria meningitidis* (serogroups A and C) to undergo refractive changes and swelling, which are detected by light microscopy. Serum or CSF can be tested.

7. The *Limulus* **lysate assay** is used to detect gram-negative bacterial infection. Minute quantities of bacterial endotoxin cause the gelation of an extract from amebocyte lysate of *Limulus polyphemus*. This test can also be used to support the diagnosis of gram-negative bacterial infection, especially septicemia or meningitis.

8. The **bentonite flocculation test** is a slide flocculation test in which antigen-coated bentonite particles are added to the patient's serum, and agglutination is read microscopically. The results are read as negative to a maximum of 4 +. At maximum levels all particles are agglutinated. The test is used in the diagnosis of echinococcosis, trichinosis, schistosomiasis, visceral larva migrans, and filariasis.

IV. **Delayed hypersensitivity skin testing** (Table 18-2) is the most accessible means available for the clinical evaluation of cellular immunity.

A. **Skin tests** routinely used to assess delayed hypersensitivity include purified protein derivative (PPD), *Trichophyton,* and *Candida* (see Chap. 17).

B. Diseases or therapy associated with **diminished delayed hypersensitivity** (anergy) include the following:
1. Congenital or acquired **immunodeficiency.**
2. Acute **viral diseases,** including mumps, rubella, measles, varicella, influenza, and mononucleosis.
3. **Fungal diseases** such as coccidioidomycosis, cryptococcosis, and aspergillosis.
4. **Bacterial diseases,** including tuberculosis, meningitis, and pneumonia.
5. **Malignancies.**
6. **Viral immunizations.**
7. **Corticosteroid** and **immunosuppressive therapy.**

C. The skin tests are administered and interpreted as follows:
1. Clean the area.
2. Use a 1-ml tuberculin syringe with a 0.5-in., 27-gauge needle, and inject 0.1 ml of solution intradermally.
3. Encircle the area with an indelible marking pencil.
4. Read and record the skin test results in 24–72 hours depending on the test (see Table 18-2).
5. Measure the diameter of the erythema and induration of the skin test site in two directions, and record (in millimeters).

D. Measurement of delayed hypersensitivity by diagnostic skin tests is dependent on the antigen used. Specific antigen responses are presented in Table 18-2.

V. **Diagnosis of viral diseases.** The diagnosis of viral diseases can be made in four ways: by **isolation** of the viral agent in **cultures** from infected tissues (the most accurate method of identification), by demonstration of **viral inclusions or giant cells** in stained smears of skin lesions, by the demonstration of a **fourfold or greater antibody titer rise** in the serum to a specific virus during an illness, and by the demonstration of the presence of virus or its antigens in tissues, body fluids, or excretion using rapid diagnosis techniques.

A. **Appropriate culture specimens for viral isolation** can be obtained from the throat, nasopharynx, sputum, urine, stool, blood, cerebrospinal fluid, exudates, or biopsy specimens. The specimen is collected by aseptic technique and placed in a suitable sterile container for transport to a properly equipped clinical laboratory. Special precaution and equipment are required for obtaining specimens of viruses classified as hazardous; such specimens are handled by the Centers for Disease Control.

Table 18-2. Measurement of delayed hypersensitivity by diagnostic skin tests

Disease	Material	Intradermal dose	Description of positive test	Comments
Bacterial				
Tuberculosis	Tuberculin purified protein derivative (PPD), intermediate, 5 tuberculin units (TU)	0.1 ml	Read at 48–72 hr; < 5 mm induration is negative, 5–10 mm doubtful. Repeat in 1 mo if tuberculosis is suspected. Induration of ≥ 10 mm is positive.	Positive 2–10 wk after onset of infection *Other strengths:* Use 1 TU when history indicates previous markedly positive PPD. Use 250 TU when suspicious of tuberculosis with negative PPDs. Between 5 and 10 mm induration with 5 TU is possible cross-reaction with atypical mycobacteria.
Fungal				
Aspergillosis	Protein fraction of aqueous extracts of *Aspergillus fumigatus*, 1 mg/ml	0.02 ml	Immediate reaction (wheal and erythema) ≥ 5 mm in 15–20 min; Arthus reaction in 4–8 hr.	Immediate reaction is suggestive of atopic (IgE) allergy. Delayed (Arthus) reaction is suggestive of immune complex hypersensitivity. Epicutaneous test should be done prior to intradermal skin test.
Blastomycosis	1:100 dilution of filtrate from mycelial phase of *B. dermatitidis*	0.1 ml	Read at 24–48 hr; ≥ 5 mm induration.	Cross-reacts slightly with histoplasmosis and coccidioidomycosis. Unreliable test; no correlation with complement-fixation tests

Table 18-2. (continued)

Disease	Material	Intradermal dose	Description of positive test	Comments
Fungal (cont.)				
Candidiasis	*Candida albicans* "Dermatophyton 0" 1:100 dilution	0.1 ml	Read at 24–48 hr; ≥ 5 mm induration.	Use 1:10 dilution in nonreactors to 1:100. Not useful to diagnose disease; used for testing delayed hypersensitivity only.
Coccidioidomycosis	1:100 dilution of filtrate from mycelial phase of *Coccidioides immitis*	0.1 ml	Read at 24–48 hr; ≥ 5 mm induration.	Occasionally cross-reacts with blastomycin. Test becomes positive at 48–72 hr in 99% by second week of illness. Repeat in 2–3 wk if skin test is negative and coccidioidomycosis is suspected. Skin test conversion is pathognomonic of disease.
Histoplasmosis	1:100 dilution of filtrate from mycelial phase of *H. capsulatum*	0.1 ml	Read at 48 and 72 hr; ≥ 5 mm induration.	Cross-reacts with blastomycin and coccidioidin. Not a valuable test; often induces false-positive serologic test results.
Viral				
Cat-scratch fever	Heat-treated suspension of pus from a lymph node of a patient with cat-scratch fever	0.1 ml	Read at 48 hr; ≥ 5 mm induration.	Reliable but not commercially available. Positive in 90% with cat-scratch fever; false-positive in 4–8%.

	Material	Amount	Reaction	Comments
Mumps	Inactivated mumps vaccine	0.1 ml	Read at 48–72 hr; ≥ 15 mm erythema.	Frequently cross-reacts with other antigens; therefore, test is unreliable to predict protection. Used to test delayed hypersensitivity
Parasitic				
Trichinosis (*Trichinella spiralis*)	1:10,000 dilution of dried ground trichina in saline (control is saline)	0.1 ml antigen, 0.1 ml control	Immediate wheal and erythema of ≥ 5 mm, maximum in 15–20 min. Control ≤ 3 mm. Delayed 24–48 hr, 10–30 mm induration	Appears 2–3 wk after infection. Frequent false-positive reactions occur; therefore, test is unreliable.
Echinococcosis (*Echinococcus granulosus*)	Injection of inactivated hydatid cyst fluid from humans or animals (Casoni test)	0.025 ml	Immediate wheal and erythema, ≥ 5 mm in 15–20 min. Delayed 24–48 hr, ≥ 5 mm induration	Many false-positive reactions. Antigen not available commercially.
Chlamydia				
Lymphogranuloma venereum (LGV)	Killed lymphogranuloma venereum agent (Frei test). Antigen is derived from injected yolk sacs of chick embryos.	0.1 ml	Induration ≥ 6 mm in 48–72 hr	May become positive 10–30 days after infection. Positive test is presumptive evidence of LGV. Frequent false-positives make test unreliable. Remains positive for life.

B. Directions for preparation of smears of vesicular lesions for staining
1. Incise the vesicle peripherally with a scalpel.
2. Lift the top of the lesion back and remove excess fluid by gentle blotting.
3. Scrape the base of the lesion thoroughly with a scalpel blade, but do not cause bleeding.
4. Spread the cellular material collected on the edge of the blade over two separate 5- to 10-mm areas on clean microscope slides.
5. Dry the slides in air and fix in alcohol.
6. A Giemsa stain examination or, alternatively, a fluorescent antibody test can be done.
7. For best results, collect a minimum of **three** smears.

C. The immune response to a viral agent can be measured serologically by serum neutralization tests, hemagglutination-inhibition tests, complement fixation, or enzyme-linked immunosorption (ELISA). A blood sample should be collected early in the course of the disease (acute serum) and again 2–3 weeks later (convalescent phase). Remove the serum from the blood sample collected (2–10 ml of whole blood), place it in a sterile tube, and refrigerate until it is transported to the clinical laboratory (or store at −20°C [−4°F]). **A fourfold rise in antibody titer must occur to ensure an accurate serologic diagnosis of a specific viral illness.** The serologic tests commonly used for viral diagnosis (Table 18-3) are the following:
1. **Complement fixation** occurs when antibody-antigen complexes bind serum complement and leave insufficient amounts of complement for hemolysis of sensitized sheep red blood cells. Dilutions of serum, mixed with a standard amount of viral antigen, are incubated to permit the formation of antibody-antigen complexes.
2. **Serum neutralization,** a highly specific virus-antibody reaction, can measure antibody levels against specific viruses and can determine the capacity of a serum to neutralize or interfere with viral infectivity in the susceptible host. The test is performed by mixing dilutions of the patient's serum with a predetermined amount of a known virus.
3. **Hemagglutination-inhibition** measures the inhibition of agglutination of antigen-coated red blood cells by homologous antigen. It is a highly specific and sensitive test for detecting small quantities of soluble antigen in blood or tissue fluids. Certain viruses adsorb to human blood type O cells or chicken erythrocytes, causing them to agglutinate. This test measures the ability of the patient's serum to prevent agglutination by prior reaction to the virus.

D. Rapid viral diagnosis by serology using known antibody
1. Radioimmunoassay (RIA).
2. Immunofluorescence.
3. ELISA.

E. Specific serologic tests for infectious mononucleosis. Infectious mononucleosis is an acute viral disease of children and young adults characterized by fever, sore throat, lymphadenopathy, splenomegaly, and an increase in peripheral blood lymphocytes. The disease is associated with the Epstein-Barr (EB) virus, but a similar illness is seen with cytomegalovirus, early rubella, brucellosis, glandular tularemia, acquired toxoplasmosis, and, occasionally, leukemia and lymphoma. Specific serologic tests detect immune response to the EB virus.
1. **Heterophile antibodies** are IgM agglutinins reactive with several groups of antigens (heterophile antigens) occurring in unrelated animals (e.g., humans, sheep, cows). They appear in about 90% of patients with the characteristic clinical and laboratory findings of infectious mononucleosis. They also can appear in lower concentration in normal persons.
   a. The **detection of heterophile agglutinins for sheep erythrocytes** is the classic laboratory reference method for the diagnosis of infectious mononucleosis. Differential absorption with guinea pig kidney cells or beef erythrocytes distinguishes the cross-reacting Forssman (in normal serum) and serum sickness heterophiles (Table 18-4). A heterophile ti-

Table 18-3. Types of serologic tests commonly used in viral diagnosis

Type of virus	Complement fixation	Hemagglutination inhibition	Neutralization	Fluorescent antibody	Radioimmunoassay	Enzyme-linked immunosorbent assay	Immunoelectrophoresis
DNA viruses							
Adenovirus	1	1	1			1	
Poxvirus: smallpox and vaccinia	1	1		2			
Herpesviruses							
Herpes simplex	1		1	2		1	
Varicella-zoster	1			2		1	
Cytomegalovirus[b]	1	2	2	2		1	
Epstein-Barr	2			1			
Hepatitis B					1[c]		
RNA viruses							
Reovirus	1	1					
Enterovirus (poliovirus, coxsackievirus, echovirus)	1	1	1				
Rhinovirus				1			
Arbovirus	1	1[d]	2				
Myxovirus							
Influenza A and B	1	1	2				
Parainfluenza	1	1					
Mumps	1	1					
Respiratory syncytial virus	1	1	2				
Rubeola	1	1					
Rabies	1		1	1		1	
Rubella	1	1	2	2		1	
Rotavirus[e]						1	
Hepatitis A					1[c]	1	
Human immunodeficiency virus						1	2

Key: 1 = most commonly used serologic test; 2 = less commonly used serologic test.

[a]Paired specimens are usually necessary, acute, and convalescent serums obtained 4 weeks apart.

[b]Cytomegalovirus IgM fractionation is available by immune adherence hemagglutination.

[c]RIA is the most sensitive and specific method, but ELISA and immune electron microscopy can be used.

[d]Western equine encephalitis only.

[e]Diagnosis can be made by electron microscopy.

ter of 1:128 to 1:256 is considered diagnostic in most laboratories. Levels are usually detectable within 3–4 weeks of illness (false-positives occur with leukemia, viral hepatitis, cytomegalovirus, Burkitt's lymphoma, rheumatoid arthritis, and with the use of horse antisera). Titers do not reflect the degree of illness, but sequential titer determinations are useful in following the clinical course.

  b. The **Mono-Test*** (Mono-spot Test) is a rapid, highly specific screening test that detects infectious mononucleosis heterophile antibody (agglutination of stabilized horse erythrocytes) without differential absorption.

2. **Specific serologic tests** are needed to identify heterophile-negative cases of infectious mononucleosis caused by EB virus. Often, in children with primary infections, no heterophile antibody is produced. The following specific tests are indicated:

  a. **Viral capsid antigens (VCAs)** are measured by immunofluorescence. The IgM fraction appears and peaks early in the disease (2 weeks) and lasts 2–3 months; the IgG fraction remains detectable for life and appears to be associated with permanent immunity.

  b. The **EB early antigen (EA)** measures antibody by immunofluorescence to the D (diffuse) and R (restricted) components of the early antigen complex of the EB virus. This antibody peaks in the early acute phase of the illness (2–3 weeks).

  c. Cell **membrane antigen (MA)**, measured by immunofluorescent techniques, is intermediate in onset and remains for life.

  d. The **EB nuclear antigen test (EBNA)** utilizes an anticomplement immunofluorescence technique. Antibody to EB nuclear antigen appears around the fourth week of infectious mononucleosis and persists in all patients throughout life.

  e. **Epstein-Barr virus–induced early antibodies** are measured by immunofluorescence. Antibody to EB virus appears early; titers rapidly decrease to low or nondetectable levels, and the antibodies disappear following recovery from infection.

  f. **Complement-fixation test.** Complement-fixation antibody titers to EB virus persist for years and have no diagnostic value in acute infections.

F. **Specific serologic tests for viral hepatitis.** Viral hepatitis is a systemic infection manifested by liver inflammation and necrosis. The two known, major etiologic agents are designated **type A** and **type B viruses.** A third viral agent termed **non-A, non-B virus** is documented, although other viruses such as cytomegalovirus, E-B virus, adenovirus, and varicella are also associated with hepatitis.

1. **Hepatitis A virus (HAV)** is a small-sized (27-nm) RNA virus. The most specific, diagnostic serologic method of identification, measurement of specific IgM antibody in the blood by either **radioimmunoassay** or **ELISA** confirms recent hepatitis A virus infection. The diagnosis can also be made by immune adherence hemagglutination, demonstrating a fourfold or greater rise in antibody titer in 4 weeks. Immune electron microscopy has been used diagnostically. Anti–hepatitis A virus (anti-HAV) is used to measure hepatitis A, IgG antibody.

2. **Hepatitis B virus (HBV)** is a double-stranded DNA virus composed of a 27-nm nucleocapsid core (HbcAg) surrounded by an outer coat, the surface antigen HbsAg. HBV consists of an outer coat and an inner core, each expressing antigenic specificity. The coat or surface antigen (HbsAg) appears in the blood up to 6 weeks before clinical symptoms and may continue in some patients with or without disease (chronic HbsAg carrier). HbsAg is present in 90–95% of early clinical cases of hepatitis B. The core antigen (HbcAg) appears during active disease, and its detection in a single, serum specimen is presumptive evidence of active hepatitis B. Antibody to HbsAg

---

*Wampole Laboratories, Division of Carter-Wallace, Inc., Cranbury, NJ 08512.

Table 18-4. Differential absorption of heterophile agglutinins

Agglutinin	Sheep erythrocyte absorption	Guinea pig kidney absorption	Beef erythrocyte absorption
Infectious mononucleosis	Absorbed, increased serum concentration	Absorbed	Not absorbed
Serum sickness	Absorbed, increased serum concentration	Not absorbed	Not absorbed
Forssman (normal serum)	Absorbed	Not absorbed	Absorbed

(anti-Hbs) may be detected in the blood from 2–26 weeks after HbsAg disappears; the presence of anti-Hbs suggests clinical recovery and the development of specific immunity.

A third antigen (HbeAg) usually appears late in the incubation period or after the onset of disease (in HbsAg positive sera) and after the appearance of HbsAg. Its presence in the blood suggests active disease and its persistence represents chronic infectivity (chronic hepatitis). Antibody to HbeAg (anti-Hbe) may be detected after the disappearance of HbeAg. Its presence in the blood is indicative of recovery or, with the continuing presence of HbsAg, a healthy carrier. (An HbsAg carrier with HbeAg-positive sera has a 10-fold greater incidence of infectivity than an HbsAg carrier with HbeAg-negative, anti-Hbe positive sera.) Antibody to HbcAg (anti-Hbc) may be detected in the serum after the disappearance of HbcAg, and its presence correlates with the persistence of HbsAg after recovery (chronic, infective HbsAg carrier).

Patient infectivity (transmissibility) is best determined by the presence of both HbsAg and HbeAg in the blood.

The following serologic tests are used to detect hepatitis B antigens and antibodies.

   a. **Radioimmunoassay** is the most sensitive, specific method for detection of HbsAg, anti-Hbs, HbcAG, and anti-Hbc. False-positive tests occur, especially with commercially available test kits.

   b. **Enzyme immunoassay (EIA)** is available in kit form for all hepatitis B markers except core antigen.

   c. **Agar gel diffusion** is used to detect the presence of HbsAg. The test is convenient, but slow and less sensitive than other methods.

   d. **Counterimmunoelectrophoresis** is faster and more sensitive than agar gel diffusion for detection of HbsAg.

   e. **Rheophoresis,** a technique similar to the agar gel diffusion, provides increased sensitivity similar to counterimmunoelectrophoresis. At present, it is used for detection of HbeAg and anti-Hbe.

   f. **Reversed passive latex agglutination** is a rapid and simple test used to detect HbsAg. Frequent false-positive reactions occur and require confirmation by other methods.

   g. **Hemagglutination tests,** either passive hemagglutination or reversed passive hemagglutination, are rapid, simple, sensitive tests performed in a microtiter plate. False-positive tests occur and require confirmation by other methods.

3. Hepatitis B delta antigen is a small defective RNA that replicates only in patients with chronic hepatitis B virus infection. This virus is primarily found in drug addicts, homosexual males, and hemophiliacs. There is no available serologic test at present.

4. Non-A, non-B hepatitis is a common form of hepatitis and accounts for 90% of transfusion hepatitis. No serologic test is available for the detection of non-A, non-B hepatitis. Presumptive diagnosis is made by clinical assess-

ment, elevation of liver enzymes, and the failure to detect the presence of HAV, HBV, or other viral agents. Non-A, non-B virus is most commonly associated with post-transfusion hepatitis.

G. The **human immunodeficiency virus (HIV)**, a retrovirus, is the determined cause of the acquired immunodeficiency syndrome (AIDS) (see Chap. 17). Two types of serologic tests are available to detect the presence of HIV in patients' blood.

  1. An **ELISA test** (available in kits*) measures nonspecific viral antigens. In low-risk populations the test has a false-positive rate of up to 90%. This rate is significantly less in higher risk populations. The frequency of false-positive reactions probably relates to nonspecific reactions to antigens in cell culture materials. Test kits from different manufacturers have varying sensitivities.

  2. The **Western Blot Test** is a highly specific immunoelectrophoresis test that detects serologic reactions to the viral core antigen complex or the viral envelope antigen complex or both. The test is primarily available in reference laboratories, and each laboratory establishes its own standard of positivity.

The ELISA test is currently used to screen all blood donors and is also used to screen women at risk for HIV infection who are pregnant or plan to become pregnant and for individuals who have received blood products between the years of 1978 and 1985. The test can also be used as an adjunct in the diagnosis in symptomatic individuals suspected of having AIDS. The application of this test for routine screening of high-risk asymptomatic individuals is not established at this time. A positive ELISA test should be repeated. A repeat positive ELISA should be confirmed by a positive Western Blot Test before the individual is notified. A repeat positive ELISA test verified by a positive Western Blot Test is considered to be a true positive test for the presence of the HIV.

VI. **Diagnosis of mycoplasma diseases.** Mycoplasma are the smallest free-living organisms. They are distinct from viruses in their ability to grow on cell-free media and are distinct from bacteria in lacking cell walls. The primary mycoplasma infective for humans is *Mycoplasma pneumoniae*, a respiratory pathogen that causes primary atypical pneumonia in children, adolescents, and young adults. *Mycoplasma hominis* and *Ureaplasma urealyticum* also cause infections in humans, particularly in the reproductive system.

Specimens from infected tissue can be cultured in agar and require about 2–4 weeks for growth.

The **serologic tests** for mycoplasma include the following:

A. **Cold agglutinins,** IgM antibodies reactive in a cold environment, are present in the sera of patients with a variety of diseases. Generally, if a patient has pneumonia and a cold agglutinin titer of 1:32 or more, or if a fourfold rise in specific antibody titer occurs, the diagnosis of *Mycoplasma pneumoniae* can usually be made.

B. The **complement-fixation test** is the most useful method of detecting antibody to *Mycoplasma*. A fourfold or greater antibody-titer rise from acute to convalescent sera is diagnostic. High titers ($\geq 1:256$) are suggestive of recent infection. Antibody titers can remain at low levels for years.

C. The **metabolic inhibition test** measures the ability of *Mycoplasma* antibody to inhibit the growth of the organism. The end point can be lower when fewer test organisms are used. Interpretation of the test is also influenced by antibiotic in the serum sample, since it will inhibit growth of the test organism.

D. The **indirect immunofluorescence test** is performed by immunofluorescent staining of infected chick embryo lung tissue sections. It is highly specific and sensitive but is unavailable in most clinical laboratories.

E. **ELISA**—now available in many commercial laboratories.

*Abbott Laboratories, N. Chicago, IL 60659; ElectroNucleonics, Columbia, MD 21045; and Litton Bionetics (Organon Teknika), Charleston, SC 29402.

VII. Diagnosis of bacterial diseases
  A. Serologic tests for the diagnosis of streptococcal disease
    1. Screening test (Streptozyme test).* A commercial product, Streptozyme (STZ) can be used for screening purposes only. The test contains multiple group A streptococcal antigens adsorbed on sheep red blood cells, which agglutinate in the presence of antistreptococcal antibody. Agglutination ($\geq$ 100 STZ units) is a positive reaction suggesting a recent streptococcal infection and occurs in 20% of patients with negative antistreptolysin O (ASO) titers. The STZ antibodies increase more rapidly and appear earlier than the ASO antibodies.
    2. Specific tests. Group A beta-hemolytic streptococci produce several intracellular and extracellular antigens. These stimulate the production of antibody that can be detected by serologic tests.
      a. The **ASO test,** the most frequently used test for group A beta-hemolytic streptococci, is available in most clinical laboratories. It is a neutralization test based on the ability of reduced enzyme streptolysin O to lyse erythrocytes.
        (1) An **elevation** of the ASO titer usually indicates a recent infection with group A beta-hemolytic streptococci and is also useful in the diagnosis of acute rheumatic fever and acute glomerulonephritis.
        (2) Low titers can be associated with skin infection.
        (3) False-positive titers are associated with liver disease and the growth of certain bacteria in the serum specimen.
        (4) The ASO titer reaches a peak about 3–5 weeks after infection and falls to negative within 6–12 months of infection. Antibiotic therapy can depress the antibody response.
        (5) A fourfold rise in titer between the acute and convalescent state specimens is considered to be significant; a single ASO titer of 1:240 or greater is suggestive of recent infection with any strain of group A streptococcus.
      b. Antideoxyribonuclease B test (anti-DNase B). Streptococci produce DNase enzymes that are shared between the various streptococcal groups. Because DNase B is found predominantly in group A beta-hemolytic streptococci, it is helpful for the detection of group A infections. **This test is the best single method for the serologic identification of streptococcal infection.** False-positive titers are rare. Titer rises to anti-DNase B occur later than with ASO, reach a peak 4–6 weeks after infection, and remain elevated for a longer period than the ASO titer. Antibiotic therapy can suppress the height of the titer and cause it to decline more rapidly. Significant serologic titers are 1:80 or greater in preschool children, 1:240 or greater in school-age children, and 1:120 or greater in adults. A fourfold titer rise between acute and convalescent specimens is significant.
      c. Antistreptococcal hyaluronidase (ASH) titer. A titer of 1:128 to 1:256 is equivocal; 1:512 or greater is positive.
      d. Rapid diagnostic tests for group A hemolytic streptococcal pharyngitis are available commercially using a number of methods for the detection of streptococcal antigens. These antigen detection tests employ a simple extraction process to remove specific group A streptococcal antigens from throat swab specimens and a subsequent reaction with antigen-specific antibody on a solid phase particle for detection. In one series the sensitivity of this method (Culturette Group A Strep ID Test, Marion Scientific, Kansas City, MO) when compared with the recovery of group A streptococci from a duplicate throat swab ranged from 77–95%, and specificity ranged from 88–100%. The rapidity of diagnosis and the suit-

---

*Wampole Laboratories, Division of Carter-Wallace, Inc., Cranbury, NJ 08512.

ability to an office laboratory make these tests popular. Several test kits are available, and reliability is widely variable.

B. Anthrax bacillus is a large, gram-positive spore-forming microorganism. An **indirect hemagglutination test** is available from the Centers for Disease Control in Atlanta, Georgia.

C. Brucella. Brucellosis is an acute or chronic illness with primary manifestations of chills, fever, and weakness. **Febrile agglutinins** will detect antibody to *Brucella.* Three specific serologic tests are available:

1. The **standard tube agglutination test,** generally available in local laboratories, is the most sensitive test and usually becomes positive in the first week of the illness. A standard antigen must be used. Titers greater than 1:160 usually occur within 3 weeks of onset and remain positive for years.

2. The *Brucella* **card test** is a rapid and sensitive agglutination test that detects antibody in up to 92% of patients by 9–15 days of illness. It becomes negative in 80% of patients after 1 year and in 90% by 6 years.

3. A **complement-fixation test** is available in some state laboratories and from the Centers for Disease Control. Cross-reactions occur with *Vibrio cholerae* immunization (100%), *Francisella tularensis* (4%), and *Yersinia enterocolitica* (1–2%). At best, the test is positive in 71% of the patients.

D. Listeria monocytogenes, the infecting agent in listeriosis, is a gram-positive organism. Listeriosis presents with several clinical forms: meningeal, oculoglandular, typhoidal, endocardial, and cutaneous. *Listeria* commonly infects newborn infants. Serologic tests include the following:

1. **Agglutination test.** Acute and convalescent titers are obtained. A single high-titer serum is suggestive of disease, while a fourfold or greater titer rise constitutes a presumptive diagnosis.

2. A **tube agglutination test** is available at the Centers for Disease Control. Paired sera are required.

E. Tularemia, caused by the organism *Francisella tularensis,* presents in several forms (cutaneous, pneumonic, typhoidal, and oculoglandular). A **tularemia agglutination test** is an available, reliable test. Agglutinins appear within 10–14 days. A titer of 1:40 is strongly suggestive, but must be confirmed by a greater than fourfold rise. Antibody titers in excess of 1:1280 occur between the fourth and eighth week of illness. A minor cross-reaction with *Brucella* can occur, but titers are much lower.

F. Yersinia

1. *Yersinia enterocolitica* is associated with enterocolitis, mesenteric adenitis, and an illness similar to acute appendicitis. An **agglutinin titration (Widal reaction)** against the *Yersinia* antigen is the most widely used test. A single agglutinin titer greater than 1:160 is suggestive of infection; a single titer of 1:1280 or a fourfold greater titer rise in paired sera is diagnostic of infection.

2. *Yersinia pseudotuberculosis* **agglutinin (Widal reaction)** levels are high in the acute phase of the disease. A titer of 1:160 or higher is indicative of actual infection.

3. *Yersinia pestis* causes bubonic plague, presenting as pneumonic, septicemic, meningeal, or pharyngeal forms. A presumptive plague diagnosis is made with a single elevated fluorescent antibody titer; a confirmed plague diagnosis is made with a fourfold rise in specific antibody titer. Specific antibody tests include the following:

   a. **Passive agglutination** with sensitized sheep erythrocytes. This is the recommended serologic test. An antibody titer of 1:256 is evidence of plague.

   b. The **indirect hemagglutination test.** This can be performed by the Centers for Disease Control.

   c. A **fluorescent antibody test.** This sensitive test is becoming more widely used.

   d. The **ELISA test** is most commonly used.

G. **Diphtheria.** An **indirect hemagglutination test** is available at the Centers for Disease Control.

H. *Neisseria meningitidis.* Capsular polysaccharides are the basis for classifying meningococci into serologic subgroups. Four serologic tests are commonly used in the diagnosis of meningococcal infection: passive hemagglutination, latex agglutination, serum bactericidal, and indirect fluorescent antibody tests. Individual laboratories determine their own positive titers. Generally, a fourfold antibody titer rise in paired sera indicates infection.

1. The **passive hemagglutination test** is a simple, specific serologic test primarily for the detection of the **IgM antibody** response from either infection with *N. meningitidis* or polysaccharide immunization. The test is based on the ability of antibodies to agglutinate erythrocytes coated with polysaccharide antigen. Peak serum antibody titers occur 1–3 weeks after infection or immunization. After natural infection, antibody titer falls rapidly, usually within 2 months. However, after vaccination, antipolysaccharide titers remain high for many years. A passive hemagglutination antibody response to infection or immunization occurs in 90% of subjects.

2. The **latex agglutination test** has the advantage of commercial availability and standardization. However, it is less sensitive than the passive hemagglutination test, even though it is based on the same principle (except for the nature of the insoluble particle). The test is positive in response to infection or immunization in 90% of those tested and primarily measures IgM antibody.

3. The **serum bactericidal test** measures the ability of the serum to kill viable bacteria and requires an exogenous source of complement. Both IgG and IgM antibodies participate in the meningococcal bactericidal reaction. Although cumbersome, this test is useful in evaluating patients with suspected immunodeficiency or recurrent meningitis since it measures functional opsonizing capability.

4. **Indirect fluorescent antibody test.** Titers of 2+ or greater by the indirect immunofluorescence test are considered positive. Paired sera are necessary for proper interpretation of the results; a fourfold or greater rise in titer is significant.

5. *Neisseria gonorrhoeae* complement-fixation test is done commercially. A negative result is a titer less than 1:2.

I. *Salmonella* infections are best diagnosed by **isolation of the organism** from the blood, urine, or stool. Serologic tests include the following:

1. **Febrile agglutinins.** This test detects serum agglutinins to *Salmonella* flagella H, somatic O, and Vi antigens, as well as paratyphoid A, B, and C antigens. These serologic studies can be used as a presumptive diagnostic test to implicate a particular organism if attempts to culture the bacterium have failed. The agglutination reaction usually becomes positive during the second week after typhoid fever infection. Paired acute and convalescent phase sera are collected 1–2 weeks apart; a fourfold or greater titer rise is usually considered significant. Febrile agglutinins may be elevated in narcotic addicts and after typhoid vaccination or febrile illnesses. Early effective treatment of *Salmonella* infection can prevent high titer rises. A *Salmonella typhi* O antibody titer of 1:160 or greater is indicative of *Salmonella* infection in patients who have not had a recent typhoid immunization (typhoid vaccine antibody titer remains elevated for several years). *S. typhi* H antibody titers of 1:80 or greater are also suggestive. Paratyphoid A, B, or C antibody titers of 1:160 or greater indicate paratyphoid infection.

2. **Tube agglutination** titers can be helpful in the diagnosis if the culture for *Salmonella* is negative.

3. **Hemagglutination** antibody titers are available through the Centers for Disease Control. Typhoid immunization elevates the titer.

4. The **anti-Vi hemagglutination test,** although thought to be helpful in the

detection of typhoid carriers, has a high incidence of false-positive and false-negative reactions.

J. Tetanus. The **indirect hemagglutination test** is available through the Centers for Disease Control.

K. Cholera. The most practical and easily performed serologic tests for cholera involve measurement of antibodies against the somatic O antigen of *V. cholerae* by agglutination or vibriocidal antibody assays.

    1. Agglutination test. A fourfold convalescent titer rise will occur in 90% of patients when live antigens are used in the test.

    2. The **vibriocidal test** depends on the bacterial effect of somatic O antibody in the presence of complement on *V. cholerae*. Of patients with bacteriologic evidence of cholera, 90–95% will have a fourfold or greater antibody titer rise.

L. Pertussis agglutination tests are valuable for epidemiologic surveillance but are not routinely used in individual patients. A **fluorescent antibody test** can be obtained through the Centers for Disease Control.

M. *Legionella pneumophila* is a gram-negative bacillus that is implicated as the causative agent in patients with fever, weakness, malaise, anorexia, cough, and radiographic evidence of pneumonia. Cases often occur in clusters and are termed **Legionnaire's disease.** Isolation of the organism is diagnostic.

Demonstration of a fourfold or greater rise in direct immunofluorescent antibody titer, or titers of 1:128 or greater, are good evidence for diagnosis of the disease. A titer rise is usually evident in the first week of illness.

An ELISA test is being evaluated for this disease.

N. Mycobacterium tuberculosis is a pleomorphic, nonmotile, weakly gram-positive rod that is easily demonstrated microscopically by "acid-fast" stain. The organism has been associated with infection in the lungs, heart, connective tissue, bone, skin, and central nervous system as well as generalized infection. Diagnosis is usually made by visualization of the organism in acid-fast stain. The organism takes 4–8 weeks to grow in culture. Recently, an antibody to the organism has been demonstrated by the ELISA method and may soon be available commercially.

VIII. Diagnosis of spirochetal diseases

    A. Syphilis. The response in humans to infection by *Treponema pallidum* leads to production of multiple antibodies of two basic types.

        1. Nontreponemal tests measure nonspecific nontreponemal antibodies (reagins), which react with the lipid antigens of the treponemal organism or with other, similar lipid antigens (e.g., beef heart) prepared from normal tissue. These tests for antibody (reagins) are of two general types: flocculation and complement fixation. Since antigens used in these tests are found in normal tissues, false-positive tests are common; thus, a reactive test should be confirmed by a specific treponemal antigen test.

            a. The **Venereal Disease Research Laboratory (VDRL) test** is the most commonly used flocculation test. The test is a microscopic slide flocculation test utilizing cardiolipin antigen (beef heart), which reacts with reagin (antibody). An antibody titer of 1:8 or greater is reactive, and a quantitative test should be performed. The VDRL usually becomes reactive 1–3 weeks after the primary chancre appears. The VDRL titer can be negative, low, or high in primary syphilis, usually high in secondary syphilis, and variable in late (tertiary) disease. It can be reactive in low titer or nonreactive in the late stages of syphilis. A fourfold or higher rise in antibody titer is significant.

            The VDRL test on cerebrospinal fluid (CSF) consists of a microscopic examination of a slide flocculation as in the serum VDRL test except that one part of antigen is diluted with one part of 10% saline. Although false-positive reactions occur commonly in serum VDRL analysis, they are rare in CSF specimens.

            b. Several rapid reagin tests have been developed as screening procedures: the Plasma Crit, Unheated Serum Reagin, the RPR Teardrop card test and the automated reagin test (ART). These tests are more sensitive but less specific than the VDRL test. If a screening test is positive, it must be rechecked by the VDRL test or a specific treponemal test.

   c. The **Kolmer test** is the most common complement-fixation test for syphilis in use.

2. **Specific treponemal tests**

   a. The *T. pallidum* **immobilization test** measures the ability of antibody and complement to immobilize a suspension of living treponemes (extracted from rabbit testes and visualized with a dark-field microscope). The test is expensive and time consuming, but is accepted as the treponemal test of reference. Two-thirds of patients with primary syphilis and one-third with secondary syphilis have negative test reactions. The test does not distinguish syphilis from other treponematoses (bejel, yaws, pinta).

   b. The **Reiter test** is a modification of the complement-fixation test, employing a nonpathogenic treponeme (Reiter) as the antigen. This test is rarely used and is reactive in only 50% of patients with late syphilis.

   c. **Fluorescent treponemal antibody absorption (FTA-ABS).** In this test, the patient's serum is treated to remove nonspecific antibody to *T. pallidum,* thereby allowing specific antitreponemal antibody present in the serum to combine with treponemal antigen. These complexes are detected by the addition of antihuman globulin labeled with fluorescein isothiocyanate.

      (1) The results are recorded by intensity of fluorescence from 0 to 4 + : 0 is negative; less than 1 is borderline; 1 + is minimally reactive; 2 + is moderately reactive; 3 + is strongly reactive; and 4 + is very strongly reactive. The test is reactive in most cases of syphilis and other treponemal infections, including bejel, yaws, and pinta. In most laboratories, this test is done on all reactive VDRL sera.

      (2) The FTA-ABS test is the most sensitive serologic test in all stages of syphilis. Its diagnostic accuracy is 86% in primary syphilis, 100% in secondary syphilis, and in 99% of early latent, 96% of late latent, and 97% of tertiary syphilis. The test is not helpful in serial evaluation of patients with syphilis. Once positive, it remains positive for many years, at times for life. Although false-positive reactions are rare, patients with systemic lupus and other collagen vascular diseases, and occasionally old age, drug addiction, and pregnancy, can produce borderline false-positive reactions. If a patient has a reactive reagin test and weakly positive FTA-ABS, the test should be repeated monthly; a fourfold rise in titer is significant. The FTA-ABS test does not distinguish between syphilis and bejel, yaws, and pinta. The diagnosis of central nervous system syphilis may be made by a CSF cell count of more than 5 mononuclear cells/mm^3, a total protein greater than 40 mg/dl, and a reactive CSF-VDRL. Response to therapy is best followed by observing a fall in serial CSF cell counts. Infants suspected of congenital syphilis should have serial VDRL test on their serum. If antibody is maternal, the titer will fall; if infection is present, the titer will increase.

   d. The *T. pallidum* **hemagglutination assay** requires less technical skill than the FTA-ABS.

B. **Nonsyphilitic treponematoses**

   1. **Bejel** is a treponemal disease of children, nonvenereally acquired and characterized by cutaneous and mucocutaneous lesions on the lips, tongue, palate, and larynx. Bony involvement, with gumma formation, can occur. Serologic tests for syphilis are positive and do not distinguish this disease from other treponematoses.

   2. **Yaws** is a nonvenereally transmitted treponemal disease characterized by early benign skin lesions. A latent period is followed by destructive lesions of the skin and bones lasting for months to years. Serologic tests for syphilis

are reactive several weeks after onset and do not differentiate the disease from syphilis. Diagnosis can be made by positive dark-field examination of lesions.

3. **Pinta** is a chronic, nonvenereally transmitted treponemal disease associated with characteristic skin lesions that include late depigmentation. Serologic tests for syphilis may become positive relatively late in the disease (at about 4 months) and may remain positive for life. No specific serologic test can confirm the diagnosis. Diagnosis is made by dark-field examination of lesions.

4. **Lyme disease,** first described in 1975 in Lyme, Connecticut, is characterized by erythematous skin lesions (erythema chronicum migrans), arthritis, and at times central nervous system and cardiac symptoms. A spirochete isolated from ticks has been implicated as the causative agent. Serologic testing is available in some laboratories and through the Centers for Disease Control.

C. **Relapsing fever,** a febrile illness associated with spirochetes of the genus *Borrelia,* is transmitted by body lice or ticks. *Borrelia* are spiral-shaped organisms that can be visualized by aniline dyes. The diagnosis of relapsing fever is made by demonstration of the spirochete in a Wright-stained or Giemsa-stained thin or thick smear of peripheral blood. Serologic evidence for infection in louse-borne relapsing fever includes the following: *Proteus* OX-K agglutinins are positive in 90% of patients at a titer of 1:40 or greater; the *Borrelia* complement-fixation test is positive in 50% of cases; and the serum borreliolysin test is positive in 50–60% of the cases at a titer of 1:100 or greater.

D. **Leptospirosis** is transmitted from animal reservoirs and can present as a subclinical illness or as an acute, fatal febrile illness. The following three serologic tests are employed in its diagnosis:

1. The **microscopic agglutination test,** the standard procedure used in most laboratories for the diagnosis of leptospirosis, is highly sensitive and specific, although specific *Leptospira* serotypes with live organisms as antigens must be used. Agglutinins begin to appear in 6–12 days and reach a maximum in 3–4 weeks.

2. The **macroscopic agglutination test,** a slide test using killed organism antigen pools, is used to screen sera for detecting current infection.

3. The **indirect hemagglutination test,** a simple qualitative screening test, becomes positive early in the course of infection. Positive test specimens can be sent to the Centers for Disease Control for confirmatory testing by the agglutination test.

E. *Spirillum* is a spiral-shaped organism associated with rat-bite fever. Diagnosis is made by positive culture.

IX. **Diagnosis of fungal diseases.** Serologic procedures provide presumptive, rapid evidence of fungal infection and can help to evaluate the effects of therapy. A positive serologic reaction at high antibody titer is diagnostic. Early in disease, antibody titers can be low or negative.

Collect specimens for serologic tests aseptically by venipuncture or by lumbar puncture. Remove serum after the blood has clotted, and refrigerate or freeze the specimens. Fungal infection is indicated by a fourfold antibody titer rise.

In some fungal diseases, delayed cutaneous hypersensitivity is measured by specific skin test material administered intradermally by injecting 0.1 ml of properly diluted antigen into the volar surface of the forearm (see Table 18-2). A positive skin test is demonstrated in a sensitized person by measurement of induration and erythema at the injection site after 48–72 hours. Skin tests become positive in 2–10 weeks after infection has occurred. Serologic tests usually become reactive before the delayed hypersensitivity skin test response.

A. *Aspergillus* can act as an antigen (asthma and allergic bronchopulmonary aspergillosis) or as an invasive agent, especially in patients on immunosuppressive therapy. Two serologic tests are available.

1. The **immunodiffusion test** is an effective and very specific method for the diagnosis of systemic disease. Precipitating antibodies are found in 90% of

patients with fungal infection and 70% of patients with allergic bronchopulmonary aspergillosis. This test is available in many clinical laboratories and through the Centers for Disease Control. These antibodies have also been identified by ELISA and RIA techniques in selected laboratories.

2. The **complement-fixation test** is less specific but useful for detecting active or recent aspergillosis. It is available in most laboratories.

B. **Blastomycosis** is manifested by either cutaneous or systemic symptoms. Three serologic tests are available.

1. The **immunodiffusion test** is the most specific (80% specificity). A negative test does not exclude the diagnosis.

2. The **complement-fixation test,** less specific because of lack of specific antigens, can cross-react with sera from patients with coccidioidomycosis, histoplasmosis, and paracoccidioidomycosis. Titers of 1:8 to 1:16 are suggestive of infection, and greater than or equal to 1:32 is diagnostic. A negative complement-fixation test does not exclude the diagnosis.

3. The **fluorescent antibody test** is used for the yeast phase but not for the mycelial phase of the disease.

C. **Candidiasis.** Serologic tests are indicated both in patients with systemic diseases (e.g., endocarditis, urinary tract infection, malnutrition, malignancy, and primary and secondary immunodeficiencies) and in patients on immunosuppressive therapy when secondary *Candida* infection is suspected. A fourfold change in agglutinin titer is presumptive evidence of systemic candidiasis, colonization, or transient candidemia. Three serologic tests are available.

1. The **latex agglutination test** detects 90% of proved cases. However, there are false-positive cross-reactions with cryptococcosis, torulosis, and tuberculosis.

2. The **immunodiffusion test** has a sensitivity of 88% and is the most specific test. However, it cross-reacts with *Torulopsis glabrata*. Patients with antibody titers of 1:4 or greater who demonstrate precipitating antibodies in the immunodiffusion test may have early disease or *Candida* colonization. Precipitating antibodies may be found in 20% of normal individuals.

3. The **complement-fixation test** is of little value because of frequent false-positive results.

D. **Coccidioidomycosis** is suggested by characteristic pulmonary, meningeal, or systemic symptoms or by x-ray findings in a person living or traveling in an endemic area. The intradermal **coccidioidin skin test** is a valuable test for screening purposes. It becomes positive in 2–3 weeks after the onset of symptoms and can remain positive for years. Patients with disseminated disease are often anergic.

1. The **complement-fixation test** is the most widely used serologic test. Antibody titers can persist for years.

a. A 1:64 titer is presumptive evidence of active infection. The test can be performed on serum, CSF, plasma, and pleural and joint fluids. It can be negative in asymptomatic patients with coccidioidomycosis. If infection is suspected and the titer is low, repeat the test in 3 weeks.

b. A positive complement-fixation test in a titer of 1:2 to 1:8, with a positive immunodiffusion test, suggests recent or active infection. These should be repeated in 3 weeks.

c. A complement-fixation titer of 1:32 or greater indicates disseminated disease. The test can be negative in cavitary coccidioidomycosis and in asymptomatic pulmonary infection.

d. The CSF titer is positive in 75% of patients with meningeal coccidioidomycosis; a falling titer can be used to follow the success of therapy.

e. The serum complement-fixation titer is serially monitored to determine disease progression or success of therapy.

2. A **tube precipitin test** effectively detects early primary infection or exacerbations of existing disease. The test measures IgM antibody and becomes positive in 53% of infections during the first week, and 91% during the second and third weeks.

    3. As does the tube precipitin test, **latex particle agglutination** measures IgM antibody response, but is more sensitive and convenient. It is often positive within the first 2–3 weeks of infection.

    4. The **immunodiffusion test** is a valuable adjunctive test for diagnosis of coccidioidomycosis. It is often used in combination with the latex particle agglutination test (93% positive in combination).

    5. **Counterimmunoelectrophoresis** is a rapid test but needs further evaluation and is not in common use.

    6. A **fluorescent antibody test** has been developed but is not widely used.

E. **Cryptococcosis** is manifested by both pulmonary and meningeal involvement. Disseminated disease involves the skin, bone, and viscera. The disease can be primary but usually occurs in immunocompromised persons. Four serologic tests are available.

    1. The **immunofluorescent antibody test** is reactive with less than 50% of sera from proved cases and has a specificity of 79%.

    2. The **tube agglutination test** measures circulating antibody. It is 95% specific for *Cryptococcus*. Agglutinins in the serum are detected in early central nervous system infection and systemic disease.

    3. The **latex slide agglutination test** for cryptococcal circulating antigen is a specific test for the diagnosis of active systemic or meningeal cryptococcosis. Rare false-positive reactions occur in adults with rheumatoid arthritis, and a rheumatoid factor test should be performed. Titers parallel the severity of infections; increasing titers indicate a poor prognosis. A positive test of CSF is found in 95% of patients with cryptococcal meningitis.

    4. A **fluorescent antibody test** has been developed but is not widely used as yet.

F. **Histoplasmosis** is characterized by respiratory symptoms, hepatosplenomegaly, and/or meningeal infection. Serologic tests are performed on serum, plasma, peritoneal fluid, or CSF. Antibodies appear 2–4 weeks after fungal exposure. **Intradermal skin testing interferes with serologic data.** Therefore, it should **not** be done in patients who are being evaluated for active disease. Five serologic tests are available. The **complement-fixation test** is the most commonly used test for histoplasmosis and is widely available. Of patients with the disease, 90% have positive tests. Yeast phase antigen is more sensitive than mycelial phase antigen in this test (it can cross-react with sera from patients with blastomycosis and coccidioidomycosis). Titers of 1:32 or greater are highly suggestive of histoplasmosis. Other less commonly used serologic tests for histoplasmosis include **immunodiffusion, counterimmunoelectrophoresis,** histoplasmin **latex slide agglutination,** and **fluorescent antibody** tests.

G. **Paracoccidioidomycosis,** endemic in Latin America, presents as a chronic disease with pulmonary symptoms, ulcerative mucosal lesions, and cutaneous lymphadenopathy. Three serologic tests are available.

    1. The **complement-fixation test** is usually diagnostic and detects antibodies in 80–90% of cases. A titer greater than 1:8 (range, 1:8–1:4096) is presumptive evidence of paracoccidioidomycosis. Low titers suggest localized or reticuloendothelial involvement; high titers suggest pulmonary or disseminated disease.

    2. **Immunodiffusion** is a specific test that, when used in conjunction with the complement-fixation test, can provide an initial diagnosis in 95% of cases.

    3. A **fluorescent antibody test** is available but is not widely used.

H. **Sporotrichosis,** manifested clinically by skin lesions, subcutaneous nodules, bone lesions, lymphadenopathy, or pulmonary disease, is often contracted by persons working with thorny plants or garden moss. Three serologic tests are available.

    1. The **latex agglutination test** is a rapid, specific, positive test in 94% of cases. Titers of 1:4 or greater are presumptive evidence of sporotrichosis.

    2. The **tube agglutination test** is 94% sensitive, but produces false-positive results at low titers (1:8 and 1:16) in patients with leishmaniasis.

    3. A **fluorescent antibody test** is available but is not widely used.

X. Diagnosis of *Chlamydia* diseases. *Chlamydia* are bacterialike organisms that contain both RNA and DNA. Both *C. trachomatis* and *C. psittaci* are associated with disease in humans. *C. trachomatis* is the etiologic agent in lymphogranuloma venereum (LGV), a sexually transmitted disease, and inclusion conjunctivitis (trachoma), which occurs worldwide. It is the most common agent associated with nongonorrheal urethritis, cervicitis, and salpingitis. Recently, it has been associated with inclusion conjunctivitis and pneumonitis in infants less than 3 months of age. *C. psittaci* is the causative agent of the lung disease psittacosis, which is transmitted by some species of birds (e.g., parrots).

A delayed hypersensitivity skin test with killed lymphogranuloma venereum agent (Frei test) is unreliable. Serologic methods available include the complement-fixation, the neutralization, and the microimmunofluorescence test. However, diagnosis is more accurately made by culture of the organism.

The diagnosis of *psittacosis* is made by suggestive history and a rise in acute and convalescent complement-fixation antibody titers. In LGV, diagnosis may be made by culture of lymph node aspirate or rectal biopsy. A rise in complement-fixation antibody titer greater than or equal to 1 : 16 is presumptive. Serologic diagnosis of infection by *C. trachomatis* can be measured by a neutralization test. A commercial test is available using indirect immunofluorescence to measure specific IgM antibody.

XI. Diagnosis of parasitic disease. Specific serologic tests are particularly valuable in the diagnosis of amebiasis, echinococcosis, toxoplasmosis, and trichinosis. They also are helpful in diagnosing cysticercosis, filariasis, and visceral larva migrans. These tests include complement-fixation, precipitin, and agglutination tests. More recently developed methods include indirect immunofluorescence, double diffusion, immunoelectrophoresis, counterimmunoelectrophoresis, and the enzyme-linked immunosorbent assay (ELISA).

Reagents, including antigens, antisera, and diagnostic kits for serologic immunodiagnosis, are commercially available.*

A. Serologic diagnosis of protozoan parasitic disease

1. **Amebiasis** is an infection due to *Entamoeba histolytica* and is transmitted by the ingestion of fecally contaminated food or water or by direct fecal-oral contact. The disease has variable expressions, from asymptomatic infection to dysentery to hematogenous spread with abscess formation in the liver or brain. Asymptomatic disease evokes a weak or negligible antibody response; tissue invasion usually involves a strong antibody response. The serologic tests are sensitive and specific with invasive amebiasis and efficacious in detecting the asymptomatic cyst carrier, but they are less sensitive with amebic dysentery.

   a. The **indirect hemagglutination test** is highly specific for the detection of antibody. However, the presence of antibody cannot be equated with active disease because antibody can persist for many years after treatment. The incidence of seropositivity in the United States is 2–5%. Titers of 1 : 128 or greater are considered positive; 87–100% are positive in liver abscess, 85–100% are positive in acute amebic dysentery, and 44% are positive in endemic areas.

   b. **Immunofluorescence test.** A significant titer is 1 : 64; 99% of patients with extraintestinal infection and 95% with intestinal amebiasis have positive tests. Sensitivity occurs in 15% of asymptomatic cyst passers.

   c. **Counterimmunoelectrophoresis** is a reliable method. Positive titers suggest active, invasive clinical amebiasis. A commerical kit is available.

   d. By **immunoelectrophoresis,** 97% of patients with extraintestinal amebiasis and 83% of patients with intestinal amebiasis have positive reactions.

*Information regarding these kits can be obtained from local and state health departments or the Centers for Disease Control, Parasitic Section, Atlanta, GA 30333.

2. **Babesiosis** usually occurs in animals, but humans occasionally develop infection with fever, malaise, and anemia. The disease is caused by sporozoan intraerythrocytic parasites of animals transmitted by a tick bite. A serologic test is available from the Centers for Disease Control.

3. **African trypanosomiasis** usually starts as a mild systemic illness that later progresses to meningoencephalitis. The etiologic agents *Trypanosoma gambiense* and *T. rhodesiense* are transmitted by the tsetse fly. Diagnosis in the acute stage is by observation of the parasite in blood smears. Later diagnosis is serologic. **Complement fixation** and **hemagglutination** tests are available. The latter test is positive in the CSF of affected patients. Extremely high serum and CSF-IgM titers are usually found.

4. **American trypanosomiasis (Chagas' disease),** an acute or chronic disease caused by *Trypanosoma cruzi,* is transmitted to humans through reduviid bugs that carry the parasite. It is associated with fever, malaise, lymphadenopathy, achalasia, megaesophagus, megacolon, hepatosplenomegaly, and cardiomyopathy. Serologic diagnostic tests for the disease have a high degree of sensitivity and specificity. The three commonly used tests are **complement-fixation, indirect hemagglutination,** and **immunofluorescence.** Antibody titers become positive within 30 days of the onset of infection.
The complement-fixation test is the most sensitive; an antibody titer of 1:8 is considered positive. Neither indirect hemagglutination nor immunofluorescence is specific, but both are useful in epidemiologic studies. A significant titer is 1:128 in the indirect hemagglutination test and 1:64 in the immunofluorescence test.
Other serologic tests include latex agglutination, counterimmunoelectrophoresis, and ELISA.

5. **Leishmaniasis** results from an intracellular parasite (carried by the sandfly) that infects macrophages of the skin or viscera. Three forms occur: cutaneous, visceral, and mucocutaneous. The **leishmanin skin test,** which is positive within 3 months of the appearance of active disease, is helpful in the diagnosis of all forms of the disease. Leishmaniasis is diagnosed serologically by the **indirect hemagglutination test** (performed by the Centers for Disease Control). A titer of 1:64 to 1:128 is significant. A **complement-fixation test** demonstrates antibodies in the blood of patients with active kala-azar, a visceral form of leishmaniasis infection. Fluorescent antibodies also appear early and persist for about 3 years. Cutaneous and mucocutaneous leishmaniasis can be diagnosed by demonstration of the parasite in skin biopsy specimens and a positive leishmanin skin test.

6. **Malaria** is caused by species of the protozoan parasite *Plasmodium,* which is transmitted by the *Anopheles* mosquito. The four *Plasmodium* species infectious for humans are *P. falciparum, P. vivax, P. malariae,* and *P. ovale.* The diagnosis is usually made when a high index of suspicion prompts a search for the parasite in thick or thin blood smears. Serologic tests are not generally available in most hospital laboratories. **Indirect immunofluorescence (IIF)** is the test of choice for the serologic diagnosis of malaria. A titer of 1:64 is suggestive of recent infection. The **indirect hemagglutination (IHA) test** is used primarily for serologic population studies. A significant IHA titer is 1:16 and can distinguish species of malarial parasites in newly acquired infections.

7. The protozoan parasite *Pneumocystis carinii* is associated with interstitial pneumonia, usually found in newborns or in patients with immunodeficiency states or malignancy or taking immunosuppressive drugs. The diagnosis is usually made by microscopic visualization of the silver methenamine-stained organism, which is obtained either by transtracheal aspiration, bronchoscopy, or open lung biopsy. Specific tests include the CF and IIF tests, which detect about 85% of patients with the parasite, but are of little clinical value.

8. **Toxoplasmosis** is a parasitic infection of humans caused by the protozoan

Toxoplasma gondii. Although the disease is often asymptomatic, its manifestations can include fever, splenomegaly, and lymphadenopathy. Congenital infection is the result of acute infection acquired by the mother during gestation. The parasite can be contracted by ingestion of raw meat or from exposure to oocysts from infected cats. Diagnosis is usually made serologically. Of the many serologic tests employed for toxoplasmosis, the **indirect immunofluorescence (IIF) test** and the **indirect hemagglutination test** are the most commonly used. A fourfold antibody titer rise in any test is considered diagnostic for *Toxoplasma.* Also available are the ELISA and the fluoroimmunoassay (FIA) techniques, which measure specific IgM antibody. Antibodies appear in 1–6 weeks and persist for 6–8 weeks.

   a. The **indirect hemagglutination test,** a commonly used method, is simple, accurate, and economical. The antibody titer becomes positive at 1:16 or greater, rises to 1:1000 or greater, and can persist for years. In most laboratories a titer of 1:256 or greater is considered significant.

   b. **Indirect immunofluorescence antibody test (IIF)** is the most widely available procedure. Antibody titers parallel those of the dye test, appear in 1–2 weeks, peak at 1:600 or greater in 6–8 weeks, and can persist for life. An antibody titer of 1:64 or greater is considered significant.

   c. IgM antibody specific for *T. gondii* can be measured by IIF, ELISA, and fluoroimmunoassay (FIA) techniques.

   d. **Complement fixation** is used infrequently and is not standardized for routine use. A titer of 1:4 or greater is positive. With acute infection the titer usually rises to 1:32 and can persist for months or even years.

   e. **Sabin-Feldman dye test.** Antibody appears within 2 weeks after acute infection, peaks in 6–8 weeks, and gradually declines to low titers that can persist for life. A fourfold or greater rise in titer is diagnostic. With acute disease, titers are usually 1:1000 or greater. This test is now rarely used.

B. Diagnosis of intestinal nematode disease is primarily made by examination of stool specimens for ova and parasites. Diagnosis of some tissue helminths can be made serologically.

   1. Filariasis consists of a group of infections caused by nematode roundworms (filariae) transmitted to humans by the bite of infected insect vectors. Since immunologic tests are not highly specific, direct parasite observation is preferred for the diagnosis. Serologic tests are available through the Centers for Disease Control.

   a. **Immunofluorescent antibody** is found in 25% of patients with filariasis. Although antibody titers correlate with the presence of disease, there is a lack of sensitivity, cross-reactivity can occur with other nematodes, and correlation of the serologic responses with the intensity of infection is poor.

   b. The **indirect hemagglutination test,** available through the Centers for Disease Control, is significant at titers of 1:16.

   2. Trichinosis is a nematode infection acquired by ingestion of infective larvae of *Trichinella spiralis* in uncooked or poorly cooked meat, particularly pork. Serologic tests include **complement-fixation, indirect hemagglutination, double diffusion, flocculation,** and **immunofluorescence tests.**

   a. The **bentonite flocculation test,** the most effective and specific test for the infection in humans, is positive after 3 weeks. A titer of 1:5 or greater is significant; a fourfold rise in antibody titer is diagnostic, and elevations may remain for 2–3 years.

   b. The **immunofluorescence test** is very sensitive, demonstrating antibody in pigs with slight infection.

   c. A **complement-fixation test** is available and can detect specific antibody earlier than 3 weeks of infestation.

   3. Toxocariasis is a parasitic infection primarily of preschool children who ingest dirt contaminated with larval eggs. The clinical syndrome, termed

visceral larva migrans, is associated with extraintestinal migration of larval nematodes through human tissue. The primary causative agent of visceral larva migrans is the common dog roundworm, *Toxocara canis,* but *Toxocara cati, Ascaris lumbricoides, Capillaria hepatica, Angrostrongylus cantonensis, Gnathostoma spinigerum,* and species of *Dirofilaria* also infect humans. Common symptoms include fever, pallor, seizures, cough, wheezing, and hepatomegaly associated with eosinophilia, hyperglobulinemia, and elevation in isohemagglutinin (anti-A, anti-B erythrocyte antibody) titers. Because eggs rarely appear in the feces, a definitive diagnosis is made by the demonstration of specific antibody in serum. Three serologic tests are available.

  a. The **enzyme-linked immunosorbent assay (ELISA),** a sensitive test, is the most commonly used test in the United States.

  b. The **bentonite flocculation test** is measured with antigen prepared from adult *T. canis* worms. It has poor specificity.

  c. The **indirect hemagglutination test** is about 66% sensitive but has poor specificity.

C. Serologic diagnosis of trematode and cestode disease

  1. Clonorchiasis and fascioliasis are caused by the liver flukes *Clonorchis* and *Fasciola,* which are often asymptomatic clinically. Abdominal pain and diarrhea may occur. Several serologic tests for these diseases are employed, including **complement-fixation, indirect hemagglutination, and immunoelectrophoresis, latex agglutination, and indirect immunofluorescence.**

  2. Paragonimiasis is a chronic pulmonary infection caused by flukes living in the human lung. Precipitin tests and complement-fixation tests are of limited usefulness because of cross-reactions with other trematode infections.

  3. Schistosomiasis is an acute or chronic illness associated with trematodes (flukes) of the genus *Schistosoma.* The diagnosis is most often made by finding eggs in the urine *(S. hemaetobium)* or stools *(S. mansoni* and *japonicum).*

  a. The **immunofluorescence test,** using cryostat sections of adult worm antigen, is the most sensitive technique.

  b. The **bentonite flocculation test** shows a sensitivity of 70% with sera from patients with proved schistosomiasis. There is a 15% false-positive rate.

  c. A **radioimmunoassay** is currently available and appears to be more sensitive than the other serologic tests.

  4. Although **cysticercosis** is a worldwide disease in humans, associated with migration of larval forms of certain cestodes to muscles, central nervous system, eyes, and other sites, there is no readily available serologic test. CF, IHA, and double immunodiffusion reactions have been used. Recently, CEP, IE, and IF have been used. An **indirect hemagglutination antibody test** is available at the Centers for Disease Control. The results are positive in 85% of patients with proved disease. A significant titer is 1:32. Cross-reactions with *Echinococcus* can occur.

  5. Echinococcosis is caused by *Echinococcus granulosus,* a tapeworm parasite of dogs and goats. Humans are infected by ingestion of the cestode eggs. The serologic tests of choice in this disease are the **latex agglutination, indirect hemagglutination, immunofluorescence,** and **immunoelectrophoresis** tests. All have a high degree of sensitivity. A titer of 1:32 is significant. An IHA titer of 1:256 is positive in people with hepatic cysts. These tests are performed by the Centers for Disease Control.

XII. Diagnosis of congenital intrauterine infection. Maternal viral and parasitic infections during pregnancy can incidentally infect the fetus and persist for long periods of time. Such intrauterine infections include rubella, cytomegalovirus, *Herpesvirus hominis,* syphilis, and toxoplasmosis. These infections can range from a silent, subclinical course to a syndrome with multiple-organ involvement at birth or later. The immune response by the infant is reflected in the cord blood predominantly as

IgM antibody. Levels of IgM in cord blood greater than 20 mg/dl are elevated and suggest intrauterine infection. However, IgM elevation in cord blood may result from maternal blood contamination and a repeat determination of the IgM concentration in a sample from the newborn is required.

A. The diagnosis of **congenital rubella** is suggested by a history of serologically proved rubella or a rubellalike rash during the first trimester of pregnancy, together with associated clinical manifestations of rubella in the infant at birth (e.g., microcephaly, cataracts, congenital heart disease, hepatosplenomegaly). The diagnosis is confirmed by the following:

   1. Isolation of the virus by culture of the anterior nares, urine, or both.

   2. A cord IgM level of 20 mg/dl or greater.

   3. **Hemagglutination-inhibition** antibody titers measure passively acquired maternal IgG antibodies. If a child has congenital rubella, the antibody titer can remain elevated after 6 months of age.

   4. Rubella IgM antibody titers are short lived and often disappear during the first year of life. The presence of rubella IgM antibodies in early infancy indicates rubella infection.

B. Congenital cytomegalovirus

   1. The diagnosis is best made by culture of fresh urine or pharyngeal swab.

   2. Paired cord and postpartum sera for cytomegalovirus antibody titers indicate active disease if a fourfold rise in titer occurs. A fall in titer indicates passive maternal antibody.

   3. Cord cytomegalovirus serologic tests are experimental.

C. Herpesvirus hominis

   1. Skin lesions should be cultured for the virus.

   2. A fourfold rise in acute and convalescent antibody titers is considered significant. A fourfold decrease indicates the presence of passive maternal antibody.

D. The diagnosis of **congenital syphilis** can be made if typical clinical signs are present (rhinitis, rash, anemia, and hepatosplenomegaly). Without these signs, reactive VDRL and FTA-ABS tests in cord blood (IgG antibody) may signify passive maternal antibody (in such a case the cord serum may be lower in titer than the maternal serum). Treatment of the asymptomatic infant can be delayed and the VDRL repeated in 1 month to look for a fourfold or greater rise in titer, which indicates infection in the infant. An IgM–FTA-ABS test, measuring infant IgM antibody to syphilis, is currently not a standard test.

   1. Elevated **VDRL** and **FTA-ABS** titers on cord blood cannot differentiate maternal and infant infection.

   2. The **cord IgM antibody test** for syphilis infection in the infant is experimental and not in routine use as yet. If the mother has reactive VDRL and FTA-ABS tests and has no history of therapy or has had inadequate therapy, a lumbar puncture should be performed on the infant. If the CSF-VDRL is positive, the infant should receive therapy for central nervous system syphilis.

   3. If the diagnosis is suspected but not proved, serial VDRL titers should be done monthly for 3 months. If a fourfold rise in VDRL occurs, the infant should be treated with penicillin.

E. Congenital toxoplasmosis is the result of acute infection, often asymptomatic, acquired by the mother during pregnancy. The lowest incidence occurs during the first trimester; the highest in the third trimester. A positive Sabin-Feldman dye test or indirect fluorescent antibody test in the serum of a neonate can represent passively acquired maternal IgG antibody and can persist for 6–12 months. The diagnosis of congenital toxoplasmosis is based on the clinical findings of the disease and the following serologic criteria:

   1. A cord serum IgM antibody titer 20 mg/dl or greater.

   2. Persistent high antibody titers with the indirect fluorescent antibody test on serial testing.

   3. An elevated IgM-IFA test titer equal to or greater than 1:2 in the absence of a placental leak.

Table 18-5. Interpretation of the Weil-Felix test used
in the diagnosis of rickettsial disease

Group	Rickettsial disease	OX-19	OX-2	OXK
I	Louse-borne typhus	3 +	1 +	0
	Murine typhus	3 +	1 +	0
II	Rocky Mountain spotted fever	3 +	1 +	0
	Tick typhus	3 +	3 +	0
	Rickettsialpox	0	0	0
III	Scrub typhus	0	0	3 +
IV	Q fever	0	0	0

Key: 0 = no response; 1 + = weakly positive; 3 + = strongly positive.

XIII. Diagnosis of rickettsial infection. Rickettsial species, which are small coccobacilli that function as intracellular parasites, are transmitted by arthropod bite and multiply in the endothelial cells of blood vessels. The Weil-Felix test is the most commonly employed test in the diagnosis of the rickettsial diseases (Table 18-5). Antibody response to OX-19, OX-2, and OXK strains of *Proteus vulgaris* can be evoked by epidemic, murine, or scrub typhus and the spotted fever group.

   A. The **complement-fixation test** is the single most useful test for all rickettsial diseases except scrub typhus. Complement-fixation antibody titers ($\geq 1:128$) usually appear in 7–14 days after the onset of disease and fall slowly to low levels, which can remain for years.

   B. The rickettsial **agglutination test** is more species-specific than the complement-fixation test. Agglutinins are more readily demonstrated, appear earlier, rise to higher titers, and decline more slowly to low levels that persist for years.

Selected Readings

CDC: Provisional Public Health Service Interagency. Recommendations for screening donated blood and plasma for antibody to the virus causing acquired immunodeficiency syndrome. *M.M.W.R.* 34:1, 1985.

Lennette, E. H., et al. (eds.). *Manual of Clinical Microbiology* (4th ed.). Washington, DC: American Society for Microbiology, 1985.

Lobel, H. O., and Kagan, I. G. Seroepidemiology of parasitic diseases. *Annu. Rev. Microbiol.* 32:329, 1978.

Rose, N. R., and Friedman, H. (eds.). *Manual of Clinical Immunology* (3rd ed.). Washington, DC: American Society for Microbiology, 1986.

Stites, D. P., et al. (eds.). *Basic and Clinical Immunology.* Los Altos, CA: Lange, 1984.

Voller, A., Bartlett, A., and Bidwell, D. E. The use of the enzyme-linked immunosorbent assay in the serology of viral and parasitic diseases. *Scand. J. Immunol.* 8:125, 1978.

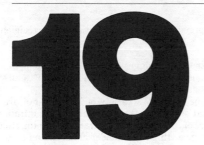

Immunizations and Immunoprophylaxis

Hemant H. Kesarwala

Immunization, either by naturally contacting the disease or by use of a vaccine, is a process that renders the body temporarily or permanently resistant to an infectious disease. The goal of **immunoprophylaxis,** using vaccines or hyperimmune sera, is to confer such resistance without producing the disease itself.

Immunoprophylaxis

I. **Active and passive immunization**

   A. **Active immunization** is accomplished by administration of an antigen to stimulate a normal immune response and provide protection against disease. It produces immunity and allows a booster response with repeat immunization. In diseases with long incubation periods (e.g., rabies), active immunization can also provide protection after exposure.

   B. **Passive immunization** introduces preformed serum antibodies titered against specific antigens to provide temporary immunity when active immunization is not possible. These sera, raised in humans or animals, provide immediate but variable, short-lived protection (1–6 weeks), allow no booster effect, and are often associated with adverse reactions. Passive immunization is primarily used for postexposure prophylaxis.

II. **Types of vaccines**

   A. **Bacterial vaccines** may contain live or killed organisms. In live vaccines the pathogenicity of the organism is altered, but its immunogenicity is retained. Organisms can also be pathogenic by virtue of toxin production, which can be neutralized by antitoxin antibodies. **Toxoids** are antigenic, nontoxic derivatives of toxins that produce antitoxin antibodies.

   B. **Viral vaccines** also may contain live or killed organisms. Live virus vaccines resemble the natural disease in that they produce longer immunity; killed vaccines require more frequent booster doses to maintain immunity. Care in the production of live virus vaccines is necessary to decrease the pathogenicity while retaining immunogenicity.

III. **Vaccine combinations.** Antigenic competition exists when two or more antigens are administered simultaneously. Diminished antibody response occurs to a weak antigen when it is given concurrently with a strong antigen. Vaccine combinations whose safety and efficacy have not been demonstrated in combination should not be routinely used. Single live virus vaccines should be given 1 month apart to avoid interference with the immune response (such interference has been documented between live measles and yellow fever vaccines).

   The following vaccine combinations have proved efficacy and safety. Triple oral poliovirus vaccine (TOPV); diphtheria-tetanus-pertussis (DTP); diphtheria-tetanus (DT) (for pediatric use); tetanus-diphtheria (Td) (for adult use); triple oral poliovirus vaccine and diphtheria-tetanus-pertussis; measles-mumps-rubella (MMR); mumps-rubella; and measles-mumps-rubella and the third or fourth dose of triple oral poliovirus vaccine. The simultaneous administration of MMR, DPT, and OPV produces satisfactory protective responses without increasing side effects. If the return of a vaccine recipient is doubtful, simultaneous administration of all vaccines appropriate to age (depending on the previous vaccination status of the recipient) is recommended.

IV. Techniques of administration

    A. For injectable vaccines, use disposable syringes and needles. Use a ⅝-in.-long, 25-gauge needle for subcutaneous or intradermal injection. For intramuscular injection, use a 1¼-in.-long, 22-gauge needle.

    B. Subcutaneous injections can be given in a variety of locations but are best given in the extensor or lateral surface of the upper arm. Give **intradermal** injections on the anterior surface of the forearm and **intramuscular** injections in the anterolateral aspect of the upper thigh or, in older children and adults, in the deltoid muscle. **Multiple injections** should be given at different sites. In the past, the upper, outer quadrant of the buttocks was often selected as the site for immunization administration. This area is no longer recommended, except for large volume administration (e.g., gamma globulin in some instances). When this site is used, care must be exercised in avoiding injury to the sciatic nerve; a site well into the upper outer mass of the gluteus maximus and away from the central region of the buttocks should be selected.

    C. Prior to the injection of the vaccine, the syringe plunger should be pulled back to see if blood appears; if so, the needle should be relocated.

    D. A separate, disposable needle and syringe should be used for each immunization. Used needles and syringes should be disposed of in specially labeled containers to prevent accidental inoculation or theft.

V. Vaccine storage. Improper handling of vaccine results in loss of potency and efficacy. Follow manufacturers' guidelines for vaccine storage and handling. The following are guidelines for commonly used vaccines.

    A. Unless otherwise specified, vaccines are stored at 2–8°C and should not exceed 10°C during shipment. **Do not freeze.**

    B. Store **trivalent oral poliovirus vaccine** in the freezer compartment. Frozen vaccine should go through no more than 10 freeze-thaw cycles. The thawing temperature should not exceed 8°C, and the total cumulative thawing period should not exceed 24 hours; if this period is exceeded, use the vaccine within 30 days (during this 30-day period the storage temperature should not exceed 8°C).

    C. Measles, mumps, and rubella vaccines should be protected from light. Use only the diluent supplied by the manufacturer for reconstitution because it is free of preservatives and antiviral substances, which can inactivate live attenuated viruses. Use as soon as possible after reconstitution.

VI. Side effects and adverse reactions. Most vaccination-associated side effects are mild and consist of **local** reactions (induration and pain at the injection site). Occasionally, massive local reactions occur, with marked induration, tenderness, and erythema. These reactions, especially with repeat doses of tetanus toxoid and typhoid vaccines, are abnormal, and repeat vaccinations generally should be avoided.

Systemic reactions include fever, arthralgia, arthritis, skin rashes, and fainting episodes. Low-grade fever is common but requires only symptomatic management and antipyretics. Allergic reactions include sensitivity to the vaccine itself or to egg proteins, antibiotics, or mercury preservatives contained in the vaccines. (For adverse reactions to specific vaccines, see Table 19-3).

In recent years, the use of pertussis vaccine has become controversial. An analysis of its cost-benefit ratio reveals that continued use of the current vaccine is appropriate when properly used. The following adverse reactions occurring after DPT or single antigen pertussis vaccination are **absolute contraindications** to further vaccination with a vaccine containing pertussis antigen: (1) allergic hypersensitivity (rare); (2) fever of 40.5°C (104.9°F) or greater, unexplained by another cause within 48 hours; (3) collapse or shocklike state (hypotonic-hyporesponsive episode) within 48 hours; (4) persistent, inconsolable crying or screaming lasting 3 hours or more or an unusual, high-pitched cry occurring within 48 hours; (5) convulsion(s) with or without fever occurring within 3 days (all children with convulsions, especially those with convulsions occurring within 4–7 days of receipt of DPT, should be fully evaluated to better clarify their medical and neurologic status before a decision is made whether to initiate or continue vaccination with DPT); and (6) encephalopathy occurring within 7 days (including severe alterations in consciousness with generalized or focal neurologic signs) (*M.M.W.R.* 34:27, 1985; and the American Academy of Pediatrics, *Report of the Committee on Infectious Diseases,* Evanston, IL, American Academy of Pediatrics, 1986. P. 272.)

VII. Precautions and contraindications. No vaccine is completely safe and free of adverse reactions to its use. It is given when the benefits of immunization outweigh the risks. Clinical situations that usually contraindicate immunization include the following:

A. Acute febrile illness. However, upper respiratory tract symptoms without fever are not a contraindication.

B. Patients with **immunodeficiency disorders** should not be given **live vaccines** until their immune status has been completely evaluated. Killed virus vaccines or toxoids may be given.

C. Patients taking **immunosuppressive agents** (corticosteroids, radiation therapy, antimetabolites, cytotoxic agents, alkylating agents, antilymphocyte serum) should not receive live vaccines.

D. Live vaccines should not be given to **pregnant women** or to patients with **leukemia, lymphoma,** or other related disorders.

E. Recent **gamma globulin therapy, blood transfusions,** or **plasma transfusions** are **temporary** contraindications. Immunizations can be given **8 weeks** after transfusion or gamma globulin administration.

F. Concurrent administration of single vaccines should not be given unless the **efficacy** and **safety** of the combination have been determined.

G. A history of prior **allergic reaction** to the same or a related vaccine contraindicates immunization to that particular vaccine. Patients with proved allergy to eggs, chicken, or duck (e.g., systemic reactions after egg ingestion) should not receive vaccines grown on **chick or duck embryos.** These vaccines include yellow fever and influenza. Although vaccines grown on **chick or duck fibroblast tissue cultures** (measles, mumps) are generally free of egg albumin and yolk components, isolated cases of anaphylaxis following administration of measles vaccine in egg-allergic individuals have been reported. In highly allergic patients, skin testing with the vaccine and desensitization in sensitive patients are indicated (J. J. Herman, R. Radin, and R. Schneiderman. Allergic reactions to measles (rubeola) vaccine in patients hypersensitive to egg protein. *J. Pediatr.* 102:196, 1983.)

In suspected cases of allergy to proteins used for growing the virus, an alternative source of the vaccine can be used (if available). Alternatively, skin testing for vaccine sensitivity can be done.

1. Test allergic patients with the vaccine (1:10 dilution in normal saline) using a scratch or prick technique. Wait 20 minutes and observe for a wheal-and-flare reaction (see Chap. 2 for skin testing techniques).

2. If there is no reaction, perform intradermal testing with 0.02 ml of a 1:100 dilution.

3. If there is no reaction to the 1:100 dilution, use 0.02 ml of a 1:10 dilution intradermally.

4. If no reactions occur, the vaccine can be given. (Carefully observe the patient for 30 minutes after full dose is given.)

VIII. Pregnancy and immunization

A. Avoid administration of live virus vaccines (measles, smallpox, rubella, poliovirus, mumps, and yellow fever) in pregnant women. In rare circumstances (unavoidable exposure during foreign travel), **yellow fever** vaccine can be given.

B. Inactivated viral vaccines (rabies and influenza) can be given during pregnancy when there are specific indications: bite of an animal with proved rabies or heavy exposure to influenza in a patient with cardiac or respiratory disease. Tetanus and diphtheria toxoids can be given during pregnancy and are recommended for the nonimmunized.

    C. A child with a pregnant mother can receive **all** immunizations, including live virus vaccines. A mother's pregnancy does not contraindicate immunization o her child.

IX. Immunization schedules for infants and for older children not immunized in in fancy appear in Tables 19-1 and 19-2, respectively. These schedules are appropriate for premature and low-birth-weight infants and can be given during any season of the year.

X. Immunizations in the adult. Adequate immunization in the pediatric age group, followed by a booster of tetanus-diphtheria (adult type) every 10 years, constitutes adequate adult immunization. No other immunization is required routinely. The schedule in Table 19-2 can be modified for use in the adult with no previous immunizations or history of naturally acquired disease.

XI. Immunization for foreign travel. The majority of United States citizens who travel abroad do not need additional immunizations if their routine immunization statu is up-to-date according to the requirements of the United States Public Health Service. No vaccinations are required for travel in Europe, Canada, Mexico, Australia, New Zealand, and the Caribbean or when returning from these countries to the United States. However, standards of health care and hygiene can vary considerably in the countries of Africa, Asia, South or Central America, the South Pacific, and the Middle and Far East. Travel to these areas requires individual consideration along the following guidelines:

    A. Know the **immunization requirements** of each country. Obtain this information from the Centers for Disease Control's publication "Health Information for International Travel" (revised annually; can be purchased from the Superintendent of Documents, U.S. Printing Office, Washington, DC 20402) and local or state health departments. If you have questions, call the Centers for Disease Control (Atlanta, GA) or the consulate of the country in question.

    B. Immune serum globulin (ISG, gamma globulin) administration is recommended for hepatitis A exposure for travelers who visit rural areas of developing countries and other areas where the risk of hepatitis is increased. This is repeated at 6 months. Residence for more than 1 year in such areas results in subclinical infection and active immunity, so that ISG is no longer required.

    C. Consider not only the countries on the itinerary but also the order in which they are visited and the areas of the country to be visited (rural versus urban).

    D. Plan ahead to allow for adequate time for vaccination and obtaining the required international certificates of vaccination.

XII. Interruption of an immunization schedule does not interfere with the final immunity achieved. This includes the primary immunization of infancy. **Do not start the**

Table 19-1. Recommended immunization schedule for normal infants and children

Age	Vaccine
2 mo	DTP, TOPV
4 mo	DTP, TOPV
6 mo	DTP (TOPV optional)
15 mo	Measles,* rubella, mumps
18 mo	DTP, TOPV
24 mo	HBPV
4–6 yr	DTP, TOPV
14–16 yr	Td (repeat every 10 yr)

Key: DTP = diphtheria-tetanus-pertussis; TOPV = trivalent oral poliovirus; Td = tetanus-diphtheria vaccine (adult type); HBPV = *Haemophilus* b polysaccharide vaccine.
*A tuberculin test can be administered prior to or simultaneously with measles vaccine.
Source: American Academy of Pediatrics. Recommended Schedule for Active Immunization of Normal Infants and Children. 1986 Redbook. With permission.

Table 19-2. Recommended primary immunizations
for children not immunized in early infancy

Age	Vaccine
Less than 7 yr old	
First visit	DTP, TOPV, MMR (if ≥ 15 mo old), tuberculin test
Interval after first visit:	
1 mo	HBPV (for children 24–60 mo)
2 mo	DTP, TOPV
4 mo	DTP, TOPV (optional)
10–16 mo or preschool	DTP, TOPV (TOPV not given if third dose given earlier)
At age 14–16 yr	Td (repeat every 10 yr)
7 yr old or older	
First visit	Td, TOPV, MMR, tuberculin test
Interval after first visit:	
2 mo	Td, TOPV
8–14 mo	Td, TOPV
At age 14–16 yr	Td (repeat every 10 yr)

Key: DTP = diphtheria-tetanus-pertussis vaccine; TOPV = trivalent oral poliovirus vaccine; Td = tetanus-diphtheria vaccine (adult type); HBPV = *Haemophilus* b polysaccharide vaccine; MMR = mumps, measles, rubella. See Table 19-3 regarding polio immunization in adults.
Source: American Academy of Pediatrics. Primary Immunization for Children Not Immunized in Early Infancy. 1986 Redbook. With permission.

series again. The remainder of the schedule can be completed regardless of the length of interruption.

Vaccines for Active Immunizations

Vaccines currently available for active immunization are summarized in Table 19-3. Dosage, route of administration, efficacy, and side effects are listed.
Vaccines in various stages of development are available from the Centers for Disease Control for special purposes.

Agents for Passive Immunoprophylaxis

I. **Human immune serum globulin (ISG) (gamma globulin)**
   A. **Preparations for intramuscular administration.** The antibody-rich fraction of pooled plasma from normal donors consists mainly of IgG antibodies and traces of immunoglobulins IgM and IgA and other serum proteins. The IgG concentration is 165 mg/ml (16.5% solution). Immune serum globulin preparations are stored at 2–8°C. **Do not freeze.**
      1. Give **intramuscularly** deep into a large muscle mass with an 18- or 20-gauge needle. Avoid inadvertent intravenous administration. Ordinarily, do not give more than 5.0 ml in one site in an adult or large child (lesser amounts, e.g., 1.0–3.0 ml for small children and infants). No more than 20 ml should be given at one time, even in an adult. Do not give to patients with severe thrombocytopenia or any coagulation disorder that precludes intramuscular injection. Normal dosage guidelines according to the specific indications for treatment are given in Table 19-4.

Table 19-3. Vaccines for active immunization

Disease	Vaccine	Route	Dose[a]	Efficacy	Indications	Side effects
Diphtheria	*DTP*, *DT*, *dT* (toxoid)	IM	3 primary, 1 booster (0.5 ml/dose)	Excellent	Routine immunization	Local pain, tenderness
Tetanus	*DTP*, *DT*, or *dT* (toxoid)	IM	3 primary, 1 booster (0.5 ml/dose)	Excellent	Routine immunization Booster every 5 yr for "tetanus-prone" wounds (e.g., puncture wounds, neglected wounds, necrotizing wounds)	Local pain, tenderness
Pertussis	*DTP* (inactivated bacteria)	IM	3 primary, 1 booster (0.5 ml/dose)	Fair to good	Routine immunization Not given after 6 yr of age except in exceptional circumstances	**Commonly,** local induration, pain, fever. **Rarely,** high fever, prolonged crying, convulsions, encephalopathy, shocklike state or thrombocytopenia purpura. **Do not repeat dose after severe reactions** (see p. 408)

		Route	Dose	Efficacy	Recommendations	Reactions
Rubeola (measles)	MMR (Live attenuated virus chick embryo)	SC	1 dose (0.5 ml)	Very good	Routine immunization Patients who may have received inactivated vaccine (1962–1968 in United States) should receive live vaccine. If given immediately after exposure, it may provide some protection.	Mild fever, rash Rarely, anaphylaxis in egg-sensitive individuals
Rubella (German measles)	MMR (Live attenuated virus—human diploid cell cultures)	SC	1 dose (0.5 ml)	Very good	Routine immunization Contraindicated in pregnancy When given to women of childbearing age, a medically acceptable method of contraception is needed for 3 mo after pregnancy has been ruled out.	Commonly, fever and rash; less commonly, arthralgia, arthritis, lymphadenopathy, headache in adolescents and adults; rarely, peripheral neuritis–like symptoms
Smallpox (variola)	Live attenuated vaccinia virus (calf lymph or chick embryo)	Intradermal	1 drop	Very good	Not routinely recommended For exposed laboratory workers Vaccine not available for civilian use	Local induration is common. Rarely, encephalitis, vaccinia necrosum, or eczema vaccination occurs.

Table 19-3. (continued)

Disease	Vaccine	Route	Dose[a]	Efficacy	Indications	Side effects
Yellow fever	Live attenuated virus (chick embryo)	SC	1 dose	Very good	Recommended for travel to endemic areas	In 5–10% of recipients, mild headache, myalgia, and low-grade fever; contraindicated in egg-sensitive persons
Mumps	*MMR* (Live attenuated virus—chick embryo)	SC	1 dose (0.5 ml)	Very good	Routine immunization for young children or susceptible persons nearing puberty	Local pain, redness, and induration are uncommon. Rarely, fever or parotitis occurs.
Poliomyelitis	Trivalent oral (OPV) Live attenuated virus (types I, II, III) grown on monkey kidney	PO	3 primary (0.5 ml/dose), 1 booster	Very good	Routine immunization for young children and adolescents (to age 18) Immunization in adults (e.g., foreign travel, epidemic) only after explanation of risks (for previously nonimmunized adults, inactivated vaccine [IPV] indicated)	Risk of paralytic poliomyelitis is 1 in 10 million after OPV (increased risk in adults). Risk of paralytic poliomyelitis in a nonimmunized person with close contact (fecal contamination) with a current (1–2 wk) OVP recipient is 1 in 6 million (increased in immunodeficiency patients).

| Inactivated poliovirus (IPV) | SC | 4 primary doses, first 3 at intervals of 1–2 mo, fourth after 6–12 mo
Booster every 4–5 yr | Very good | Routine immunization for susceptible persons over 18 yr or maintenance of immunity (booster) in previous recipients of IPV. Use in susceptible adults for foreign travel to endemic areas (4 wk before departure), health workers, household exposure to current OPV recipient (relative indication after evaluation of risk), pregnancy, and immunodeficiency with increased risk of exposure. | Hypersensitivity to antibiotics in the vaccine (neomycin and streptomycin) |

Table 19-3. (continued)

Disease	Vaccine	Route	Dose[a]	Efficacy	Indications	Side effects
Rabies	Inactivated virus (human diploid cell vaccine [HDCV])	IM	Preexposure: 1 ml on first day of treatment and repeat doses at 7 and 28 days Postexposure: 1 ml on first day of treatment and repeat doses at 3, 7, 14, and 28 days	Good	Each rabies exposure must be considered individually: species of animal; circumstances of bite; vaccination status of animal; and presence of rabies in the area. **Preexposure** prophylaxis only for occupationally exposed persons (veterinarians, animal handlers, spelunkers, etc.) and persons traveling abroad and exposed to field conditions.	**HDCV vaccine:** local reactions; fever; nausea, headache, dizziness, and systemic reactions including hives
Tuberculosis	**BCG**, live attenuated mycobacteria	Intradermal	1 dose Newborns, 0.05 ml Older children, 0.10 ml	Fair to good	For high-risk groups with negative PPD and in presence of endemic exposure **Do not give** to immunoincompetent or pregnant patients.	**Commonly,** local ulceration, regional adenopathy **Rarely,** osteomyelitis and dissemination

Typhoid	Inactivated bacteria	SC	2 doses at 4-wk intervals (adult, 0.5 ml; children, 0.25 ml)	Fair to good	Recommended only for travel to endemic area or exposure to a **household** contact. Addition of paratyphoid not required	Local reaction and pain, headache, malaise, and fever
Cholera	Inactivated bacteria	SC or IM	2 doses, 1 wk apart (0.2–0.5 ml/dose)	Fair	May need for international travel	Local induration, malaise, fever, headache
Influenza	Inactivated virus vaccine (whole virion or subvirion)	SC or IM	Age 6–35 mo, 2 doses (subvirion only), 4 or more wk apart[b] Age 3–12 yr, 2 doses (subvirion only), 4 or more wk apart[b] > 12 yr, 1 dose (0.5 ml), whole or subvirion	Good	Antigenic composition varies each year; for high-risk groups (≥ 65 years, chronic cardiac, pulmonary, or neurologic disease) Contraindicated in egg-sensitive patients	**Commonly,** local erythema, induration, fever, malaise, neuralgia **Rarely,** Guillain-Barré syndrome
Meningococcus	Polysaccharide vaccine Quadravalent (A, C, Y, W135)	SC	1 dose	Good	For military recruits, in epidemic situations and high-risk groups (e.g., anatomic or functional asplenia), and in hyperendemic areas.	Localized erythema for 1–2 days
Plague	Inactivated *Yersinia pestis* organisms	IM	3 doses at 4-wk intervals (0.5, 0.5, and 0.2 ml)	Fair	For occupational exposure to potentially infected rodents or travel to Vietnam, Cambodia, or Laos	Mild pain, erythema, induration, fever, headache, sterile abscesses

Table 19-3. (continued)

Disease	Vaccine	Route	Dose[a]	Efficacy	Indications	Side effects
Pneumococcus	Multivalent vaccine (23 serotypes)	SC	0.5 ml	Good	For high-risk groups (e.g., SS disease, splenectomy)	Erythema and mild pain locally
Haemophilus influenzae infections	*Haemophilus* b polysaccharide (HBPV)	SC	0.5 ml	Good (above 2 yr of age) Fair (18–24 yr) Ineffective (below 18 mo)	Routine immunizations beyond 24 mo (children at 18 mo with high risk of disease, e.g., day care attendance)	Fever, local reactions
Hepatitis B	Hepatitis B vaccine (plasma-derived)	IM (deltoid preferred site of injection)	3 doses, 10 μg/dose (< 10 yr of age), 20 μg/dose (> 10 yr of age); second and third doses 1 and 6 mo after first dose	Very good	High-risk groups: patients often exposed to blood products, health care workers, homosexuals, percutaneous drug users, hemodialysis patients, those with a large no. of heterosexual contacts	Local soreness
Hepatitis B	Hepatitis B vaccine (recombinant)	Same as plasma-derived vaccine (anterolateral thigh in children)	3 doses, 5 μg/dose (< 10 yr of age), 10 μg/dose (> 10 yr of age); second and third doses 1 and 6 mo after first dose	Same as plasma-derived vaccine	Same as plasma-derived vaccine	Local soreness

[a] See Tables 19-1 and 19-2 for primary immunization schedules.

[b] Check package insert for dose recommendations of each vaccine after initial immunization of 2 doses. Subsequent yearly immunization is usually accomplished by 1 dose.

Table 19-4. Indications for dosage of standard human immune serum globulin

Disease	Goal	Dose	Comments
Antibody deficiency (IgG)	Treatment	1.4 ml/kg initially, then 0.7 ml/kg every 2–4 wk	For patient comfort, divide and give at different sites.
Hepatitis A	Prevention after exposure	0.02–0.04 ml/kg	Give as soon as possible after exposure (not indicated 2 wk after exposure).
	Prevention in continuous exposure	0.06–0.12 ml/kg; repeat in 4–6 mo	
Hepatitis B	Prevention	0.12 ml/kg, repeated in 1 mo; for infants, 0.6 ml/kg	Use only if hepatitis B immune globulin is unavailable.
Measles	Prevention	0.25 ml/kg	Give as soon after exposure as possible; give vaccine in 12 wk for permanent protection.
Rubella	Prevention	0.55 ml/kg	**Of limited value.** Obtain rubella titers to determine immunity and need for ISG.*

*Documented exposure in the first trimester of pregnancy in the nonimmune woman who refuses therapeutic abortion is the only indication for ISG.

2. There are no reports or evidence of transmission of the AIDS agent, human immunodeficiency virus, by immune serum globulin or specific (hyperimmune) immune serum globulins.

3. **Do not** use ISG for recurrent colds, asthma, or allergies unless a **proved IgG antibody deficiency** state coexists. Indiscriminate use of ISG can lead to sensitization and possible severe systemic reactions.

4. The **systemic side effects** of ISG administration include anaphylactoid reactions, especially with inadvertent intravenous injection (aggregates of IgG activate the complement cascade). **Local reactions** include pain and tenderness, sterile abscesses, muscle fibrosis, and possible sciatic nerve injury.

B. **Preparations for intravenous administration.** Because of limitations of standard gamma globulin given intramuscularly, efforts have been made to develop soluble intravenous gamma globulin products. Three intravenous gamma globulin preparations are currently available in the United States for replacement therapy of antibody deficiency states. Gamimune N (Cutter Biologicals) is a gamma globulin reduced by alkylation to render it suitable for intravenous use. Sandoglobulin (Sandoz) uses mild acid treatment at pH 4 to render the immunoglobulin free of anticomplementary activity while retaining its biologic properties. Gammagard (Travenol) is obtained by subjecting plasma to a series of filtration and adsorption procedures.

These products have been shown to provide adequate replacement therapy in immunoglobulin deficiency states (see Chap. 17). For certain preparations (con-

Table 19-5. Indications for and dosage of human hyperimmune serum immunoglobulins

Disease	Agent	Indications	Dosage	Comments
Hepatitis B	Hepatitis B immune globulin (HBIG)	For **prevention** after exposure (e.g., puncture with contaminated needle, splashing of infected blood onto mucous membranes, pipetting accident), give immediately and repeat dose in 28 days. For sexual contact, single dose within 14 days of sexual contact.	0.06 ml/kg in children (5 ml for an adult), 0.12 ml/kg to newborn of mother with hepatitis B or carrier of HbsAg	No value for **treatment** of ongoing infection; not generally recommended for hospital or school exposure. Large doses of HBIG (0.5 ml/kg) may be given if patient is transfused **(in retrospect)** with HbsAg blood.
Rabies	Rabies immune globulin (RIG)	After exposure, for wild carnivore bite, bat bite, and domestic animal bite when animal cannot be observed	20 IU/kg, one-half IM, one-half locally to bite site	Give rabies vaccine concurrently.
Rh hemolytic disease of newborn	Rh₀ (D) immune globulin (RhIG)	For prevention of sensitization of Rh₀ (D)-negative persons exposed to Rh-positive blood by full-term delivery, miscarriage, abortion, ectopic pregnancy, amniocentesis, abdominal trauma in second or third trimester, or transfusion accidents	After full-term pregnancy,[a] give 1 vial to mother. After miscarriages, etc. (before 12 wk of gestation), a smaller dose can be given (MICRhoGAM). After mismatched blood transfusion, give 1 vial for each 15 ml of blood transfused	Give within 72 hr. **Do not give to the infant.**
Tetanus	Tetanus immune globulin (TIG)	For **prevention** in nonimmunized persons For neglected wounds (> 24 hours) and for tetanus-prone wounds (e.g., wounds contaminated with animal excreta, puncture wounds, necrotizing wounds) in immunized persons	250–500 IU IM	Give alum-precipitated toxoid at same time but at different site. Complete immunization series in nonimmunized patients.

		For **treatment** of clinical tetanus	3000–6000 units IM. Infiltrate portion around wound.	In severe cases, intravenous equine antitoxin can be given. **Do not give TIG intravenously.**
Smallpox, vaccinia	Vaccinia immune globulin (VIG)	For prevention and modification in nonimmunized persons exposed to smallpox. For accidental vaccination or autoinoculation of eye, eczema vaccinatum, severe generalized vaccinia, and vaccinia necrosum. **Not indicated** for established smallpox infections, postvaccinia encephalitis, or hypersensitivity rashes after vaccination	0.3 ml/kg for smallpox or vaccinia exposure in susceptible patients; 0.6 ml/kg for vaccinia complications	For expert advice and help in obtaining VIG, consult Centers for Disease Control (404-329-3914 or after business hours, 404-329-2888)
Zoster, varicella (chickenpox)	Zoster immune globulin (ZIG)[b]	For **prevention** of chickenpox or herpes zoster in newborns of mothers with varicella and in exposed, high-risk, susceptible patients with leukemia, lymphoma, primary immunodeficiency, or taking immunosuppressive agents	125 units/10 kg; maximum, 625 units. Give within 72 hours of exposure.	**Of no value** in established varicella or zoster infections

[a] Consult *Physicians' Desk Reference* for specific indications and recommended dosage.
[b] Now distributed by the American Red Cross through 13 regional blood centers (see *Morbidity and Mortality Weekly Report* 30:2 (Jan. 23, 1981).

Table 19-6. Indications for and dosage of animal antisera and antitoxins

Disease	Agent	Indications	Dosage	Comments
Botulism	Trivalent ABE equine antitoxin, bivalent AB antitoxin, or type E antitoxin*	Give trivalent antitoxin to **symptomatic** patients immediately. Other agents can be used if the toxin type is known. **Prophylactic** use for patients who ingested food containing the toxin may be given	1 vial IV and 1 vial IM. Repeat in 2–4 hr as needed.	Antitoxin not ordinarily indicated in infant botulism.
Diphtheria	Equine diphtheria antitoxin	Give immediately to **symptomatic** patients. Use for routine prophylaxis is not recommended.	20,000–120,000 units IV, depending on toxicity and extent of disease	Asymptomatic, unimmunized household contacts should be given antibiotic prophylaxis and diphtheria toxoid and observed for 7 days.
Rabies	Equine antirabies serum	After exposure to wild carnivore bite, bat bite, and domestic animal bite when animal cannot be observed	40 IU/kg with infiltration of a portion of the serum locally	Use equine antiserum (40% have allergic reactions) only if human rabies immune globulin treatment will be delayed.
Black widow (*Latrodectus mactans*) spider bite	Equine black widow antiserum	Treatment immediately after exposure	1 vial (2.5 ml) IM; may repeat in 3 hr if necessary. In severe cases or in children under 12 give IV in 10–50 ml saline.	Anaphylaxis and serum sickness are common. Give supportive therapy; corticosteroids and calcium gluconate are helpful.

| Snakebite | Equine coral snake (*Micrurus fulvius*) antivenom
Equine *Crotalidae* (vipers) polyvalent antiserum | Treatment immediately after exposure | Give 2–15 or more vials (20–150 ml or more of antiserum) IV depending on severity of envenomation. | Anaphylaxis and serum sickness are common. |
| Tetanus | Equine tetanus antitoxin | For treatment and prophylactic use **only if human tetanus immune globulin is not available** | For **treatment:** 50,000 units. In severe clinical tetanus, give 100,000 units: 20,000 units IV and 80,000 units IM.
For prophylaxis, 3000–5000 units in a person who has had less than 2 doses of DPT or in an immunized person with wounds neglected for 24 hr or more and grossly contaminated | |

*Available from the Centers for Disease Control, Atlanta, GA.

sult package inserts), intravenous immunoglobulin has been used in idiopathic thrombocytopenic purpura (ITP) to increase platelet counts (see Chap. 15).

II. Hyperimmune serum immunoglobulins. Special ISG preparations, obtained from immunized or convalescing donors and standardized according to specific antibody content, are available for the prevention and treatment of specific infectious diseases (Table 19-5). The major advantage of human preparations is the diminished incidence of side effects compared with those from animal antisera. For best results, give these agents as soon as possible after exposure. The duration of protection is short-lived; give tetanus or rabies vaccine with the specific hyperimmune serum globulin.

III. Plasma transfusions. Fresh-frozen plasma for transfusion is available in units of 200–250 ml. The **indications** for plasma transfusion include the following: for volume expansion in shock; to supply immunoglobulins when immune serum globulins cannot be given (dose of 20 ml/kg/month); and to supply specific plasma factors in deficiency states, e.g., antihemophilic globulin in hemophilia and C1-esterase inhibitor in hereditary angioedema. (Dose must be individualized.)

The **advantages** of plasma are intravenous injection, which obviates the pain and discomfort of intramuscular injection, and supplementation of other plasma proteins (e.g., IgA, IgM, complement factors) not found in appreciable amounts in human immune serum globulin. **Disadvantages** include possible disease transmission, volume overload, possible sensitization to plasma proteins, and possible graft-versus-host reactions with nonirradiated plasma in T cell–deficient patients.

IV. Animal antisera and antitoxins

A. Use in situations **in which only** animal antisera are available, because of a high incidence of reactions as compared with human antisera. **Adverse immunologic reactions** to the administration of heterologous serum consist of anaphylaxis, exaggerated local reactions resembling Arthus reactions, and serum sickness. **Serum sickness,** which occurs in approximately 20% of patients who receive horse serum, is more likely with a higher dose of serum, is unpredictable by prior immunologic testing, and may be diminished in frequency and intensity by prophylactic treatment with antihistamines. Table 19-6 lists the available animal antisera and antitoxins, the indications for their use, and dosages.

B. Observe the following **precautions** for optimal safety:

1. Use only for **unequivocal** indications.

2. Obtain a **careful history** of previous allergic reactions to animal serum use. A positive history of sensitivity to horse dander is an indication of the need for extreme caution. Even in patients with no history of sensitivity, any administration of heterologous serum must be preceded by appropriate sensitivity tests.

3. First perform a scratch or prick test with a 1:100 dilution of serum (dilute with normal saline). If there is no reaction after 30 minutes, proceed to intradermal testing with 0.02 ml of a 1:1000 dilution of serum.

4. If the intradermal skin test is negative after 30 minutes, proceed with an intramuscular injection. A negative skin test, however, is not an absolute guarantee of the absence of sensitivity and does **not** obviate the need for caution. If the skin tests are positive, proceed to desensitization (see **7**).

5. If the serum is to be used intravenously, give as slowly as possible a preliminary dose of 0.5 ml of serum in 10 ml of saline or 5% glucose, and observe for reactions over one-half hour. If no reaction occurs, infuse a 1:20 dilution at a rate not to exceed 1 ml/minute. Observe the usual precautions against anaphylaxis (Chap. 10).

6. Be aware that animal antisera and antitoxins can also produce acute febrile reactions and delayed serum sickness–type reactions.

7. A **positive history** of systemic reactions or a **positive skin test reaction** to animal antisera indicates the need for **desensitization.**

   a. Have available a syringe loaded with epinephrine and a tourniquet. Start an intravenous infusion with normal saline. No single "desensitization" schedule is appropriate for all patients. Published recommendations can serve as guides for the desensitization procedure (American Academy of Pediatrics, *Report of the Committee on Infectious Diseases* (20th ed.) (the "Redbook"). Evanston, IL: American Academy of Pediatrics, 1986. Pp. 29–34).

b. If a reaction occurs at a given dose, and the heterologous serum is considered absolutely essential, the following measures are recommended:

(1) Treat with intramuscular epinephrine (0.3–0.5 ml 1:1000; 0.01 ml/kg in children).

(2) Wait 15–30 minutes.

(3) Use the dose that did not cause a reaction, and proceed carefully as before.

c. Pretreatment with antihistamines and corticosteroids may be beneficial but gives **no guarantee** that anaphylaxis will not occur. Methylprednisolone, 1–2 mg/kg, and diphenhydramine, 1.5 mg/kg (up to 50 mg), can be given parenterally 2 hours before the next desensitization dose.

Selected Readings

American Academy of Pediatrics, Report of the Committee on Infectious Diseases. Elk Grove Village, IL: American Academy of Pediatrics, 1986.

Prevention and control of influenza. (Recommendations of the Immunization Practices Advisory Committee, ACIP.) *M.M.W.R.** 35:317, 1986.

Update: Prevention of *Hemophilus influenzae* type B disease. (Recommendations of the Immunization Practices Advisory Committee, ACIP.) *M.M.W.R.* 35:170, 1986.

Diphtheria, tetanus, and pertussis: Guidelines for vaccine prophylaxis and other preventive measures. *M.M.W.R.* 34:405, 1985.

Meningococcal vaccines. (Recommendations of the Immunization Practices Advisory Committee, ACIP.) *M.M.W.R.* 34:255, 1985.

Polysaccharide vaccine for prevention of *Hemophilus influenzae* type B disease. *M.M.W.R.* 34:201, 1985.

Adult immunization. *M.M.W.R.* 33(Suppl.):15, 1984.

Feigin, R. D., and Cherry, J. D. (eds.). *Textbook of Pediatric Infectious Diseases*. Philadelphia: Saunders, 1987. (Two volumes.)

*Morbidity and Mortality Weekly Report is published weekly and can be obtained from the U.S. Department of Health and Human Services, Public Health Service, Centers for Disease Control, Atlanta, GA 30333. Refer to these reports for recent updates.

Appendixes

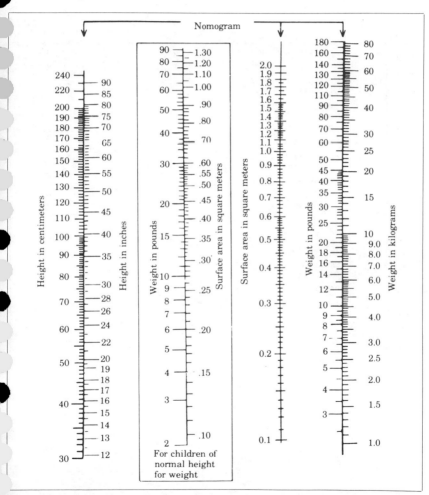

Surface area is indicated where a straight line connecting the height and weight intersects the surface area column; or, in a person of normal proportions, from weight alone (enclosed column). (From C. D. West. Electrolyte Imbalance and Parenteral Fluid Therapy. Procedures in use at Children's Hospital Medical Center, Cincinnati, OH.)

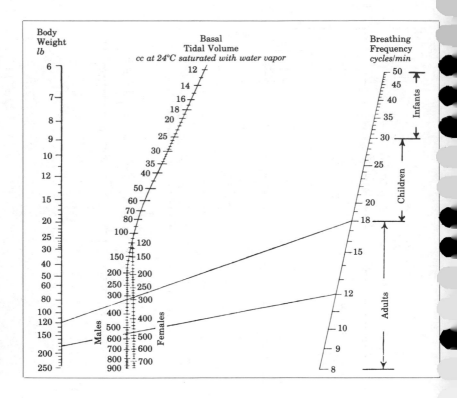

*Corrections to be applied to tidal volume as required: Daily activity, add 10%; fever, add 5% for each degree F above 99° (rectal); altitude, add 5% for each 2000 ft above sea level; tracheotomy and endotracheal intubation, subtract a volume equal to half the body weight. From E. P. Radford, et al. Clinical use of a nomogram to estimate proper ventilation during artificial respiration. Reprinted by permission of the *New England Journal of Medicine* (251:877, 1984).

A. Examination of Nasal Secretions

I. Collection of specimen. Instruct the patient to blow his or her nose into a piece of wax paper (6 × 6 in.). Place a glass microscope slide on top of the mucus, or apply and spread the mucus from the paper to the slide with a cotton-tipped applicator. Alternatively, place a cotton-tipped applicator into the anterior nasal cavity and leave in place for 2–3 minutes. Then remove and smear the adherent mucus on a glass microscope slide.

II. Staining of the nasal smear. Conjunctival mucus and sputum can be similarly stained.
- **A.** Allow the smear to air-dry.
- **B. Hansel's stain** (preferred for demonstration of eosinophils)
  1. Cover the slide with methyl alcohol and allow to dry
  2. Flood the slide with Hansel stain* (methanol 95%, eosin, methylene blue, glycerine 5%) and allow the stain to incubate for 30 seconds.
  3. Add a small volume of distilled water (5 drops) for 30 seconds (may mix by gentle blowing to dilute the stain, where a sheen of "oil" appears on the surface).
  4. Pour off the stain and wash with distilled water.
  5. Flood with methyl alcohol to decolor (until specimen appears to have a pale green color).
  6. Air-dry.
- **C. Wright's stain** (used alternatively)
  1. Flood the slide with Wright's stain (eosin and sodium bicarbonate diluted in methyl alcohol and added to methylene blue) and incubate for 2–3 minutes.
  2. Layer on phosphate buffer (pH 6.4) and blow gently to mix. Allow to stand for 2–3 minutes.
  3. Wash with distilled water.
  4. Air-dry.

III. Examination of the smear. Examine with a microscope under low power (100×) first to determine the adequacy of the specimen and the areas of interest. Then examine under a high-power lens and oil immersion (1000×). Count the number of eosinophils (pink cytoplasmic granules with blue, bilobed nuclei) and the total number of polymorphonuclear leukocytes (PMN) (which have pale-pink cytoplasm and blue, multilobed nuclei) in five separate fields. Express as the ratio of eosinophils to PMNs. Nasal epithelial cells have unlobulated, blue nuclei and abundant pale-blue cytoplasm.

IV. Interpretation
- **A.** If there are 10% or more eosinophils, allergic rhinitis is suggested.
- **B.** A predominance of PMNs suggests infection (eosinophils can be present in moderate amounts).
- **C.** Acellular specimens without predominance of eosinophils or PMNs suggest vasomotor rhinitis.

*Lide Laboratories, 515 Timberwyck, St. Louis, MO 63131.

B. Examination of Nasal or Conjunctival Epithelium Specimens

Alfredo A. Jalowayski and
Robert S. Zeiger

I. Collection of specimens. Instruct the patient to clear the nose of excess secretions. In infants, a rubber bulb may be used to aspirate excess mucus. Using a disposable plastic curette (e.g., Rhino-probe*) or a similar device, and under direct illumination and visualization of the nasal cavity, sample the medial or inferior portion of the inferior turbinate posteriorly, avoiding the anterior bulb area. Gently press the cupped tip of the probe on the mucosal surface and move outward 2–3 mm (see below). Repeat the motion twice and withdraw the probe without touching the nasal vestibule to prevent contamination. To obtain conjunctival specimens, invert the inferior lid, have the patient look up, and gently scrape the palpebral conjunctiva 1–2 mm with the same type of probe used to obtain mucosal epithelial cells. A topical ophthalmic anesthetic (e.g., Ophthetic†) can be used for the sensitive patient. The specimen is gently spread over a small area of a microscope slide and fixed quickly in a jar containing 95% ethyl alcohol for 1 minute or until stained.

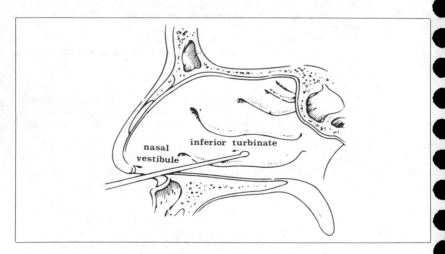

II. Staining of the epithelial specimens. Staining may be achieved with the Wright-Giemsa Dip Method as described below. Hansel's stain can be used if eosinophils are the only cells of interest. Wright's stain may be used for eosinophils and metachromatic cells with variable results. See Appendix II. A.

    A. Remove the slide(s) from the jar and drain excess alcohol, but do not allow the cells to air-dry.

    B. Dip the slide(s) in Wright-Giemsa (e.g., Volu-Sol*) stain for 10–15 seconds.

    C. Drain the excess stain, then dip the slide(s) in Volu-Sol buffer for 15–30 seconds.

*Synbiotics Corporation, San Diego, CA 92127.
†Allergan Pharmaceuticals, Inc., Irvine, CA 92715.

D. Drain the excess buffer, then dip the slide(s) in Volu-Sol Hematology Rinse for 4–5 seconds, using quick dips.

E. Drain the excess rinse and air-dry the specimens.

III. Examination of nasal and conjunctival cytograms. Examine with a microscope under low power (100×) first to determine the adequacy of the specimens and the areas of interest. Grade the cytogram under a high-power lens and oil immersion (1000×) quantitatively as the mean number of cells/10 high-power fields examined, or grade qualitatively, on a scale of 0 to 4+, as suggested in section IV. Normal epithelium consists of numerous epithelial cells (ciliated columnar, nonciliated columnar, goblet, and basal cells) stained light blue, and contains no eosinophils or metachromatic cells (basophils or mast cells); however, a few neutrophils and bacteria can usually be seen.

IV. Grading of nasal cytograms

Quantitative Analysis[a]

Grade[b]	Eosinophils, neutrophils	Metachromatic cells (basophils/mast cells)	Goblet cells[c]
0	0–1.0	0–0.3	
1+	1.1–5.0	0.4–1.0	
2+	6.0–15.0	1.1–3.0	
3+	16.0–20.0	3.1–6.0	
4+	>20.0	>6.0	

Qualitative Analysis[d]

Grade	Eosinophils, neutrophils, metachromatic cells (basophils/mast cells)
0	No cells seen
1+	Few cells seen
2+	Moderate number of cells seen
3+	Many cells seen
4+	Large number of cells seen

[a] Mean number of cells/10 high-power fields (1000×).
[b] Comparative reference for qualitative analysis.
[c] Ratio of goblet cells to epithelial cells, expressed as a percent. The presence of over 50% goblet cells on the nasal cytogram is considered increased.
[d] See relative numbers of cells in quanitative analysis above.

V. Interpreting nasal cytograms

Cellular type	Suggested disorder
Increased eosinophils[a]	Allergic rhinitis, eosinophilic non-allergic rhinitis (ENR) or non-allergic rhinitis with eosinophils (NARES), rhinitis associated with non-IgE-mediated asthma, aspirin sensitivity, Churg-Strauss syndrome, nasal polyps
Increased metachromatic cells (basophils/mast cells)	Conditions listed for increased eosinophils, nonallergic basophilic rhinitis, or primary nasal mastocytosis
Increased neutrophils[a] with:	
1. Intracellular bacteria	Infectious nasopharyngitis or sinusitis
2. Ciliocytophoria[b]	Viral upper respiratory tract infection (URI)

3. No bacteria	Viral URI, irritant rhinitis, or chemically induced rhinitis or sinusitis (or both), may be associated with eosinophils in allergic rhinitis
Increased goblet cells[c]	Allergic rhinitis, infectious rhinitis, or possibly vasomotor rhinitis

[a]1+ or greater quantitatively or qualitatively.
[b]Epithelial cells with clumping of chromatin material.
[c]Greater than 50%.

VI. Interpreting conjunctival cytograms

The presence of inflammatory cells within the conjunctival mucosa (superficial epithelial scraping) suggests certain disorders depending on the specific cell types present.

Cellular type	Suggested disorder
Eosinophils, metachromatic cells, (basophils/mast cells)	Allergic, vernal, or giant papillary conjunctivitis or keratoconjunctivitis
Neutrophils	Infectious (bacterial) or irritant conjunctivitis, may be associated with eosinophils in allergic conjunctivitis
Lymphocytes	Viral conjunctivitis

Total Eosinophil Count

The total eosinophil count determines the number of eosinophils/mm^3 of blood.

I. Technique

  A. Use fresh fingertip whole blood or oxalated whole blood (not over 4 hours old).
  B. Draw up blood to the 1.0 mark on a standard white cell pipette (alternatively, commercial kits* are available).
  C. Then draw up eosinophil diluting fluid (Phloxine diluting fluid, Pilot's solution, or Tannen's diluting fluid) to the 11.0 mark.
  D. Allow the pipette to stand for 15 minutes.
  E. Shake the pipette for 2–3 minutes.
  F. Discard the first 4 drops.
  G. Now add to **both** sides of a standard counting chamber. ("Adding to **both** sides of the counting chamber" means to add to the side used for the white cell count and also the side used for the red cell count.)
  H. Place the counting chamber on the stage of a microscope.
  I. Using the 10× (16-mm) objective, bring the cells into view. (It makes no difference which side of the counting chamber is used to start the count.)
  J. Scan several fields, and note that the eosinophils are red in color.
  K. The eosinophils are counted in the entire ruled area of the counting chamber (both sides).
  L. Add the counts from each side of the counting chamber.
  M. Divide the total count by 2 to get the average count on each side.
  N. Multiply the average count by 11, which **gives the total eosinophil count in cubic millimeters.** (The figure 11 represents two correction factors. First, the blood was diluted 1 in 10, dilution correction factor of 10. Second, the cells were counted in a volume of 0.9 mm^3, and the report is to be given as the number in 1.0 mm^3, a volume correction factor of 1.0:0.9. Multiplying the dilution correction factor of 10 by the volume correction factor of 1.0:0.9 gives the figure 11.)

II. Expected normal values

Age	Eosinophils/mm^3	
	Mean	Range
Newborn	400	20–850
One-year-old child	300	50–700
Adult	200	0–450

*Unopette, Becton-Dickinson and Co., Rutherford, NJ 07070

IV

The paper radioimmunosorbent test (PRIST) is a test system designed to quantitate the total amount of IgE antibody in blood samples. The test is a direct radioimmunoassay using paper disks as a solid phase. Anti-IgE, covalently coupled to the paper disk, is allowed to react with the IgE in the sample during the first incubation. After washing, a fixed amount of immunosorbent purified ^{125}I-labeled antibodies against IgE is added, forming a complex with the IgE molecules bound to the antibodies on the paper disk during the previous incubation. Bound and free radioactivity are separated by washing the disk. The radioactivity of the complex is then measured in a gamma counter. The amount of bound activity is directly proportional to the concentration of IgE antibody in the sample.

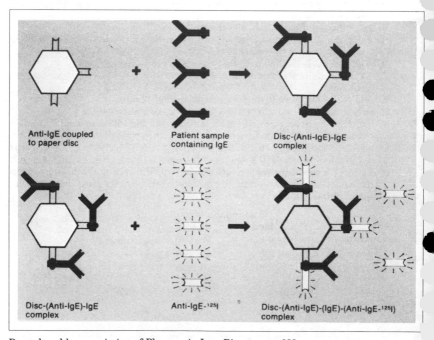

Reproduced by permission of Pharmacia Inc., Piscataway, NJ

V

A. Radioallergosorbent Test

The radioallergosorbent test (RAST) is a test system designed to quantitate the amount of circulating allergen specific IgE antibody in blood samples. The allergen of interest, covalently coupled to a paper disk, reacts with the specific IgE antibody in the patient's serum sample. After nonspecific IgE is washed away, radioactively labeled antibodies against IgE are added, forming a complex. The radioactivity of this complex is easily measured in a gamma counter. The more bound radioactivity that is found, the more specific IgE antibody is present in the sample. The counts are compared directly with the count rates obtained with reference samples run in parallel with the unknowns, thus enabling a classification of the test results. RAST scoring is usually divided into 6 classes, 0 and 1 to 5, corresponding to known standards with increasing numbers of counts. Class 0 is negative and classes 1 to 5 are increasingly positive with class 5 being the most significantly positive.

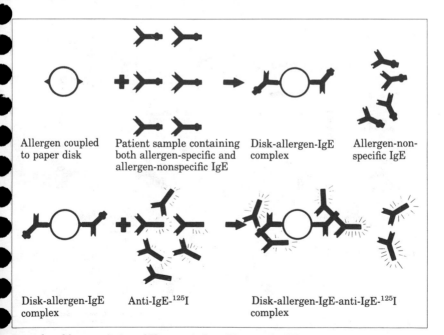

Allergen coupled to paper disk

Patient sample containing both allergen-specific and allergen-nonspecific IgE

Disk-allergen-IgE complex

Allergen-non-specific IgE

Disk-allergen-IgE complex

Anti-IgE-^{125}I

Disk-allergen-IgE-anti-IgE-^{125}I complex

Reproduced by permission of Pharmacia Inc., Piscataway, NJ

B. Enzyme-Linked Immunosorbent Assay (Enzyme RAST) Test

The enzyme-linked immunosorbent assay (enzyme RAST) is a test system designed to quantitate the amount of circulating allergen specific IgE antibody in blood samples. The allergen of interest, covalently coupled to a paper disk, reacts during the first incubation with the specific IgE antibodies in the patient's serum sample. After washing, which removes nonspecific IgE, a disk-allergen/IgE complex remains. Anti-IgE antibody conjugated with enzyme (e.g., β-galactosidase) is added and the complex disk-allergen/IgE/anti-IgE–enzyme is formed. Excess of enzyme-anti-IgE is removed by washing the disk. The enzyme is then released by a reducing substance (e.g., glutathione) and reacts with a substrate (e.g., o-nitrophenyl-β-galactosidase) to form a colored product. The amount of allergen-specific IgE antibody is then quantitated by the amount of colored product detected with a photometer and compared with reference samples run in parallel.

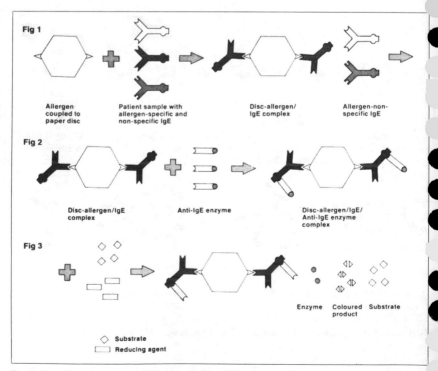

C. IgG-Radioallergo-sorbent Test (IgG-RAST)

The IgG-radioallergosorbent (IgG-RAST) test is a test system designed to measure the amount of allergen-specific IgG antibody in the circulating blood. The principal application of this test is in the determination of specific IgG-blocking antibody produced in Hymenoptera-sensitive individuals on venom immunotherapy.

The allergen of interest, covalently coupled to a paper disk, reacts with the specific IgG antibodies in the patient's sample. After washing, a fixed amount of immunosorbent purified ^{125}I-labeled anti-IgG antibody is added, forming a complex with the IgG antibodies bound to the allergen on the paper disk during the previous incubation. Bound and free radioactivity is separated by washing the disk. The radioactivity of the complex is then measured in a gamma counter. The amount of bound activity is proportional to the concentration of specific IgG antibodies in the sample, which is compared with reference samples run in parallel.

Reproduced by permission of Pharmacia Inc., Piscataway, NJ.

D. IgE Fluoroallergosorbent (IgE FAST*) Test

The IgE fluoroallergosorbent (IgE FAST) test is an assay system designed to quantitate the amount of allergen specific IgE antibody in the circulating blood. The allergen of interest is immobilized on the inner surface of a microtitration well. The patient's serum is added to the well and allowed to incubate. The well is then washed, leaving allergen-specific IgE antibodies bound to the immobilized allergen. An enzyme labeled (alkaline phosphatase) anti-IgE antibody (monoclonal antihuman IgE mouse antibody) is added to the well that binds to the patient's IgE antibody. The well is washed and a fluorogenic substrate (4-methylumbelliferyl phosphate) is added with a buffer and is caused to fluoresce by enzyme activation. The amount of allergen-specific IgE antibody is then quantitated by the amount of fluorescence detected with a fluorometer and compared with reference samples.

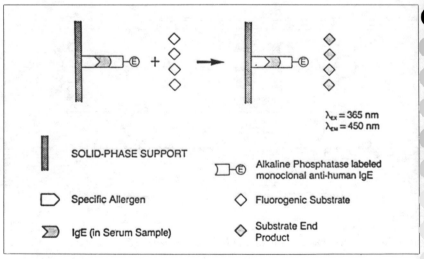

$\lambda_{ex} = 365$ nm
$\lambda_{em} = 450$ nm

SOLID-PHASE SUPPORT

Alkaline Phosphatase labeled monoclonal anti-human IgE

Specific Allergen

Fluorogenic Substrate

IgE (in Serum Sample)

Substrate End Product

From Y. G. Tsay, et al. IgE fluoroallergosorbent (IgE FAST) test: Concept and clinical applications. *Immunol. Allergy Pract.* 6:169, 1984. With permission.

*Allergenetics, Mountain View, CA 94042.

E. Multiple Allergen RAST Variants

Systems are available commercially to detect multiple allergens with a single test particle. These systems utilize solid particles with multiple allergens fixed to a single particle surface and use an anti-IgE detection method similar to RAST. Individual systems differ in the solid particle and the type of tracer attached to the anti-IgE protein. Two commercially available systems are the multiple allergosorbent test (MAST)*, which utilizes cellulose threads contained in a pipette chamber as the solid phase and a chemiluminescent assay for IgE detection, and the Ventrex allergosorbent test (VAST) Allergy Microscreen†, which utilizes a paper disk as the solid phase and an enzyme-visable product for IgE detection. Manufacturers claim results similar to RAST testing for allergen-specific IgE detection.

*MAST Immunosystems, Mountain View, CA 94043.
† Ventrex Laboratories, Inc., Portland, ME 04103.

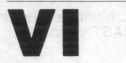

Age	Geometric mean (units/ml)	Geometric mean + 1 SD	Geometric mean + 2 SD
0 days	0.22	0.53	1.28
6 wk	0.69	2.05	6.12
6 mo	2.68	6.60	16.26
12 mo	3.49	7.29	15.22
2 yr	3.03	9.46	29.48
3 yr	1.80	5.51	16.86
4 yr	8.58	24.31	68.86
7 yr	12.89	45.60	161.32
10 yr	23.66	116.20	570.61
14 yr	20.07	62.58	195.18
Adults	14.00	41.30	122.00

Source: Adapted from N. I. M. Kjellman, S. G. O. Johansson, and A. Roth. Serum IgE levels in healthy children quantified by a sandwich technique (PRIST). *Clin. Allergy* 6:51, 1976.

Levels of Immunoglobulins in Sera of Normal Subjects, By Age

Age	IgG		IgM		IgA		Total immunoglobulin	
	mg/dl	Percent of adult level	mg/dl	Percent of adult level	mg/dl	Percent of adult level	mg/dl	Percent of adult level
Newborn	1031 ± 200*	89 ± 17	11 ± 5	11 ± 5	2 ± 3	1 ± 2	1044 ± 201	67 ± 13
1–3 mo	430 ± 119	37 ± 10	30 ± 11	30 ± 11	21 ± 13	11 ± 7	481 ± 127	31 ± 9
4–6 mo	427 ± 186	37 ± 16	43 ± 17	43 ± 17	28 ± 18	14 ± 9	498 ± 204	32 ± 13
7–12 mo	661 ± 219	58 ± 19	54 ± 23	55 ± 23	37 ± 18	19 ± 9	752 ± 242	48 ± 15
13–24 mo	762 ± 209	66 ± 18	58 ± 23	59 ± 23	50 ± 24	25 ± 12	870 ± 258	56 ± 16
25–36 mo	892 ± 183	77 ± 16	61 ± 19	62 ± 19	71 ± 37	36 ± 19	1024 ± 205	65 ± 14
3–5 yr	929 ± 228	80 ± 20	56 ± 18	57 ± 18	93 ± 27	47 ± 14	1078 ± 245	69 ± 17
6–8 yr	923 ± 256	80 ± 22	65 ± 25	66 ± 25	124 ± 45	62 ± 23	1112 ± 293	71 ± 20
9–11 yr	1124 ± 235	97 ± 20	79 ± 33	80 ± 33	131 ± 60	66 ± 30	1334 ± 254	85 ± 17
12–16 yr	946 ± 124	82 ± 11	59 ± 20	60 ± 20	148 ± 63	74 ± 32	1153 ± 169	74 ± 12
Adults	1158 ± 305	100 ± 26	99 ± 27	100 ± 27	200 ± 61	100 ± 31	1457 ± 353	100 ± 24

*One standard deviation.

Source: Adapted from E. R. Stiehm, and H. H. Fudenberg. Serum levels of immune globulins in health and disease: A survey. *Pediatrics* 37:715, 1966. Copyright American Academy of Pediatrics, 1966.

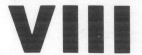

VIII

**Important Pollens
and Molds in
the United States
and Canada**

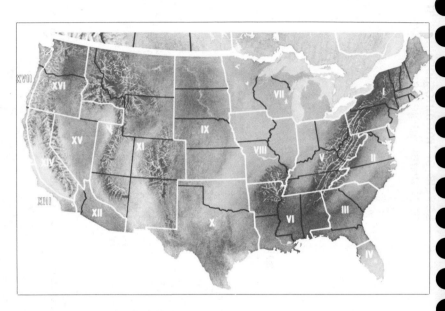

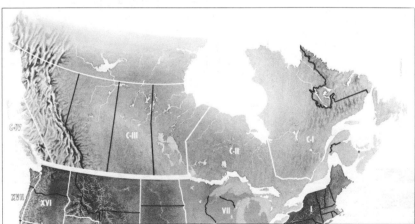

Floristic regional zones in the United States (top) and Canada (bottom). Adapted from *Pollen Guide for Allergy*. Spokane: Hollister-Stier Laboratories, 1978. Copyright 1978, Hollister-Stier.

444

A. Principal Pollens, by Region

Region I (North Atlantic)

Connecticut, Maine, Massachusetts, New Hampshire, New Jersey, New York, Pennsylvania, Rhode Island, Vermont

Trees (pollinating season: late winter through spring)
Box elder/maple (*Acer.* spp.)
Birch (*Betula* spp.)
Oak (*Quercus* spp.)
Hickory (*Carya ovata*)
Ash (*Fraxinus americana*)
Pine (*Pinus strobus*)
Sycamore (*Platanus occidentalis*)
Cottonwood/poplar (*Populus deltoides*)
Elm (*Ulmus americana*)

Grasses (pollinating season: spring through early summer)
Redtop (*Agrostis alba*)
Orchard (*Dactylis glomerata*)
Fescue (*Festuca elatior*)
Timothy (*Phleum pratense*)
Bluegrass/June grass (*Poa* spp.)

Weeds (pollinating season: summer through early fall)
Lamb's-quarters (*Chenopodium album*)
Ragweed, giant and short (*Ambrosia* spp.)
Cocklebur (*Xanthium strumarium*)
Plantain (*Plantago lanceolata*)
Dock/sorrel (*Rumex* spp.)

Region II (Mid-Atlantic)

Delaware, District of Columbia, Maryland, North Carolina, Virginia

Trees (pollinating season: late winter through spring)
Box elder/maple (*Acer* spp.)
Birch (*Betula nigra*)
Cedar/juniper (*Juniperus virginiana*)
Oak (*Quercus* spp.)
Hickory/pecan (*Carya* spp.)
Walnut (*Juglans nigra*)
Mulberry (*Morus* spp.)
Ash (*Fraximus americana*)
Cottonwood/poplar (*Populus deltoides*)
Hackberry (*Celtis occidentalis*)
Elm (*Ulmus americana*)

Grasses (pollinating season: spring through early summer)
Redtop (*Agrostic alba*)
Vernal grass (*Anthoxanthum* spp.)
Bermuda grass (*Cynodon dactylon*)
Orchard grass (*Dactylis glomerata*)
Ryegrass (*Elymus* and *Lolium* spp.)
Timothy (*Phleum pratense*)
Bluegrass/June grass (*Poa* spp.)
Johnson grass (*Sorghum halepense*)

Weeds (pollinating season: summer through early fall)
Pigweed (*Amaranthus retroflexus*)
Lamb's-quarters (*Chenopodium album*)
Mexican firebush (*Kochia scoparia*)
Ragweed, giant and short (*Ambrosia* spp.)
Cocklebur (*Xanthium strumarium*)
Plantain (*Plantago lanceolata*)
Dock/sorrel (*Rumex* spp.)

Region III (South Atlantic)
Florida (north, above Orlando), Georgia, South Carolina
  Trees (pollinating season: late winter through spring)
    Box elder/maple (*Acer* spp.)
    Birch (*Betula nigra*)
    Cedar/juniper (*Juniperus virginiana*)
    Oak (*Quercus* spp.)
    Hickory/pecan (*Carya* spp.)
    Walnut (*Juglans nigra*)
    Mesquite (*Prosopis juliflora*)
    Mulberry (*Morus* spp.)
    Ash (*Fraxinus americana*)
    Cottonwood/poplar (*Populus deltoides*)
    Hackberry (*Celtis occidentalis*)
    Elm (*Ulmus americana*)
  Grasses (pollinating season: spring through early summer)
    Redtop (*Agrostis alba*)
    Sweet vernal grass (*Anthoxanthum* spp.)
    Bermuda grass (*Cynodon dactylon*)
    Orchard grass (*Dactylis glomerata*)
    Ryegrass (*Elymus* and *Lolium* spp.)
    Fescue (*Festuca elatior*)
    Timothy (*Phleum pratense*)
    Bluegrass/June grass (*Poa* spp.)
    Johnson grass (*Sorghum halepense*)
  Weeds (pollinating season: summer through early fall)
    Lamb's-quarters (*Chenopodium album*)
    Ragweed, giant and short (*Ambrosia* spp.)
    Sagebrush (*Artemisia* spp.)
    Cocklebur (*Xanthium strumarium*)
    Plantain (*Plantago lanceolata*)
    Dock/sorrel (*Rumex spp.*)
Region IV (Subtropic Florida)
Southern Florida (below Orlando)
  Trees (pollinating season: winter through spring)
    Box elder (*Acer negundo*)
    Cedar/juniper (*Juniperus virginiana*)
    Oak (*Quercus* spp.)
    Pecan (*Carya pecan*)
    Privet (*Ligustrum lucidium*)
    Palm (*Cocos plumosa*)
    Australian pine (beefwood) (*Casuarina equisetifolia*)
    Sycamore (*Platanus occidentalis*)
    Cottonwood/poplar (*Populus deltoides*)
    Elm (*Ulmus americana*)
    Brazilian peppertree (Florida holly) (*Schinus terebinthifolius*)
    Bayberry (wax myrtle) (*Myrica* spp.)
    Melaleuca (*Melaleuca* spp.)
  Grasses (pollinating season: spring through early summer)
    Redtop (*Agrostis alba*)
    Bermuda grass (*Cynodon dactylon*)
    Salt grass (*Distichlis* spp.)
    Bahia grass (*Paspalum notatum*)
    Canary grass (*Phalaris minor*)
    Bluegrass/June grass (*Poa* spp.)
    Johnson grass (*Sorghum halepense*)
  Weeds (pollinating season: summer through early fall)
    Pigweed (*Amaranthus spinosus*)
    Lamb's-quarters (*Chenopodium album*)

Ragweed, giant and short (*Ambrosia* spp.)
Sagebrush (*Artemisia* spp.)
Marsh elder/poverty weed (*Iva* spp.)
Dock/sorrel (*Rumex* spp.)
Plantain (*Plantago lanceolata*)
Region V (Greater Ohio Valley)
Indiana, Kentucky, Ohio, Tennessee, West Virginia
  Trees (pollinating season: late winter through spring)
    Box elder/maple (*Acer* spp.)
    Birch (*Betula nigra*)
    Oak (*Quercus rubra*)
    Hickory (*Carya ovata*)
    Walnut (*Juglans nigra*)
    Ash (*Fraxinus americana*)
    Sycamore (*Platanus occidentalis*)
    Cottonwood/poplar (*Populus deltoides*)
    Elm (*Ulmus americana*)
  Grasses (pollinating season: spring through early summer)
    Redtop (*Agrostis alba*)
    Bermuda grass (*Cynodon dactylon*)
    Orchard grass (*Dactylis glomerata*)
    Fescue (*Festuca elatior*)
    Ryegrass (*Lolium* spp.)
    Timothy (*Phleum pratense*)
    Bluegrass/June grass (*Poa* spp.)
    Johnson grass (*Sorghum halepense*)
  Weeds (pollinating season: summer through early fall)
    Waterhemp (*Acnida tamariscina*)
    Pigweed (*Amaranthus retroflexus*)
    Lamb's-quarters (*Chenopodium album*)
    Ragweed, giant and short (*Ambrosis* spp.)
    Sagebrush (*Artemisia* spp.)
    Cocklebur (*Xanthium strumarium*)
    Dock/sorrel (*Rumex* spp.)
    Plantain (*Plantago lanceolata*)
Region VI (South Central)
Alabama, Arkansas, Louisiana, Mississippi
  Trees (pollinating season: late winter through early spring)
    Box Elder/maple (*Acer* spp.)
    Cedar/juniper (*Juniperus virginiana*)
    Oak (*Quercus* spp.)
    Hickory/pecan (*Carya* spp.)
    Walnut (*Juglans nigra*)
    Ash (*Fraxinus americana*)
    Sycamore (*Plantanus occidentalis*)
    Cottonwood/poplar (*Populus deltoides*)
    Elm (*Ulmus americana*)
  Grasses (pollinating season: spring through early summer)
    Redtop (*Agrostis alba*)
    Bermuda grass (*Cynodon dactylon*)
    Orchard grass (*Dactylis glomerata*)
    Ryegrass (*Lolium* spp.)
    Timothy (*Phleum pratense*)
    Bluegrass/June grass (*Poa* spp.)
    Johnson grass (*Sorghum halepense*)
  Weeds (pollinating season: summer through early fall)
    Pigweed (*Amaranthus retroflexus*)
    Lamb's-quarters (*Chenopodium album*)
    Ragweed, giant and short (*Ambrosia* spp.)

Sagebrush (*Artemisia* spp.)
Cocklebur (*Xanthium strumarium*)
Dock/sorrel (*Rumex* spp.)
Plantain (*Plantago lanceolata*)

Region VII (Northern Midwest)
Michigan, Minnesota, Wisconsin
Trees (pollinating season: late winter through spring)
Box elder/maple (*Acer* spp.)
Alder (*Alnus incana*)
Birch (*Betula* spp.)
Oak (*Quercus rubra*)
Hickory (*Carya ovata*)
Walnut (*Juglans nigra*)
Ash (*Fraxinus americana*)
Sycamore (*Platanus occidentalis*)
Cottonwood/poplar (*Populus deltoides*)
Elm (*Ulmus americana*)
Grasses (pollinating season: spring through early summer)
Redtop (*Agrostis alba*)
Brome (*Bromus inermis*)
Orchard grass (*Dactylis glomerata*)
Fescue (*Festuca elatior*)
Ryegrass (*Lolium* spp.)
Canary grass (*Phalaris arundinacea*)
Timothy (*Phleum pratense*)
Bluegrass/June grass (*Poa* spp.)
Weeds (pollinating season: summer through early fall)
Waterhemp (*Acnida tamariscina*)
Lamb's-quarters (*Chenopodium album*)
Russian thistle (*Salsoal kali*)
Ragweed, giant and short (*Ambrosia* spp.)
Marsh elder/poverty weed (*Iva* spp.)
Cocklebur (*Xanthium strumarium*)
Dock/sorrel (*Rumex* spp.)
Pigweed (*Amaranthus retroflexus*)
Plantain (*Plantago lanceolata*)

Region VIII (Central Midwest)
Illinois, Iowa, Missouri
Trees (pollinating season: late winter through spring)
Box elder/maple (*Acer* spp.)
Birch (*Betula nigra*)
Oak (*Quercus* spp.)
Hickory (*Carya ovata*)
Walnut (*Juglans nigra*)
Mulberry (*Morus* spp.)
Ash (*Fraxinus americana*)
Sycamore (*Platanus occidentalis*)
Cottonwood/poplar (*Populus deltoides*)
Elm (*Ulmus americana*)
Grasses (pollinating season: spring through early summer)
Redtop (*Agrostis alba*)
Bermuda grass (*Cynodon dactylon*)
Orchard grass (*Dactylis glomerata*)
Ryegrass (*Lolium* spp.)
Timothy (*Phleum pratense*)
Bluegrass/June grass (*Poa* spp.)
Johnson grass (*Sorghum halepense*)
Corn (*Zea mays*)

Weeds (pollinating season: summer through early fall)
    Pigweed (*Amaranthus retroflexus*)
    Lamb's-quarters (*Chenopodium album*)
    Mexican firebush (*Kochia scoparia*)
    Russian thistle (*Salsoa kali*)
    Ragweed, giant, short, and western (*Ambrosia* spp.)
    Marsh elder/poverty weed (*Iva* spp.)
    Plantain (*Plantago lanceolata*)
    Dock/sorrel (*Rumex* spp.)
    Water hemp (*Acnida tamariscina*)
Region IX (Great Plains)
Kansas, Nebraska, North Dakota, South Dakota
  Trees (pollinating season: later winter through spring)
    Box elder/maple (*Acer* spp.)
    Alder (*Alnus incana*)
    Birch (*Betula* spp.)
    Hazelnut (*Corylus americana*)
    Oak (*Quercus macrocarpa*)
    Hickory (*Carya ovata*)
    Walnut (*Juglans nigra*)
    Ash (*Fraxinus americana*)
    Cottonwood/poplar (*Populus deltoides*)
    Elm (*Ulmus americana*)
  Grasses (pollinating season: spring through early summer)
    Quack grass/wheatgrass (*Agropyron* spp.)
    Redtop (*Agrostis alba*)
    Brome (*Bromus inermis*)
    Orchard grass (*Dactylis glomerata*)
    Ryegrass (*Elymus* and *Lolium* spp.)
    Fescue (*Festuca elatior*)
    Timothy (*Phleum pratense*)
    Bluegrass/June grass (*Poa* spp.)
  Weeds (pollinating season: summer through early fall)
    Water hemp (*Acnida tamariscina*)
    Pigweed (*Amaranthus retroflexus*)
    Lamb's-quarters (*Chenopodium album*)
    Mexican firebush (*Kochia scoparia*)
    Russian thistle (*Salsola kali*)
    Ragweed, false, giant, short, and western (*Ambrosia* spp.)
    Sagebrush (*Artemisia* spp.)
    Marsh elder/poverty weed (*Iva* spp.)
    Cocklebur (*Xanthium strumarium*)
    Plantain (*Plantago lanceolata*)
    Dock/sorrel (*Rumex* spp.)
Region X (Southwestern Grasslands)
Oklahoma, Texas
  Trees (pollinating season: late winter through spring)
    Box elder (*Acer negundo*)
    Cedar/juniper (*Juniperus virginiana*)
    Oak (*Quercus virginiana*)
    Mesquite (*Prosopis juliflora*)
    Mulberry (*Morus* spp.)
    Ash (*Fraxinus americana*)
    Cottonwood/poplar (*Populus deltoides*)
    Elm (*Ulmus americana*)
  Grasses (pollinating season: spring through early summer)
    Quack grass/wheatgrass (*Agropyron* spp.)
    Redtop (*Agrostis alba*)

Bermuda grass (*Cynodon dactylon*)
Orchard grass (*Dactylis glomerata*)
Fescue (*Festuca elatior*)
Ryegrass (*Lolium* spp.)
Timothy (*Phleum pratense*)
Bluegrass/June grass (*Poa* spp.)
Johnson grass (*Sorghum halepense*)
Weeds (pollinating season: summer through early fall)
Water hemp (*Acnida tamariscina*)
Careless weed/pigweed (*Amaranthus* spp.)
Saltbush/scale (*Atriplex* spp.)
Lamb's-quarters (*Chenopodium album*)
Mexican firebush (*Kochia scoparia*)
Russian thistle (*Salsola kali*)
Ragweed, false, giant, short, and western (*Ambrosia* spp.)
Sagebrush (*Artemisia* spp.)
Marsh elder/poverty weed (*Iva* spp.)
Cocklebur (*Xanthium strumarium*)
Dock/sorrel (*Rumex* spp.)
Plantain (*Plantago lanceolata*)
Region XI (Rocky Mountain Empire)
Arizona (mountainous), Colorado, Idaho (mountainous), Montana, New Mexico,
Utah, Wyoming
Trees (pollinating season: late winter through spring)
Box elder (*Acer negundo*)
Alder (*Alnus incana*)
Birch (*Betula fontinalis*)
Cedar/juniper (*Juniperus scopulorum*)
Oak (*Quercus gambelii*)
Ash (*Fraxinus americana*)
Pine (*Pinus* spp.)
Cottonwood/poplar (*Populus deltoides, P. sargentii*)
Elm (*Ulmus* spp.)
Grasses (pollinating season: spring through early summer)
Quack grass/wheatgrass (*Agropyron* spp.)
Redtop (*Agrostis alba*)
Brome (*Bromus inermis*)
Bermuda grass (*Cynodon dactylon*)
Orchard grass (*Dactylis glomerata*)
Ryegrass (*Elymus* and *Lolium* spp.)
Fescue (*Festuca elatior*)
Timothy (*Phleum pratense*)
Bluegrass/June grass (*Poa* spp.)
Weeds (pollinating season: summer through early fall)
Water hemp (*Acnida tamariscina*)
Pigweed (*Amaranthus retroflexus*)
Saltbush/scale (*Atriplex* spp.)
Sugarbeet (*Beta vulgaris*)
Lamb's-quarters (*Chenopodium album*)
Mexican firebush (*Kochia scoparia*)
Russian thistle (*Salsola kali*)
Ragweed, false, giant, short, and western (*Ambrosia* spp.)
Sagebrush (*Artemisia* spp.)
Marsh elder/poverty weed (*Iva* spp.)
Cocklebur (*Xanthium strumarium*)
Plantain (*Plantago lanceolata*)
Dock/sorrel (*Rumex* spp.)

Region XII (The Arid Southwest)
Arizona, Southern California (southeastern desert)
    Trees (pollinating season: winter through spring)
        Cypress (*Cupressus arizonica*)
        Cedar/juniper (*Juniperus californica*)
        Mesquite (*Prosopis juliflora*)
        Ash (*Fraxinus velutina*)
        Olive (*Olea europaea*)
        Cottonwood/poplar (*Populus fremontii*)
        Elm (*Ulmus parvifolia*)
    Grasses (pollinating season: spring through early summer)
        Brome (*Bromus* spp.)
        Bermuda grass (*Cynodon dactylon*)
        Salt grass (*Distichlis* spp.)
        Ryegrass (*Elymus* and *Lolium* spp.)
        Canary grass (*Phalaris minor*)
        Bluegrass/June grass (*Poa* spp.)
    Weeds (pollinating season: summer through early fall)
        Careless weed (*Amaranthus palmeri*)
        Iodine bush (*Allenrolfea occidentalis*)
        Saltbush/scale (*Atriplex* spp.)
        Lamb's-quarters (*Chenopodium album*)
        Russian thistle (*Salsola kali*)
        Alkali blite (*Suaeda* spp.)
        Ragweed, false, slender, and western (*Ambrosia* spp.)
        Sagebrush (*Artemisia* spp.)
        Silver ragweed (*Dicoria canescens*)
        Burro brush (*Hymenoclea salsola*)
Region XIII (Southern Coastal California)
    Trees (pollinating season: late winter through spring)
        Box elder (*Acer negundo*)
        Cypress (*Cupressus arizonica*)
        Oak (*Quercus agrifolia*)
        Walnut (*Juglans* spp.)
        Acacia (*Acacia* spp.)
        Mulberry (*Morus* spp.)
        Eucalyptus (*Eucalyptus* spp.)
        Ash (*Fraxinus velutina*)
        Olive (*Olea europaea*)
        Sycamore (*Platanus racemosa*)
        Cottonwood/poplar (*Populus trichocarpa*)
        Elm (*Ulmus* spp.)
    Grasses (pollinating season: spring through early summer)
        Oats (*Avena* spp.)
        Brome (*Bromus* spp.)
        Bermuda grass (*Cynodon dactylon*)
        Orchard grass (*Dactylis glomerata*)
        Salt grass (*Distichlis* spp.)
        Ryegrass (*Elymus* and *Lolium* spp.)
        Fescue (*Festuca elatior*)
        Bluegrass/June grass (*Poa* spp.)
        Johnson grass (*Sorghum halepense*)
    Weeds (pollinating season: summer through early fall)
        Careless weed/pigweed (*Amaranthus* spp.)
        Saltbush/scale (*Altriplex* spp.)
        Lamb's-quarters (*Chenopodium album*)
        Russian thistle (*Salsola kali*)
        Ragweed, false, slender, and western (*Ambrosia* spp.)

Sagebrush (*Artemisia* spp.)
Cocklebur (*Xanthium strumarium*)
Plantain (*Plantago lanceolata*)
Dock/sorrel (*Rumex* spp.)
Region XIV (Central California Valley)
Sacramento Valley, San Joaquin Valley
  Trees (pollinating season: late winter through spring)
    Box elder (*Acer negundo*)
    Alder (*Alnus rhombifolia*)
    Birch (*Betula fontinalis*)
    Cypress (*Cupressus arizonica*)
    Oak (*Quercus lobata*)
    Pecan (*Carya pecan*)
    Walnut (*Juglans* spp.)
    Ash (*Fraxinus velutina*)
    Olive (*Olea europaea*)
    Sycamore (*Platanus acerifolia*)
    Cottonwood/poplar (*Populus fremontii*)
    Elm (*Ulmus* spp.)
  Grasses (pollinating season: spring through early summer)
    Redtop (*Agrostis alba*)
    Oats (*Avena* spp.)
    Brome (*Bromus* spp.)
    Bermuda grass (*Cynodon dactylon*)
    Orchard grass (*Dactylis glomerata*)
    Salt grass (*Distichlis* spp.)
    Ryegrass (*Elymus* and *Lolium* spp.)
    Fescue (*Festuca elatior*)
    Canary grass (*Phalaris minor*)
    Timothy (*Phleum pratense*)
    Bluegrass/June grass (*Poa* spp.)
    Johnson grass (*Sorghum halepense*)
  Weeds (pollinating season: summer through early fall)
    Pigweed (*Amaranthus retroflexus*)
    Saltbush/scale (*Atriplex* spp.)
    Sugarbeet (*Beta vulgaris*)
    Lamb's-quarters (*Chenopodium album*)
    Russian thistle (*Salsola kali*)
    Ragweed, false, slender, and western (*Ambrosia* spp.)
    Sagebrush (*Artemisia* spp.)
    Cocklebur (*Xanthium strumarium*)
    Plantain (*Plantago lanceolata*)
    Dock/sorrel (*Rumex* spp.)
Region XV (Intermountain West)
Idaho (southern), Nevada
  Trees (pollinating season: late winter through spring)
    Box elder (*Acer negundo*)
    Alder (*Alnus incana*)
    Birch (*Betula fortinalis*)
    Cedar/juniper (*Juniperus utahensis*)
    Ash (*Fraxinus americana*)
    Sycamore (*Platanus occidentalis*)
    Cottonwood/poplar (*Populus trichocarpa*)
    Elm (*Ulmus* spp.)
  Grasses (pollinating season: spring through early summer)
    Quack grass/wheatgrass (*Agropyron* spp.)
    Redtop (*Agrostis alba*)
    Brome (*Bromus inermis*)
    Bermuda grass (*Cynodon dactylon*)

Orchard grass (*Dactylis glomerata*)
Salt grass (*Distichlis* spp.)
Ryegrass (*Elymus* and *Lolium* spp.)
Fescue (*Festuca elatior*)
Timothy (*Phleum pratense*)
Bluegrass/June grass (*Poa* spp.)
Weeds (pollinating season: summer through early fall)
Pigweed (*Amaranthus retroflexus*)
Iodine bush (*Allenrolfea occidentalis*)
Saltbush/scale (*Atriplex* spp.)
Lamb's-quarters (*Chenopodium album*)
Mexican firebush (*Kochia scoparia*)
Russian thistle (*Salsola kali*)
Ragweed, false, slender, and western (*Ambrosia* spp.)
Sagebrush (*Artemisia* spp.)
Marsh elder/poverty weed (*Iva* spp.)
Cocklebur (*Xanthium strumarium*)
Plantain (*Plantago lanceolata*)
Dock/sorrel (*Rumex* spp.)
Region XVI (Inland Empire)
Oregon (central and eastern), Washington (central and eastern)
Trees (pollinating season: late winter through spring)
Box elder (*Acer negundo*)
Alder (*Alnus incana*)
Birch (*Betula fontinalis*)
Oak (*Quercus garryana*)
Walnut (*Juglans nigra*)
Pine (*Pinus* spp.)
Cottonwood/poplar (*Populus trichocarpa*)
Willow (*Salix lasiandra*)
Grasses (pollinating season: spring through early summer)
Quack grass/wheatgrass (*Agropyron* spp.)
Redtop (*Agrostis alba*)
Vernal grass (*Anthoxanthum* spp.)
Brome (*Bromus inermis*)
Orchard grass (*Dactylis glomerata*)
Ryegrass (*Elymus* and *Lolium* spp.)
Velvet grass (*Holcus lanatus*)
Timothy (*Phleum pratense*)
Bluegrass/June grass (*Poa* spp.)
Weeds (pollinating season: summer through early fall)
Pigweed (*Amaranthus retroflexus*)
Saltbush/scale (*Atriplex* spp.)
Lamb's-quarters (*Chenopodium album*)
Mexican firebush (*Kochia scoparia*)
Russian thistle (*Salsola kali*)
Ragweed, false, giant, short, and western (*Ambrosia* spp.)
Sagebrush (*Artemisia* spp.)
Marsh elder/poverty weed (*Iva* spp.)
Plantain (*Plantago lanceolata*)
Dock/sorrel (*Rumex* spp.)
Region XVII (Cascade Pacific Northwest)
California (northwestern), Oregon (western), Washington (western)
Trees (pollinating season: late winter through spring)
Box elder (*Acer negundo*)
Alder (*Alnus rhombifolia*)
Birch (*Betula fontanalis*)
Hazelnut (*Corylus cornuta*)
Oak (*Quercus garryana*)

Walnut (*Juglans regia*)
Ash (*Fraxinus oregona*)
Cottonwood/poplar (*Populus trichocarpa*)
Willow (*Salix lasiandra*)
Elm (*Ulmus pumila*)
Grasses (pollinating season: spring through early summer)
Bent grass (*Agrostis maritima*)
Sweet vernal grass (*Anthoxanthum* spp.)
Oats (*Avena* spp.)
Brome (*Bromus inermis*)
Bermuda grass (*Cynodon dactylon*)
Orchard grass (*Dactylis glomerata*)
Salt grass (*Distichlis* spp.)
Ryegrass (*Elymus* and *Lolium* spp.)
Fescue (*Festuca elatior*)
Velvet grass (*Holcus lanatus*)
Canary grass (*Phalaris arundinacea*)
Timothy (*Phleum pratense*)
Bluegrass/June grass (*Poa* spp.)
Weeds (pollinating season: summer through early fall)
Pigweed (*Amaranthus retroflexus*)
Saltbush/scale (*Atriplex* spp.)
Lamb's-quarters (*Chenopodium album*)
Russian thistle (*Salsola kali*)
Ragweed, false, giant, short, and western (*Ambrosia* spp.)
Sagebrush (*Artemisia* spp.)
Cocklebur (*Xanthium strumarium*)
Plantain (*Plantago lanceolata*)
Dock/sorrel (*Rumex* spp.)
Region C-I (Atlantic Provinces and Quebec)
New Brunswick, Newfoundland, Nova Scotia, Prince Edward Island, Quebec
Trees (pollinating season: late winter through spring)
Box elder (*Acer negundo*)
Hard maple (sugar) (*Acer saccharum*)
Tag alder (speckled) (*Alnus incana*)
Paper birch (white) (*Betula papyrifera*)
Beech (*Fagus grandifolia*)
White ash (*Fraxinus americana*)
Green ash (*Fraxinus pennsylvanica*)
Butternut (*Juglans cinerea*)
Sycamore (*Platanus occidentalis*)
Balsam poplar (*Populus balsamifera*)
Trembling aspen (*Populus tremuloides*)
Bur oak (*Quercus macrocarpa*)
Black willow (*Salix nigra*)
American elm (*Ulmus americana*)
Grasses (pollinating season: spring through early summer)
Quack grass/couch grass (*Agropyron repens*)
Redtop (*Agrostis alba*)
Brome (*Bromus* spp.)
Orchard grass (*Dactylis glomerata*)
Ryegrass (*Elymus* and *Lolium* spp.)
Timothy (*Phleum pratense*)
Bluegrass (*Poa* spp.)
Weeds (pollinating season: summer through early fall)
Pigweed (*Amaranthus retroflexus*)
Ragweed (*Ambrosia* spp.)
Lamb's-quarters (*Chenopodium album*)
Plantain (*Plantago lanceolata*)

Dock/sorrel (*Rumex* spp.)
Russian thistle (*Salsola kali*)
Region C-II (Ontario)
  Trees (pollinating season: late winter through spring)
    Box elder (*Acer negundo*)
    Hard maple (sugar) (*Acer saccharum*)
    Tag alder (speckled) (*Alnus incana*)
    Paper birch (white) (*Betula papyrifera*)
    Beech (*Fagus grandifolia*)
    White ash (*Fraxinus americana*)
    Green ash (*Fraxinus pennsylvanica*)
    Butternut (*Juglans cinerea*)
    Sycamore (*Platanus occidentalis*)
    Balsam poplar (*Populus balsamifera*)
    Aspen (*Populus tremuloides*)
    Bur oak (*Quercus macrocarpa*)
    Black willow (*Salix nigra*)
    American elm (white) (*Ulmus americana*)
    Chinese elm (Siberian) (*Ulmus pumila*)
  Grasses (pollinating season: spring through early summer)
    Quack grass (couch grass) (*Agropyron repens*)
    Redtop (*Agrostis alba*)
    Brome (*Bromus* spp.)
    Orchard grass (*Dactylis glomerata*)
    Ryegrass (*Elymus* and *Lolium* spp.)
    Timothy (*Phleum pratense*)
    Bluegrass (*Poa* spp.)
  Weeds (pollinating season: summer through early fall)
    Pigweed (*Amaranthus retroflexus*)
    Ragweed (*Ambrosia* spp.)
    Lamb's-quarters (*Chenopodium album*)
    English plantain (*Plantago lanceolata*)
    Dock/sorrel (*Rumex* spp.)
    Russian thistle (*Salsola kali*)
Region C-III (Prairie Provinces and Eastern British Columbia)
Alberta, British Columbia (eastern), Manitoba, Saskatchewan
  Trees (pollinating season: late winter through spring)
    Box elder (*Acer negundo*)
    Tag alder (speckled or mountain) (*Alnus incana*)
    Paper birch (white) (*Betula papyrifera*)
    Green ash (*Fraxinus pennsylvanica*)
    Balsam poplar (*Populus balsamifera*)
    Trembling aspen (*Populus tremuloides*)
    Bur oak (*Quercus macrocarpa*)
    Willow (yellow) (*Salix* spp.)
    Chinese elm (Siberian) (*Ulmus pumila*)
  Grasses (pollinating season: spring through early summer)
    Quack grass (couch grass)/wheatgrass (*Agropyron* spp.)
    Redtop (*Agrostis alba*)
    Common wild oats (*Avena fatua*)
    Brome (*Bromus* spp.)
    Orchard grass (*Dactylis glomerata*)
    Ryegrass (*Elymus* and *Lolium* spp.)
    Timothy (*Phleum pratense*)
    Bluegrass (*Poa* spp.)
  Weeds (pollinating season: summer through early fall)
    Pigweed (*Amaranthus retroflexus*)
    Ragweed (*Ambrosia* spp.)
    Lamb's-quarters (*Chenopodium album*)

Sagebrush (*Artemisia* spp.)
Marshelder/poverty weed (*Iva* spp.)
English plantain (*Plantago lanceolata*)
Dock/sorrel (*Rumex* spp.)
Russian thistle (*Salsola kali*)

Region C-IV (Western British Columbia and Vancouver Island)
Trees (pollinating season: late winter through spring)
Box elder (*Acer negundo*)
Red alder (*Alnus rubra*)
Sitka alder (*Alnus sinuata*)
Paper birch (white) (*Betula papyrifera*)
Sycamore (*Platanus occidentalis*)
Black cottonwood (*Populus trichocarpa*)
Trembling aspen (*Populus tremulides*)
Dougls fir (*Pseudotsuga menziesii*)
Garry's oak (*Quercus garryana*)
Yellow willow (Pacific) (*Salix lasiandra*)
Chinese elm (Siberian) (*Ulmus pumila*)
Grasses (pollinating season: spring through early summer)
Quack grass/couch grass (*Agropyron repens*)
Redtop (*Agrostis alba*)
Tall oats grass (*Arrhenatherum elatius*)
Common wild oats (*Avena fatua*)
Brome (*Bromus* spp.)
Orchard grass (*Dactylis glomerata*)
Ryegrass (*Elymus* and *Lolium* spp.)
Timothy (*Phleum pratense*)
Bluegrass (*Poa* spp.)
Weeds (pollinating season: summer through early fall)
Pigweed (*Amaranthus retroflexus*)
Ragweed (*Ambrosia* spp.)
Lamb's-quarters (*Chenopodium album*)
Marshelder/poverty weed (*Iva* spp.)
English plantain (*Plantago lanceolata*)
Dock/sorrel (*Rumex* spp.)
Russian thistle (*Salsola kali*)

Alaska
Trees (pollinating season: spring)
Alder (*Alnus incana*)
Aspen (*Populus tremuloides*)
Birch (*Betula papyrifera*)
Cedar (*Thuja plicata*)
Hemlock (*Tsuga hetrophylla*)
Pine (*Pinus contorta*)
Balsam poplar (*Populus balsamifera*)
Spruce (*Picea sitchensis*)
Willow (*Salix* spp.)
Grasses (pollinating season: late spring and summer)
Bluegrass/June grass (*Poa* spp.)
Brome (*Bromus inermis*)
Canary grass (*Phalaris arundinacea*)
Fescue (*Festuca rubra*)
Orchard grass (*Dactylis glomerata*)
Quack grass/wheatgrass (*Agropyron* spp.)
Redtop (*Agrostis alba*)
Ryegrass (*Lolium perenne*)
Timothy (*Phleum pratense*)
Weeds (pollinating season: summer)
Bulrush (*Scirpus* spp.)

Dock/sorrel (*Rumex* spp.)
Lamb's-quarters (*Chenopodium album*)
Nettle (*Urtica dioica*)
Plantain (*Plantago lanceolata*)
Sagebrush/wormwood (*Artemisia* spp.)
Sedge (*Carex* spp.)
Spearscale (*Atriplex patula*)

Hawaii (all islands) (pollinating season: less defined than for continental regions)

Trees

Acacia (*Acacia* spp.)
Australian pine (beefwood) (*Casuarina equisetifolia*)
Cedar/juniper (*Juniperus* spp.)
Monterey cypress (*Cupressus macrocarpa*)
Date palm (*Phoenix dactylifera*)
Eucalyptus (gum) (*Eucalyptus globulus*)
Mesquite (*Prosopis juliflora*)
Paper mulberry (*Broussonetia papyrifera*)
Olive (*Olea europaea*)
Privet (*Ligustrum* spp.)

Grasses

Bermuda grass (*Cynodon dactylon*)
Corn (*Zea mays*)
Finger grass (*Chloris* spp.)
Johnson grass (*Sorghum halepense*)
Love grass (*Eragrostis* spp.)
Bluegrass/June grass (*Poa* spp.)
Redtop (*Agrostis alba*)
Sorghum (*Sorghum vulgare*)

Weeds

Cocklebur (*Xanthium strumarium*)
Plantain (*Plantago lanceolata*)
Kochia (*Kochia scoparia*)
Pigweed (*Amaranthus* spp.)
Ragweed, slender (*Ambrosia* spp.)
Sagebrush (*Artemisia* spp.)
Scale (saltbush) (*Atriplex* spp.)

Source: Adapted from *Pollen Guide for Allergy*. Spokane: Hollister-Stier Laboratories, 1978. Copyright Hollister-Stier, 1978.

B. Incidence of Individual Molds in the United States[a]

Type of mold	Northeast[b] Indoor (%)	Northeast[b] Outdoor (%)	Southeast[c] Indoor (%)	Southeast[c] Outdoor (%)	Central[d] Indoor (%)	Central[d] Outdoor (%)
Hormodendrum	56.7	66.8	66.8	96.5	63.3	81.8
Penicillium	37.0	25.1	31.5	22.8	30.1	27.3
Alternaria	23.4	48.2	18.0	54.3	39.1	72.3
Aspergillus	20.0	7.3	14.7	7.9	16.0	6.3
Pullularia	9.5	19.6	5.4	10.5	4.1	9.1
Geotrichum	11.5	5.5	19.4	8.8	6.1	3.4
Fomes	7.1	16.3	5.8	8.8	5.0	18.2
Epicoccum	6.1	12.6	7.0	20.2	4.1	6.8
Fusarium	5.7	15.1	7.0	21.9	6.4	17.6
Sterile Mycelia	5.4	12.3	10.3	12.3	8.1	8.5
Phoma	2.8	12.3	1.4	8.8	3.1	9.7
Rhodotorula	5.3	3.3	4.0		1.7	2.3
Cephalosporium	4.6	9.8	7.2	11.4	3.7	7.4
Stemphylium	4.0	2.5	2.1	3.5	4.0	
Streptomyces	2.4	7.8		8.8	1.2	13.6
Botrytis	3.9	5.0		6.1		
Mucor		7.5	2.8	9.6	1.2	6.3
Poria	3.8	2.8	1.9		2.7	1.7
Trichoderma	2.1	5.0		7.0	2.3	4.0
Helminthosporium	3.6	3.5	5.8	10.5	1.8	4.0
Tetracoccosporium		2.3				
Sporobolomyces	3.1	1.5	1.2		2.0	1.7
Rhodosporium				1.8		
Polyporaceae	1.5					1.7
Curvularia			4.9	6.1		
Nigrospora				1.8		
Rhizopus				1.8	2.3	1.7
Spondylocladium						
Verticillium						
Fusidium						
Chaetomium						
Acremonium						
Monosporium						
Unidentified yeast						
Polyporus						
Pleospora						

[a] Expressed as the percentage of total exposures when a given fungal genus was recovered.
[b] Delaware, Maryland, Connecticut, Massachusetts, New Jersey, Pennsylvania, New York, Maine, New Hampshire, Rhode Island, and Vermont.
[c] Florida, Georgia, South Carolina, North Carolina, West Virginia, Virginia, Kentucky, Alabama, Arkansas, Louisiana, and Tennessee.
[d] Ohio, Michigan, Wisconsin, Minnesota, Illinois, Missouri, Iowa, and Indiana.
Source: Adapted from *The Role of Molds in Allergy*. Spokane: Hollister-Stier Laboratories, 1977.

South Central[e]		Northwest[f]		Southwest[g]		West[h]	
Indoor (%)	Outdoor (%)	Indoor (%)	Outdoor (%)	Indoor (%)	Outdoor (%)	Indoor (%)	Outdoor (%)
78.6	92.9	62.5	69.6	63.8	93.0	74.5	68.4
25.2	32.1	41.4	40.6	31.9	35.7	35.1	35.9
41.7	85.7	21.1	27.5	42.6	64.3	39.7	47.0
21.3	17.9	15.1	8.7	4.3	7.1	10.1	11.1
1.9		8.0	11.6	6.4	7.1	6.3	12.8
13.6	3.6	6.8	2.9	6.4		2.9	
		2.0	1.4			1.7	5.1
11.7	10.7	2.0	4.3		7.1	16.6	17.1
5.8	46.6	1.2	10.1	4.3	21.4	4.0	11.1
23.3	25.0	4.0	15.9	4.3		7.7	3.4
	7.1	4.8	10.1	6.4	28.6	2.9	8.5
		2.8	7.2	2.1	7.1	2.2	
5.8	21.4	5.2	5.8	4.3	7.1	7.2	4.3
6.8		5.6	11.6	19.1	21.4	10.1	10.3
1.9	17.9	6.8	17.4		35.7	2.9	13.7
		2.4		2.1		4.3	9.4
		3.2	8.7	2.1		3.4	9.4
		1.2	2.9				
		5.2	13.0	2.1			1.7
28.2	25.0	3.6		6.4	14.3	6.3	8.5
		1.2		6.4		1.4	
	32.1	1.6					1.7
4.9	10.7			2.1			
1.9		2.4		6.4	7.1	3.1	5.1
1.9							
	3.6						2.6
	3.6						
			1.4				
				2.1			
				2.1			
					14.3		
						1.2	1.2
							5.1

[e] Oklahoma and Texas.
[f] Nevada, New Mexico, Idaho, Colorado, Montana, and Utah.
[g] California.
[h] Oregon and Washington.

IX

Normal Pulmonary Values

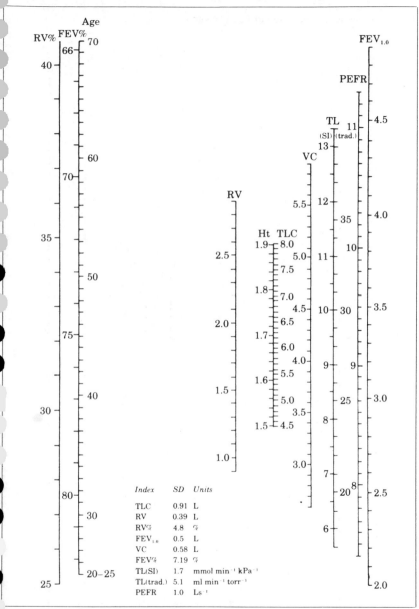

Nomogram relating indices of pulmonary function to height and age for healthy adult men. Ht = height in meters, TLC = total lung capacity, RV = residual volume, RV% = percentage residual volume (RV/TLC × 100), $FEV_{1.0}$ = forced expiratory volume in 1 second, VC = vital capacity, FEV% = percentage expired ($FEV_{1.0}$/FVC × 100), TL(SI) = transfer factor of gas exchange (international system of measurement), TL (trad.) = transfer factor of gas exchange (traditional system of measurement), PEFR = peak expiratory flow rate, SD = standard deviation. The RV% and the FEV% are related only to age, and the TLC only to height. (From J. E. Cotes. Lung Function at Different Stages in Life. In *Lung Function*. London: Blackwell, 1975.)

B. Normal Pulmonary Function in Adult Women

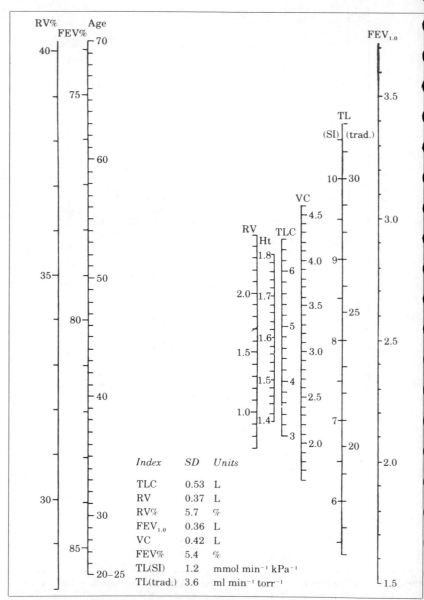

Nomogram relating indices of lung function to height and age for healthy adult women (see Appendix IX.A for terminology). The RV% and the FEV% are related only to age, and the TLC only to height. (From J. E. Cotes. Lung Function at Different Stages in Life. In *Lung Function*. London: Blackwell, 1975.)

C. Normal Lung Volumes for Male Children (function of height in centimeters)

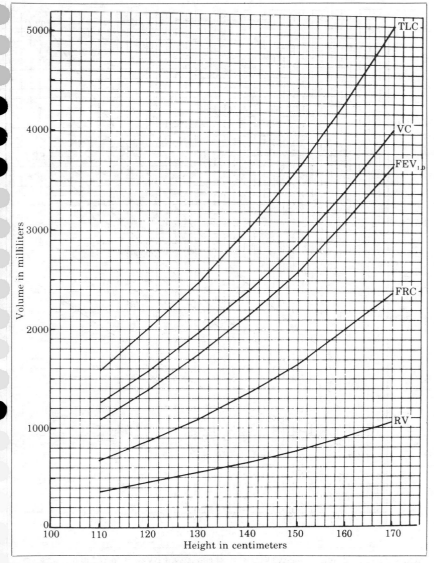

Key: TLC = total lung capacity, VC = vital capacity, $FEV_{1.0}$ = forced expiratory volume in 1 second, FRC = functional residual capacity, RV = residual volume. (From G. Polgar and V. Promadhat. Standard Values. In *Pulmonary Function Testing in Children: Techniques and Standards*. Philadelphia: Saunders, 1971.)

D. Normal Lung Volumes for Female Children (function of height in centimeters)

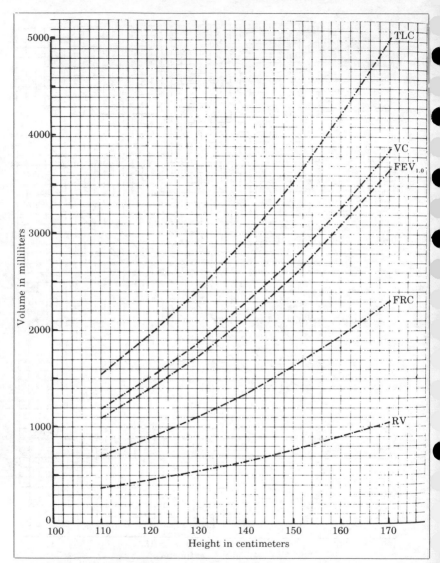

Key: TLC = total lung capacity, VC = vital capacity, $FEV_{1.0}$ = forced expiratory volume in 1 second, FRC = functional residual capacity, RV = residual volume. (From G. Polgar and V. Promadhat. Standard Values. In *Pulmonary Function Testing in Children: Techniques and Standards*. Philadelphia: Saunders, 1971.)

E. Normal Pulmonary Flow Rates for Male and Female Children (function of height in centimeters)

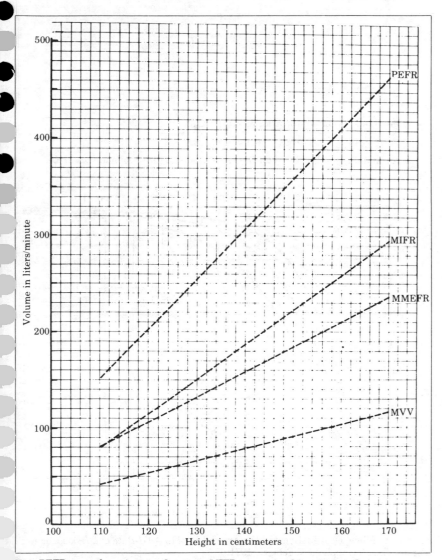

Key: PEFR = peak expiratory flow rate, MIFR = maximal inspiratory flow rate, MMEFR = maximal midexpiratory flow rate, MVV = maximal voluntary ventilation. (From G. Polgar and V. Promadhat. Standard Values. In *Pulmonary Function Testing in Children: Techniques and Standards*. Philadelphia: Saunders, 1971.)

Oxygen Values

A. Prediction Equation for Arterial PO$_2$ (PaO$_2$)*

$$PaO_2 = 109 - 0.43 \times \text{age (years)} \pm 4.1 \text{ (S.D.)}$$

B. Normal Oxygen Dissociation Curves in Humans (pH-dependent at 37°C)

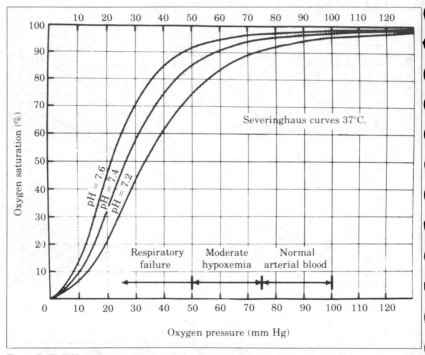

From G. F. Filley. Oxygenation and the Arterial PO$_2$. In *Acid-Base and Blood Gas Regulation*. Philadelphia: Lea & Febiger, 1971.

*At sea level; assumes PaCO$_2$ = 38–42 mm Hg.

XI

Growth Charts

The National Center for Health Statistics (NCHS) has prepared percentiles for assessing physical growth of children in the United States. The NCHS percentiles are based on accurate measurements made on large, nationally representative samples of children. Several groups of experts in physical growth, pediatrics, and clinical nutrition identified the need for new reference data and agreed on the appropriateness of the data used to generate the NCHS percentiles. Seven NCHS percentiles (5th, 10th, 25th, 50th, 75th, 90th, and 95th) are available for two age intervals: birth to 36 months and 2–18 years. For the younger age interval, percentiles are presented for body weight for age, length for age, weight for length, and head circumference for age (**A–D**). Data used in generating these percentiles are from the Fels Research Institute, Yellow Springs, Ohio. For the 2–18 years age interval, body weight for age and stature for age percentiles are presented (**E** and **F**).

The NCHS percentiles provide reliable, up-to-date reference data for assessment of physical growth. Comparison of the measurements for an individual child against NCHS percentiles indicates where the child ranks relative to all contemporary children in the United States of the same age and sex. Measurements outside the extreme percentiles may be indicative of health or nutritional problems sufficiently severe to affect growth. On the other hand, measurements within the central or intermediate percentiles are indicative that growth is within normal limits by current standards.

Use of the NCHS percentiles results in accurate anthropormorphic classification of a child only if the measurement technique is the same as that used to obtain the reference data. Key points regarding the birth to 36 months interval are that body weight should be measured with the infant nude, and length should be measured in the recumbent position. For the 2–18 years interval, the child may wear light garments during measurement of body weight, and upright stature is measured in stocking feet. It is necessary to know the age of the child for proper interpretation of measurements. However, weight for stature percentiles are assumed to be independent of age before pubescence and are applicable to most children before, but not after, the appearance of secondary sex characteristics such as breast development or the presence of axillary or pubic hair, regardless of chronologic age.

A. NCHS Percentiles for Length and Weight for Age, Boys, Birth to 36 Months

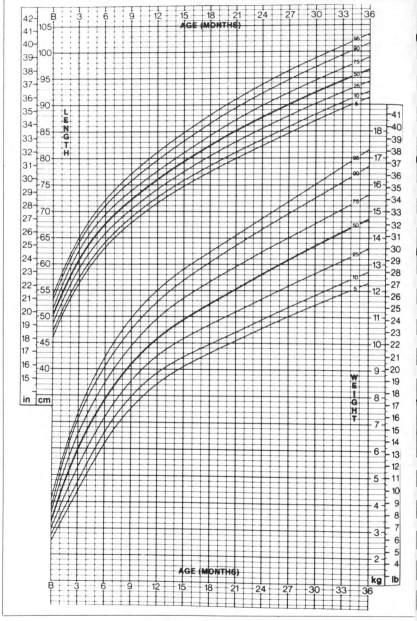

Fig. XI-A. Courtesy of Ross Laboratories, Columbus, OH.

B. NCHS Percentiles for Weight for Length, Boys, Less Than 4 Years, and for Head Circumference, Boys, Birth to 36 Months

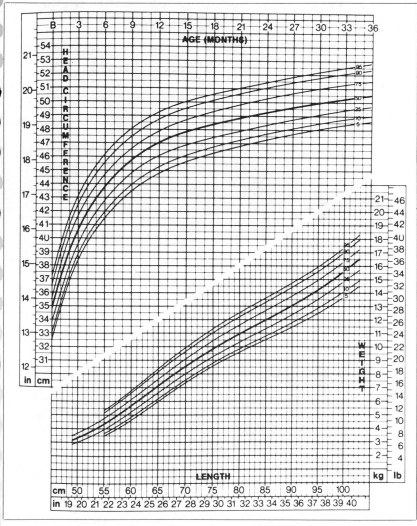

Fig. XI-B. Courtesy of Ross Laboratories, Columbus, OH.

C. NCHS Percentiles for Length and Weight for Age, Girls, Birth to 36 Months

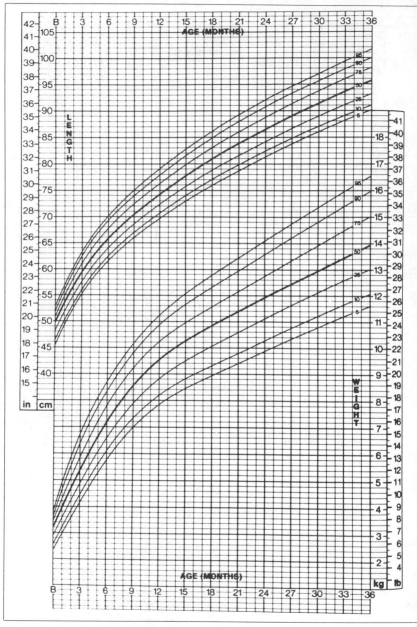

Fig. XI-C. Courtesy of Ross Laboratories, Columbus, OH.

D. NCHS Percentiles for Weight for Length, Girls, Less Than 4 Years, and for Head Circumference, Girls, Birth to 36 Months

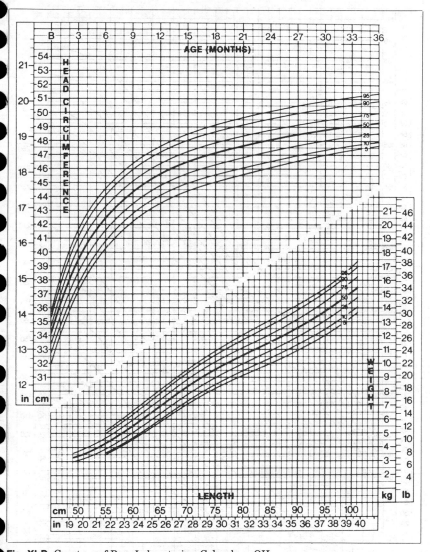

Fig. XI-D. Courtesy of Ross Laboratories, Columbus, OH.

E. NCHS Percentiles for Stature and Weight for Age, Boys, 2 to 18 Years

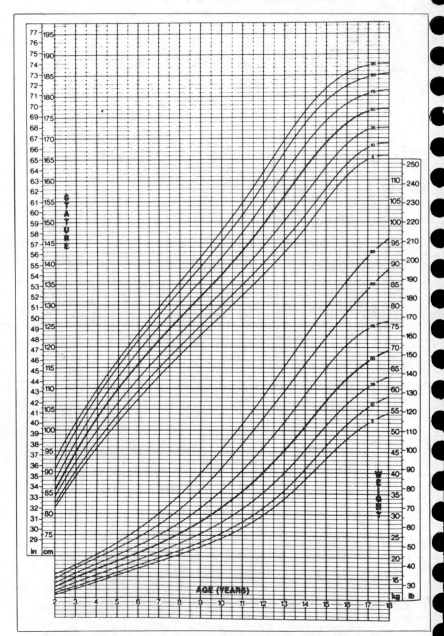

Fig. XI-E. Courtesy of Ross Laboratories, Columbus, OH.

F. NCHS Percentiles for Stature and Weight for Age, Girls, 2 to 18 Years

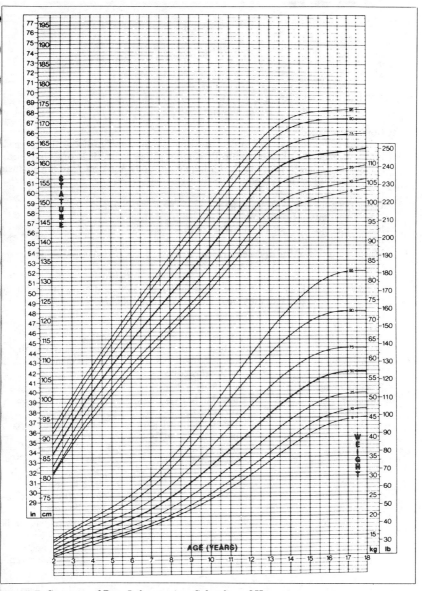

Fig. XI-F. Courtesy of Ross Laboratories, Columbus, OH.

XII

Allergy Elimination
Diets

A. Cow's milk-free diet*

All cow's milk and cow's milk products are eliminated from the diet. Although cow's milk and goat's milk are antigenically similar, patients allergic to cow's milk occasionally can tolerate goat's milk. **All labels on foods must be read** for products containing milk or milk products:

Instant non-fat dry milk powder	Margarine
	Casein
Milk solids	Casein hydrolysate
Butter	Ice cream
Whey	Cheese
Curd	Lactose

Read every label, since it is impossible to list all sources of milk. The composition of any food product may be changed without notice.

Types and amounts of food	Include	Omit
Soups As desired	Bouillon, broth, consommé, plain or made with allowed foods	Cream soups and all soups made with milk or milk products
Meat and meat substitutes 2–3 servings (5 oz total)	Beef, chicken, ham, kidney, lamb, liver, pork, turkey, veal, fish Sausage and luncheon meats made without milk products Eggs, peanut butter	Cheese, cottage cheese Sausage products, such as wieners or bologna, containing milk products Breaded or creamed meat, fish, or poultry Eggs cooked with milk or milk products Egg substitutes, such as Egg Beaters
Potato and potato substitutes 1 or more servings (¼ cup each)	White and sweet potatoes, macaroni, noodles, rice, spaghetti	Any prepared with milk or milk products, such as mashed potatoes or macaroni and cheese

---

*Brand names are used for clarification only and do not constitute an endorsement.

We wish to thank Jean Lakness, M.Ed., R.D., Clinic Dietitian at Children's Hospital Medical Center, Cincinnati, OH, for her help in supplying these diets.

474

Types and amounts of food	Include	Omit
Vegetables 2 or more servings (¼ cup each)	All (includes 1 serving dark-green or deep-yellow vegetable daily for a source of vitamin A)	Any prepared or creamed with milk or milk products (such as creamed spinach)
Breads 3 or more servings	French, Italian, or Vienna bread Breads made without milk (most breads contain non-fat dry milk) Ry-Krisp	Any made with milk or milk products: dough-nuts, pancakes, waffles, hot breads, biscuits, crackers, rolls, rusk, zwieback, teething biscuits
Cereals 1 or more servings (½ cup)	Cooked cereals prepared without milk or milk products Ready-to-serve cereals (served with formula)	All precooked and pre-pared with added milk solids High-protein cereals
Fats 3 or more servings (1 tsp each)	Kosher margarine Margarine without added milk solids Vegetable oil Shortening, oil and vinegar salad dress-ing, meat fat, lard, bacon Milk-free gravy	Butter, cream, mar-garines containing milk solids Salad dressings and mayonnaise contain-ing milk or milk products Milk gravy
Fruits and fruit juices 2 or more servings (4 oz juice or ¼ cup fruit each)	All prepared or served without milk or cream (Include 1 serving citrus fruit or juice daily for a source of Vitamin C.)	None
Desserts In moderation	Angel food cake, fruit ices, fruit whips, gela-tin, meringues Homemade products from allowed ingre-dients, such as cakes, pies, cookies, pud-dings	Any prepared with in-gredients not allowed Commercial cakes, cookies, pies, pud-dings, ice cream, sherbet, yogurt, pre-pared mixes
Milk 2 or more servings (8 oz each)	Soy formulas: Isomil Isomil SF Nursoy ProSobee RCF Soyalac	Cow's milk, skim milk, nonfat dry milk, evaporated milk, con-densed milk, yogurt Standard prepared in-fant formulas Cocoa prepared with cow's milk Ovaltine
Beverages	Water as desired Weak tea, carbonated beverages, fruit drinks	Milk beverages, such as eggnog, cocoa, milkshakes, malts

Types and amounts of food	Include	Omit
Miscellaneous	Salt (iodized), sugar, honey, corn syrup, hard candy, pure chocolate, pure cocoa, jelly Spices, herbs, pepper, catsup, mustard Nuts, olives, pickles Popcorn prepared with allowed ingredients	Milk chocolate Cream sauce Au gratin dishes Curd, whey Foods fried in butter or batter Imitation chocolate chips

B. Egg-free diet

All egg and egg products are eliminated from the diet. **All labels on foods must be read** for products containing eggs, egg powder, dried egg, or albumin. **Read every label, since it is impossible to list all sources of eggs, and the composition of any food product may be changed without notice.**

Types and amounts of food	Include	Omit
Soups As desired	Broth or cream soups prepared with allowed ingredients	Mock turtle and egg noodle soup, any stock soup cleared with egg, i.e., consommé, bouillon, etc.
Meat and meat substitutes 2–3 servings (5 oz total)	Meat, poultry, cheese, fish, seafood prepared without eggs Meats breaded with egg-free breading	Any prepared using egg as a binding agent, such as sausage, hamburger, meatloaf, croquettes, or casseroles Breaded foods in which egg is used in the breading Meat and fish sauces containing egg batter for deep fat frying Cheese soufflé, cheese fondue, cheese puffs
Eggs	None	Eggs in any form, e.g., poached, scrambled, baked, creamed, fried, deviled, hard- or soft-boiled, omelet, soufflés, egg salad, egg sandwich, egg sauces, meringues Dried or frozen eggs Egg substitutes, such as Egg Beaters
Potato and potato substitutes 1 or more servings (¼ cup)	White or sweet potatoes, macaroni, rice, spaghetti	Duchess potatoes, potato cakes, potato puffs, egg noodles

Types and amounts of food	Include	Omit
Vegetables 2 or more servings (¼ cup each)	All fresh, frozen, dried, or canned (Include 1 serving dark-green or deep-yellow vegetable daily for a source of vitamin A.)	Vegetables combined with egg sauces, such as hollandaise, corn custard, spinach, soufflé
Breads 3 or more servings	Plain enriched white, rye, whole wheat bread, Ry-Krisp, hamburger and weiner buns, biscuits made from egg-free baking powder (Some contain egg white or albumin—read the label.) Any homemade breads made from egg-free recipes (Many commercial breads and rolls contain eggs, dried eggs, or egg powders or are brushed with egg white to glaze the top.) Plain crackers	Commercially prepared muffins, pancakes, French toast, popovers, doughnuts, waffles Prepared mixes for pancakes, muffins, waffles, etc.
Cereals 1 or more servings (½–¾ cup)	All	None
Fats 3 or more servings (1 tsp each)	Butter, margarine, cream, gravy, vegetable oil, shortening Oil and vinegar salad dressings, eggless mayonnaise French dressing Bacon	Mayonnaise, commercial salad dressing, Thousand Island dressing, tartar sauce, or any prepared with egg
Fruits and fruit juices 2 or more servings (4 oz juice or ¼ cup fruit each)	All (Include 1 serving citrus fruit or juice daily for a source of vitamin C.)	Fruit served with custard sauces Fruit whips
Desserts In moderation	Homemade frostings, cakes, cookies, pastries, pies, puddings, ice cream, sherbet prepared without egg Gelatin, fruit crisp, popsicles, fruit ice	Commercially prepared frosting, cakes, cookies, pastries, pies, puddings, ice cream, sherbet (Check ingredient label —some may be egg-free.) Piecrust brushed with egg Custard, marshmallow, meringue

Types and amounts of food	Include	Omit
Milk 4 or more servings (8 oz each)	All	Eggnog Malted cocoa drinks Any milk beverages prepared with egg or egg products
Beverages	Water as desired Fruit drinks, weak tea, carbonated beverages	Coffee or wine cleared with egg white or eggshells Root beer to which egg is added as foaming agent
Miscellaneous	Salt (iodized), sugar, honey, molasses, table syrups, jam, jelly, marmalade, hard candy, gum drops Nuts, popcorn, coconut, vinegar, pepper, yeast, olives, pickles, catsup, chili sauce, herbs, spices, flavoring	Baking powder that contains egg white or albumin Divinity fudge, nougat, marshmallows (Many commercial candies made without eggs are brushed with egg white to give them luster.) All prepared mixes, frozen dinners, etc., unless label clearly indicates absence of egg

C. Wheat-free diet

All wheat and products made from wheat are eliminated from the diet. This includes any wheat flour (cake, whole wheat, etc.), graham flour, wheat germ, bran, farina, bread crumbs, cracker meal, or flour used as a thickening agent. **All labels on foods must be read** for products containing wheat or wheat products.

Types and amounts of food	Include	Omit
Soups As desired	Bouillon, broth, consommé Cream soups made with allowed ingredients and thickened with cornstarch or rice flour	Soups containing noodles, alphabets, dumplings, spaghetti, or thickened with wheat flour
Meat and meat substitutes 2–3 servings (5 oz total)	Beef, ham, lamb, liver, pork, veal, chicken, turkey Fish, cheese, peanut butter "All meat" wieners or luncheon meat Dried beans or peas Eggs	Floured or breaded meat or poultry Meats containing filler, such as meatloaf, wieners, bologna, luncheon meats
Potato and potato substitutes 2 or more servings (½ cup each)	White or sweet potatoes, rice	Noodles, macaroni, spaghetti Potatoes or rice prepared with wheat flour, such as escalloped potatoes

Types and amounts of food	Include	Omit
Vegetables 2 or more servings (¼ cup each)	All Any prepared with allowed flours (Include 1 serving dark-green or deep-yellow vegetable daily for a source of Vitamin A.)	Any breaded or prepared with wheat flour
Breads 3 or more servings	Breads made from arrowroot, corn, rice, rye, potato, barley, or oat flour Ry-Krisp Rice sticks	Bread or bread crumbs made from wheat flour Wheat crackers Matzos Doughnuts, muffins, biscuits, rolls, dumplings, pancakes, French toast Bread and cracker stuffing Rye bread or corn bread with wheat flour
Cereals 1 or more servings (1 cup each)	Cereals made from corn, oats, or rice and to which no wheat has been added in manufacture	Cereals containing wheat
Fats 3 or more servings (1 tsp each)	Butter, margarine, cream, vegetable oil, shortening, lard Pure mayonnaise Gravy made with cornstarch	Commercially prepared salad dressings, thickened with wheat flour Commercial gravy Gravy made with wheat flour
Fruits and fruit juices 2 or more servings (¼ cup each)	Fresh, frozen, or canned fruits Fruit juice (Include 1 serving citrus fruit or juice daily for a source of vitamin C.)	Strained fruits with added cereals
Desserts In moderation	Custard, fruit ice, gelatin, cornstarch or rice puddings Homemade cookies, cake, pie from allowed ingredients Homemade ice cream, sherbet, popsicles	All products made with wheat flour: cake, cookies, pie, pastries, ice cream cones Commercial ice cream, sherbets Frosting Prepared mixes Packaged puddings
Milk 3 or more servings (8 oz each)	Homogenized milk, low fat, skim Evaporated or dry milk powder Buttermilk	None
Beverages	Water as desired Weak tea, carbonated beverages, fruit drinks	Postum Beer, whiskey

Types and amounts of food	Include	Omit
Miscellaneous	Salt (iodized), sugar, honey, jelly, syrup, hard candy, chocolate, cocoa	Sauces thickened with wheat flour
		Pretzels
		Accent
	Catsup, mustard, pepper, spices, herbs	Many commercial candies contain wheat products: candies with cream centers, prepared chocolates
	Pickles, olives, popcorn, vinegar, cornstarch	Some brands of yeast, soy sauce (read label)

Substitutions for 1 tablespoon of wheat flour:
½ tbsp cornstarch
½ tbsp potato starch flour
½ tbsp arrowroot starch
½ tbsp rice flour
2 tsp quick-cooking tapioca

Substitutes for 1 cup of wheat flour:
½ cup barley flour
1 cup corn flour
¾ cup oatmeal (coarse)
1 scant cup cornmeal (fine)
⅝ cup potato flour
⅞ cup rice flour
1¼ cup rye flour
1 cup rye meal
1⅓ cup ground rolled oats

The combination of any two of the following also can be substituted for 1 cup of wheat flour:
1. ½ cup rye flour plus ½ cup potato flour
2. ⅔ cup rye flour plus ⅓ cup potato flour
3. ⅝ cup (10 tbsp) rice flour plus ⅓ cup rye flour
4. 1 cup soy flour plus ¾ cup potato starch flour

When substituted for wheat flour, a combination of flours often produces a more palatable product than one flour. Products made with rice flour and cornmeal have a grainy texture. To obtain a smoother texture, the rice flour or corn meal may be mixed with liquid called for in the recipe, brought to a boil, and then cooled before adding to other ingredients. Soy flour cannot be used as the only flour; it must be combined with another. Baked products made with flour other than wheat require long and slow baking, particularly when made without milk and eggs. Coarse flours or a combination of several flours need not be sifted before measuring. A combination of flours should be thoroughly mixed with other dry ingredients.

Coarse meals and flours require more leavening than wheat flour. 2½ tsp of baking powder is recommended for each cup of coarse flour. Batter made with flours other than wheat often appears thicker or thinner than wheat-flour batters. Products made of flours other than wheat often have a better texture when made in individual portions, e.g., muffins and biscuits rather than loaves of bread. Cake made with flours other than wheat are apt to be dry. Frosting and storing in a closed container tend to preserve moisture. Dry cereals such as rice flakes or corn flakes, when crushed, make an excellent breading for chicken, chops, or fish.

D. Gluten-free diet

This diet excludes all products containing gluten. Gluten is in wheat, rye, oats, and barley. These grains and products containing these grains must be omitted from the diet. Gluten may also be present as an incidental ingredient. **It is important to read all labels.** Omit any food or seasoning that lists the following as ingredients: hydrolyzed vegetable protein; flour or cereal products; vegetable protein; malt and malt flavorings; and starch, unless specified as corn or other allowed starch. Flavorings, vegetable gum, emulsifiers, and stabilizers may be derived from or contain wheat, rye, oats, or barley. Foods of unknown composition should be omitted or the manufacturer contacted for complete ingredient information. When dining out, choose foods prepared simply, such as broiled or roasted meats, plain vegetables, and plain salads. Since flour and cereal products are often used in the preparation of foods, it is important to be aware of the methods of preparation as well as the foods themselves. For this reason, all breaded, creamed, or escalloped foods, meatloaf, and gravies are omitted. If these foods are prepared at home using the allowed grains and flours, however, they may be consumed.

Types and amounts of food	Include	Omit
Soups As desired	Homemade broth and unthickened vegetable soups Cream soups prepared with cream, cornstarch, rice, potato, or soybean flour	Noodle soup, canned soups,* bouillon, dehydrated soup mixes
Meat and meat substitutes 3 or more servings	Fresh meat, poultry, seafood, plain unbreaded frozen meats, fish, poultry Fish canned in oil or brine Swiss cheese, cream cheese, cheddar cheese, Parmesan cheese, pure peanut butter, plain dried beans or peas Eggs	Prepared meats that contain wheat, rye, oats, or barley, such as sausage,* weiners,* bologna,* luncheon meats,* chili,* meatloaf,* hamburger with cereal filler,* sandwich spreads,* pasteurized cheese spreads* Canned baked beans* Soufflés unless prepared with allowed flours Cottage cheese*
Potato and potato substitutes 1 or more servings	White potato, sweet potato, yams, rice, hominy	Creamed or escalloped potatoes unless prepared with allowed flours Macaroni, noodles, spaghetti, lasagna, vermicelli Commercial potato salad,* packaged rice mixes*
Vegetables 1 or more servings	All plain, fresh, canned (Include a dark-green or deep-yellow vegetable daily for a source of vitamin A.)	Breaded, creamed, or escalloped vegetables unless prepared with allowed flours Commercially prepared vegetables or salads*

*Some may be used if checked with manufacturer and found to be gluten-free.

Types and amounts of food	Include	Omit
Breads 3 or more servings	Bread or muffins made from: rice flour, cornstarch, tapioca flour, potato flour, soybean flour, and/or arrowroot flour Rice wafers or sticks (usually available at Oriental specialty stores) Pure corn meal tortillas, gluten-free bread mix	All bread and bread products containing wheat, rye, barley, oats, bran, or graham, wheat germ, malt, millet, kasha, or bulgar All crackers, Ry-Krisp, rusks, zwieback, pretzels Bread or cracker crumbs Wheat starch
Cereals 1 or more servings	Only puffed rice, pure corn meal, rice, hominy grits or hominy, cream of rice, Kellogg's Puffed Rice, Post's Rice Krinkles, Nabisco Rice Honeys	Snack cereal foods, bran cereals, cream of wheat, farina, Grapenuts, oatmeal, shredded wheat, puffed wheat, Ralston, wheatena, pablum, wheat germ, buckwheat, Rice Krispies, corn flakes* Cereals with malt added
Fats As desired	Butter, cream, margarine, vegetable oil, vegetable shortening, animal fat, pure mayonnaise, homemade salad dressings and gravies prepared with allowed ingredients Bacon	Commercially prepared salad dressings and gravies containing gluten stabilizers or thickened with gluten-containing flours* Nondairy creamers
Fruits 2 or more servings	Fresh, frozen, canned or dried fruits and fruit juices (Include 1 serving citrus fruit or juice daily for a source of Vitamin C.)	Fruits prepared with wheat, rye, oats, or barley
Desserts As desired	Homemade cakes, cookies, pastries, pies, puddings (cornstarch, rice, tapioca) prepared with allowed ingredients Gelatin desserts, meringues, custard, fruit ices, whips	Commercial cakes, cookies, pies, doughnuts, pastries, puddings, pie crust, ice cream cones, prepared mixes containing wheat, rye, oats, or barley Icing mixes, ice cream and sherbet containing gluten stabilizers*

*Some may be used if checked with manufacturer and found to be gluten-free.

Types and amounts of food	Include	Omit
Milk 2 or more cups	Fresh, dry, evaporated, or condensed milk, sweet or sour cream	Malted milk, some commercial chocolate drinks, yogurt* Ovaltine
Beverages As desired	Sanka, pure instant coffee, coffee, tea, carbonated beverages, fruit juices (fresh or frozen), pure cocoa powder, frozen lemonade concentrate	Fruit punch powders, cocoa powders, ale, beer, gin, whiskey, root beer, Postum, instant coffee*
Miscellaneous As desired	Salt (iodized), sugar, honey, jelly, jam, molasses, pure cocoa, coconut, olives, pure fruit syrup, herbs, extracts, food coloring, cloves, ginger, nutmeg, cinnamon, cornstarch, yeast, sodium bicarbonate, cream of tartar, nuts, dry mustard, monosodium glutamate, cider vinegar, wine vinegar, pure chili pepper	Chili seasoning mix, gravy extracts, starch,* malt, natural flavoring (may contain malt), hydrolyzed vegetable protein,* chewing gum,* catsup,* mustard,* soy sauce,* curry powder,* horseradish, vegetable gum Emulsifiers and stabilizers* may be derived from or contain wheat, rye, oats, or barley Vinegar,* distilled vinegar, malt vinegar Pickles* Chili powder*

E. Soy-free diet

All soybeans and soybean products are eliminated from the diet. **All labels on foods must be read** for products containing soy or ingredients that may contain soy. Soy is used freely as a filler and often is not marked on packages. Possible sources of soy in foods include vegetable protein, lecithin, flour, and vegetable oil. **Read every label,** since it is impossible to list all sources of soy. The composition of any food product may be changed without notice. For nebulous ingredients such as "vegetable protein," check with the food manufacturer for possible soy.

Types and amounts of food	Include	Omit
Soups As desired	Soups prepared without soy or soy products	Soups containing soy or soy products
Meat and meat substitutes 2–3 servings (5 oz total)	Beef, chicken, ham, kidney, lamb, liver, pork, turkey, veal, fish Sausage and luncheon meats made without soy filler Eggs, peanut butter Cheese, cottage cheese	Cold cuts or sausages containing a soy additive Hamburger with soy protein "Vege burgers" made with textured vegetable protein Products fried in soy oil Fish canned in soy oil

*Some may be used if checked with manufacturer and found to be gluten-free.

Types and amounts of food	Include	Omit
Potato and potato substitutes 1 or more servings (¼ cup each)	White and sweet potatoes, macaroni, noodles, rice, spaghetti	Spaghetti made with soy flour Products cooked with soy oil or soy margarine
Vegetables 2 or more servings (¼ cup each)	Any canned, cooked, frozen or raw vegetables (Include 1 serving dark-green or deep-yellow vegetable daily for a source of vitamin A.)	Soybeans, soybean sprouts Vegetables prepared with soy sauce
Breads 3 or more servings	Breads and rolls prepared without soy-bean flours	Soy bread "Cornmeal bread" Breads containing soy oil
Cereals 1 or more servings (½ cup)	Cooked or ready-to-eat cereals without soy	Cereals containing soy flour, soy oil, vegetable protein
Fats 3 or more servings (1 tsp each)	Butter, cream, bacon, margarine, shortening or oils that do not contain soy	Soybean oil, margarine or shortening, salad dressing containing soybean oil as an ingredient
Fruits and fruit juices 2 or more servings (4 oz juice or ¼ cup fruit each)	All (Include 1 serving citrus fruit or juice daily for a source of vitamin C.)	None
Desserts In moderation	Gelatin, custard, corn-starch puddings Homemade ice cream, sherbet, cake, cookies, pastries, pie	Commercial ice cream Most commercial bakery products (Soybean flour is often added to bakery products to keep them moist.)
Milk 3 or more servings (8 oz each)	Milk, 2% milk, skim milk, evaporated milk, non-fat dry milk powder	Soy milks such as Isomil, ProSobee, Nursoy, Soyalac Commercial milkshakes
Beverages	Water as desired, tea, carbonated beverages, fruit drinks, coffee	Excessive use of sugared and caffeinated drinks
Miscellaneous	Salt (iodized), sugar, honey, jelly, syrup, chocolate, cocoa Catsup, mustard, olives, pickles, vinegar, pepper, herbs, spices	Lecithin (derived from soybeans, often used in candy) Soy sauce, Worcestershire sauce, steak sauce Toasted soybeans Caramel candies Excessive use of salt or sugar

F. Corn-free diet

All corn and corn products are eliminated from the diet. **All labels on foods must be read** for products containing corn or corn products. The following are some of these products:

Corn syrup	Popcorn
Corn oil	Grits
Corn meal	Hominy
Cornstarch	Corn sugars (dextrose, Dyno,
Vegetable oil	Cerelose, Puretose, Sweetose, glucose)
Maize	Margarine

Read every label, since it is impossible to list all sources of corn. The composition of any food product may be changed without notice. Paper containers (boxes, cups, plates, milk cartons) may contain corn, and the inner surface of plastic food wrappers may be coated with cornstarch.

Type and amounts of food	Include	Omit
Soups As desired	Broth, homemade soups prepared without corn	Vegetable soup Commercial soups*
Meat and meat substitutes 2–3 servings (5 oz total)	Beef, lamb, liver, pork, veal, chicken, turkey Fish, cheese, eggs, dried beans or peas	Peanut butter* Cold cuts,* ham,* wieners,* sausage* Breaded or fried foods* Cheese* Chili,* chop suey,* chow mein* Cheese spreads* Fish sticks*
Potato and potato substitutes 1 or more servings (¼ cup each)	White and sweet potatoes, macaroni, noodles, rice, spaghetti	Coated rice Potatoes or rice fried in corn oil
Vegetables 2 or more servings (¼ cup each)	All except corn (Include 1 serving darkgreen or deep-yellow vegetable daily for a source of vitamin A.)	Corn, hominy, mixed vegetables,* succotash Harvard beets, canned peas, frozen vegetables,* pork and beans,* creamed vegetables*
Breads 3 or more servings	White or whole-grain bread, provided cornmeal is not used in the baking process Saltine crackers	Any bread containing a corn product or dusted with cornmeal Graham crackers Baking powder biscuits Baking mixes, corn fritters, pancakes,* English muffins, tacos, tamales, tortillas
Cereals 1 or more servings (½ cup)	Cooked or ready-to-eat cereals made from wheat, rye, oats, barley, rice	Cornflakes, corn cereals, grits, hominy, presweetened cereals,* polenta

*Some may be used if checked with the manufacturer and found to be corn-free.

Types and amounts of food	Include	Omit
Fats 3 or more servings (1 tsp each)	Butter, cream, soy oil, safflower oil, peanut oil	Corn oil, vegetable oil,* gravy,* shortening,* margarine,* bacon,* salad dressing*
Fruit and fruit juices 2 or more servings (4 oz juice or ¼ cup fruit each)	Fresh fruits or juices Unsweetened fruit juices (Include 1 serving citrus fruit or juice daily for a source of vitamin C.)	Canned or frozen fruits or juices with "sugar added"* Dates, confection
Desserts In moderation	Homemade cakes, cookies, pies, artificially sweetened gelatin	Ice cream,* sherbet,* gelatin,* cakes,* cookies,* pies,* pastries,* puddings,* frosting*
Milk 3 or more servings (8 oz each)	Homogenized, low fat, skim milk Evaporated milk Nonfat dry milk powder, buttermilk	Chocolate milk,* milkshakes,* soy milks,* eggnog*
Beverages	Water as desired, tea, coffee, diet soda	American wines,* whiskey, gin, carbonated beverages,* 7-Up, Coca-Cola, ale, beer, instant coffee,* lemonade*
Miscellaneous	Beet or cane sugar, lactose, maltose, sucrose, fructose, honey, pure maple syrup Baker's unsweetened, semisweet, and German sweet chocolate Spices, herbs, pepper	Corn sugar, glucose, dextrose, corn syrup, Karo syrup, powdered sugar, confectioner's sugar, pancake syrup, jelly, jam, candy*
		Salt,* white distilled vinegar, monosodium glutamate
	Baking soda, pure extracts, unbleached flour, pure yeast, baker's yeast, arrowroot	Cornstarch, baking powder, cake yeast,* vanillin, bleached flour*
		Chewing gum,* catsup,* popcorn, potato chips,* corn curls, Fritos, pickles*
		Sauces, Chinese food,* maize
		Gelatin capsules, adhesives (envelopes, stamps, stickers)
		Toothpaste,* vitamin preparations,* medications* taken as tablets, capsules, or liquids
		Laundry starch

*Some may be used if checked with the manufacturer and found to be corn-free.

G. Foods often containing tartrazine (FD&C dye no. 5)

Certain breakfast cereals
Aproten (low-protein pasta products)
Refrigerated rolls and quick breads
Cake mixes
Commercial pies
Commerical gingerbread
Chocolate chips
Butterscotch chips
Commercial frostings
Ready-to-eat canned puddings
Certain instant and regular puddings
Certain ice creams and sherbets
Certain candy coatings
Candy drops and hard candies
Colored marshmallows
Flavored carbonated beverages
Flavored drink mixes

H. Common substances that contain or may contain sulfiting agents*

Foods

Restaurant salads (lettuce, to-matoes, carrots, peppers, and dressings)
Fresh fruit
Dried fruits (e.g., apricots)
Wine, beer, and cordials
Alcohol (all sparkling grape juices, including nonalcoholic)
Fruit juices and soft drinks (especially outside of USA)
All bottled lemon and lime juice
Packages of lemons (plastic)
Gelatin
Glucose, syrup and solid
Corn bread or muffin mix

Potatoes (e.g., French fries, chips)
Sausage meats (especially outside of USA)
Cider and vinegar
Pickles
Dehydrated vegetables
Cheese and cheese mixtures
Hot peppers (jar)
Sauces and gravies used on meats and fish
Shrimp and other seafood
Clams, canned and jarred
Clam chowder
Fresh fish
Soups (canned or dried)
Avocado dip (guacamole)

Bronchodilator solutions†

Adrenalin chloride 1:1000 (Parke-Davis)
Alupent solution (Boehringer-Ingelheim‡
Bronkosol (Breon)
Metaprel solution (Dorsey)

Isuprel hydrochloride solution (Breon)
Mironefrin solution (Bird)
Vapo-iso solution (Fisons)
Vaponefrine solution (Fisons)

Other parenteral agents

Amikacin (Amikin)
Betamethasone phosphate (Celestone, Schering)
Demerol
Dexamethasone phosphate (Decadron, MDS)

Dopamine (Intropin)
Etiocaine hydrochloride with epinephrine (Duranest, Astra)
Eye drops (Pred-mild, Pred-Forte, Sulfacetamide, Prednisol, Dexamethasone)

*Food and medication sulfite content subject to change with changing FDA regulations (see p. 151).
†Not contained in metered-dose inhalers.
‡Not contained in Alupent solution unit-dose vials.

Other parenteral agents (cont.)

Garamycin (Schering)
Gentamycin injectable (Wyeth)
Lidocaine with epinephrine (Xylocaine, Astra)
Mepivacaine (Carbocain, Cook-Waite)
Metarminol (Aramine, MSD)
Metoclopramide (Reglan, Robins)

Morphine sulfate
Norepinephrine (Levophed, Breon)
Procaine hydrochloride (Novocain, Breon)
Prochlorperazine (Compazine, SKF)
Promethazine (Phenergan, Wyeth)
Tetracaine (Pontocaine, Breon)
Tobramycin (Nebcin)

Sulfitest (Center Laboratories, Inc., Port Washington, NY 95380) paper test strips are available for testing suspected foods for the presence of sulfites. False-negative results are common and certain foods, depending on color, acidity, or presence of other chemicals, cannot be tested. Thus, the test is not an absolute indicator of the presence or absence of sulfites.

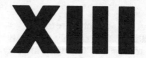

XIII

Antibodies Reactive to Human Tissue Used in Medical Diagnosis*

Antibody	Antigen	Interpretation
Acetylcholine receptor binding antibody	Antibody directed to acetylcholine receptors at neuromuscular junctions of skeletal muscle	Elevated in myasthenia gravis
Acetylcholine receptor blocking antibody	Antibody directed to acetylcholine receptors that block binding of ^{125}I alpha-bungarotoxin	Elevated in one-third of patients with myasthenia gravis. Indicated when acetylcholine receptor binding antibodies are not elevated
Antiadrenal cortex antibody	Antibody directed to adrenal cortex cells	Elevated in 75% of patients with autoimmune hypoadrenal corticism
Anticardiolipin antibody	Antibody directed to cardiolipin	Present in systemic lupus erythematosus (SLE) associated with arterial and venous thromboses and in patients with placental infarcts in early pregnancy with or without SLE. Elevation may be predictive of risk of thrombosis or recurrent spontaneous abortions of early pregnancy
Anticentromere antibody	Antibody directed to chromosome centromeres	Elevated in the CREST syndrome; also elevated in 30% of patients with Raynaud's disease

*Tests are used to support medical diagnosis. Sensitivity and specificity are variable. Method of detection and reference standards vary among laboratories. Interpretation should be confirmed with the laboratory performing the test.

Antibody	Antigen	Interpretation
Antiglomerular basement membrane antibody	Antibody directed to renal glomerular basement membrane	Presence suggests Goodpasture's syndrome and autoimmune glomerulonephritis
Antiintrinsic factor antibody	Antibody directed to intestinal intrinsic factor	Presence indicates pernicious anemia
Antimitochondrial antibody	Antibody directed to components of cell mitochondria	High titer suggests primary biliary cirrhosis. Low titers occur in other forms of liver disease
Antimyocardial antibody	Antibody directed to myocardial tissue	Presence suggestive of rheumatic fever or cardiac injury (Dressler syndrome)
Antiparietal cell antibody	Antibody directed to gastric parietal cells	Presence seen with gastritis. Present in 75% of patients with pernicious anemia
Antiplatelet antibody	Antibody directed to blood platelets	Present in immune thrombocytopenia
Antiskin antibody	Antibody directed to intercellular substances of skin	Present in pemphigus
Antismooth muscle antibody	Antibody directed to components of smooth muscle	High titer suggests autoimmune chronic active hepatitis. Also seen in viral infections (e.g., infectious mononucleosis)
Antistriated muscle antibody	Antibody directed to components of striated muscle	Presence suggestive of myasthenia gravis with thymoma, but can occur with each separately
Antithyroglobulin antibody	Antibody directed to thyroid globulin protein	Presence suggests autoimmune thyroiditis
Antithyroid antibody	Antibody directed to thyroid microsomal components	Presence suggests autoimmune thyroiditis

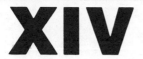

XIV

Manufacturers of Allergenic Extracts for Diagnosis and Treatment

ALK America, Inc., 132 Research Drive, Milford, CT 06460

Allergy Laboratories, Inc., Suite 204, Plaza Court Building, 1100 Classen Drive, Oklahoma City, OK 73103

Allergy Laboratories of Ohio, Inc., 623 East 11th Avenue, Columbus, OH 43211

Berkeley Biologicals, 1831 Second Street, Berkeley, CA 94701

Center Laboratories, Inc., 35 Channel Drive, Port Washington, NY 11050

Dome Laboratories, 400 Morgan Lane, West Haven, CT 06516

Greer Laboratories, Inc., P.O. Box 800, Lenoir, NC 28645

Hollister-Stier Laboratories, Box 3145 T.A., Spokane, WA 99220

Nelco Laboratories, Inc., 50-B Brook Avenue, Deer Park, NY 11729

Index

ABO incompatibility, 331–332
N-Acetylcysteine, in asthma, 146, 164
Acoustic reflex threshold, 110, 111
Acquired Immunodeficiency syndrome. *See*
    AIDS.
Adenoidectomy
  in immunodeficiency, 370
  in otitis media, 112
Adrenergic drugs, 52–63
  in allergic rhinitis, 100–101
  alpha agonists, 52, 55, 62
  alpha antagonists, 62
  in asthma, 64–67, 131–136, 148
  beta agonists, 62–63
  in food allergy, 278
  intermittent positive pressure breathing with,
    134
  as nasal decongestants, 59–61
  in urticaria and angioedema, 222
Aeroallergens, 36–44
  epidermal, 43
  house dust, 43
  house dust mite, 43
  insect parts, 43–44
  mold, 40–43
  orris root, 43
  pollen, 39–40
  pyrethrum, 43
  sampling techniques for, 36–38
    gravitational methods, 36–37
    interpretation of data from, 37–38
    volumetric methods, 37
  seeds, 43
  sources and sizes of, 36
  vegetable gums, 43
African trypanosomiasis, 402
Agglutination, red blood cell, 324
Agglutination test, in infectious disease, 383
Agglutinins, heterophile, 388–390, 391
AIDS, 375–379
  as transfusion complication, 339–340
  categoric stratification of, 377
  classification system in, 378
  clinical findings in, 376
  diagnosis of, 376
  epidemiology of, 375
  immunity abnormalities in, 378
  laboratory abnormalities in, 377, 378
  in newborn, 376–377
  pediatric, 376–377
  proposed therapy in, 379
  risk of transmission in, 379

  virus in, 375
AIDS-related complex, 376
Air cleaners, 46–47, 48
Air conditioners, 46
Air pollution, 44
  control of, 50
  in neoplasia, 344
Airway. *See* Bronchial airway.
Albay single venom preparation, 240
Albumin, transfusion of, 342
Albuterol, in asthma, 66, 136
Allergen
  immunochemical quantitation of, 38
  sensitization by, 16, 17, 18
  for skin tests, 28
Allergen inhalation challenge test, in
    hypersensitivity pneumonitis, 169
Allergenic extracts, 88–91. *See also*
    Immunotherapy.
  manufacturers of, 491
Allergic crease, 26, 97
Allergic facies, 26
Allergic reactions, classification of, 13–14
Allergic salute, 26, 97
Allergic shiners, 97
Allergoid, 89
Allergy elimination diets, 474–488
Alpha-adrenergic agonists, 52, 55, 62
  adverse effects of, 55, 62
  clinical indications for, 52
  dosage and route of administration of, 52, 55
Alpha-adrenergic antagonists, 62
Alpha fetoprotein, as tumor marker, 347–349
Alpha heavy-chain disease, 338
Alpha-1–antitrypsin deficiency, asthma vs, 130
Alveolar gas equation, 124–125
Amebiasis, 401
American trypanosomiasis, 402
Aminophylline
  in anaphylaxis, 231
  in asthma, 139–140, 148
  chemical structure of, 63, 68
  intravenous dosages for, 139
  in status asthmaticus, 159–160
Anaphylactic shock, mast cell activation in,
    16
Anaphylactoid reaction, 14, 225
  classification of, 226
  urticaria and angioedema in, 214, 215–216
Anaphylaxis, 23–24, 225–232
  acute, H_1 antihistamines in, 51
  aminophylline in, 231

216